Textbook of Evolutionary Psychiatry and Psychosomatic Medicine

The origins of psychopathology

SECOND EDITION

Martin Brüne

Professor of Psychiatry, Department of Psychiatry, Division of Cognitive Neuropsychiatry and Psychiatric Preventive Medicine
Ruhr-University of Bochum, Germany

OXFORD
UNIVERSITY PRESS

OXFORD
UNIVERSITY PRESS

Great Clarendon Street, Oxford, OX2 6DP,
United Kingdom

Oxford University Press is a department of the University of Oxford. It furthers the University's objective of excellence in research, scholarship, and education by publishing worldwide. Oxford is a registered trade mark of Oxford University Press in the UK and in certain other countries

First Edition published in 2008
Second Edition published in 2016

Impression: 1

Published in the United States of America by Oxford University Press
198 Madison Avenue, New York, NY 10016, United States of America

British Library Cataloguing in Publication Data
Data available

Library of Congress Control Number: 2015934706

ISBN 978–0–19–871794–2

Printed in Great Britain by
Clays Ltd, St Ives plc

For Moritz, Svea, Anna, and Ute

Foreword to the first edition

Russell Gardner, Jr, MD
Madison, Wisconsin, USA

In the title of his innovative and authoritative *Textbook of Evolutionary Psychiatry*, Martin Brüne of the University of Bochum has combined the term 'evolution' with instruction on psychiatry. Although the adjective 'evolutionary' may seem to indicate that this is a subfield or subspecialty of psychiatry—like child psychiatry, for instance—don't let that fool you. The book, in fact, provides a fully informed scientific underpinning for the entire medical specialty, and moreover helps psychiatry to enter the domain of medicine more fully than has been the case to date. Brüne brings forth vistas of modern biological science into fresh understandings of the perplexing disorders of psychiatry, making it easier for the beginner as well as for the experienced clinician to gain useful perspectives.

For that matter, I expect the book will be of help to readers other than clinicians, including those with patient status, or a patient's family or friends—and given the prevalence of psychiatric disorders, that may include everyone! The information in this book may alleviate some of the distressing mystery illnesses elicit in the self, and others that feel as though they have arisen 'out of the blue'. This book suggests the disorders exist for reasons—and adaptive ones at that—not always fully understood *yet*, but that will be understandable at some point. Several twentieth-century models presented one-size-fits-all accounts that didn't work, such as the idea that difficulties result solely from bad parenting (although, of course, parents make an enormous difference) or that molecular accidents of nature have caused the condition (although, of course, molecules and their functions have central roles at that level of the functioning organism).

Brüne, instead, tells us about the importance of the social functions of the human brain at all levels of analysis—functions that are often trivialized in other nineteenth- and twentieth-century discussions (Bakker et al. 2002). Descriptions may focus on the brain as though communicational functions weren't basic to it, but merely taken-for-granted epiphenomena. Mental model descriptions may fail to refer to the brain at all, or may not show social functions as central to how the mind operates. Both extremes for considering brain and behaviour imply that the idea of a stand-alone, socially isolated individual suffices to understand how the mind works or how the therapies that bear on it do their job. But, even for a recluse or hermit, people necessarily pervade the person's social brain: parents, siblings, and other people from the past including friends, foes, and pets that populate memory and anticipations. Only death divorces us personally from all such contacts, although the person gone remains in the consciousness of those left.

Brüne instructs us on the various 'orders' that lie behind psychiatric dis-orders, and achieves greater coherence because he assumes the responsibility of a single integrating author. Careful guide and mentor, he shepherds us along with helpful summary highlights and artfully uses chapter 'after thoughts'. He goes well beyond the narrow conceptual foci that typified contemporary psychiatry of the last century, namely, that one's malady stems from misplaced or inadequate molecules and that one regains good health if one can only find the correct medication and dose, or that a particularly insightful therapy interpretation may solve the person's conflict-determined neurosis, or—most recently—that a technique followed faithfully in machine-like fashion may accomplish repair.

Indeed, I suggest his graciousness and tact will help to repair the damage remaining from the conceptual wars that unfortunately characterized psychiatry over the last half of the twentieth century—at least, as I have experienced them over the decades in the USA, where I live, and which I understand (through participation in the World Psychiatric Association, for instance) have also occurred in other parts of the world. Certainly, the anthropologist Tanya Luhrman documented the conflict in a number of US locations with extensive direct observations and interviews in medical and psychiatric educational settings (Luhrman 2000). Major conflict often hinged around the term 'biology' in departments that felt obliged to employ on the faculty people who held polar extreme views, who then felt demonized—or who combatively themselves made demonizing advances towards 'the enemy'. Their different perspectives, covertly as well as openly argued, caused problems for students and trainees akin to those endured by the offspring of conflict-ridden parents.

Biology turns up in the present book as a word Brüne barely or only incidentally uses—perhaps he omits it tactfully—owing to the limited meaning given to the term by the molecularly focused proponents of one side of the conflict. Biological psychiatry, of course, labels a redundancy. As psychiatry has clearly assumed the status of a medical specialty, the importance of the body in illness causation can be taken for granted—despite the fact that the word 'psyche' indicates a non-corporeal entity (think of it translated as 'soul-iatry').

The bio-word advocates used the added emphasis to distinguish themselves not for any religious implications but to combat the *theory* of psychoanalysis. Untestable theory not only failed to help, they felt, but also involved a retreat to superstition and conjecture based on authority. They wished instead to foster a science that was truly data based and to enhance a back-to-basics empiricism that would replace insufficiently supported speculation. They strove for a greater resemblance to the rest of medicine, from which they discerned a distance that had in turn stemmed from the free-wheeling enterprise of psychoanalysis and its invasion of the American medical school establishment after World War II, when persuasive followers of Freud came to the USA, occupied professorial and administrative academic positions, and dominated funding patterns.

After all, Freud did not refer to the actual brain after 1900, despite his training as a researcher and neurologist (indeed, he had previously authored books on aphasia and childhood paralysis). For him, brain science at that time lagged too far behind his clinical observations and he hoped for a later linkage, but he and his followers proceeded without empirical check. 'Biological' critics correctly discerned that an empirical verification did not exist for the therapy he originated; no formal studies with adequate controls justified his method of therapy. Results of psychoanalytic treatment depended on testimonials, not data—anathema to modern medicine.

So, biological psychiatry galloped to the rescue, but along the way jettisoned pathophysiology (the understanding of how disease deviates from a normal system)—think of how we understand heart disease as involving deviations from normal cardiac functioning. Freud, in fact, meant his psychoanalytic models of symptom causation to possess pathophysiologic functions, but they had so little foundation in brain realities that a pathogenesis-baby disappeared along with the bathwater (not only for psychoanalysis, but also for psychiatry). In the rest of medicine, the diagnosis and treatment of disease, for instance of the heart, gut, or kidney, is of course rationalized from knowledge of the normal organ and its functions. Thus the absence of a normal psychiatric physiology contrasts dramatically with practice in the rest of medicine (Gardner 1997).

On the other hand, fortunately and very importantly, major emphases in psychotherapy outcome research have produced a vast outpouring of well controlled, carefully performed, studies. Bruce Wampold's review and synthesis of these shows that such treatment is of striking help, but also that no one approach performs better than any other—countering specificity hypotheses. He also shows that treater warmth accounts for much of the result (Wampold 2001).

Biological psychiatry assumed that pathophysiology would happen, along the way—eventually, probably at the molecular level—almost contemptuous of the organismic level of conception, but at the same time forming a parallel with how Freud thought brain science would catch up with his conceptions. Both parties in the conflict failed to realize the hypothesis-generating potential of the 'social brain', along with its real-world testability. The following finding has commanded amazingly little interest for clinicians: in vervet monkeys, social rank causes large differences in blood serotonin level, whereas a serotonin-enhancing drug causes a low ranker to assume dominance (Raleigh et al. 1991). Contrastingly, Brüne discusses relational and communicational functions that invariably go awry in people with psychiatric disorders.

Remaining stuck in the twentieth century, the American Psychiatric Association's *Diagnostic and Statistical Manual* depicts 'disorders' as independent of normal system functioning, with the 'orders' from which they deviate never mentioned at all. The importance of Brüne's book hinges on his matter-of-factly moving forward into the next century and millennium, and along the way nudging psychiatry towards a fully medical realization, unapologetically bringing its social dimensions together with its organ, cellular, and molecular facets. He also links pathogenesis with empiric results.

Despite his sparing use of the word 'biology', by including the adjective 'evolutionary' in the title of his book Brüne brings biology into the front and centre stage of his reframed view of psychiatry and the basic sciences underlying it. As we recall from our earlier schooling, the full and usual meaning of biology addresses the science of all living things. Biology encompasses zoology and botany; both use classifications that name and characterize the whole organism, hardly limiting themselves to the cellular–molecular level alone. Biology as a term—and concept—stretches back only two centuries. Before 'biology', things seemed only incidentally lifeless *versus* living. How amazing to think of that now, given how much our understanding of the world (and of ourselves) has been helped by now pervasive biological ideas, ranging from Darwin's and Mendel's inheritance conceptions to those of Watson and Crick who in the mid twentieth century cracked the genetic code.

Curiously, in an early reference to the new term made in the first decade of the 1800s, the meaning of 'biology' referred only to humans—self-centred creatures that we are! Stop for a moment! In the previous sentence I found myself using the word 'creatures' to describe human beings, but I leave in the drafted word to reflect with you that even in writing this foreword on evolution—the antithesis of creationism—religious terminology has managed to creep in! Additional to such habits of thought and expression, formal resistances to Brüne's term will stem from those who remain ensconced in the molecular–psychoanalytic wars of the psychiatry of the late twentieth century. And not only them: religious fundamentalists in various regions of the world (certainly in the USA!) vigorously articulate their beliefs and oppose any other consideration. For them, and for many others, evolution persists as a hot button issue.

'Evolution', the term that typically labels Darwin's natural selection theory—'descent with modification'—connects all humans with animal entities that had come before, and relates us also to other animals that evolved in parallel with us. Interestingly though, Darwin initially rejected the term evolution and used it only belatedly in later editions of *The Origin of Species*. His early distress with it involved the nineteenth-century meaning of evolution, which implied perfection—think of a rose bloom 'evolved to perfection' because nature designed it to do so.

Contrariwise, Darwin felt the enormous burden of convincing the world that the 'perfect' human form did not originate from Mother Nature as a steam-engine-making engineer (a popular nineteenth-century machine metaphor), artistic designer, or other kind of encompassing god, but rather from the blind operations of reproducing entities impacted by natural selection. Of course, aging human males know all too well that the location of the prostate shows that Nature (what kind of mother is she?) managed to allow design flaws in the human urinary and reproductive system.

Darwin did accomplish his persuasion with extraordinarily detailed compilations of evidence, observation, and careful reason. But his ideas flew in the face of his wife's religious beliefs and those of many others in our present day—'belief', for them, holding out over the approach of hypothesis formation and testing, data collection, and rational analysis of results.

It was not only Darwin who toppled humans from a pyramid of perfection: psychiatric disorders do as well, as they represent insults to the human self-image wish for perfection. In psychiatry we work with 'imperfections' of the human mind and brain, such as strange thoughts, convictions, attitudes, emotions, interaction tendencies, too much or too little of good things, like too much enthusiasm in those with mania or too little attention in those with attention deficit disorders, and the poor social interactions of schizoid people, autistics, or those with anxiety disorders.

These interested Darwin, too, who knew about them from the observations of a young psychiatrist, James Crichton Browne, later a co-founder of the journal *Brain*. The clinician provided Darwin with descriptions of hospitalized mental patients that the older writer then used in his landmark book on emotions, precisely a century before European ethologists won the Nobel Prize for Medicine and Physiology after employing behaviour observations in the context of Darwin's natural selection ideas.

In his emotions book, Darwin used early photography to show continuities between the emotional expression of non-human animals, such as dogs, and that of humans. He implied that communicational features existed in the common ancestor of humans and dogs. Social brains typify mammalians. Darwin—and now Brüne—underline that seemingly aberrant characteristics may in fact serve adaptive functions. Freud did too, although he limited himself to within-the-individual nineteenth-century machine models. Publishing in 2001, Wampold shows for psychotherapy, in all its variations, that people help people if the effort happens with warmth and respect (Wampold 2001). Overall, adaptation—about which you will learn much from Dr Brüne—means the survival of genes down the generations, and for humans this happens better when cooperating in-group members help one another.

So, let me pause now from these nineteenth- and twentieth-century preoccupations to point you instead towards those of the twenty-first century. Martin Brüne, with warmth and respect, guides you through new horizons for psychiatry. Enjoy the learning experience.

References

Bakker C, Gardner R, Koliatsos V, et al. (2002). The social brain: a unifying foundation for psychiatry. *Academic Psychiatry*, **26**, 219.

Gardner R (1997). Sociophysiology as the basic science of psychiatry. *Theoretical Medicine*, **18**, 335–56.

Luhrman TM (2000). *Of Two Minds: The Growing Disorder in American Psychiatry*. Alfred A. Knopf, New York.

Raleigh MJ, McGuire MT, Brammer GL, Pollack DB, and Yuwiler A (1991). Serotonergic mechanisms promote dominance acquisition in adult male vervet monkeys. *Brain Research*, **559**, 181–90.

Wampold B (2001). *The Great Psychotherapy Debate: Models, Methods, and Findings*. Lawrence Erlbaum, Mahwah, New Jersey.

Preface to the first edition

The idea to write this book dates back several years ago when (in 2003) I spent a 1-year fellowship at the Centre for the Mind, a joint venture of the Australian National University and the University of Sydney. During that time of freedom from clinical routine with the privilege of enjoying intellectual liberty in a stimulating environment, my initial plan was to compile a volume on the existing evolutionary hypotheses on psychiatric disorders. Then it dawned on me that the book ought to be different from the ones that were already on the market, a book less 'exotic' and easily accessible to the interested medical student, clinical practitioner, and researcher alike. In fact, the thought was growing that it should be more in the format of a standard introductory textbook of psychiatry, but with the difference that the book would include an evolutionary perspective as one of several essential dimensions that contribute to the understanding of psychopathological conditions.

In fact, a number of excellent books about evolutionary psychiatry have been published over the last few decades, including *Sociobiology and Mental Disorder* (1984) and *Sociobiological Psychiatry* (1990) by Brant Wenegrat; *Evolutionary Psychiatry* (1996) by Anthony Stevens and John Price; and *Darwinian Psychiatry* (1998) by Michael T. McGuire and Alfonso Troisi; as well as textbooks on evolutionary psychotherapy, such as *Exiles from Eden* by Kalman Glantz and John Pearce (1989) and *Genes on the Couch*, edited by Paul Gilbert and Kent Bailey (2000). These books are real quarries, full of details and important background information, for those who have a special interest in evolutionary thinking in relation to psychiatric and psychotherapeutic matters.

However, my experience is that while colleagues are often interested in evolutionary ideas regarding psychopathology and psychiatric disorders, most of them do not regard knowledge in evolutionary aspects of psychiatry as absolutely essential for diagnosing and treating mental disorders. In other words, many specialists and registrars in psychiatry see people who have a special interest in evolution with regard to psychiatric disorders as a sort of 'bird of paradise'—extravagant, at best offering an interesting, though more or less superfluous perspective on mental disorders. This view needs a radical revision. If psychiatry wants to survive as a medical discipline at the interface of neuroscience and the social sciences, it can no longer be satisfied with a knowledge base that covers just 50 percent of what is needed for a full comprehension of psychopathological conditions. This is, however, exactly what currently happens: psychiatry has leaped forward in understanding the proximate causes of psychopathology, that is, (patho)physiology, genetics, and ontogenetic factors contributing to psychiatric disorders. The other 50 percent is largely ignored—ultimate causes of cognition, emotion, and behaviour, that is, the phylogeny of human make-up and the adaptive value of evolved mechanisms, of which psychiatric conditions often represent extremes of variation.

This book is therefore arranged in three major parts. Part I comprises five introductory chapters, which are intended to provide a theoretical basis for the understanding of the clinical chapters and special topics. Part II comprises the major psychiatric disorders as they are grouped in the Diagnostic and Statistical Manual of Mental Disorders version IV-TR, and International Classification of Diseases Version 10. The clinical chapters are organized according to Nikolaas Tinbergen's famous four questions, which address both the proximate and the ultimate causes of cognition, emotion, and behaviour. The main reason for keeping the traditional classification of psychiatric disorders was to facilitate accessibility for readers unfamiliar with evolutionary thinking. Theoretically, it would have been more advisable to group 'disorders' according to their functional meaning (e.g. defence strategies, assertive strategies, etc.) or genetic basis, but such an approach would perhaps have been too radical as to provide common ground for clinicians and researchers. As far as therapeutic issues are concerned, I have included the URLs of the latest treatment guidelines of the American Psychiatric Association (APA), the Royal College of Psychiatrists (RCP), and the Royal Australian and New Zealand College of Psychiatrists (RANZCP) (I have borrowed the idea of integrating URLs from Matthew Rossano's excellent book *Evolutionary Psychology*). Part III comprises several special topics that in my impression were insufficiently covered by the clinical part. Each chapter of Part I and Part III contains an Afterthought in which I have tried to provide additional information that may be helpful in rounding off the topic of the respective chapter. All chapters close with suggestions of up to 30 references for further reading, the selection of which is, however, highly subjective. An exhaustive list of references is provided at the end of the book. Throughout, I have sought to strip-off most of the biological jargon to make access to the field easier.

The book has several advantages (hopefully) associated with a 'one-man' authorship. One advantage could be that the organization of each chapter follows the same logic. In terms of theoretical conceptualizations, I have been strongly influenced by classic ethology, sociobiology, evolutionary ecology, evolutionary psychology, and attachment theory. I am indebted to many important thinkers and researchers whose work has greatly inspired my thinking about psychopathology and psychiatric disorders. I would also like to acknowledge the writings of Richard Alexander, John Allman, Jay Belsky, David Buss, Richard Byrne, Leda Cosmides, Richard Dawkins, Irenäus Eibl-Eibesfeldt, Peter Fonagy, Chris and Uta Frith, Russell Gardner Jr, Sarah Blaffer Hrdy, Randolph Nesse, Jaak Panksepp (from whom I adopted the idea of having an Afterthought added to the theoretical chapters), John Tooby, Robert Trivers, Andrew Whiten, and George Williams, as well as those who have passed away, including William Hamilton, Paul MacLean, Konrad Lorenz, Ernst Mayr, Detlev Ploog, and Nikolaas Tinbergen. Further, to me an ingenious key note speech on 'theory of mind' in autism delivered by Simon Baron-Cohen at the 1998 biennial conference of the International Society for Human Ethology in Vancouver was an eye-opener regarding the importance of social cognition for the understanding of psychopathology and for negotiating social affairs such as the patient–doctor relationship and psychotherapy. This assemblage of scholars who have influenced my thinking about psychopathology is certainly not exhaustive. I have always been surprised how much of what is currently being confirmed by empirical work has already been envisioned by Charles Darwin, but listing all people who since Darwin's times have contributed to current conceptualizations of psychiatric disorders in evolutionary perspective would probably be impractical.

Special thanks go to my colleagues and friends Wulf Schiefenhövel and Hedda Ribbert with whom I have had the opportunity to exchange and discuss ideas for far more than a decade, and to my wife Ute Brüne-Cohrs for her continuing support in realizing this project.

I am also grateful to Petra Nengelken for drawing the figures and for her support in organizing the reference list, as well as to Daniel Hartelt who helped me gather heaps of literature.

Large parts of the book were written in times full of clinical and academic obligations, which helped me stay in touch with 'real-life' psychiatry. I should also be grateful to Eric Clapton who over so many years has composed such beautiful music that helped me keep my concentration during many late-night writing sessions and the inventors of the iPOD shuffle who made it possible for me to enjoy the music without bothering my family.

To me, among all medical disciplines, psychiatry is by far the most exciting one. A psychiatrist needs a profound knowledge of internal medicine and neurology—psychiatry is at the core of human experience and behaviour, not only in terms of deficiency and impairment, but also in terms of resource activation, encouragement, and support to develop perspectives for a patient's life. Helping patients cope with stressful life events and mental illness is central to all psychiatric treatment. I strongly believe that an evolutionary synthesis of the proximate and ultimate causes of mental disorders can greatly contribute to this endeavour.

Martin Brüne, October 2008.

Preface to the second edition

The new edition of this book presents several notable changes and additions. One is that the clinical chapters are now adapted to the new (fifth) version of the Diagnostic and Statistical Manual of Mental Disorders (DSM-5). Even though DSM-5 is no more compatible with evolutionary thinking than its predecessors, I felt that the best way to familiarize clinicians and researchers with evolutionary conceptualizations of psychiatric conditions would be to utilize an existing framework that is known best and widely distributed.

Content-wise, all chapters have been extensively revised. In contrast to the first edition, chapters are now fully referenced and the 'selected further reading' sections have been discarded. Moreover, I introduced or elaborated on several concepts that—in my view—have profound impact on our understanding of psychiatric disorders. Chapter 1 now contains a new section on the concept of 'differential genetic susceptibility', suggesting that the same genetic variation (or allele) can promote vulnerability to disorder (if associated with adverse early experiences) or protect against psychiatric illness (if associated with favourable environmental contingencies). Ignorance of this fundamental concept is perhaps one of the most important scientific omissions of contemporary psychiatry. Chapter 2 now includes a description of the evolution of the autonomic nervous system (ANS), because persistent alterations of the ANS due to early life stress may have prognostic implications, are easily accessible electrophysiologically, and may even offer a window to monitor therapeutic progress. Chapter 3 now covers a more detailed description of life-history theory and life-history strategies. This extension was necessary to highlight the fact that most psychiatric problems can be seen as pathological extremes of life-history strategies. It is hoped that readers are able to identify 'fast' and 'slow' life-history patterns, as reflected in psychiatric conditions, more easily when referring to individual differences in life-history strategies as they emerge from complex gene–environment interaction. Where appropriate, I have touched upon life-history theory in the clinical chapters. In addition, in Chapter 4 I have elaborated on the relationship of (early) stress to immune function and how this may affect psychological well-being. Immunological aspects are also included in the clinical chapters.

While Part I still comprises five chapters, the clinical section (Part II) now consists of 14 chapters. Specifically, affective disorders are now split into two chapters, one on depression and the other on bipolar affective disorder. Similarly, obsessive-compulsive disorder (OCD) is no longer part of the anxiety disorders in DSM-5, so a separate chapter on OCD and related disorders is included. By the same token, I have included a new chapter on trauma and stressor-related disorders, which largely focuses on post-traumatic stress disorder. Moreover, a new chapter deals with the new DSM-5 category of somatic symptom and related disorders. Likewise, a new chapter concerns sexual dysfunction disorders.

Finally, the chapter on feeding and eating disorders has been expanded by a discussion of obesity (which is not included in DSM-5 but shares important features with the 'classic' eating disorders, anorexia nervosa and bulimia). Part III contains a new chapter about issues concerning evolutionary considerations of pharmacological treatment.

In light of these manifold changes, I considered it appropriate to change the book title to *Textbook of Evolutionary Psychiatry and Psychosomatic Medicine: The Origins of Psychopathology* in order to acknowledge the broader ramifications of the book to psychiatric as well as psychosomatic topics.

In general, I have retained the structure of the chapters as described in the Preface to the first edition. In addition to the scholars whom I mentioned and acknowledged in the latter, I would like to express my gratitude to several others from whom I have learned so much and who shared their insights with me and provided me with the latest literature, much of which I might have overlooked, given the explosion in the number of articles dealing with evolutionary aspects of health and disease. So, I am indebted to Riadh Abed, Mohammed Abbas, Karl-Jürgen Bär, Bernard Crespi, Bruce Ellis, Horacio Fabrega, Jay Feierman, and the World Psychiatric Association (WPA) Group of Evolutionary Psychiatrists, Sir Paul Gilbert, Simone Shamay-Tsoory, Dan Stein, Paul St John-Smith, James Anderson ('Andy') Thomson, Alfonso Troisi, Dan Wilson, and many others. I also gratefully acknowledge my good colleague and friend Erwin Geerts, who tragically died in a road accident in 2010, and whose work on ethological aspects of psychiatric disorders has profoundly influenced both my research and my clinical work. Finally, I would like to thank my former PhD students Christine Heinisch, Elliot C. Brown, Cumhur Tas, and Cristina Gonzalez-Liencres for their enthusiasm and discussions of evolutionary topics in psychiatry.

Stephanie Czyganowski, Bettina Finger, Petra Nengelken, and Birgit Zander helped me collect and organize the many new references.

I would finally like to thank my patients from whom I have learned a great deal about life-history strategies in 'real life' and what may help them cope with the predicaments that emerged from past and present adversity. I very much hope that the new edition of this book may provide some useful insights for both researchers and clinicians.

Martin Brüne, September 2015.

Contents

Introduction

1 Definition

Psychiatry and psychosomatic medicine are two related medical fields that are concerned with the assessment, description, prevention, and treatment of psychiatric and psychosomatic conditions. Both are interdisciplinarily situated at the interface of the social and the biological sciences (Engel 1977; Fabrega 2007). Psychiatry and psychosomatic medicine utilize insights from psychology, philosophy, and ethics, as well as from neuroscience, biology, pharmacology, neurology, internal medicine, and other medical specialties. Contemporary psychiatry can be divided into several subspecialties, including biological psychiatry, social and community psychiatry, consultation and liaison psychiatry, emergency psychiatry, child and adolescence psychiatry, old age or geriatric psychiatry, cross-cultural psychiatry, and forensic psychiatry. Moreover, psychotherapy is an integral part of any psychiatric and psychosomatic treatment. Various 'schools' of psychotherapy exist, of which several focus on learning theory (e.g. behaviour therapy), whereas others work more specifically with the patient's autobiographical material (e.g. psychodynamic psychotherapy).

2 Epistemological issues

The epistemological foundations of modern psychiatry and psychosomatic medicine (including most psychotherapies) are clearly rooted in naturalism. That is, the only scientifically valuable understanding of psychiatric disorders refers to cognitive, emotional, and behavioural phenomena as being the consequence of neural activity in the central nervous system. More specifically, it is tacitly acknowledged that human beings have not only a personal history (ontogeny), but also a phylogenetic history. In other words, over aeons, natural and sexual selection have shaped brain mechanisms through which an individual effectively communicates with his or her inner and outer environment. Mental life with all its facets is an adaptation to environmental conditions to which humans have been exposed, including those environmental contingencies that lay in the remote past of our species and ancestral species from which we evolved. Importantly, psychiatric conditions reside at the extremes of variation, rather than being qualitatively distinct from 'normalcy'. Put another way, virtually all signs and symptoms that may qualify a psychiatric condition can be found in weaker expression in the general population (van Os et al. 1999, 2000).

Since humans are essentially gregarious, many of the mechanisms represented in the human brain evolved to deal with social matters. One can, therefore, pointedly speak of the human brain as a 'social brain'(Brothers 1990a, 1990b; Dunbar 1998, 2003). This strongly suggests that the way we currently use the term 'biological' with regard to psychiatry is greatly impoverished. The entire biological heritage of our species is so inevitably linked with sociality that virtually all interpersonal matters have a biological dimension. Such a vantage point does by no means downplay the importance of placing psychiatric conditions including therapeutic approaches in a biocultural context, without which the 'meaning' of a psychiatric condition or syndrome cannot be fully understood (Fabrega 2006). In any event, for various reasons the phylogenetic perspective has not yet been fully recognized by contemporary psychiatry, and evolutionary theory has never formally entered medical curricula, which may be considered a major impediment for therapeutic progress (Nesse et al. 2006, 2008; Nesse et al. 2010; Stearns et al. 2010b). Some of the reasons for disregarding evolution in current psychiatric conceptualizations are sketched in the next section.

3 Historical notes

The term 'psychiatry' was coined by Johann Christian Reil (1759–1813) in 1808. At that time, the treatment of the mentally ill was poorly integrated in medicine. Mental illness was seen as the result of personal spiritual or moral failure, or punishment by God, rather than caused by brain dysfunction or adverse experiences. Many mentally ill were therefore incarcerated and exposed to cruelty.

In France, Philippe Pinel (1745–1826) and his pupil Jean Etienne Dominique Esquirol (1772–1840) were the first who challenged the common view that mental illness could not be cured and that mentally ill people had to be confined for their unpredictable behaviour and protection of society. Instead, they introduced the *traitement morale*, characterized by empathy and compassion, and developed the first scientifically grounded psychiatric nosology. In Germany, Wilhelm Griesinger (1817–1868) became one of the leading authorities in psychiatry. In 1845, he published one of the first scientific textbooks of psychiatry (*Die Pathologie und Therapie der psychischen Krankheiten*), in which he emphasized the necessity to adopt a naturalistic perspective in psychiatry and to characterize mental illness as 'disorders of the brain'. Griesinger assumed, for example, that psychotic disorders would go through different stages of deterioration of cognitive functioning, but form a continuum with mental health. This view of 'unitary psychosis' was found unsatisfactory by many of his contemporaries who, in analogy to other medical branches, sought to distinguish 'natural disease entities' based on current phenomenology and changes of the symptomatology during the 'natural' course of the disease. In methodological terms, Karl Ludwig Kahlbaum (1828–1899) developed the 'clinical method' comprising unprejudiced behavioural observation and a thorough recording and description of all psychic and somatic (physical) signs and symptoms. Kahlbaum's intention was to link the empirically acquired clinical material with neuropathological correlates, an aim that remained unsuccessful in his time. Kahlbaum's most famous publications on 'catatonia'('tension insanity'; 1874) and 'hebephrenia'('juvenile insanity'; 1871; written by Kahlbaum's colleague and pupil Ewald Hecker (1843–1909) on behalf of Kahlbaum) were later adopted by Emil Kraepelin who included the two clinical pictures in his concept of 'dementia praecox'. Kahlbaum had already made the attempt to categorize psychiatric illnesses according to Carl von Linné's classification of animals and plants (*Die Gruppirung der psychischen Krankheiten und die*

Eintheilung der Seelenstörungen; 1863), another idea that was espoused and developed further by Kraepelin. The Swiss psychiatrist Eugen Bleuer (1857–1939) later replaced the term 'dementia praecox' by 'schizophrenia', partly to highlight the fact that not all patients had a poor prognosis associated with inevitable cognitive deterioration.

Interestingly, many psychiatrists of the second half of the nineteenth century and early twentieth century saw strong implications of evolutionary theory for psychiatry. This was, in part, based on the growing acceptance of philosophical monism and abandonment of mind–body dualism. On the other hand, the confusion of biological evolution with steady progress led to the view that mental illnesses were the result of abolishment of the forces of natural selection (for a critique of the false interpretation of biological evolution in psychiatry see Afterthought to Chapter 1). For example, towards the end of his career Kraepelin wrote:

> The development [phylogeny] of human personality has been perfected only after a process characterized by infinitely small, barely perceptible forward steps; retrograde steps have also occurred. Detours have been followed and then left behind. The end result of this unpredictable progress naturally retains traces and vestiges of the various stages of development, even if the vast majority of once-formed then superseded mechanisms have been completely lost. If we therefore try today to fit the expressions of insanity to the individual stages of personality development, then we find the necessary evidence conspicuous only by its absence. Should such attempts ever be successful, it will be necessary to trace back manifestations of our psychological life to their roots in the psyche of the child, of primitive man and of animals. In this way we can discover to what extent certain illnesses reflect a recrudescence of emotions hitherto concealed in our individual or phylogenetic developmental history. Prospects for this seem to me encouraging, despite the poverty of our current knowledge. From this endeavour we may receive help towards our foremost and hardest task: the clinical understanding of disease forms.
>
> (Emil Kraepelin (1920) The Manifestations of Insanity (translated by Dominic Beer)

Even earlier, James Crichton-Browne (1840–1938) had hypothesized that 'it seemed not improbable that the cortical centres which are last organised, which are most highly evolved and voluntary, and which are located on the left side of the brain, might suffer first in insanity'(Crichton-Browne 1879, p.42). As a young man, Crichton-Browne supported Charles Darwin in publishing his book on *The Expression of the Emotions in Man and Animals* (1872), to which Crichton-Browne contributed several drawings. Crichton-Browne was befriended to John Hughlings Jackson (1835–1911) who developed the idea of disease-associated dissolution of the nervous system in reverse steps of its evolutionary development. Jackson proposed a hierarchical organization of the brain, with the capacity for self-reflection being localized in the most recently evolved part of the brain, the prefrontal cortex. In similar ways, Henry Maudsley (1835–1918) referred to brain evolution as a crucial aspect for the understanding of psychopathology, however, without belittling the impact of the social environment for both the manifestation and therapy of mental disorders (Maudsley 1867, p.421).

Thus, many important concepts emerging in the new medical discipline of psychiatry were, at least in part, rooted in evolutionary thinking (as was early psychoanalysis; see Chapter 22). However, as the unit of selection was unclear, and the rules of inheritance unknown, psychiatric nosology and the search for 'natural disease entities' remained elusive. Moreover, even though the Mendelian rules of inheritance were rediscovered at the turn of the twentieth century by de Vries, Tschermak, and Correns (independently of each other), many psychiatrists remained oblivious to these important findings and held the view that acquired characters could be inherited. Likewise, at that time the view prevailed that selection would take place at the species level, and it took many more decades until the mechanisms of selection at the level of the individual organism were discovered. More importantly, however, during the late nineteenth and early twentieth century, psychiatry was concerned by the observation of a large-scale increase in number of psychiatric in-patients. By the outgoing nineteenth century, thousands of patients across Europe and the USA were treated, or all too often merely institutionalized, in large asylums. The sky-rocketing number of mentally ill led psychiatrists to conclude that the abolishment of natural selection had induced a degeneration of the population, a popular idea that curiously met the then prevailing cultural pessimism.

On his journey to Java, Kraepelin observed, for example, that mental disorders were comparably rare in 'primitive' races, and that the prognosis of mental illness was more favourable than in the developed world, which Kraepelin interpreted as the result of greater resistance against disease in people from developing countries. Kraepelin's opinion that mental illnesses were the result of a domestication-induced degeneration strongly influenced psychiatric nosology, which grossly neglected poverty, poor hygiene, and lack of education as possible causes of psychiatric illness. Consequently, as effective pharmacological treatment of mental disorders was unavailable, many countries introduced eugenic measures to prevent further increase of prevalence rates of mental illnesses, including compulsory sterilization. Many psychiatric authorities who approved such means saw themselves as advocates of mental hygiene at the population level (with several clearly having racial hygiene in mind), rather than medical doctors who dealt with individuals.

The introduction of Social Darwinist ideas in psychiatry and the poor quality of care for psychiatric patients in mental hospitals certainly contributed to psychiatry's bad reputation, and to the rejection of evolutionary theory as a powerful tool to understand psychiatric disorders. (As a side-note, it should be emphasized that the term 'Social Darwinism' must not be misunderstood in a way that suggests that Charles Darwin promoted the application of evolutionary theory to social politics. On the contrary, Darwin was reluctant in that matter.)Moreover, the abuse of psychiatry for political purposes, especially in Nazi Germany and other totalitarian systems, still plays a fundamental role in how psychiatry is recognized in the public today.

4 Ethical issues

The aftermath of the atrocities of Nazi human experimentation brought a desperately needed ethics codex for human experimentation, known as the Nuremberg Code. In 1964, the World Medical Association issued the Declaration of Helsinki, which since then unambiguously regulates the recognition of individual rights including respect to the individual, self-determination, and informed consent to treatment and research.

In 1977, the World Psychiatric Association approved the Declaration of Hawaii, which sets the ethical guidelines for the practice of psychiatry. It covers patient examination, constant medical education and update of knowledge, human dignity and patient rights, confidentiality, and research ethics. The 1996 Madrid revision of the Declaration also includes guidelines on specific situations, including the psychiatrist's refusal to participate in euthanasia, torture, death penalty, sex selection, and ethnic or cultural discrimination. It also defines rules of conduct for psychiatrists concerning organ transplantation, media relations, genetic research and counselling, conflict of interest with industry and third-party payers, and psychotherapy, including violation of trust and boundaries between psychiatrists and patients.

The full text has been made available by the World Psychiatric Association at <http://www.wpanet.org/>.

5 Conceptual issues

For decades, psychiatrists had to struggle with divergent ways of conceptualizing psychiatric illnesses, depending on the underlying focus of attention. As pointed out, the late nineteenth and early twentieth century witnessed a first wave of biologizing mental disorders (Roelcke 1997), based on false biological premises and an almost complete lack of acknowledging social factors as causative for mental disorders. The pendulum swung back in the 1950s, when psychoanalytic theory became the dominating framework in psychiatry. During this period, the view prevailed that psychiatric disorders were exclusively rooted in repressed thoughts and feelings, as well as in an unfavourable mother–child dyad, culminating in concepts such as 'the schizophrenogenic mother'. Since the 1980s, with the advent of new diagnostic tools, there is again a growing interest in the genetic underpinnings of psychiatric disorders, in anatomical brain abnormalities, and in abnormal neurotransmission as correlates of abnormal cognition, emotions, and behaviour.

Still, there has been a strong movement that sought to reformulate insights from psychoanalysis (and behaviourism) into a new concept of the understanding of psychiatric disorders as being caused by adverse early experiences. However, in the conceptual perspective, biological causes (genetics and neurotransmission) and psychological causes (adverse interpersonal factors) have long been treated as diametrically opposite approaches to the understanding of psychiatric disorders. Thus, not only in clinical terms but also with regard to research issues, these two camps have led quite solitary lives, mainly because the overarching conceptual framework—based on evolutionary theory—has been insufficiently appreciated (Nesse and Jackson 2006).

To overcome difficulties in diagnosing psychiatric disorders—all the more as psychiatry lacks sufficient knowledge regarding the aetiology and reliable laboratory tests of most psychiatric disorders—psychiatry has formalized the diagnostic process. The most widely used manuals are the Diagnostic and Statistical Manual of Mental Disorders (DSM) and the International Classification of Diseases (ICD). These manuals have the advantage to improve reliability of diagnosis, though at the cost of reducing the complexity of clinical phenomena. Although claimed to be largely 'atheoretical', they represent compromises between various 'schools' of psychiatry. Moreover, they seem to suggest the existence of discrete disease entities (although the manuals explicitly state otherwise), which is not supported by any scientific evidence. For students and residents in psychiatry, the impression that there are distinct diagnostic categories in psychiatry may give them a false sense of certainty about diagnosis and treatment, yet psychiatric disorders emerge along continua from normalcy, and dimensional or gradual differences even between disorders are the rule, not the exception.

Thus, purely descriptive manuals help to reach diagnostic consensus between clinicians but should be used with caution due to their arbitrariness. What DSM and ICD insufficiently reflect are differences between the sexes in presentation of signs and symptoms, as well as cross-cultural issues. Our diagnostic systems are too narrow for a valid cross-cultural comparison (Fabrega 2002), presumably because they largely originated in a small geographical area of western Europe (Burton-Bradley 1979).

We are now at a point at which the integrity of psychiatry is jeopardized by its subspecialties drifting apart. Biological, social psychiatry and psychotherapy need an integrative framework that is suitable for both clinicians and researchers. For example, clinicians who see patients don't have access to the patients' genetic make-up or neurotransmitter receptor profiles, nor do they have their activation patterns during functional brain imaging at hand. The clinicians' task is to understand patients' cognition, emotions, and behaviour in a face-to-face setting. By contrast, researchers increasingly need to abandon the nosological systems in order to make scientific progress. The contributions of genetic variation of individual genes, or the activation pattern during functional brain imaging, are at best symptom-specific, rather than specific to a syndrome (or disorder). In keeping with the descriptive approach, disorders need to be understood in terms of their symptomatology, epidemiology, genetic and environmental factors, pathophysiology, and gene–environment interaction, whereby 'life-history theory' can act as a guide to integrate these sources of information (Ellis and Del Giudice 2014).

All this aims at understanding the function of an individual's cognitions, emotions, and behaviours, which is difficult enough in what we call normal functioning, but much harder in disordered states. Psychiatric disorders clearly reflect states of abnormal and maladaptive functioning, to the extent that the presentation of signs and symptoms may at times appear functionally meaningless. However, in light of the dimensional perspective suggesting that psychopathological signs and symptoms are distinct from 'normalcy' by degree, not by kind, the analysis of the corresponding adaptive mechanisms may shed light on the communicative aspects of abnormal mental phenomena.

Another crucial aspect in the understanding of psychiatric disorders resides in observations that many psychiatric conditions affect the whole body, not just the brain. This seems to be most obvious for eating disorders and somatic symptom disorder. However, growing evidence indicates that epigenetic dysregulation of stress physiology and immunological reactions are important aspects of all major psychiatric conditions (McEwen 2002; Ottaviani 2011). In summary, it is essential that psychiatric conditions, like other medical conditions, are holistically analysed from the perspective of Darwinian medicine (Nesse and Williams 1994) or 'Hamiltonian' medicine (Crespi et al. 2014). These issues are dealt with in the next chapters.

Part I

Theoretical background to evolutionary psychiatry and psychosomatic medicine

Chapter 1

Principles of evolutionary theory, evolutionary psychopathology, and genetics

Abstract

Darwin's work on evolution by natural and sexual selection is the central scientific framework in biology that explains how life developed through adaptation to changing environments. Evolution has been the driving force that has shaped the human brain and mind in the same way as it has formed somatic traits. Many adaptations pertaining to human cognition, emotions, and behaviour emerged in ancestral environments of evolutionary adaptedness, from which modern living conditions deviate in one way or another. Such 'mismatches' of evolved traits and current environments may cause vulnerability to dysfunctional operation of cognitive, emotional, and behavioural traits. Genes and environment interact in manifold ways, yet genetic plasticity may not only convey vulnerability to dysfunction. Instead, the very same genetic variants that may lead to dysfunction when associated with environmental adversity exert protective effects against dysfunction when environments are more favourable. These insights have yet to be acknowledged by psychiatry and psychosomatic medicine.

Keywords

natural selection, sexual selection, environment of evolutionary adaptedness, genetic plasticity, gene–environment interaction

1.1 Introductory remarks to evolutionary theory, evolutionary psychopathology, and genetics

Traditionally, the causes of psychiatric and psychosomatic disorders as well as their underlying psychopathological and somatic signs and symptoms are conceptualized in terms of developmental disruptions during foetal development and adverse events during infancy, early childhood, or adolescence. At the neurobiological level, they are described in terms of malfunctioning of neural circuits, dysbalanced neurotransmission, or genetic vulnerability. For example, depression can be seen as the result of adverse events during infancy, such as separation from an attachment figure, as a serotonin deficiency syndrome, or be associated with allelic variation of the serotonin transporter gene. There is no doubt that research into the behavioural and neurobiological roots of psychological dysfunction has greatly improved our understanding of psychopathology, but from a broader biological perspective this is only half of the story.

A common misconception of psychiatry and psychosomatic medicine is to assume that an understanding of an individual's early developmental conditions and the neurochemistry or molecular level of brain function is sufficient to understand the pathology of cognitive-emotional-behavioural systems or somato-psychic systems. This is as incorrect as it would be to assume that ontogeny and physiology alone were sufficient to understand the nature of animal behaviour. Nikolaas Tinbergen, one of the great ethologists of the last century, referred to these levels as the proximate or immediate causation of behaviour (Tinbergen 1963). The proximate causes of behaviour comprise ontogenetic development and physiological mechanisms. Proximate causes of behaviour (and pathology) can change during an individual's life-time. However, for a full understanding of behaviour, as Tinbergen pointed out, it is essential to also acknowledge the ultimate level of behaviour. The ultimate or evolutionary level embraces the reconstruction of the phylogenetic development of behaviour, that is, the attempt to trace back the evolutionary roots of behaviour by studying closely related species, and to analyse the selective advantage or adaptive value of a given trait. Taken together, these four 'why' questions, namely ontogeny, physiological mechanism, phylogeny, and adaptive value, constitute the key components of a complete understanding of behaviour. The proximate and evolutionary (ultimate) levels are by no means mutually exclusive. On the contrary, they are essentially complementary (Nesse 2013; Brüne 2014b).

Proximate mechanisms (ontogeny and physiology) and ultimate causes (phylogeny and adaptive function) are complementary dimensions that are considered essential for the understanding of behaviour.

From this perspective, human cognition, emotion, and behaviour can only be understood if all four questions have been addressed, and the explicit understanding that maladaptive traits have to be analysed in the same way constitutes the main thread of this book (Nesse 2013; Brüne 2014b). However, this is not to say that any psychopathological sign or symptom represents an adaptation. Conversely, signs and symptoms are genuinely maladaptive in both the common understanding of the term and its evolutionary meaning. Psychopathological signs and symptoms reflect the extremes of variation that have become dysfunctional due to their abnormal frequency, intensity, or inappropriateness in current context (Brüne 2002). For example, fear is an ancient adaptive trait that signals threat to the individual and helps to avoid environmental hazards. Pathological anxiety, by contrast, is considered maladaptive because it occurs in circumstances that pose no 'real' threat, although an affected individual may subjectively perceive a particular situation as dangerous. Fear responses are usually easily elicited because it makes evolutionary sense to keep the

Psychopathological signs and symptoms can be analysed accordingly, with the understanding that they constitute dysfunctional extremes of variation of adaptive traits.

releasing threshold low. If too high, a fearless individual probably lost his life very early and thus did not leave surviving offspring.

Throughout evolutionary times, it has therefore been 'cheaper' to be sometimes unnecessarily frightened than to be fearless once in real danger (Nesse 2001). This could be one reason why fear and anxiety are part of so many psychopathological conditions. Moreover, the case of fear and anxiety may be exemplary of the difficulty to draw a clear line between physiology and pathology, as well as between adaptedness and maladaptedness. It is necessary to emphasize, however, that depression is not just exaggerated sadness; likewise, a persecutory delusion is not merely akin to extreme suspiciousness. In addition, psychopathological signs and symptoms reflect the extremes of adaptive traits, whose maladaptedness is expressed by the limited ability or failure of the organism to recover spontaneously, that is, without medical and/or psychotherapeutic aid. The impairment of self-healing capacity can be caused by many distinct factors, ranging from early experiences of neglect or abuse (which may be associated with malfunction of the stress system; Brody et al. 2013), intoxicating effects of psychotropic substances, perpetual entrapment in interpersonal conflict, and unattainable biosocial goals, which natural selection has insufficiently equipped the human mind to cope with.

Psychopathological signs and symptoms reflect extremes of adaptive traits, whose maladaptedness is expressed by the limited ability or failure of the organism to recover spontaneously, that is, without medical and/or psychotherapeutic aid. Similar to fever and cough, which are natural defence mechanisms against pathogenic agents, psychological defence can break down if systems are exhausted or overwhelmed by the 'virulence' of the causal event.

Similar to fever and cough, which are natural defence mechanisms against pathogenic agents, psychological defence can break down if systems are exhausted or overwhelmed by the 'virulence' of the causal event. According to this analogy, while sadness may be seen akin to fever, depression could be likened to septic shock. These brief examples give rise to a number of important questions such as: 'To what kind of circumstances did our species adapt?' 'What were the environmental conditions that shaped the human mind?' 'What were the evolutionary costs of the emergence of the *conditio humana*?' 'Why isn't the mind better adapted to cope with adversity?' (Gilbert 1998; Brüne 2014b).

Accordingly, if we want to understand the dysfunction of complex cognitive-emotional-behavioural systems, we need to comprehend its function at all levels, as proposed by Tinbergen. The next sections summarize basic evolutionary concepts that are essential for the understanding of the evolutionary (ultimate) causes of psychological mechanisms and pathological variants.

1.2 **Definition of evolution**

Evolution is a historical process that cannot directly be observed. It has to be inferred from observation; nevertheless, there is no doubt that evolutionary processes have shaped human cognition, emotion, and behaviour in the same way as anatomy and physiology (Barkow et al. 1992; Garcia 1996). Evolution by common descent is a highly conservative and rather slow process. The

Evolution by natural and sexual selection is a historical process that has shaped human cognition, emotion, and behaviour.

molecular similarities between chimpanzees and humans, for instance, suggest that the two lineages split from a common ancestor some 5–7 million years ago (mya) (Kaessmann and Pääbo 2002), which adds up to differences in around 35 million single nucleotides (Varki and Altheide 2005), but even yeast and humans have several genes in common.

Evolution takes place in potentially interbreeding individuals of a species at the population level and reflects the genetic turnover of individuals. Evolution is so slow, because stabilizing selection over hundreds or thousands of generations has the tendency to reduce the interindividual variance within populations, thereby driving the population close to the optimal genotype that is adapted to a certain ecological niche (Mayr 2001). Within populations there is nevertheless genetic and phenotypic variation between individuals, which is necessary for producing the 'raw material' on which selection can operate (Abecasis et al. 2012). By definition, those individuals who successfully reproduce are considered the best adapted to current environmental conditions (Darwin 1859; misleadingly epitomized as 'survival of the fittest'). Since most new variations that arise from mutations—copy errors of the deoxyribonucleic acid (DNA)—are disadvantageous, selection largely acts as an elimination process of less well-adapted variations (negative selection). Positive selection may, however, occur if a newly developed trait increases an individual's reproductive fitness and leads to fixation in the gene pool of a population. Together, this suggests that selection operates at the level of the individual phenotype (Mayr 2001), where a more radical view is that selection can act on individual genes and that genes can compete with one another (Dawkins 1976). The debate about the level at which selection acts has not entirely been settled. In contrast to former propositions, however, the assumption that selection takes place at the species level has been discarded, and group selection may play a role in cases where a particular trait benefits a population of individuals that outcompetes another group lacking that trait (Boyd et al. 2003).

Stabilizing selection tends to reduce interindividual differences within interbreeding populations, yet even small differences between individuals contribute to differential reproductive success.

Most mutations are deleterious; hence selection is largely a process of elimination. Occasionally, however, positive selection may lead to a rapid spread of the respective trait within populations.

Selection largely takes place at the individual level. Most adaptations are not optimal by design, but represent compromises. This partly explains why some maladaptive traits (including those we associate with psychopathology) are not removed by selection.

Evolution through natural selection is a 'thrifty' process. This means that adaptations are not optimal by design, but represent compromises between benefit and costs in terms of economy and reliability of adaptive traits (Williams 1966). This is crucial to keep in mind when addressing the question why pathologies (including *psycho*pathologies) exist and have not been removed by selective forces (Nesse and Williams 1994; see Chapter 4).

It is important to note that the individual phenotype not only consists of its structure and physiology, but also of its cognitive, emotional, and behavioural make-up, referred to as the 'extended' phenotype (Dawkins 1982). The extended phenotype can be the target of selection, which is of particular importance for the study of human psychological characteristics.

In humans, both individual and group selection may have contributed to the evolution of cooperation, morality, and social cognitive abilities.

Group selection is a mechanism that can occur in highly cooperative species, if the net fitness advantage of the group surpasses the arithmetic mean of all individual fitness values. In humans, individual selection and group selection are complementary. For example, cooperation between genetically unrelated individuals can benefit the group in terms of survival and reproduction (Boyd et al. 2003). It has, in turn, also shaped individual cognitive and emotional adaptations, such that the ability to detect 'free-riders' and to impose moral punishment of violations of group standards has emerged (Boyd et al. 2003). This is particularly important for the understanding of the specialization of the human brain on processing information from the social environment ('social brain hypothesis'; see Chapter 2) and for the understanding of certain pathologies such as hypervigilance towards deception, the extremes of which are reminiscent of (in psychiatric terminology) syndromes involving 'persecutory delusions' (Zolotova and Brüne 2006).

1.2.1 Natural and sexual selection

Evolutionary processes can theoretically be divided into traits that emerge from natural selection and others that originate from sexual selection (Darwin 1859, 1871). Generally speaking, natural selection favours those characteristics that help the individual to survive. For example, to escape a predator, it can be advantageous to be a fast runner (or, alternatively, to camouflage), such that the fastest runners are on average more likely to produce surviving offspring than slower runners. Predatory species are likewise exposed to selection, because the most skilled hunters are those that are most likely to reproduce. This competitive principle in nature is probably one reason why anagenesis, that is, the tendency in evolution towards increasing complexity and body size, can be observed (Mayr 2001). Evolutionary theorists have called this a co-evolutionary 'arms race' or Red Queen Principle (after Lewis Carroll's *Alice in Wonderland*) as a metaphor for the observation that increasing complexity is a necessity to at least stay in the same place (and not become extinct; Dawkins and Krebs 1979).

Natural and sexual selection are two separate processes that drive the evolution of species. 'Arms races' between and within species contribute to the speed of adaptive modifications.

Evolutionary 'arms races' occur between as well as within species. In humans, for instance, selection towards increasing cooperation between genetically unrelated individuals may have exerted considerable pressure towards the evolution of many social cognitive abilities such as 'theory of mind' or 'mentalizing', that is, the ability to cognitively represent one's own and others' mental states, and empathic concern for others (for details see Chapter 2). Naturally selected traits are basically the same in both sexes. In contrast, characteristics that are dissimilar between male and female individuals of the same species are the product of sexual selection.

Before Charles Darwin discovered sexual selection as the second (and at least equally important) evolutionary force, he was confused by the fact that some traits, mostly found in males, obviously represent survival *dis*advantages (Darwin 1871; Hiraiwa-Hasegawa 2000). The tail of the peacock, for example, is so conspicuous and heavy that it impedes particularly those individuals with the largest tails from escaping predators. However, it is these individuals that are preferentially chosen by females as mates. Two hypotheses may account for the evolution of such exaggerated morphological features in males. One is called 'genetic drift', a mechanism by which random changes in allele frequency in small breeding populations increase the frequency of a certain characteristic through so-called runaway selection. Runaway selection is understood as a mechanism by which a trait that is by chance preferred by females leads to overexpression of this trait by males in successive generations and, in turn, to even stronger preference in females (this could also apply for some human psychological traits; Nesse 2007). The other one refers to the 'good genes' hypothesis or 'handicap principle'. In the peacock, for instance, a large tail may indicate good genes, because an individual that can 'afford' to grow it is likely resistant against pathogens (Alcock 2001; Rossano 2003). Furthermore, males' attractiveness for females is also a matter of symmetry. It has been proposed that 'good genes' are associated with diminished fluctuating asymmetry, because disease processes, particular during early ontogeny, may lead to greater asymmetry, which is perceived as less attractive (a hypothesis that has been put forth regarding schizophrenia; Yeo et al. 1999; see Chapter 8).

Sexual selection has long been a puzzle to Charles Darwin, because some traits such as the peacock's tail obviously convey fitness disadvantages in terms of survival. Sexually selected traits may emerge due to 'genetic drift' or signify superior genetic quality.

In most species males compete with one another (intrasexual competition) for access to females (Buss 1988a). Thus, selection favours greater body size and strength in males compared with females, known as sexual dimorphism, at least in species in which one male dominates multiple females. Intrasexual competition over territories may be resolved by not only body size or physical power but also weaponry such as antlers or large canines by which males create dominance hierarchies. A special type of intrasexual competition occurs if males have more or less equal access to females. In such instances the amount and quality of sperm may decide over which male fathers offspring of an inseminated female; thus this represents another level at which intrasexual competition can take place. Some individuals even produce so-called 'kamikaze sperm', sperm cells that appear highly dysmorphic but may be toxic to other sperm (Baker and Bellis 1995; for further details see section 1.2.2.2).

Intrasexual competition between males for access to fertile females has led to body sexual dimorphism and the evolution of sperm competition. By contrast, in most species (including humans) it is the female that chooses her mate based on the evaluation of the male's mate quality.

There is also competition between the sexes, referred to as intersexual competition. The principle of female choice has already been mentioned. The reason why females are more discriminating in terms of mate choice than males is that in most species females invest more in potential offspring than males (see section 1.2.2.2). In other words, females have much more to lose in regard to their reproductive fitness compared to males if they did not thoroughly choose the best mate available. The logic behind female choice is that reproductive fitness is determined not only by the mere number of offspring, but more so by the genetic quality of the next generation. It is therefore in the interest of the female to pick a genetically high-quality male (Buss 1998). In monogamous species like many birds, females quite frequently engage in extra-pair copulation. Conversely, males are usually highly vigilant to prevent their mates' infidelity (Buss and Shackelford 1997). In our own species men may have evolved strategies such as physical violence towards spouses, and even rape (Wilson and Daly 1996; MacDonald 2000; Thornhill and Palmer 2000). These mechanisms have profound implications for the behaviour of males and females, depending on the species' social structure and genetic relatedness to others.

1.2.2 Inclusive fitness theory

The modern synthesis of evolutionary theory has discovered that individual reproductive success is the central theme of differential evolutionary development. Inclusive fitness theory proposes that reproductive success does not solely depend on an individual's number of offspring (classical fitness), but also on the reproductive success of genetically related individuals (Hamilton 1964). Thus, it can be advantageous—in terms of fitness—to support the reproductive effort of close kin. In other words, inclusive fitness is the sum of an individual's reproductive success plus the success of relatives weighted by their degree of relatedness (e.g. a brother or sister is more closely related than a cousin). Selection should favour behaviours that maximize reproductive success, because from a genetic point of view it is in the interest of an organism to pass on its genes to the next generations. Thus, genetically motivated altruistic behaviour should be confined to kin, and indeed altruistic acts are widespread in the animal kingdom, including social insects and other species with similar social structures, such as naked vole rats (Trivers and Hare 1976). In contrast, in human societies, mutual help can often be found among genetically distantly or unrelated individuals (Hill et al. 2011). This requires an explanation, because it seemingly contradicts inclusive fitness theory. Decision-making about selfish versus altruistic behaviour involves conflict over resource allocation, which may arise among not only genetically unrelated individuals but also individuals of the opposite sex. This is so because their strategies to maximize reproductive success may be fundamentally different. Conflict even occurs between parent and offspring generation, because a parent shares, on average, only 50 percent of genetic material with an individual offspring. These areas of conflict have been pinpointed by Robert Trivers in three seminal papers.

Inclusive fitness theory suggests that an individual's fitness is the sum of the individual's own reproductive success and the reproductive success of genetically related individuals.

1.2.2.1 Reciprocal altruism

Reciprocal altruism can be described as a form of altruism between genetically unrelated individuals that provides a benefit to one organism (the recipient) at the expense of another (the organism performing the altruistic act), whereby future reciprocation of the altruistic act is uncertain (Trivers 1971). Food sharing is one such behaviour that occurs in many species. Reciprocal altruism can only work properly if the individual who behaves altruistically possesses psychological mechanisms for memorizing the scenario and the individual who benefited from it. Moreover, an essential feature of reciprocality is to be able to recognize if the beneficiary individual refuses to reciprocate. The detection of cheating is one cognitive mechanism that must have been selected in the human lineage to counteract deceptive behaviour, because otherwise genes favouring cheating tendencies would have spread in the population and a system of mutual aid would have collapsed (Trivers 1971).

The theory of reciprocal altruism proposes that altruism between genetically unrelated individuals can only persist if altruistic behaviour is being reciprocated, and if mechanisms exist that are suitable to detect non-cooperative behaviour and to reinforce reciprocation.

The problems associated with reciprocal altruism were so pervasive in ancestral (and surely modern) human societies because the opportunities for exchange are greatest in long-lived species with low dispersal rates and a high degree of mutual dependence, including parental care over an extended period of time (Bell 2001). Thus, reciprocal assistance in times of danger, food sharing, helping sick, very old, or very young individuals, and sharing implements and knowledge are altruistic behaviours that can be observed in every human culture (Trivers 1971). Trivers has identified several cognitive and emotional characteristics that evolved in humans to maintain reciprocal altruism among individuals belonging to a social group or tribe. Positive emotions such as friendship, sympathy, and gratitude may have evolved as emotional rewards in altruistic partnerships; in contrast, negative emotions including moralistic aggression may reduce cheating tendencies and prevent continuing altruistic behaviour in the absence of reciprocation; if attempts of cheating are being detected, emotions such as guilt or shame (on the side of the cheater) may help restore reciprocal partnership. At the cognitive level, one may, however, pretend moralistic aggression, sympathy, or feelings of guilt to induce altruistic behaviour in others. Such subtle cheating mechanisms may in turn have led to the selection of abilities to discriminate between honest and hypocritical behaviour. The emotions of trust and suspiciousness may have directly evolved in relation to the problem of reciprocal altruism. There is also evidence to suggest that forgiveness evolved as a mechanism to reinstall cooperation when violation of social norms has occurred. Along similar lines, donating to a common good may serve the purpose of strengthening group cohesion (McCullough et al. 2013). Furthermore, maintaining reciprocity probably also contributed to the evolution of autobiographical memory, which allows recalling personally salient social interaction after years or even decades (Suddendorf 2013).

In humans several of the social emotions such as sympathy, shame, and guilt presumably evolved in response to problems associated with reciprocality. In addition, forgiveness evolved as a mechanism to reinstall cooperation when violation of social norms has occurred.

Group selection may in addition have favoured collective punishment of cheaters (Boyd et al. 2003). In light of the extraordinary extensive mutual dependence of individuals in early hominid groups, it becomes clear why group cohesion and obedience to social rules and norms were targets of selective forces. There is abundant evidence that humans are even willing to take additional costs to punish non-cooperative behaviour of group members (Fehr and Rockenbach 2004).

In terms of psychopathology, two aspects have face value in association with the problems of reciprocal altruism: one is the extreme of variation of suspiciousness, that is, paranoid ideation, which may eventually lead to delusions of persecution or delusions of reference. Interestingly, the content of persecutory delusions is almost always such that the affected individual is convinced that somebody else has malicious intents (i.e. wants to cheat on him). Benevolent intentions as content of persecutory delusions are the exception (for details see Chapter 8). The other is the extreme of variation of cheating, that is, psychopathy. Psychopathy has been interpreted as a cheater morph that may prevail in populations at low prevalence levels. Current conceptualizations suggest that psychopathy does not represent a pathology per se, even though there is overlap with antisocial personality disorder (Mealey 1995; Troisi 2005; for details see Chapter 19).

Psychopathological syndromes such as persecutory delusions can be seen as an extreme of variation of a mechanism involved in the detection of cheating behaviour. By contrast, psychopathy reflects a behavioural tendency that makes excessive use of deceiving others for one's own benefit.

Furthermore, neuroeconomic approaches to the understanding of cooperation, reciprocality, trust, and fairness norms offer new insights into the environmental contingencies that impact on these complex social behaviours and alterations of social decision-making associated with psychiatric illness (Wischniewski et al. 2009; Kishida et al. 2010).

1.2.2.2 Parental investment and sexual selection

Sexual reproduction has several disadvantages compared to asexual reproduction. Sexual reproduction is expensive in terms of time and energy to find a suitable mate; it also wastes genetic material, because only 50 percent of an individual's genes are passed on to offspring. The reason why sexual reproduction evolved resides in the fact that it counterbalances the effects of accumulating deleterious mutations by the recombination of genes. In a similar vein, sexual reproduction is the most important mechanism by which organisms improve their defence systems against rapidly evolving pathogenic germs and parasites (Ridley 2004). Sexual reproduction is particularly important for long-lived species with a slow turnover of genetic material. Evolution has produced two kinds of gametes: one large gamete (egg) that requires considerable metabolic resources, and (in energetic terms) much 'cheaper' gametes (sperm) that are produced in very large numbers. By convention, these different kinds of gametes are referred to as 'female' (egg) and 'male' (sperm). Differences between male and female gametes have important ramifications for the amount of parental investment in offspring and reproductive strategies.

Sexual reproduction has the advantage over asexual reproduction of counterbalancing the accumulation of deleterious mutations and better fending off threats from rapidly evolving pathogenic germs.

Trivers defined parental investment as 'any investment by the parent in an individual offspring that increases the offspring's chances of survival (and hence reproducing) at the cost of the parent's ability to invest in other offspring' (Trivers 1972). In mammals, pregnancy, lactation, nurturing, and protection of offspring are expenditures of female organisms, whereas in most species males invest little more than fertilization. It follows from this prediction that the sex that invests more in potential offspring (usually females) will be more discriminating in terms of mate choice, and that the sex that invests less (usually males) competes intrasexually for access to the higher investing sex, but is less discriminating with regard to the mate's reproductive fitness (Buss and Schmitt 1993). The reason for this is that reproduction is expensive in terms of energy, resources, and time, and that these constraints are more important for females, because their reproductive success is limited by the number of fertile eggs. In contrast, the reproductive success of males is (theoretically) limited only by the number of accessible fertile females. In other words, the sex that invests the most in producing offspring becomes a limiting resource over which the other sex will compete (Buss 1999).

In primates, and humans in particular, reproductive success is constrained by an additional number of factors, including the vastly extended juvenile period, advanced age at reproduction, singleton births, and long birth intervals. As a consequence, selection has favoured human males who are willing to invest heavily in offspring. Accordingly, in most human societies (most likely including ancestral ones; Walker et al. 2011) men usually have one or few wives (polygyny), which is directly linked to the greater paternal investment of human males relative to most other primates (Møller and Thornhill 1998). Very rarely polyandry can be observed. Still, human mothers, on average, invest more in children than do fathers, and it must have been in the interest of women to choose mates who were willing and have the resources to pursue long-term partnerships, in order to get support from their mates in raising children (Hrdy 2000). Conversely, it would follow from parental investment theory that it should be in the interest of human men to mate with more than one woman.

In most mammals, females invest much more in potential offspring than do males. Consequently, females are more discriminative in terms of mate choice (female choice principle).

In primates, including humans, reproductive success is constrained by an extended juvenile period, late reproduction, and long birth intervals, which favoured an increase of paternal investment relative to many other mammals.

In line with these predictions, selection has favoured a number of emotional, cognitive, and physiological adaptations, including mate guarding, emotions of jealousy (Wiederman and Kendall 1999; Buss 2000a, 2000b), concealed ovulation, and perhaps sexual coercion (to circumvent the 'female choice' principle; Voland 1998; Buss 1999). These adaptations are, at the behavioural level, not unique to primates or humans, but the subjective emotional dimension probably is. Jealousy is an important emotion in both men and women, but perhaps for different reasons (Daly et al. 1982). Women may be more emotionally jealous because they may be afraid of being

The relatively large amount of both male and female parental investment in humans has selected for emotional adaptations such as jealousy to ensure paternity and emotional commitment.

abandoned by their mates for another woman. Men, by contrast, are expected to be more sexually jealous, because they face the problem of uncertain paternity (Wiederman and Allgeier 1993; Sheets et al. 1997). That is, a woman can always be 100 percent sure that she is the mother of her children; fathers cannot be equally certain. In fact, cuckoldry is widespread in many species, including monogamous birds, in which the phenomenon has intensively been studied. In modern human societies, up to 10 percent of children are not biologically related to their fathers. Experimental studies have shown that men have been selected to compensate for the risk of uncertain paternity by producing more sperm after separation from their partners (Baker and Bellis 1995). Moreover, the anatomical form of the *glans penis* has been interpreted as an adaptation to remove (another man's) sperm from the vagina while at the same time inserting own sperm. These mechanisms may relate to so-called 'sperm competition', that is, the post-copulatory deferral of intrasexual competition between males (Baker 1993).

Monogamy is, however, perhaps not the only possible mating strategy evolved in humans (Rutberg 1983; Brewer et al. 2000). In experimental conditions young women close to ovulation prefer (unconsciously) the body odours of symmetrical men and facial features of masculine men, whereas their actual mate choice may be influenced by a man's willingness to pursue a long-term relationship. A closer look at our closest relatives may illustrate how selection has operated differentially on mating systems (McGrew et al. 1996). Gorillas, for example, are characterized by large differences in body size between males and females (called sexual dimorphism). However, testes size is small (about 30 g) in gorillas relative to body size. This has to do with the social structure of gorillas which can best be described as unimale polygyny. In contrast, in chimpanzees sexual dimorphism is relatively small. Yet a male chimpanzee—although only one-third of the size of an adult silverback gorilla—has comparably huge testes of about 120 g. The evolutionary explanation for this discrepancy is that chimpanzees live in multimale–multifemale groups, and females behave 'promiscuously' in the sense that they mate with multiple males when sexually receptive. Thus, intrasexual competition among male chimpanzees is shifted to post-copulation by variation in the amount of sperm males are able to place in a female's vaginal tract (sperm competition). Female chimpanzees may play an active role in the process of sperm competition, however, by accepting sperm from multiple males to ensure that the sperm reaching the egg is competitive (thus indicating the 'good genes' of its producer; Baker and Bellis 1995).

Human physical characteristics tell a different story. Sexual dimorphism is relatively small (men are about 10–15 percent larger), testes size is small (about 40 g), and women, in contrast to chimpanzees, have no visible signs indicating ovulation. Concealed ovulation may have evolved to solve various adaptive problems, including securing resources from males (the 'sex-for-food' hypothesis), protecting offspring from male infanticide, and enhancing pair bonding (Moller and Thornhill 1998). Male infanticide is

The mild sexual dimorphism, small testes size, and concealed ovulation support the hypothesis that humans under ancestral conditions have lived in societies in which monogamy or mild polygyny prevailed.

common in many mammalian species including primates and occurs if a new adult male manages to assume the alpha position of the social hierarchy, where the alpha male sires most offspring. From the male's perspective it makes sense to kill all offspring he has not fathered, because females become receptive again much faster and the time the male may enjoy the alpha position is likely to be short. Whether this has been an issue in early humans remains controversial; however, research in modern societies and hunter-gatherer cultures has shown that infants are at much greater risk of being maltreated or even killed by step-fathers than by biological fathers (Daly and Wilson 1988; Overpeck et al. 1998; for a divergent view see Temrin et al. 2000).

Differences in the amount of parental investment of males and females are also reflected in the survival ratio between the sexes. In primates there is mostly a female advantage throughout the entire lifespan, but in species in which the male carries the offspring, the difference in survival advantage disappears or is even reversed in favour of males. In apes, males contribute relatively little to the care for offspring; thus there is a large survival advantage for females. The figure of female to male survival is approximately 1.4 in chimpanzees and roughly 1.2 in gorillas. It decreases in humans to 1.05–1.08, which indicates the relatively large amount of paternal care for children compared with other apes (Allman 1999).

As already shown, many of these biological factors have shaped behaviour and particularly mate choice in humans. An extensive body of research has shown that, on average, women prefer slightly older socially high-ranking men as mates, whereas men prefer younger women whose attractiveness is indicated by her waist-to-hip ratio and breast size (Buss et al. 1990). Both men and women prefer partners with low fluctuating asymmetry (asymmetry between bilateral characters), because high fluctuating asymmetry has been shown to be associated with greater mutation load, parasitic infections, or other environmental stressors. Thus, the reproductive 'quality' of a potential mate is largely unconsciously evaluated. Moreover, there is evidence that mate choice is also influenced by the degree of similarity (both physical and psychological) of partners and not entirely random (called 'assortative mating'; Buston and Emlen 2003).

Psychopathological syndromes such as delusional jealousy and erotomania are distortions of adaptive mechanisms involved in human mating behaviour.

Psychopathological correlates as extremes of variations of mechanisms that emerged as sexually selected human traits are abundant. Advertising one's qualities as a potential partner is perhaps one critical aspect of manic episodes or histrionic personality disorder. Mate guarding is pathologically exaggerated in cases of delusions of jealousy, which is typically seen in men. The pathological variation of the 'female choice' principle is probably reflected in erotomania, the delusional conviction of being loved by another person, most often observed in women (for details see Chapters 8 and 19).

1.2.2.3 Parent–offspring conflict

Conflicting interests between parents and offspring exist over the amount and duration of parental investment in individual offspring. There is overlap between a parent's and an offspring's genetic interests; however, interests are not identical. At some point during the ontogenetic development of the offspring, it is in the interest of the parent to invest in other progeny, because, from a gene-centred point of view, a parent shares only 50 percent with his or her descendant, such that it makes sense to produce more offspring in order to maximize reproductive success. Conversely, it is in the interest of the offspring to secure a greater amount of investment than the parent is willing to give, yet only to the point at which it becomes more than twice as costly for the parent to nurse that particular offspring, because full siblings also share 50 percent of genes. At this point, therefore, selection should operate on both parent (here, the mother) and offspring to end investment (Trivers 1974). This simple rule applies to all sexually reproducing species. In mammals, however, parent–offspring conflict may be an issue already during pregnancy. Foetal genes, for example, may be selected to extract more resources from the mother's organism than is in the mother's interest. The mother's sensitivity to insulin, for example, is downregulated by placental hormones such that her blood sugar level rises and increases the energy supply to the foetus. EPH (oedema, proteinuria, and hypertension) gestosis can been seen as the extreme (and pathological) variant of this conflict (Schuiling 2000). EPH gestosis causes severe health problems for the mother, partly due to a dysregulation of the foetus's and mother's optimal blood sugar level (Haig 1993).

Due to the amount of shared genetic material, conflict between parent and offspring generation has produced a variety of adaptations to limit parental investment (on the parent's side) and to increase parental investment (on the offspring's side).

Another parent–offspring conflict typical of mammals is weaning. Usually, the infant is selected to demand greater and longer investment (here, in terms of milk supply) than the mother is selected to provide. Parent–offspring theory also predicts that the weaning conflict aggravates if an infant's future siblings are genetically more distantly related to him/her than full siblings. In other words, if future siblings are half-siblings, because they are fathered by a different male, weaning conflict is intensified. Thus, in humans, where different fatherhood is probably the exception, the weaning conflict may actually be weaker compared with other mammalian species. However, it has been suggested that breast-fed infants may extend their mothers' amenorrhoea by extending the period of night waking, perhaps partly mediated by imprinted genes from the paternal side (whereas maternally imprinted genes may favour more consolidated sleep; Haig 2014).

Parent–offspring conflict can arise at different developmental stages of the offspring, ranging from the intrauterine environment (over the amount of energy supply) to adolescence and early adulthood (over the offspring's mate choice). A parent–offspring conflict typical of mammals is weaning.

Along similar lines, conflict between infant and mother may arise over riding or carrying. Human children often demand being carried, even when able to walk on their own (Hrdy 2000); as a side note, it is worth mentioning that in modern societies infants are carried on their mothers' hips much less than in traditional cultures, which contributes to the problem of hip dysplasia, because riding on mother's hip is the best prevention of sub-luxation of the femur).

Infants (both human and non-human) have a variety of behaviours at hand to elicit parental investment in their parents. Since the infant is much smaller and less experienced than the parent, and the parent has control over available resources, infants have been selected to develop psychological mechanisms rather than physical means to increase the amount of parental investment (Trivers 1974). The infant cry when hungry or in perceived danger may be such an example. In species in which the offspring is particularly helpless and vulnerable, parents have been selected to respond more readily to the infant's needs. This has certainly been important throughout human evolution, because human babies are physiologically preterm at birth and thus extremely immature compared to other primate babies (see Chapter 3). A 'tactic' on the side of the offspring as it grows older could be to revert to behaviours of an earlier ontogenetic stage in order to increase parental investment. This phenomenon is well known in human psychology and referred to as 'regression'. Temper tantrums are another way to force parents to increase their investment. Under natural circumstances, the existence of temper tantrums is counterintuitive, because such blatant behaviour may attract predators and is energetically expensive. In a way, temper tantrums can be seen as a risky strategy to increase parental investment which is often highly successful. The evolutionary logic behind this is that an individual offspring that puts itself at risk of being mauled by a predator also potentially decreases the parent's fitness, because of their genetic relatedness and the potential loss of all resources already invested (Trivers 1974).

'Regression' is typical of offspring as an attempt to increase parental investment.

Interaction between siblings can also be interpreted in terms of parent–offspring theory. Parents are equally related to all individual offspring, so theoretically it is in their interest that resources are distributed equally among their offspring. From genetic relatedness it would follow, however, that an individual offspring performs an altruistic act towards a full sibling only if the benefit to the sibling is twice as large as is the cost to the donor. In other words, parents are selected to encourage altruism between siblings and to discourage selfish behaviours (Trivers 1974).

Other forms of parent–offspring conflict may arise over the adult (reproductive) role of the offspring. Trivers argued that human parents ought to be particularly interested in their children's mate choice, because it could be in the interest of parents to encourage a marriage with close kin to increase the offspring's altruism towards kin (a tendency that is counterbalanced by incest avoidance). On the other hand, there may also be situations in which the offspring wants to terminate parental investment earlier than the parent wants to. This could be the case, for instance, if parents aim at precluding an individual offspring from reproduction because they want to retain the offspring as a 'helper at the nest'. Such conflicts may be particularly difficult to resolve for children grown adult (Trivers 1974).

A special variant of parent–offspring conflict refers to the sex of the offspring. Normally, natural selection favours parents who invest equally in sons and daughters, leading to an approximate sex ratio of 50/50. However, in good conditions it may pay off for a parent to produce more sons, because the reproductive success of sons may be greater than that of daughters. In poor circumstances, however, selection may favour parents who invest more in daughters, because environmental conditions have disproportionally smaller effects on females than on males (Trivers-Willard hypothesis; Trivers and Willard 1973). These biologically determined biases have been shown to exert profound effects on intrauterine male mortality as a function of (perceived?) environmental conditions in humans and other mammals. Some mammalian species are even able to 'decide' over the sex of the offspring during pregnancy, pending the environmental conditions, and abort foetuses of the 'wrong' sex (Kumm et al. 1994). A prolonged period of parental investment, like in humans and other primates, increases the biases in differential parental behaviour towards male or female offspring; however, the role of paternal investment may modify these biases in many ways.

A special case of parent–offspring conflict is associated with differential parental investment in offspring depending on the sex of the offspring. In good environmental conditions, parents may tend to favour male offspring due to the greater reproductive potential of the latter relative to females. Poor environmental conditions may favour investment in female offspring, due to smaller effects of environmental conditions on females.

The existence of differential investment in sons versus daughters in humans is a matter of great dispute, especially if moral issues are confused with biological principles. There is evidence, however, that infanticide may be the way primates and humans postpone their adjustment in parental investment until after birth, and this has apparently not only happened in ancestral or contemporary hunter-gatherer societies (Hrdy et al. 1994; Brookman and Nolan 2006). In such instances, it is almost always neonaticide that is pursued (in the first 24 hours after birth), before maternal bonding to the newborn develops (see also Chapters 3 and 21). However, whether or not a child is accepted by his or her mother also depends on the mother's age and life circumstances. This has even a profound impact on the mother's decision on abortion in modern societies (Lycett and Dunbar 1999). Single mothers, for example, are more likely to abort a pregnancy than married women. This has to do with future prospects of women to engage in marriage and have other children, both of which are considerably higher in young women and declining with age. Consequently, older women near the end of their reproductive phase are less likely to terminate a pregnancy through abortion even when living single (Braza 2004). By contrast, there is an increase in abortion rate in older married women, especially in those who have already one or two children (Lycett and Dunbar 1999). Fear of congenital birth defects does not seem to play a leading role in decision-making, because the steep increase in abortion rate is not paralleled in single older women.

Primates and humans have postponed their decision over parental investment until after birth. Neonaticide has been a method of birth control in hunter-gatherers, and even in modern societies, single adolescent mothers sometimes abandon newborns.

A combination of problems relating to parental investment theory and parent–offspring conflict is reflected in genomic imprinting. Paternally and maternally inherited genes may compete for resources provided by the mother organism (Haig 1993). This issue is dealt with in section 1.4 on genetics.

Although expressed in the technical terminology of evolutionary biology, the potential for conflict among individuals due to their differential genetic make-up has profound implications for the understanding of human psychology and psychopathology. Examples of delusional beliefs and personality disorders have already been mentioned. Another important field in which the biologically driven conflicts emerge is psychotherapy. It cannot be overemphasized that the biological arenas of conflict are largely unconscious to the individual. They are in principle accessible to conscious awareness, but probably hard, if ever, to control. Psychotherapeutic relationships are perhaps mainly characterized by projections of parent–offspring conflict, and particularly severe personality disorders such as borderline personality disorder (BPD) may in therapy display the whole array of parental investment-inducing behaviours and rejections (for further details see Chapters 19 and 20). Similarly, psychopathological conditions characterized by defence mechanisms such as depression and anxiety disorders frequently make use of behaviours akin to 'regression', which strongly signal 'no threat' and aim at maximizing care (see Chapters 10 and 11).

Behaviours associated with parent–offspring conflict are often (unconsciously) transferred to client–therapist relationships.

1.3 Principles of evolutionary psychology and psychopathology

The central premise of evolutionary psychology is that the human mind has evolved according to the same biological laws as morphological characteristics of all living things. Thus, natural and sexual selection have shaped the way we think, feel, and behave (Buss 1999; Rossano 2003). Evolutionary psychology and related disciplines such as ethology, sociobiology, and behavioural ecology have contributed to the refutation of several false presuppositions about how the human mind works. One widespread assumption concerned the view that the mind of a newborn human infant was a 'tabula rasa' ('blank slate'). We now know from careful observation that this is not the case. For example, newborns have retained some primitive reflexes that are functionally no longer useful but deeply rooted in our primate heritage, such as the Moro reflex or grasp reflex. Moreover, newborn babies are readily able to interact with their primary care figure, usually the mother, in quite sophisticated ways, which helps to strengthen attachment and bonding. Shortly after birth, newborns are also capable of imitating simple facial movements (Meltzoff and Moore 1977). Babies have a preference for face-like shapes over geometrical shapes; they have an inborn fear of being left alone, of heights, of loud noises, etc. These abilities, among many others, are highly adapted psychological mechanisms that emerged as adaptations to our species-specific environmental conditions.

The central premise of evolutionary psychology is that human cognition, emotion, and behaviour has been shaped by natural and sexual selection in essentially the same way as anatomy.

Human babies are born with a set of evolved psychological mechanisms that help them to attach and survive.

Most psychological mechanisms are, however, highly open for experiential modification, that is, they represent 'open programmes' (as opposed to 'closed programmes', which are much more instinct-driven) that respond to learning experiences throughout the human lifespan, with some periods being critical for 'imprinting-like' processes (Mayr 2001). In other words, for psychological mechanisms to function physiologically it is essential that innate predispositions ('nature') meet adequate input from a stimulating environment ('nurture'), because otherwise they may develop in malfunctioning ways. For example, if a mild strabismus goes undetected in young children, the 'non-dominant' eye may never learn to see and remain amblyopic. In amblyopia there is no organic failure in the affected eye. Rather, the disorder arises from the developmental problem that the affected eye is not properly stimulated (Eggers and Blakemore 1978). By analogy, this may happen to many other evolved psychological mechanisms, such as language and empathy, in essentially the same way, if an individual is deprived of appropriate stimulation, viz. environmental input.

Most human psychological mechanisms are 'open programmes' that highly depend on appropriate environmental stimulation to develop properly. Accordingly, deficient environmental input may cause dysfunction.

1.3.1 Evolved psychological mechanisms and biosocial goals

Human biosocial–psychological functioning is replete with psychological mechanisms that have evolved in response to selection pressures in our evolutionary past (it must be emphasized that the term psychological *mechanism* is inelegant, because it suggests rigidity and imperviousness to modification by learning. However, this is not what the expression, coined by evolutionary psychologists, actually intends to express). More specifically, psychological mechanisms are designed by evolution to solve problems of adaptive significance (Cosmides et al. 1992). In order to do so, they need to be economic, reliable, efficient, and precise (Williams 1966). These properties are best maintained by domain-specific functioning, with the possibility that several domain-general mechanisms exist to integrate information from multiple sources. Domain specificity is assumed if an adaptive problem has recurrently been present over a considerable amount of time during evolution, thereby affecting individual reproductive success. Many psychological mechanisms can be conceptualized as mental modules that operate only on a specific class of information, largely independent of other modules (Fodor 1983). Modules are activated by decision rules or triggering algorithms that help to focus attention, emotional evaluation, and behavioural responses for swift reactions.

Many evolved psychological mechanisms are domain-specific, that is, they operate only on a particular class of information in an economical, reliable, efficient, and precise way. Modules of evolved psychological mechanisms are hierarchically organized and activated by triggering algorithms.

Modules are thought to be hierarchically organized in order to increase their efficiency (which is also pivotal in medical decision-making; Gigerenzer 1996). A basic module for threat detection, for instance, that is activated under conditions of heightened vigilance such as being alone in the dark, may follow an algorithm that focuses on the detection of a moving shape. If the moving shape is identified as self-propelled (in contrast to random movements created by air circulation), a higher-order module may be activated by an algorithm examining the direction of the movement. If the direction of the movement is oriented towards the individual, another module may be triggered by an algorithm that is concerned with the assessment of whether the moving object is an animal or human.

Evolved psychological mechanisms have been likened to the diverse functions of a Swiss army knife comprising a collection of separate devices that are designed to carry out different tasks in highly efficient ways (Cosmides et al. 1992). As with most metaphorical analogies, the comparison of the human brain with a Swiss army knife is not ideal (for example, there must be someone who purposefully handles a Swiss army knife, but the orchestrated execution of multiple tasks is another function of the human brain itself; thus, in the evolutionary perspective, there is no room for dualistic conceptualizations of the human mind). The analogy illustrates, however, that decision-making and reasoning processes are neither abstract nor logical, but best conceptualized as selected answers to recurrent problems during human evolution. One of the most important discoveries of evolutionary psychology is that many, perhaps most, human brain functions are biased towards the solution of *social* problems rather than abstract ones (Cosmides 1989). Some evolved psychological mechanisms are ridiculously illogical, at least in a strictly economic perspective, especially when the evolved mechanisms are concerned with social matters such as social rules and moral values (for further details pertaining to the social brain hypothesis see Chapter 2).

Psychological mechanisms are biased towards the solution of problems of adaptive significance, which does not necessarily invoke any logic.

Due to the outstanding significance of social life for the human species, and in light of the multiform selection pressures that have operated on the human mind, the pursuit of biosocial goals is the actual target of evolved psychological mechanisms (Gilbert 1998). It has to be emphasized that humans—like other organisms—cannot be seen as 'fitness maximizers' in the sense that one's behaviour is consciously guided towards maximization of individual reproductive fitness. Inclusive fitness can only be measured in retrospect; future reproductive success is incalculable. Thus, evolved psychological mechanisms, sometimes referred to as evolved 'strategies', operate at the proximate level, because achieving biosocial goals increases the likelihood of successful reproduction (which can be, but need not be, an indicator of fitness). Of note, the word 'strategy' does not involve conscious awareness of how to accomplish a certain biosocial goal.

The most common human biosocial goals involve the motivation and behaviour to elicit care from others, to provide care for others—mainly kin and close allies—to find a suitable mate, to form cooperative alliances, and to attain the highest social rank possible (Gilbert 1998). Biosocial goals also aim to compare one's social position with the position of others in terms of inferiority or superiority, and to negotiate relationships with higher and lower ranking individuals. Strictly speaking, biosocial goals are part of the proximate level, because they are malleable during an individual's life-time. For example, an individual can climb up or go down the social hierarchy ladder or change his or her effort in directing social support to others. Biosocial goals, therefore, take a somewhat intermediate position between the basic proximate causes of cognitions, emotions, and behaviour mediated by physiological processes, the action of genes or individual rearing conditions, and the problems

Human biosocial goals such as care-eliciting, care-giving, mating, alliance formation, etc. guide an individual's actual behaviour.

caused by genetic similarity and dissimilarity between individuals. Male and female individuals differ markedly in goal priorities, which relates to the divergent roles males and females assumed under ancestral condition (see section 1.3.2), as well as to different reproductive constraints, which have influenced reproductive issues to the present day (Voland and Dunbar 1995). Thus, for males, status and access to resources may have been more important throughout evolutionary history, whereas females may have been more oriented towards strong affiliative bonds and emotional ties.

Notably, evolved psychological mechanisms are rarely, if ever, optimally designed (Gilbert 1998); they often represent design compromises, which essentially bears the risk of failure or malfunction, because design optimality would be much too costly (metabolically) to evolve. Along similar lines, mutual dependence and the need for accommodating social relationships can create problems that may lead to psychological dysfunction. These issues and other possible sources for psychopathology are further explored in Chapter 4 and the subsequent clinical chapters.

Evolved psychological mechanisms are not optimal by design, which renders them vulnerable to dysfunction.

1.3.2 **Environments of evolutionary adaptedness**

The idea that most psychological mechanisms that make us human evolved in environmental conditions of a remote past was introduced by John Bowlby (1969). Bowlby argued that most facets of human mentality originated when our forebears lived as hunter-gatherers during a geological period called the Pleistocene (2 mya until 10,000 years ago). Research into the life of hunter-gatherers suggests that ancestral humans lived in small, partly kin-based, and mostly patrilocal tribal groups that were relatively egalitarian in social structure, with the accumulation of material goods largely absent. Recent studies of hunter-gatherer social structures indicate that a significant proportion of group members may be non-relatives, and that adult brother–sister co-residence is maintained by bisexual philopatry and dispersal (Hill et al. 2011). These models of societal structure probably prevailed for most of the history of our species, at least since the advent of anatomically modern humans some 150,000 years ago until quite recent times, when humans adopted a more sedentary lifestyle. However, a single one scenario of the environment of evolutionary adaptedness (EEA) has been criticized as too simplistic, and it is plausible to assume that several environments have impacted on selection of human physical and psychological traits (Foley 1996).

Many aspects of human mentality evolved under ancestral environmental conditions of hunter-gatherer life. Humans are adapted to live in small close-knit kin-based communities with personal acquaintances of about 150 people.

Among the most important universals, cooperation of members of the same group has been critical to secure food from game hunting and foraging. This included mutual aid between women to raise children cooperatively (thereby shortening between-birth intervals from 5–6 years down to 3–4 years; Mace and Sear 1997; Hrdy 2000), and between men to protect the group from large predators and competing human groups (Axelrod and Hamilton 1981). Ancestral human communities comprised perhaps not more than 30–40 individuals, which together with neighbouring groups or extended kin made up to 150 people who were personally acquainted with one another. Trade, but also warfare with adjacent groups, was probably prevalent throughout human history. Data from horticultural societies, which until recently lived under intense pressure to compete for scarce resources, suggest that about one in four men dies a violent death, mainly in between-group conflict (Diamond 2012). As a consequence and prime cause of human tragedy lingering to the present day, humans are—despite their high inclination towards within-group cooperation—essentially xenophobic and ingroup-biased. That is, they have a strong tendency to mistrust strangers, and act in less empathetic ways when strangers are in danger or need of help, as compared to members of their own group, a mode of action that is partly under control of oxytocin (Cikara et al. 2011; de Dreu et al. 2012; Shamay-Tsoory et al. 2013; Balliet et al. 2014). Even infants 'instinctively' develop xenophobia in their first year of life, particularly oriented towards strange males (Eibl-Eibesfeldt 1995).

Within-group cooperation and between-group competition (including warfare) prevailed over extended periods of human evolution.

Beyond adaptations that occurred in the most recent history of humans living as hunter-gatherers, the relevance of adaptations evolving prior to the Pleistocene period also needs to be taken into consideration. For example, since the human and chimpanzee lineages split around 5–7 mya, adaptations in humans to the cooling climate have included bipedalism, brain enlargement and reorganization, and, eventually, language. Long before this period occurred, primates evolved from largely nocturnal, solitary-living insectivores to diurnal, gregarious foragers. This transition was accompanied by the evolution of binocular view, colour vision, and eye–hand coordination, which further fostered the emergence of social adaptations (Allman 2000). For instance, the movement of the eyeballs from the side to the front of the skull may, on the one hand, have improved hunting skills and brachiation, however, at the cost of constricting the previously almost panoramic visual field, which reduced the ability to detect predators approaching from the rear. This may, in turn, have selectively favoured the formation of social groups and, hence, brain systems for dealing with adaptive problems from the social environment (Allman 2000; more remote adaptations are reflected in our hierarchically organized 'triune' brain; for details see Chapter 2).

Prior to the most recent adaptations, binocularity may have contributed to the evolution of sociality in primates, as constriction of the visual field required the formation of social groups.

Conversely, several adaptations are even more recent and emerged after early humans left Africa to populate the entire planet (except Antarctica). Although perhaps only a small group of humans started out, indicated by the close genetic relatedness of all humans (referred to as the 'evolutionary bottleneck' hypothesis), there were many EEAs to which local populations adapted (for example, two randomly picked humans are genetically much more closely related than any two chimpanzees of the same social group). Thus, the EEA is

All humans are genetically closely related. There are hints indicating ongoing adaptive modification of humans, some of which have been associated with the evolution of language and writing.

probably best conceptualized as a statistical composite of environmental contingencies that lasted long enough to create selection pressures on evolving humans (Hrdy 2000).

Accordingly, humans have and continue to adapt to changing environments, be they physical, biotic, or psychological in nature. For instance, allelic variation in the human ASPM gene and the FoxP2 gene family that emerged a few thousand years ago may relate to brain enlargement and the evolution of language. One such variation in the ASPM gene has been found to be as young as 5,800 years, and it has been speculated that the coincidence with the discovery of the earliest written documents did not happen by chance (Mekel-Brobov et al. 2005). Along similar lines, a gene called microcephalin, which is involved in the regulation of brain size, has undergone positive selection during human evolution (Evans et al. 2004). On the other hand, brain size and body size have declined in humans over the past 50,000 years, which has given rise to the speculation that these changes could relate to 'domestication' effects, as the result of selection towards reduced aggressiveness (Leach et al. 2003).

Even more recently, the emergence of Tay–Sachs disease, the first occurrence of which can be traced back to medieval times, when people increasingly gathered in overcrowded cities, may be associated with selection of genes associated with greater resistance against tuberculosis (Diamond 1988). These latter examples may show that even the most recent adaptations in humans did not spare the nervous system (see also Chapter 2), and that humans continue to evolve, as has been shown in a study suggesting an extension of the reproductive period at both ends (earlier menarche, later menopause) in a large cohort of women of European ancestry (Byars et al. 2010; Stearns et al. 2010a). The way selection operates in our modern environments on human cognition, emotion, and behaviour, however, has not been sufficiently understood (but caused many scientifically untenable speculations), though it may be interesting to ask if we can watch ourselves evolving, as rapidly changing environments almost certainly impact on differential reproductive success. For example, the plague epidemics in the medieval period may have created genetic bottlenecks, which unquestionably selected for changes in immune function and may also have influenced psychological adaptations. Conversely, increased population size, changing selection pressures due to modern medical achievements, and perhaps a larger number of *de novo* mutations related to increasing paternal and maternal age may contribute to a larger genetic diversity (Greenspan 2013).

Rapidly changing environments impact on differential reproductive success. The medieval plague epidemics may have created genetic bottlenecks. Conversely, recent changes in selection pressures due to modern medical achievement may contribute to a larger genetic diversity.

1.3.3 Testing evolutionary hypotheses of human cognition, emotion, and behaviour

Perhaps the most significant advantage of an evolutionary framework applied to human psychology over competing non-biological approaches is that it allows generating testable predictions about human behaviour (Buss 1999). Testing evolutionary psychological hypotheses can take a top-down approach, that is, a testable hypothesis can be derived from one of the central theories pertaining to the genetic relatedness of organisms, such as parental investment theory. One may, for instance, hypothesize that women, compared with men, are selected to seek secure partnerships with socially highly regarded mates, because of women's greater parental investment in potential offspring. A bottom-up approach, by contrast, would set out with an actual observation of behaviour, for instance, that women more often divorce if the (perceived) social rank of their partners has declined, or that men abandon their female partners more often for younger partners than women do if the female partner's fecundity decreases, for example, as a function of age (Betzig 1989). Such observations can be cast into a testable hypothesis to confirm or refute the hypothesis. See Figure 1.1.

Empirical testing of hypothesis derived from evolutionary psychological theory can be in one of two ways: the top-down approach, by which a hypothesis is directly derived from evolutionary theory; or the bottom-up (observation-driven) approach.

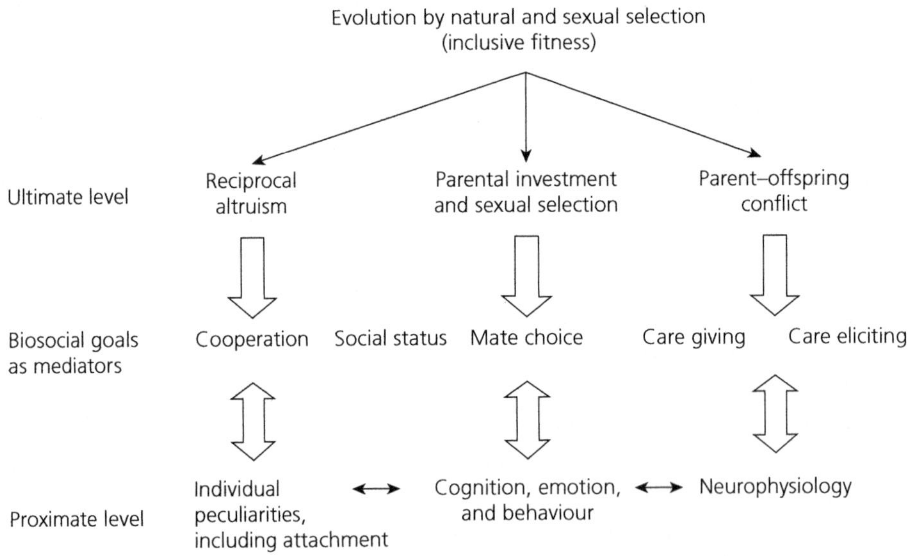

Fig. 1.1 Hierarchically structured framework for the analysis of cognition, emotion, and behaviour according to evolutionary psychology and psychopathology. The 'top-down' analysis is theory driven and focuses on creating testable hypotheses from which testable predictions can be derived. The 'bottom-up' analysis is observation-driven. Hypotheses on the adaptive function of an observed trait are cast into experimentally testable designs to confirm predictions on the basis of empirical results. In psychopathology, the 'bottom-up' approach is useful with the understanding that psychopathological signs and symptoms are extremes of variation at either end of a (hypothetical) Gaussian curve. (Reproduced from Martin Brüne, Toward an Integration of Interpersonal and Biological Processes: Evolutionary Psychiatry as an Empirically Testable Framework for Psychiatric Research, *Psychiatry: Interpersonal and Biological Processes*, 65 (1), pp. 48–57 © 2002, Taylor & Francis, with permission.)

Both bottom-up and top-down approaches can utilize diverse sources of evidence, including experimental tests to examine sex differences in cognition, emotion, and behaviour; questionnaires (which can, however, be burdened with the problem of response biases according to social expectations and desirability; Daly and Wilson 1999); archival data that have been gathered devoid of evolutionary theory; cross-cultural comparison in the search for human universals, but also to assess culture-specific modifications of evolved mechanisms; and across-species comparison among closely related species. Finally, even psychopathological signs and symptoms can be used as a viable source for understanding normal psychology. It was Konrad Lorenz who argued from an ethological point of view that pathologies of behaviour (e.g. vacuum activities, displacement activities) might even have superior explanatory power for normal functioning over analysis of the physiological function of behaviour (Lorenz 1973). Such an approach might be particularly fruitful if psychopathology is being considered as a source of evidence for the understanding of human psychology. To date, however, this prospect has greatly been neglected in evolutionary psychology (Brüne 2002).

1.4 Genetics

The information required to grow an organism is stored in the individual genome. All genetic information is encoded in a macromolecule called deoxyribonucleic acid (DNA). It is composed of monomeric deoxynucleotides that carry one of four kinds of base: adenine (A), guanine (G), cytosine (C), and thymine (T), whereby A is always paired with T, and G with C. This 'alphabet' or genetic code is identical in all living organisms. Thus, the basic design of animals, known as *bauplan* (incorrectly translated as 'body plan', because the German 'plan' better translates into 'map'), is maintained by regulatory genes that have been preserved over very long periods of time (Mayr 2001). They largely act independently of structural genes, which are the central theme of the following paragraphs.

All genetic information is stored in an individual's DNA, which consists of deoxynucleotides carrying adenine, guanine, cytosine, or thymine. The genetic code of life has been highly conservative throughout evolutionary history.

Human DNA comprises an estimated 3.5 billion base pairs. DNA consists of a mix of coding DNA and non-coding DNA (McGuffin et al. 2005). The human genome contains perhaps some 30,000 functional genes, which is a surprisingly low number, though not the least exceptional in the animal kingdom. Notably, about 55 percent of coding DNA is expressed in the human brain, suggesting that the brain is the prime target for mutations. An estimated 97 percent of the human DNA is non-coding, of which the function is not entirely known. It is, however, probably incorrect to speak of 'junk' DNA, because evolution would have eliminated superfluous DNA, since the production of DNA is too

The human genome is believed to comprise some 30,000 functional genes. A gene represents a unit or template from which messenger RNA is transcribed. About 55 percent of coding DNA is expressed in the human brain, which renders the brain the prime target of mutation-selection processes.

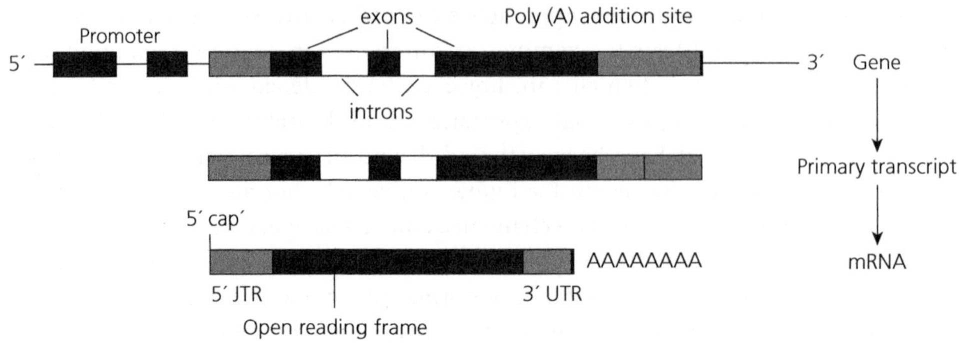

Fig. 1.2 The structure of a gene encoding messenger RNA (mRNA). Genes contain a promoter at the 5′ end, which binds RNA polymerase and initiates transcription. Although the whole gene sequence is transcribed into a primary transcript, only a proportion of the gene is represented in mRNA. Sequences present in mRNA (grey and black) are called exons. The intervening sequences are called introns (white). In producing a mature mRNA, the primary transcript undergoes RNA splicing to remove intronic sequence, is cleaved at its 3′ end, and a poly A sequence added (polyadenylation) while the 5′ end is capped. The mature RNA sequence contains a stretch of sequence (black) encoding protein that is not interrupted by a stop codon. This is called the open reading frame. The residual sequences and both 5′ and 3′ ends are called untranslated regions because they do not encode protein. (This material was originally published in *Psychiatric Genetics and Genomics* edited by Peter McGuffin, Michael J Owen, and Irving I Gottesman and has been reproduced by permission of Oxford University Press (<http://ukcatalogue.oup.com/product/9780198564867.do>). For permission to reuse this material, please visit <http://www.oup.co.uk/academic/rights/permissions>.)

expensive a process to maintain for no purpose. Part of the non-coding DNA, for instance, consists of introns that help keep the starting codons of genes (exons) apart (McGuffin et al. 2005). Put another way, it is the non-coding DNA that is responsible for the regulation of gene expression (Babbitt et al. 2010; Barrett et al. 2012).

A gene comprises the unit of DNA that serves as a template to be transcribed into messenger ribonucleic acid (mRNA) (see Figure 1.2). A gene usually consists of a start (promoter) and a stop region. These regions are important for the initiation and termination of the transcription process from DNA to RNA. A gene has both introns and exons, whereby the introns have to be removed from the primary transcript by a process called RNA splicing, which produces fully mature mRNA. RNA is similarly structured as DNA, except that T is replaced with uracil (U).

Three adjacent bases form a triplet or codon, which code for amino acids to build proteins. There are 4^3 (= 64) possible triplet combinations, which code for 20 different amino acids; thus, the DNA (RNA) code is degenerate, because there is more than one possible triplet combination per amino acid (see Figure 1.3).

Normally, DNA takes the shape of a double helix that in humans represents the basis of 23 pairs of chromosomes, two of which are the sex chromosomes X and Y. The

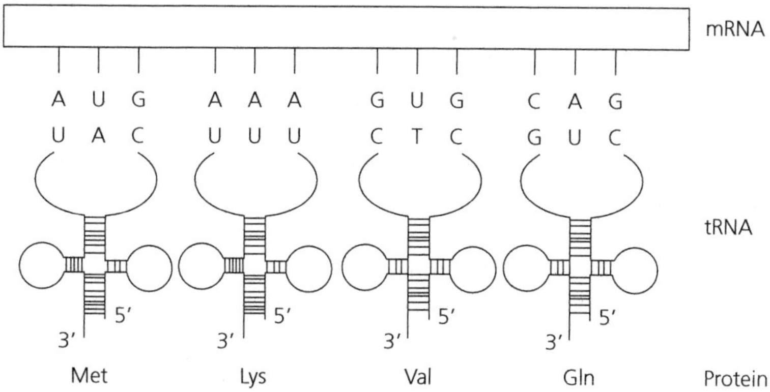

Fig. 1.3 Translation. Specific anti-codons in transfer RNA (tRNA) recognize mRNA codons by base pairing. Each tRNA brings a specific amino acid to the translational machinery consisting of an mRNA/ribosomal complex. In this way, the codon sequence is translated to an amino acid sequence. (This material was originally published in *Psychiatric Genetics and Genomics* edited by Peter McGuffin, Michael J Owen, and Irving I Gottesman and has been reproduced by permission of Oxford University Press (<http://ukcatalogue.oup.com/product/9780198564867.do>). For permission to reuse this material, please visit <http://www.oup.co.uk/academic/rights/permissions>.)

chromosomes are numbered according to size, with chromosome 1 being the largest. Compared to the great apes, which have 48 chromosomes, the 46 human chromosomes are reduced in number, but not in the amount of genetic information. At some time after the human and the chimpanzee lineages split, around 4–5 mya, chromosomes 12 and 13 of the common ancestor's chromosomes present in the gorilla and the chimpanzee merged to form the human chromosome 2 (Marks 1992). In mammals, female organisms carry two X chromosomes, whereas males carry an X and a Y chromosome. The Y chromosome—although considerably smaller than the X—determines the sex; its possession produces a male and its absence a female organism (by contrast, in birds, XX are male and XY female). The karyotype of an organism gives the number of the autosomes and sex chromosomes separately. Thus, healthy humans have 44 XX or 44 XY. Changes in the normal number of chromosomes are called aneuploidies. The most frequent example is trisomy 21 causing Down syndrome; aneuploidies of the sex chromosomes may cause Klinefelter's syndrome (47 XXY), Turner's syndrome (45 X0), or other syndromes. Aneuploidies are often associated with mental retardation and increased risk of psychosis or other behavioural abnormalities. In addition to the possibility of aneuploidies, parts of a chromosome may be lost by deletion, reinserted in the opposite direction (inversion), duplicated, or translocated to another chromosome. These rearrangements can exert a profound impact on development including mental health.

Humans possess 23 pairs of chromosomes, which carry the DNA. Two of these chromosomes, X and Y, are called sex chromosomes. Aneuploidies—deviations in the number of chromosomes—often cause behavioural abnormalities.

The chromosomes are eccentrically 'squeezed' in a region called the centromere, leading to a long (q) and a short (p) arm. The arms have microscopically visible banding patterns, which are numbered starting close to the centromere. Pairs of the same chromosomes are called homologous, a term that must not be confused with 'homozygous', which means that the information on at a given locus on both homologous chromosomes is identical (otherwise, the individual is heterozygous at that locus; McGuffin et al. 2005).

The DNA of two randomly picked humans is more than 99 percent identical. DNA is thus a highly conservative biological structure. However, theoretically, variation may occur at any locus on any chromosome, and such variation is called allelic. The most common mechanism by which allele variation is produced is mutation through replacement of a single base or nucleotide. If the frequency of at least two alleles at a given locus is greater than 1 percent of the population, these variants are called polymorphisms. Single nucleotide polymorphisms (SNP, conveniently pronounced 'snips') are common and believed to occur on average once every 1,500 bases. Since most SNPs lie in non-coding regions, they are phenotypically silent. However, SNPs can have dramatic effects if they are located in coding, promoter, enhancer, or silencer regions of the genome that may affect gene expression.

The DNA of two randomly picked humans is 99 percent identical. Variations of single nucleotides that pertain to more than 1 percent of a population are called SNPs. Insertions, deletions, and duplications of one or more bases can exert considerable phenotypic effects, if located in a coding region of the genome. The functional significance and evolutionary origin of such copy number variations (CNV), as well as 'orphan genes', is largely unknown.

Similarly, the insertion or deletion (loss) of one or more bases can have profound consequences for the functioning of the respective stretch of the genome. For example, research has shown that some human-specific deletions are associated with changes concerning anatomic features of the human penis (i.e. loss of a keratinized epidermal spine) and changes relating to forebrain structures, which are possibly linked to the generation of inhibitory interneurons (McLean et al. 2011). Insertions, deletions, duplications, and complex multisite variants have recently been subsumed under the term copy number variations (CNV) or copy number polymorphisms (CNP). Such variations are much more frequent in the human genome than previously assumed. An estimated 1,400 + regions comprising CNVs have been identified so far, covering approximately 12 percent of the human genome. The functional significance of CNVs is poorly understood, as is their evolutionary origins, including the emergence of 'orphan genes', so-called because they lack a functional equivalent in other lineages (Tautz and Damazet-Loso 2011). It can be expected, however, that research into CNV loci will ultimately have implications for psychiatry in the near future (Redon et al. 2006).

In any event, from an evolutionary point of view it is crucial to note that a variant producing a mere 1 percent fitness advantage would increase in population frequency from 0.1 percent to 99.9 percent in roughly 4,000 generations, hence, in humans within 100,000–120,000 years. In fact, there is growing evidence suggesting that accelerated evolution has occurred in a large number of loci of the human genome, some of which became rapidly fixed by positive selection, though there is some controversy about the fixation of new mutations in geographically distinct human populations (Coop et al. 2009). Among human lineage-specific genomic changes, many pertain to brain size or function, as well as immune function, some of which may be evolutionary trade-offs that render humans vulnerable to disorder or disease (O'Bleness et al. 2012). How difficult it is to judge whether or not a certain allele has produced a fitness advantage may be illustrated by the following example.

Among human lineage-specific genomic changes, many pertain to brain size or function, as well as immune function, some of which may be evolutionary trade-offs that render humans vulnerable to disorder or disease.

The homozygous valine/valine (val/val) polymorphism at position 158 in the amino acid chain of the catechol-O-methyl-transferase (COMT), a protein that is responsible for the enzymatic degradation of dopamine, works faster than the methionin/methionin (met/met) variant. In other words, the met/met variant leaves dopamine longer in the synaptic cleft, which has a measurable effect on working memory. Carriers of the val/val perform more poorly on working memory tasks than do met/met carriers, and the val/val variant has been thought to convey vulnerability to develop schizophrenia, particularly if carriers consume cannabis during early adolescence. Both homozygous variants and the heterozygous val/met allele exist at equilibrium in populations. However, the val/val allele is certainly not pathological in itself. Only in conjunction with (perhaps many) other factors that are poorly understood can such an allelic variation contribute a small amount of variance to explain the risk for schizophrenia. Recent research has in fact demonstrated that met/met carriers show increased reactivity in the limbic system and prefrontal and temporal areas to unpleasant emotional stimuli, suggesting lower resilience to negative mood states and higher emotional dysregulation (Heinz and Smolka 2006). Likewise, the presence of one met allele may convey an increased risk for obsessive-compulsive disorder (OCD) (in men; Pooley et al. 2007). In essence, these divergent findings suggest that COMT genotype variation represents a trade-off between advantageous effects on working memory and emotional responsiveness. Little is known about such trade-offs of other genetic susceptibility loci, but future research will almost certainly reveal such effects of other alleles that have prematurely been assigned the status of 'genes for' a certain disorder.

New genes can arise from duplication of existing genes and insertion in the genome close to the ancestral gene. The new gene may adopt a new function while the original remains in place. Sometimes whole chromosomes or entire genomes duplicate. Many allele variations are selectively neutral, that is, not affective for an individual's reproductive fitness. Gene flow is a process by which genes can enter or leave the gene pool of a population. It is considered a highly conservative factor in evolution, because it prevents populations from evolving into a new species. Genetic drift, by contrast, may have such an effect in small populations if alleles are lost through sampling errors (Maynard-Smith 1998).

Genes may also be differentially expressed or silenced by epigenetic mechanisms. A common mechanism by which a gene can be inactivated is methylation, which occurs especially in regions rich in cytosine (C) and guanine (G) nucleotides. Such C–phosphate–G (CpG) 'islands' are found at one end of about 50 percent of all genes, of which 60–70 percent are

Genes can be silenced by epigenetic processes, among which methylation is the most common mechanism. Methylation contributes to the silencing of one X chromosome in female organisms.

methylated. In humans, about 1 percent of DNA bases undergo methylation. DNA methylation is an important mechanism in normal cell differentiation, but has been shown to also play a role in carcinogenesis by silencing tumour suppressor genes (McGuffin et al. 2005; Jones P.A. 2012). One central dogma of molecular biology has been that no information can be transmitted from the proteins of the body to the DNA; thus inheritance of acquired characters does not occur. However, the discovery that RNA may induce gene silencing via interaction with homologous DNA sequences at loci other than the original that has coded the RNA molecule violates this rule. Moreover, animal studies have shown that non-genetic inheritance via the gametes, hormones, cytokines, and epigenetic modification may have phenotypic consequences over multiple generations (Toth 2015).

Methylation and gene silencing are also involved in the inactivation of one X chromosome, and in a process called genomic imprinting (Pfeifer 2000). Genomic imprinting results from differential methylation of male or female DNA. This can be explained in part due to different 'interests' of paternal and maternal genes represented in the embryo. From an evolutionary point of view there is arguably conflict over the amount of maternal investment between genes transmitted from the mother and genes transmitted from the father. For example, paternally inherited genes may have selected to extract a greater amount of resources than is the optimum for the mother. By contrast, maternally inherited genes may be selected to demand an amount of resources closer to the mother's optimum or even slightly below that amount (Haig 2010). Imprinted genes comprise only 1 percent of the genome, but they may exert major effects because they are often involved in growth regulation and highly pleiotropic. The target tissues for imprinted genes are the placenta and, arguably, the brain. Both placenta and brain are key organs in the process of resource transfer between genetically related individuals with partially divergent fitness interests. It can therefore be expected that dysbalanced expression of imprinted genes in the brain may cause major alterations at the functional level.

Genomic imprinting results from differential methylation of female or male DNA. Even though only 1 percent of genes are imprinted, imprinted genes may have profound effects depending on whether transmitted from the mother or the father.

In support of this hypothesis, Prader–Willi syndrome and Angelman syndrome may reflect such opposite effects due to genomic imprinting. Deletion of a particular stretch of DNA on the long arm of chromosome 15 in one of the parents or uniparental disomy in which both copies of the chromosomal region have been transmitted from one parent may lead to the expression of only maternal or paternal genes. The sole expression of maternally inherited genes causes Prader–Willi syndrome, which is characterized by poor sucking and weak cry in infants; conversely, if both copies stem from the father, the result is Angelman syndrome. Infants with Angelman syndrome display a strong but poorly coordinated sucking response.

Prader–Willi syndrome and Angelman syndrome are two known examples of genomic imprinting. Imprinting has also been discussed in autism and schizophrenia.

Recently, the process of genomic imprinting has been discussed in autism and schizophrenia as, in part, diametrically opposite manifestations of dysfunction related to the processing of social information (Badcock and Crespi 2006). Accordingly, psychosis could arise from maternally imprinted genes leading to undergrowth of certain brain areas involved in social cognition, whereas paternal imprinting could be involved in autism with a general pattern of brain overgrowth (Skuse 2000). Both extremes of variation are reflected in reduced or enhanced brain asymmetry, as well as opposite patterns of connectivity and functional correlates, respectively (for further details see Chapters 6 and 8). Recent studies in mice suggest that imprinted genes impact on adult social behaviour concerning dominance and risk-taking, though no such studies are as yet available for humans (Peters 2014).

Epigenetic mechanisms have recently been discussed in several psychiatric disorders, including addiction, depression, and schizophrenia (Tsankova et al. 2007). Interestingly, chronic stress as well as early stressful life events—important causal factors in many psychiatric disorders—may contribute to gene silencing via methylation. Moreover, animal models have shown that the intensity of maternal grooming impacts on the methylation of the glucocorticoid gene promoter (Weaver et al. 2004). Consistent with this finding, the experience of early adversity such as child abuse or maltreatment has been found to be associated with increased methylation of genes involved in stress regulation (McGowan et al. 2009; Yang et al. 2013; Kundakovic and Champagne 2015). In general, chronic stress may impact on an individual's 'allostatic load', which concerns the body's stress reactivity at several levels including the autonomic nervous system, reactivity of the hypothalamic–pituitary–adrenal (HPA) axis, body fat deposition, and immune function (McEwen 2002). Animal models suggest that these usually long-lasting effects can pharmacologically be reversed (Murgatroyd et al. 2009), a fact that will almost certainly receive greater attention in future research on psychiatric and psychosomatic conditions.

The experience of childhood adversity is associated with increased methylation of genes involved in stress regulation. Chronic stress may impact on an individual's 'allostatic load', which concerns the body's stress reactivity at several levels including the autonomic nervous system, reactivity of the HPA axis, body fat deposition, and immune function.

In very rare disorders, notably autosomal dominant transmitted diseases such as Huntington's disease, it has been observed that the severity of the disorder increases over successive generations, while the onset of the disorder is shifted to younger age. This process has become known as anticipation, which is associated with an increase in the number of repetitive trinucleotide elements during transmission from parent to child. Whether and to what extent this may play a role in other psychiatric disorders remains controversial, but anticipation has been discussed as a putative factor involved in schizophrenia, bipolar disorder, and anxiety disorders.

'Anticipation' refers to the observation that an increasing number of repetitive genetic elements may shift the onset of disorders to an earlier age. Anticipation is known to occur in Huntington's disease and has been discussed in schizophrenia, bipolar disorder, and anxiety disorders.

Finally, it is important to note that there is considerable interaction between different genes in many ways, sometimes over great distances, a process referred to as epistasis. Moreover, traits are often under the control of more than one gene, the condition being called polygenic inheritance. Conversely, a gene affecting several phenotypic aspects is called pleiotropic. These matters of

Genes may interact in complex ways, and this is referred to as epistasis. Moreover, traits that are under the control of multiple genes are called polygenic. Conversely, a gene that exerts effects on multiple traits is called pleiotropic.

fact complicate the search for allelic variations that may underlie pathological variations, but several sophisticated methods that have been refined over the years have greatly advanced the understanding of the genetic contributions to psychopathology (McGuffin et al. 2005).

1.4.1 Determining genetic contribution to psychopathology

How SNPs, complex gene interactions, additive gene effects, gene silencing and imprinting, and pleiotropic effects or anticipation contribute to psychopathology has only begun to be understood (Plomin et al. 1994). There is little doubt that an individual's genetic make-up may be associated with vulnerability to psychopathology, but the task of disentangling genetic from environmental impacts has proved extremely difficult. This is in part due to the fact that most, if not all, major psychiatric disorders do not follow a Mendelian pattern of inheritance with simple dominance–recessivity relationships (Tandon and McGuffin 2002). Moreover, it must be taken into account that genes may also variably be expressed and that penetrance, defined as the probability of a specific phenotype as a function of a certain genotype, may be incomplete. Likewise, psychopathological syndromes are quantitatively or continuously distributed in populations, rather than categorically distinct from 'normalcy'. All this requires mathematically complex and multifactorial liability-threshold models, which assume continuous liability distribution conferred by polygenetic inheritance and multiple environmental factors. Heritability is defined as the proportion of phenotypic variance that is accounted for by genetic variation relative to environmental variation. In the strict sense, heritability refers to the genetic variation in populations; it is not a valid concept at the individual level. Moreover, mathematical models have to take into account estimates of shared and non-shared environmental factors (McGuffin et al. 2005).

The genetic background of psychiatric disorders is polygenic in nature.

Heritability is defined as the proportion of phenotypic variance that is accounted for by genetic variation.

The simplest way to estimate genetic contributions to psychopathological syndromes is the study of families, as well as twin and adoption studies. They have been developed to estimate life-time expectations of a disorder and the relative contribution of common genetic make-up between closely related individuals. In family studies the life-time prevalence of a disorder can be calculated from the number of relatives who have ever been affected divided by the total number of relatives. The actual figure for the determined life-time risk, however, is lower than the actual risk, because it is unlikely that all relatives have passed through the period of risk. Moreover, family studies are unsuitable for comparing life-time risks across generations. There may also be a bias created by differential reproductive success of relatives, depending on the onset

Family, twin, and adoption studies have been used to estimate the life-time risk of developing a disorder. Studies of monozygotic (MZ) and dizygotic (DZ) twins allow an estimation of genetic and shared environmental influence on the expression of a trait. Adoption studies can contribute to differentiating between genetic and environmental causation of a disorder.

of the disorder. Twin studies, particularly comparisons between monozygotic twins (MZ) and dizygotic twins (DZ), can be more informative, because MZ share 100 percent of their genetic material compared to 50 percent in DZ. Both MZ and DZ share environmental risk factors in utero, childhood, and adolescence (if reared together) to a similar degree, although differences during pregnancy may result from not sharing a common chorion. On the other hand, siblings and even monozygotic twins occupy different 'ecological niches' within the family (with regard to siblings, in part due to birth-order effects), which has to be taken into consideration as non-shared environmental influences (Sulloway 1986; Bateson 1998).

In any event, in order to measure the genetic and environmental contributions to a disorder, adoption studies can be revealing, where biologically affected parents have adopted away children, who can be compared to adopted children from unaffected families, or where affected adoptees are compared with their unaffected adoptive relatives (Tienari et al. 2000). A special case of adoption studies is the cross-fostering design, where adoptees of adopting parents with a disorder are compared with affected adoptees with unaffected adopting parents.

Gene–environment interactions and correlations are difficult to disentangle and quantify, though. Passive gene–environment correlations may occur due to the fact that not only children inherit the genes from their parents but also parents who carry certain genes may create an environment according to their genetic make-up. For example, parents who are anxious may seek to provide their children with an environment with little or no risks. In contrast, children of parents with attention deficit/hyperactivity disorder (ADHD) may grow up in a family environment that facilitates impulsive reactions and emotional lability. Active gene–environment correlation, by contrast, refers to the possibility that children have preferences for environmental conditions that suit their genetic make-up best. For instance, children with ADHD may seek risky situations more often than anxious children do. Gene–environment interactions can therefore be defined as the sum of genetic effects, environmental effects, and gene–environment correlation (McGuffin et al. 2005).

> *Gene–environment interactions are the sum of genetic effects, environmental effects, and gene–environment correlation.*

Linkage and association analyses are methods to detect SNPs, or to test candidate genes genome-wide or located on individual chromosomes. They make use of the exponential replication of DNA by employing polymerase chain reaction (PCR). Linkage and association procedures are complementary in that they have opposite advantages and disadvantages. The method of linkage has to do with the likelihood that a crossover or recombination occurs between two points located on a chromosome. The nearer the two points are, the less likely a crossover occurs. The frequency at which crossovers take place varies between species, between male and female gametes, between individual chromosomes, and between different portions of a chromosome. Experiments

> *Linkage and association studies are suitable to detect SNPs or candidate genes in genome-wide scans. Linkage disequilibrium (LD) is a measure of how tightly linked two alleles at different loci are.*

suggest that in the human genome a crossover occurs every 1 million base pairs of DNA or 1 megabase (Mb). If the location of one or more markers is known on a chromosome, a gene that contributes to the phenotype of a disorder can perhaps be encircled in a relatively small region of interest.

Linkage is used in family analyses and is able to detect large effects over long genetic distances. Linkage analysis was originally applied to disorders that followed Mendelian inheritance, but complicated statistical procedures have become available to examine quantitative traits, which is much more appropriate for the majority of psychiatric disorders. Association studies can be applied in samples that are genetically unrelated. The simplest comparison is between an individual that has a disorder and a matched control subject. The association of a disorder with a particular allele at a certain chromosomal locus may suggest causation. Linkage disequilibrium (LD) is a measure of how tightly linked two alleles at different loci are. High LD suggests that two alleles are transmitted together, but there is great variability between loci of the same distance, such that association is only meaningful over short distances. On the other hand, association studies can detect genetic effects of comparably small statistical power. Association studies have been most successful in identifying allelic variation of candidate genes with known (patho)physiological effects such as apolipoprotein polymorphisms as a risk factor for Alzheimer's disease or dopamine transporter gene polymorphisms for ADHD.

Quantitative genetics of complex psychiatric disorders is—despite considerable progress—still in its infancy. This has to do with the complex interactions of multiple alleles at different loci such that replication of findings has often failed, with little power of individual findings to explain overall population risks. It is now widely agreed upon the fact that complex traits are not inherited via single genes, but multiple genes, each of which contributes a small amount of variance to the actual phenotype (in addition to non-genetic influences). Genes in multiple-gene systems have been referred to as quantitative trait loci (QTLs), and the contribution each QTL makes to the variation of a trait is for most characteristics unknown.

Another problem lies in the comparability of samples of different ethnic backgrounds. The most pressing difficulty is, however, that diagnostic criteria of psychiatric disorders are too vague a tool to successfully identify genes that contribute to a particular phenotype, let alone the problem that psychiatric disorders exist as extreme points along a continuum of symptom severity, with a healthy status representing the statistical norm. All this makes a thorough characterization of endophenotypes on the basis of shared biological or behavioural markers essential. An endophenotype is assumed to be genetically less complex compared to the full phenotypic variation of a disorder. Ideally, an endophenotype is heritable, and thus it cosegregates with the illness in families in which multiple individuals are affected; it can be found in unaffected relatives of an index case at higher frequencies than in the general population; and

Research into endophenotypes may be more promising than studying the full phenotypic variation of a disorder. Endophenotypes are characterized by biological and/or behavioural markers that ideally are heritable, independent of the activity of the disorder, and can be found in unaffected relatives.

an endophenotype is state independent, that is, it does not vary with illness activity (Walters and Owen 2007).

Another promising way is the incorporation of human DNA in animal (e.g. mouse) DNA, in the expectation that at least some behavioural or physiological correlates can be observed in the model animal.

However, one reason why the search for susceptibility genes for many psychiatric disorders has been frustrating so far could lie in the fact that human behaviour is so complex and influenced by hundreds, perhaps thousands of genes. From an evolutionary point of view, however, there must be an explanation why psychiatric disorders are so common in the general population (Keller and Miller 2006). High prevalence rates would rather suggest that selection had eliminated genes that predispose to psychiatric disorders. One explanation could be that genes predisposing to a psychiatric disorder had some hidden adaptive advantage during human evolutionary history, perhaps through balancing pleiotropic effects. Several psychiatric disorders, notably schizophrenia, have been likened to the example of sickle-cell anaemia (Huxley et al. 1964), which is associated with superior protection from malaria in heterozygous carriers, yet is deleterious in homozygous individuals. Although such a scenario has been proven highly unlikely for schizophrenia, a variation of the theme suggests that genes conveying adaptive advantages early in life may exert deleterious effects later in life. Such a mechanism may be plausible for disorders with late onset, that is, beyond the reproductive period, when the power of selective forces usually declines (see, for example, Chapter 18 on dementia). Balancing selection assumes that the two alleles have been of equal importance in terms of fitness over evolutionary time.

A special case of balancing selection can be made for frequency-dependent selection, which occurs when the fitness conferred by a particular allele increases as the allele becomes less frequent (Maynard-Smith 1998). Such a mechanism can parsimoniously explain the maintenance of certain traits at low frequency and may, for example, be a model for explaining antisocial behavioural tendencies, known as 'psychopathy' (for details see Chapter 19). In contrast, the possibility that alleles that increase the susceptibility for psychiatric disorders were selectively neutral (an assumption that implicitly, though erroneously, prevails in contemporary psychiatric genetics) appears implausible in light of the significant reproductive disadvantages associated with many psychiatric disorders.

Another explanation for psychiatric disorders not being eliminated by selection is that the mere sum of allelic variation renders an individual susceptible to developing a psychiatric disorder, alleles that are infrequent at any given locus in the population but that are collectively very common across loci. The 'watershed model' illustrates how several or many unfavourable SNPs at specific loci may in conjunction cause dysfunction (Keller and Miller 2006). The val/val variant of the COMT genotype may indeed lead to a high dopamine turnover in the prefrontal cortex, and this and other additive mechanisms may contribute to slightly poorer working memory functioning than in carriers of the met/met genotype. Working memory functioning together with other mechanisms may influence the cognitive phenotype, each of which, however, produces little more than noise. If enough noise is present, a threshold may be reached at which phenotypically relevant symptoms or syndromes emerge, ultimately affecting individual fitness. Estimates of how many potentially harmful alleles are present in each individual human genome arrive at numbers of 500–2,000. This and the fact that genes code for proteins and do not directly translate into cognition, emotion, or behaviour suggests that no 'gene for' a particular disorder exists. Only in close interaction with environmental factors do genes produce a certain phenotype. These important insights have to be taken into account if we want to fully understand psychopathology.

Psychiatric disorders are common in the general population, because they may reflect the additive effects of many genes, each of which has only small effects on phenotypic variation, and thus escape elimination by selection.

1.4.2 Gene–environment interaction and differential susceptibility to the environment

The idea that individuals are at elevated risk of developing a psychopathological condition due to their genetic make-up, particularly when exposed to adverse environmental conditions, known as the diathesis–stress model (Monroe and Simons 1991), has become the prevailing theoretical concept in psychiatry. According to the model, subjects who do not carry 'vulnerability' genes are less susceptible to adversity or even deemed 'resilient' (Feder et al. 2009).

The diathesis–stress model suggests that genes predispose to the development of illness if associated with unfavourable environments. Subjects who do not carry 'vulnerability' genes are less susceptible to adversity or deemed 'resilient'.

For example, it has been shown that persons who carry the low-activity variant of the monoamine oxidase A (MAO-A) enzyme are more likely to develop antisocial personality disorder when growing up under adverse environmental conditions, compared to individuals endowed with the high-activity allele. Put another way, the speed of degradation of biogenic amines such as dopamine and noradrenalin seems to determine one's vulnerability to develop ADHD, conduct disorder, or antisocial personality disorder, depending on the presence or absence of early adversity (Caspi et al. 2002). Along similar lines, it has been reported that the s-allele of the serotonin transporter gene (5-HTTLPR) predisposes to depression if accompanied by stressful life events (Caspi et al. 2003). Likewise, the 7-repeat variant of the dopamine receptor D4 gene (DRD4) increases the vulnerability for externalizing problems and ADHD in children whose mothers are insensitive to their children's needs (Bakermans-Kranenburg and van Ijzendoorn 2006). Conversely, it has been argued that the absence of adversity can compensate the genetic vulnerability, referred to as 'maternal buffering' (Suomi 2006). Moreover, some genetic variants seem to protect against the development of psychiatric conditions even in the presence of severe adversity. For example, variation at the corticotropin-releasing hormone receptor may prevent depression in subjects who as children were maltreated (Polanczyk et al. 2009).

It is therefore beyond doubt that the search for genetic contributions to psychopathology has substantially advanced our knowledge about gene–environment interaction. One problem that the diathesis–stress model faces, however, concerns the observation that many of the supposedly 'vulnerability genes' have undergone recent positive selection in human evolution. This is contradictory in itself, because it is implausible to assume that natural selection has favoured allelic variants, which increase vulnerability to adversity, particularly when considering that the EEAs were probably fraught with adverse experiences of all kinds throughout the lifespan. Instead, this strongly suggests that these genes exert hitherto undetected or overlooked beneficial effects with regard to reproductive fitness (which is not necessarily the same as 'good for health'; Ellis et al. 2011a).

Problems associated with the diathesis–stress model concern the observation that many of the supposedly 'vulnerability genes' have undergone recent positive selection in human evolution. This is contradictory in itself, because it is implausible to assume that natural selection has favoured allelic variants that increase vulnerability to adversity.

Evidence from cross-cultural genetic studies suggests, for example, that the 7-repeat variant of the DRD4 gene is the more recent allele, which emerged some 50,000 years ago in human populations, whereby the 4-repeat variant is the ancestral form (Ding et al. 2002). Notably, the long variant seems to be more prevalent in migratory, as opposed to sedentary, populations (Chen et al. 1999). Consistent with this finding, the 7-repeat allele has been (inconsistently) associated with the personality trait 'novelty-seeking', a human trait that arguably may have conferred a reproductive advantage in human history, particularly for migrating populations (Reist et al. 2007; Matthews and Butler 2011). Similarly, while carrying the s-allele of the HTTLPR may predispose to depression if associated with adverse events, the same variation is linked to superior cognitive performance in several domains and increased social conformity, which, in part, may be mediated by increased amygdala activity (Canli and Lesch 2007; Homberg and Lesch 2011). This example is prototypical for 'balanced polymorphisms', where an SNP may exert disadvantageous effects in one domain, which are compensated by advantageous effects in another domain. A balanced polymorphism also explains the frequency of a particular SNP in the general population, and why it has not been selected against.

Balanced polymorphisms are, however, implausible to account for those cases in which the compensatory effect happens to occur *in the same domain*. Accordingly, from an evolutionary point of view it has been argued that a particular genetic variation that predisposes to pathology if associated with early adversity can have beneficial effects when environmental contingencies are developmentally more supportive (Boyce et al. 1995; Belsky 1997). With regard to the assessment of the quality of environmental stimulation, several scholars have highlighted a methodological problem that is prevalent in most gene–environment interaction studies (Belsky et al. 2009; Ellis et al. 2011a). They argue that it is insufficient to equate the absence of adversity as the 'good' end of the environmental-exposure continuum. Likewise, the absence of a disorder cannot simply be likened to the 'good' end of the psychological functioning continuum. Such neglect of adequately measuring environmental variance at both ends ('good' and 'poor') may lead to the underdetection of *differential susceptibility* to environmental influence, whereby the early family environment is the key player in this regard (Belsky et al. 2009; Ellis et al. 2011a; see Chapter 3). It is therefore imperative to inquire whether the same genes that convey increased vulnerability to psychopathology under adverse environmental conditions have the potential to act in advantageous ways on psychological functioning when the environment is supportive or enriched (Belsky et al. 2009). That is, evidence supports the view that it is more accurate to speak of differential susceptibility or plasticity conferred by genetic variation—that is, responsivity to both positive and negative conditions—than focusing one-sidedly on vulnerability (Belsky and Pluess 2009).

Genetic variation that predisposes to pathology if associated with early adversity can have beneficial effects when environmental contingencies are developmentally more supportive; this is known as 'differential susceptibility'.

Consistent with this novel conceptualization, it has been demonstrated that the low-activity MAO-A variant is associated with *lower* than average prevalence of antisocial personality when children grow up in supportive environments (Widom and Brzustowicz 2006; though other studies suggest that genetic variation and environment convey independent risks; Reif et al. 2007). Likewise, the s-allele of the 5-HTTLPR confers *lower* risk for depression under favourable environmental conditions (Taylor et al. 2006). Interestingly, genetic variation of the serotonin transporter gene between more individualistic compared to collectivistic cultures seems to be associated with differences in prevalence of anxiety disorders and depression. That is, cultures that value collectivism more have a higher prevalence of the s-allele, yet lower prevalence rates of anxiety disorders and depression (Chiao and Blizinsky 2010).

Children carrying the 7-repeat variant of the DRD4 gene develop ADHD and externalizing problems *less than average* if their mothers are responsive to their children's emotional needs (Bakermans-Kranenburg and van Ijzendoorn 2006). Moreover, adult carriers of the COMTval and DRD4 7-repeat alleles show the highest responsivity to their children's needs when stress levels are low, whereas their responsivity is lower than average when stress levels are high (van Ijzendoorn et al. 2008). Taken together, these findings indicate that allelic variation involved in dopamine and serotonin turnover plays an important role in differential susceptibility to environmental conditions, possibly mediated by one's responsivity to reward and punishment, as well as stress regulation (Bakermans-Kranenburg and van Ijzendoorn 2007; Ellis et al. 2011a). There is limited evidence that this might also be the case for genes involved in oxytocin metabolism (Brüne 2012; Hammen et al. 2014). Overall, it seems that plasticity genes can have additive effects, that is, the susceptibility to the environment may increase with the number of plasticity alleles (Belsky and Beaver 2011). The potential impact of this new perspective on gene–environment interaction and behavioural consequences, as far as psychopathological conditions are concerned, can hardly be overestimated. In fact, differential susceptibility may be even unique to genes expressed in the central nervous system, as opposed to genes expressed in other organs. A false conclusion would be, however, to attempt to bolster or immunize highly susceptible individuals against adversity. Instead, it is a therapeutic imperative to supply responsive social environments to sensitive individuals from early on (Ellis et al. 2011a), which is probably a mammoth task for health care providers, especially for those concerned with prevention and early detection of psychological problems.

Plasticity genes can have additive effects, that is, the susceptibility to the environment may increase with the number of plasticity alleles.

Afterthought: on genetic determinism and the confusion of 'is' with 'ought'

Critics of an evolutionary perspective towards understanding human behaviour and psychopathology often make a couple of false claims that may cause misunderstanding or rejection of this approach. One such claim is commonly referred to as 'genetic determinism', the idea that genes could cause behaviour or determine personality. Indeed, in many articles on psychiatric genetics, phrases such as 'gene X causes disorder Y' actually represent oversimplifications of what genes really do. Genes are building blocks that are necessary to grow complex organisms. In the first place, genes code for protein synthesis, and proteins regulate growth, tissue differentiation, and other complex interactions including neurotransmission. However, genes do not do this in isolation. They can only effectively promote protein synthesis if environmental conditions are within a particular range. These conditions include temperature, pH value, supply of raw material for synthesizing amino acids, and eventually other multifactorial conditions such as parental care and nurturing, and environmental stimulation. For organisms to grow, both nature (genes) and nurture (environment) are necessary ingredients.

With regard to human cognition, emotion, and behaviour, including pathologies thereof, the nature–nurture debate has led to some confusion, because neither can solely account for a given phenotype (Schaffner 2001). It is probably correct to say that some psychiatric disorders are more, others less under genetic control. Likewise, the emergence of some disorders depends more on the presence of (adverse) environmental conditions, others less. For the majority of psychiatrically ill patients, however, the exact amount of genetic and environmental contribution to the actual phenotype is indeterminable. The evolutionary perspective, therefore, does not the least imply that a given behavioural propensity is impervious to modification. Nor does human evolutionary psychology suggest that human behaviour is largely instinctual, that is, rigid and inflexible (Gowaty 1995). On the contrary, evolution has endowed humans with the highest degree of flexibility, at the expense of an extremely protracted juvenile period, which not only delays reproduction (where reproduction certainly represents an evolutionary goal), but also renders human beings extremely vulnerable to dysfunction—*because* they critically depend on environmental input, which is, above all, provided from the social environment. These critical aspects of humanity are dealt with in Chapter 4.

Addressing all four questions, as proposed by Tinbergen (1963), pertaining to the proximate and ultimate causes of human behaviour and its extreme variants we call psychopathologies is by no means reductionist, but rather enriches the endeavour to understand the causes of psychiatric disorders by adding insights from human phylogeny. If psychiatry wants to overcome its conceptual metatheoretical weaknesses, answering all four questions should become the standard procedure in psychiatry (Nesse 2013; Brüne 2014b).

In addition, a warning sign from the history of our discipline should be brought to the attention of all students of evolutionary psychology and psychiatry, termed the 'naturalistic fallacy'. The concept refers to the erroneous notion that biological facts could translate into moral imperatives. The mere existence of biologically explicable behavioural tendencies (the 'is') must not be confused with the 'ought' of morality. For example, the biological tendency of men to mate with more than one partner should not be understood in a way that suggests that extramarital affairs are morally justified (at least not in monogamous societies). Likewise, the finding that, on average, men are more aggressive than women by no means suggests that male violence towards women is an acceptable form of behaviour. Similarly, the propensity of women to commit neonaticide, as a decision over parental investment postponed to a time after parturition, cannot simply be excused as 'natural'. This list of examples could easily be expanded. The abhorrent issue here is that psychiatrists in the not so distant past actually acted upon the naturalistic fallacy as, for example, during the Nazi regime in Germany and before. At that time, psychiatrists were concerned about what they perceived as genetic degeneration of the human species. What followed was a claim for negative eugenics (preventing those from procreation that were considered to be of minor genetic quality) and positive eugenics (breeding experiments). The former led to compulsory sterilization laws in many countries and served, in part, as scientific justification for euthanasia of many mentally ill persons. It might also have contributed to the holocaust, although the reasons that led to the untenable mass-murder of millions of innocent people were certainly not only biological in nature, but much more complex (Brüne 2001b).

If nowadays some scientists publicly declare that genetic research should be used to improve the human species, one might recall that such claims are not really new. Evolution is, however, not a directional process. It is the variation and diverseness of individual personalities that makes human life so interesting.

Psychiatry is perhaps the medical discipline that is most vulnerable to fall prey to the zeitgeist. Thus, it ought to be an obligation for all working in the field to critically review the scientific and non-scientific concepts behind our medical field. Evolutionary ideas have their place in understanding psychopathology, but, like many other scientific concepts, are prone to misuse.

Chapter 2

The human brain: anatomy, evolution, and function

Abstract

The human brain is the most complex organ that has ever evolved. It contains more neurons and synapses than any other primate brain. In relation to body weight, it is outstandingly large and distinctly convoluted. Several parts of the brain have enlarged disproportionally over evolutionary time. Those brain regions are mainly involved in emotion processing, understanding and reflecting upon one's own and other minds, memory, social decision-making, and action planning, suggesting that the human brain is adapted to dealing with social matters. The human brain is also conspicuous with regard to its slow maturation, which is linked to the huge amount of social information that needs to be learned until adulthood. Cross-talk among neurons is maintained by the action of neuromodulators and neurotransmitters, many of which are ancient and have served multiple purposes in plants and animals. They help regulate defensive and agonistic behaviour, social attachment, and inhibitory control.

Keywords

social cognition, slow maturation, social attachment, defense, agonistic behaviours, inhibitory control, neurotransmitters

2.1 Introductory remarks to the human brain

The human brain is probably the most complex organ that ever evolved. It is the 'control system' for all body functions and regulates how the human organism navigates through the environment. Environmental complexity has led to the evolution of advanced cognitive and emotional abilities, which allow a hitherto unseen and remarkable behavioural flexibility. The manifold functions that the human brain entertains are the result of a long and intricate evolutionary history. The first primitive regulatory systems—receptors and biochemical mechanisms that could propel simple organisms such as bacteria—served the purpose to buffer the organism against environmental variation, for example, in terms of avoiding toxins or

Primitive nervous systems emerged some 500 mya. They contained a number of neurons that were characterized by the presence of receptors, conductors, and effectors, as well as electrical excitability.

approaching nutrients, and this was the principal way of regulating behaviour for a couple of billion years (Allman 1999). However, these systems were not yet nervous systems. Neurons (the basis of all nervous systems) are characterized by the presence of receptors, conductors, and effectors. Neurons can be electrically stimulated, and the communication among neurons critically depends on functional connections through synapses, which probably evolved from more primitive protosynapses some 1 billion years ago (Ryan and Grant 2009). The first genuine nervous system emerged in coelenterata (e.g. jellyfish) more than 500 mya and consisted of a small aggregation of neurons. What followed was the expansion of these early nervous systems to evolve into complex hierarchically organized organs, called 'brains' (Allman 1999).

In the first place, brains probably evolved as devices to avoid hazards and, hence, threats to the organism's survival, as well as to evaluate the environment for extractable resources (food, shelter, mates). At some point during evolution, however, the brain changed its 'strategy' from preparing an organism to 'react' to environmental fluctuations in space and time to actively explore the environment. In a sense, the evolution of brains is the history of maximizing an organism's behavioural capacity to exploit and manipulate the environment (including the social environment, which is, as we will see, particularly important for social animals like ourselves) for the sake of the organism's reproductive fitness. However, the evolution of brains has always been constrained by the brain's energy consumption, because neurons are highly expensive in energetic terms. They have to maintain the ionic balance between themselves and their environment, and they need a lot of energy to synthesize transmitters for the communication between nerve cells (Fehm et al. 2006). Dendrites, for example, contain large numbers of mitochondria to maintain energy supply. Neurons communicate via neurotransmitters and electric currents called action potentials. Action potentials can travel long distances, and the evolutionary novelty of myelination greatly accelerated the information transfer from one neuron to the other (Hofman 2001). All these expensive mechanisms must have had an evolutionary advantage to be selected, otherwise brains would not exist, simply because evolutionary processes are 'thrifty' (Northcutt 2001).

Primitive brains helped organisms to avoid hazards, to seek extractable resources, and to mate. At some point during evolution, however, organisms changed their strategies by actively exploring the environment. Brain size is constrained by the large amount of energy consumption of neurons. Thus, big brains must have conveyed enormous advantages, otherwise they would not have evolved.

The human brain contains an estimated 100,000 km of connecting fibres and an estimated storage capacity of 1.25 terabytes. The mean number of cortical neurons is about 16–20 billion, which makes about 20 percent of all brain neurons. The total number of neurons of the human brain has been reported to figure at around 86 billion (Azevedo et al. 2009). It has been estimated that 1 mm^3 of human cortex contains about 44,000,000 neurons comprising 150 m of dendrites, an additional 100 m of axonal connections, and 50 million synapses. The number of glia cells is reportedly about two to ten times higher than

The human brain is unparalleled in its complexity. It contains billions of neurons and can store an estimated 1.25 terabytes. The human brain competes with other organs for energy supply. Moreover, a big brain develops slowly and requires a large amount of environmental input to mature properly.

the number of cortical neurons (Hofman 2001), whereas other reports come closer to a 1:1 ratio, which would be in line with other mammalian brains (Azevedo et al. 2009).

Such a big brain poses several biological problems because it must compete with other organs for energy supply (Fehm et al. 2006). A big brain develops slowly, because the wiring process requires a lot of environmental input over extended periods of time and thus constrains the reproductive potential of its bearer. In order to reach adulthood, an immature organism has to be protected from environmental hazards, such as predation and starvation, by adult individuals in whose genetic interest it must be that the offspring organism reproduce: in other words, the parental effort in raising offspring increases proportionally with the immaturity of descendants (Trivers 1974; Allman 1999). All these biological problems have come to a head in humans. So why does the human brain exist at all? An answer to this question shall be attempted in sections 2.2. to 2.10.

2.2 **Gross morphology of the human brain**

The human brain, like other mammalian brains, can be divided into several parts that are intensely connected with one another. The most basal part of the brain is called rhombencephalon (hindbrain or brainstem), which maintains the most basic physiological functions such as respiration, blood pressure, sleep–wakefulness rhythm, and some rather primitive behavioural responses. The middle part of the brain is called mesencephalon or midbrain. It contains the basal ganglia including many nuclei rich in neurotransmitter-producing cells such as the substantia nigra. The prosencephalon or forebrain can be divided into the diencephalon comprising the thalamus, the hypothalamus and the subthalamus that are responsible for endocrine functions and conditioned learning, and the telencephalon comprising the limbic system and the cerebral hemispheres involved in emotion regulation and cognitive functions.

The human brain is a typical mammalian brain. It comprises evolutionarily older parts such as the brainstem, the mesencephalon, and the most recently evolved telencephalon. Cortex morphology can be distinguished according to its cytoarchitecture. The allocortex comprises the hippocampal region, the entorhinal cortex, the cingulate cortex, and parts of the amygdalae. The neocortex is a six-layered structure, which covers about 96 percent of the cortical surface. The frontal and temporal lobes comprise 30 percent each, the parietal cortex another 23 percent, and roughly 15 percent belong to the occipital lobe.

The outer part of the brain is also called pallium, because it covers large parts of the more basal sections. The word pallium means 'cloak' or 'coat'. This outer part of the brain can be subdivided into the allocortex and the isocortex. Allocortex and isocortex can be distinguished on the basis of their cytoarchitecture. The isocortex or neocortex comprises a six-layered structure containing large pyramidal cells, with the exception of the motor cortex, which lacks a distinct layer IV, and the primary visual cortex, where layer IV can be subdivided into three sublayers. The primary sensory cortices receive projections from the thalamus and the geniculate bodies, and project themselves to secondary and tertiary sensory areas, which in turn send projections to the motor cortex. The phylogenetically older allocortex comprises the olfactory system (roughly equivalent to the palaeocortex, which makes up 1 percent of the total cortical surface), the hippocampal region, and entorhinal cortex, as well as the cingulate cortex, and parts of the amygdalae (equivalent to the archicortex, which makes up 3.5 percent of cortical surface). There is a stepwise transition of the cytoarchitecture from the allocortex to neocortex, where the two transition parts are called periallocortex and proisocortex (together called mesocortex). The isocortex makes up about 96 percent of the cortical surface: some 32 percent belongs to the frontal lobes, 30 percent to the temporal lobes, 23 percent to the parietal cortex, and 15 percent to the occipital lobes (Zilles 1987). Figures 2.1a and 2.1b show the lateral view of the left hemisphere and the medial view of the right hemisphere, respectively.

The cerebellum comprises two hemispheres and a midline structure called vermis. The cerebellar hemispheres are divided into four lobes. Similar to the cerebral cortex, the cerebellum is divided into an archicerebellum, palaeocerebellum, and neocerebellum according to the evolutionary origin of these structures. The cerebellum contains a large number of cells and is connected with virtually all parts of the cerebral cortex. Although

The cerebellum is largely known for its role in eye movement, vestibular control, and motor coordination. It also contributes to cognitive functions including attention, action planning, visuospatial cognition, and memory, as well as emotion regulation.

(a)

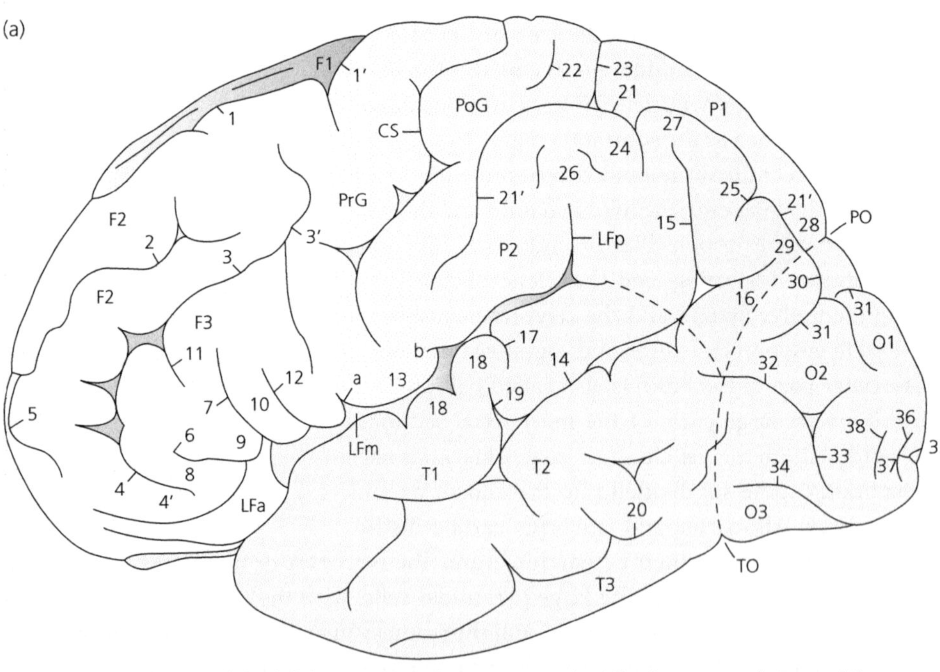

Fig. 2.1a Lateral view of the left hemisphere (brainstem and midbrain removed). Dotted lines indicate the (theoretical) boundaries between different lobes. (Reproduced from Miguel Marín-Padilla, 'Mammalian Cerebral Cortex: Embryonic Development and Cytoarchitecture', in The Human Brain, pp. 6–7, Figure 1, Copyright © 2011, Springer Science + Business Media.)

(b)

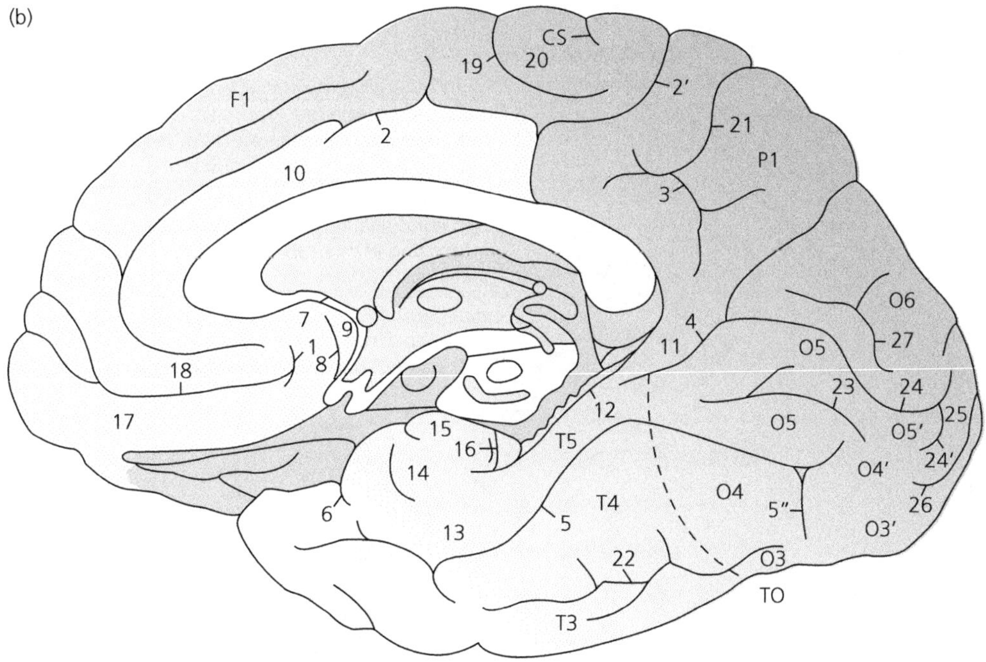

Fig. 2.1b Inferomedial view of the right hemisphere (brainstem and midbrain removed). (Reproduced from Miguel Marín-Padilla, 'Mammalian Cerebral Cortex: Embryonic Development and Cytoarchitecture', in The Human Brain, pp. 28–9, Figure 13, Copyright © 2011, Springer Science + Business Media.)

known best for its role in eye movement, vestibular control, and motor coordination, the cerebellum contributes to a variety of cognitive functions, including attention, action planning, visual-spatial cognition, memory, and emotion regulation (Katz and Steinmetz 2002).

All communication between lower (hindbrain) and higher (cortical) cerebral and cerebellar brain centres has to pass the midbrain structures; they cannot be skipped. This is a direct consequence of the evolutionary origins of the mammalian brain in distinct layers, which are hierarchically organized.

2.3 **The triune brain**

The human brain (and the brains of all mammals) can schematically be divided into three layers according to their evolutionary emergence in different classes of animals (MacLean 1990). These three layers have been termed the 'reptilian brain' or R-complex, the 'palaeomammalian brain', and the 'neomammalian brain'. Although this distinction is a (deliberate) simplification of how these three layers act in concert, the 'triune brain'

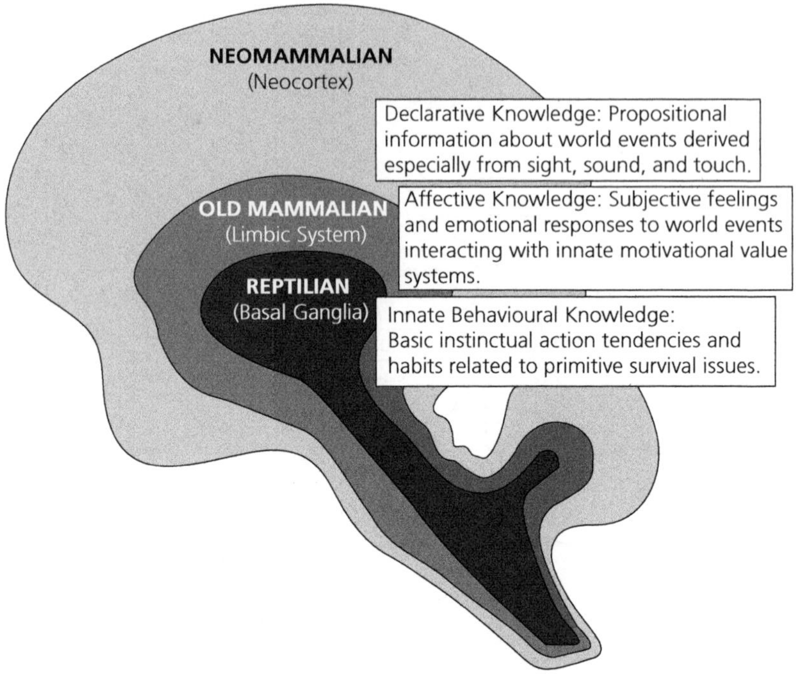

Fig. 2.2 Schematic representation of hierarchical brain organization according to MacLean's triune brain concept. (Reproduced from P.D. MacLean, The Triune Brain in Evolution: Role in Paleocerebral Functions, Plenum Press, New York, Copyright © 1990, Springer-Verlag US.)

offers a comprehensive model of the representation of functions in the brain (see Figure 2.2).

The 'triune brain' is a theoretical model to explain how complex mammalian brains evolved from more primitive stages. The reptilian brain is responsible for the regulation of the basic vital functions. The rostral parts of the reptilian brain are the seat of instinctual behaviours pertaining to mating, intrasexual aggression, and submission. The palaeomammalian brain is involved in emotion regulation, maternal care, separation distress, and playful exploration of the environment. The neomammalian brain comprises higher cognitive functions including (in humans) self-reflexive awareness.

The reptilian brain is the phylogenetically oldest structure comprising the brainstem, basal ganglia and striatum. The most ancient structures are responsible for the regulation of body temperature, blood pressure, breathing, sleep–wakefulness, and postural reflexes. The more rostral parts of the reptilian brain are the seat of largely instinctual behaviours, including ritualized social behaviours pertaining to mating, intrasexual aggression, and submission, as well as appetitive behaviours controlling food consumption, hunting, etc. Instinctual behaviours are represented in fixed action patterns with narrowly defined releasers. Conditioned learning and appetitive behaviours are maintained by striatal structures. The reptilian brain, as its name suggests, is similarly structured in reptiles and has changed relatively little during mammalian evolution (MacLean 1990) with some notable exceptions.

The autonomic nervous system (comprising the vagal and the sympathetic systems) has evolved over time to provide organisms with more flexible responses to challenges of the environment, such as predatory threat, within-species competition for social rank, and access to sexual partners. According to Porges' 'Polyvagal Theory' (1995), the most primitive threat response is immobilization or freezing behaviour which can be found in most vertebrates when escape is thwarted. Immobilization is dependent on the function of the unmyelinated vagus nerve. A phylogenetic more recent response pattern involves mobilization of fight or flight responses. This system is subserved by the action of the sympathetic nervous system. The most recent evolutionary development that occurred in mammals is functionally linked to the activity of the myelinated vagus. Porges proposes that the myelinated vagus is involved in social communication. It also acts as a break on heart rate by inhibiting the sympathetic nervous system (Porges 2007). A neurophysiological correlate of the activity of the myelinated vagus is the variability of the heart rate, which can be measured as respiratory sinus arrythmia. Dysfunction of the myelinated vagus leads to greater activity of the more primitive systems (i.e. mobilization or immobilization), which is accompanied by a reduction of the heart rate variability (i.e. failure of the vagal break on heart rate). Interestingly, the ontogenetic functional development of the myelinated vagus is dependent on environmental input. That is, intrauterine adversity (e.g. during the second trimester of gestation) can compromise the maturation of the polyvagal system, which may have profound impact not just on mental health but also on the organism's ability to regulate stress, including immunological responses (Porges 1992, 2009; Grippo et al. 2007). These aspects can have profound implications on our understanding of many psychiatric (and general medical) conditions.

Myelinated vagus fibres act as a break on heart rate by inhibiting the sympathetic nervous system. A neurophysiological correlate of the activity of the myelinated vagus is the variability of the heart rate. Intrauterine adversity (e.g. during the second trimester of gestation) can compromise the maturation of the polyvagal system.

The palaeomammalian part of the brain is roughly identical with limbic structures. The evolution of this system is closely related to the development of extensive parental care and other social emotions (Panksepp 1998). Thus, in functional terms the palaeomammalian brain regulates emotions such as fear and anger, and is involved in maternal care behaviour, expression of separation distress, and playful exploration of the environment. The selection for greater parental care and nurturance is seen as the critical correlate of the development of social emotions such as empathy and individual recognition of close relatives (Bernhardt and Singer 2012; Gonzalez-Liencres et al. 2013; Preston 2013). The palaeomammalian brain can be found in primitive mammals but has undergone some substantial changes during primate evolution. For example, it is involved in stress regulation (Morgane and Mokler 2006), as well as in interoceptive awareness of own body states (Craig 2003; see section 2.9). Accordingly, limbic structures are particularly susceptible to the influence of early

The palaeomammalian brain (limbic system) is involved in stress regulation and interoceptive awareness. Limbic structures are particularly susceptible to the influence of early life experiences and may profoundly gauge an individual's stress responsivity.

life experiences and may profoundly gauge an individual's stress responsivity (Teicher et al. 2003; Dannlowski et al. 2012).

The neomammalian brain evolved most recently and allows for much greater behavioural flexibility by integrating multimodal sensory input into modifiable concepts of the world. One of its functions is to dampen behavioural impulses from the lower brain centres, to free the organism from pursuing rigid instinctual behaviours by selecting among behavioural alternatives, to integrate information across functional domains, to plan future actions, to predict future events (foresight), and to store information (Fuster 2001; Paus 2001; Brown and Brüne 2012). Conscious awareness of what the neomammalian brain does is the exception rather than the rule, but conscious self-reflection and reflection of what others perceive is not possible without neomammalian cortical expansion. The hierarchical organization becomes immediately clear when considering that lower brain functions (e.g. breathing) may operate independent of higher functions, but not vice versa, and the functioning of the neomammalian parts of the brain depends upon an intact connection with the midbrain and hypothalamus (MacLean 1990).

The large PFC has extensive connections with other cortical regions and subcortical structures. Brain connectivity is highly dependent on early experiences.

The large prefrontal cortex (PFC) of primates is the most recently enlarged structure of the neomammalian brain. It is reciprocally connected with the brainstem, the diencephalon, and the limbic system. Afferent connections provide information about the internal environment, arousal, drives, motives, and visceral correlates of emotions. All PFC subdivisions—medial, lateral, and orbital—receive information from the amygdala and the hippocampus formation, and are connected via reciprocal projections with each other (Zilles 1987). The medial and orbital prefrontal cortices primarily carry out functions related to emotional behaviour and the control of basic drives. The lateral portion of the PFC is involved in the temporal integration of information and organization of prospective behavioural goals (Paus 2001). There are strong intrahemispheric connections between the temporal and the prefrontal lobes, and these connections are particularly relevant for the processing of social information (Hopkins and Rilling 2000). Notably, brain connectivity is highly dependent on early experiences. For example, extreme anxiety alters the connectivity between limbic (amygdala) and prefrontal brain regions (Birn et al. 2014), which may have functional implications on how the brain evaluates threat.

The neomammalian brain has undergone the most significant changes during human evolution. A comparison of brain size between humans and our closest relatives may illustrate in which parts of the brain these changes took place (Semendeferi et al. 1997; Semendeferi and Damasio 2000).

2.4 **Allometric growth curves and constraints of human brain enlargement**

Brain size varies greatly between species, even within mammals. The brain of the tiniest mammals weighs only several grams, whereas the brain of whales can weigh up to 10 kg. As a rule of thumb, brain weight of mammals is a function of body weight. Brain weight increases relative to body weight—similar to the resting energy turnover—at three quarters of body weight (Allman 1999). When plotting brain weight against body mass, however, there is considerable between-species variation in relative brain weight. The procedure by which weight or volume of an organ is normalized to body weight is called allometry. Progression indices (PI) can be obtained using this method, defined as the brain weight in a species divided by brain weight in an ancestral species or group of extant species resembling the last common ancestor. The PI therefore reflects an evolutionary trend, which, in turn, indicates the functional significance of certain brain areas relative to others (Rapoport 1990).

In mammals brain weight increases relative to body weight—similar to the resting energy turnover—at three quarters of body weight. Allometric calculations can determine the increase of an organ in size or volume relative to body size or weight by extrapolation from ancestral species of extant species resembling the last common ancestor (expressed in progression indices).

The earliest primates descended from insectivores; thus it makes sense to compare extant species that resemble ancestral species in the evolutionary transition from insectivores to early primates (e.g. tupaia), prosimians (lemurs, bushbabies, and galago), simian species (monkeys), and apes (including humans). On average, primates have two to three times larger brains than expected for their body weight compared with non-primate mammalian species. This is similar for foetal brain volumes (with the exception of toothed whales). Within the primate order, fruit eaters have on average larger brains than leaf eaters. This may be because foraging fruits may pose greater demands on computational resources due to the seasonal and spatial dispersion of ripe fruit (Allman 1999).

Early accounts have suggested an inverse correlation between brain size and gut size. Thus it can be said that the brain competes with the digestive organs for energy, because the total energy use is a function of body mass. Although the human brain has a relatively low energy consumption of about 15 W, it still consumes between 15 and 20 percent of the total energy, which is a disproportionally high amount, because its adult weight of about 1,400 g makes only 2 percent of the total body weight (Aiello and Wheeler 1995). These considerations have recently been modified to conclude that several factors have allowed for an increase in brain size during human evolution, including changing energy subsidies (cooperative breeding; see Chapter 3), improved quality of diets, and reduced energy expenditure for locomotion (i.e. bipedalism; Navarrete et al. 2011).

When comparing the size of particular parts of the brain relative to absolute brain size between closely and more remotely related species, controlling for body weight, one can get an impression of which brain areas enlarged over time during human evolution and which ones became relatively smaller. On the basis of PI, it can be concluded that the importance of the olfactory system declined in the primate lineage over evolutionary time. In insectivores, for instance, the olfactory bulb makes 18 percent of the total brain volume, in tupaias it figures around 7 percent, in the galago 4 percent, in monkeys around 0.2 percent, and in humans 0.01 percent of total brain volume (Rapoport 1990). Expressed in PI, the size of the human olfactory bulb is roughly merely 1/40 to 1/50, as expected for an insectivore of comparable body

Primate brains are on average three times larger than expected for their body weight. In humans the neocortex is over 150 times larger than expected for human body weight, whereas the olfactory bulb is roughly one fiftieth the size compared to primitive primates.

weight. By contrast, the PI of the human neocortex is 156, and in our closest extant relative, the chimpanzee, the neocortex PI is 58 (Rapoport 1990). Thus, it seems that neocortical expansion accelerated during human evolution after the split of the human lineage and the chimpanzee lineage from a common ancestor some 6 mya. The human neocortex is therefore roughly three times the size as expected for an ape of similar body size (here, in order to avoid confusion, it is essential to keep in mind that differences in brain size already exist between monkeys and apes), and hence about three times larger compared with the chimpanzee's brain (Jones et al. 1992).

Just to get an impression of how large the human brain has grown, imagine that if the human body were to grow relative to brain weight as in most primates, humans would weigh approximately 450 kg and stand 3 m tall. Or put slightly differently, the human brain grows exactly as if it was in the body of a giant ape (sometimes referred to as 'the King-Kong model'; for a different view see Herculano-Houzel 2009). Also note that the human brain continues to grow after birth at a high rate, which has to do with human immaturity at parturition (Jones et al. 1992). This characteristic reflects a design compromise due to the human pelvis anatomy (for details see Chapter 3). For an illustration see Figure 2.3.

The human neocortex is three times larger compared to other apes. If brain/body relations were similar in humans compared to other primates, humans would be expected to grow 3 m tall and weigh 450 kg.

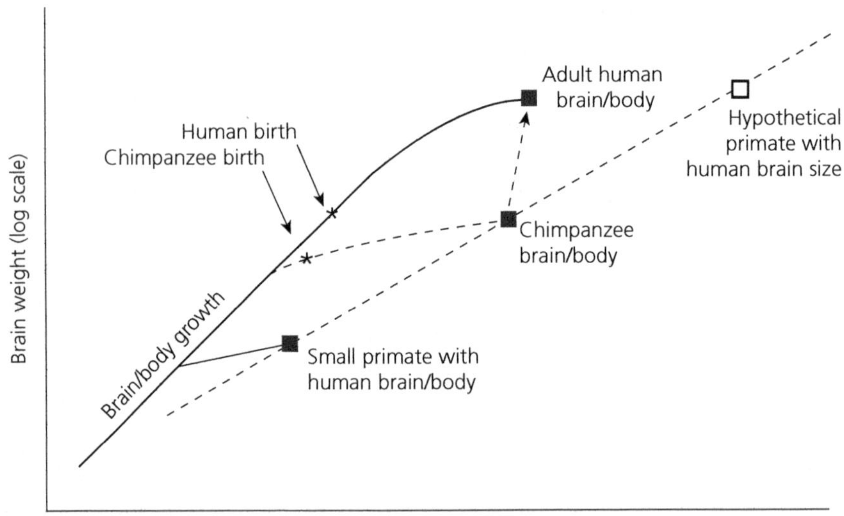

Fig. 2.3 Relationship of brain–body growth in humans compared with that of other primate species. Of note, the length of the human foetal phase (in which the brain and body grow at the same rate) is well extended into the postnatal phase as a result of premature human birth. The human brain is considerably larger than expected for a primate of human body weight. (Reproduced from Stephen Jones, Robert D. Martin, and David R. Pilbeam, The Cambridge Encyclopedia of Human Evolution, p. 118, Figure 1, Cambridge University Press, Canada, Copyright © 1994, Cambridge University Press.)

Before coming back to allometric changes within the neocortex, it is important to note that in humans several phylogenetically older parts of the brain, notably the hippocampus, the entorhinal cortex, and the amygdala, also increased disproportionally in size, reflected in PIs of 4.2, 5.5, and 3.9, respectively (Rapoport 1990). Such changes probably reflect the growing functional significance of limbic structures for emotion regulation, notably fear, aggression, attachment, and empathy, as well as the formation of autonoëtic (autobiographic) memory.

The progression indices for limbic structures are less pronounced in humans compared to neocortex enlargement, but nevertheless considerable relative to other primates.

Within the hippocampus, the CA1 region, which is most extensively connected with the neocortex, makes 44 percent of the total hippocampal formation in simians, and its PI in humans is 6.6. Notably, the dentate gyrus, as part of the hippocampal formation, is also disproportionally enlarged. Its PI is 2.6 relative to insectivores. This region is believed to be critical for adult neurogenesis, which has been considered to be a crucial neuronal correlate of behavioural plasticity and adaptive flexibility. Compromised adult neurogenesis is believed to play a role in depression, schizophrenia, and various forms of dementia (Kempermann 2012). Hippocampus and entorhinal cortex are also critical for memory function, whereby during human evolution the storage of autobiographical material has been increasingly important for social interaction. Recent animal studies suggest that the CA2 region, a small proportion of the hippocampus interposed between the larger CA1 and CA3 regions, is specifically relevant for social memory (Hitti and Siegelbaum 2014), which may stipulate further research in humans.

The amygdala is subdivided in several functional units. The cortical regions of the amygdala regulate foraging and sexual behaviours, whereas subcortical nuclei of the amygdala are involved in conditioned and observation-driven learning of defence mechanisms and aggression-associated behaviours (Allman and Brothers 1994; Amaral 2002). The amygdala is also relevant for the regulation of interpersonal space (Kennedy et al. 2009). Moreover, individual differences in amygdala size predict the size and complexity of one's social network across the lifespan (Bickart et al. 2011).

The basal ganglia also increased in size over evolutionary time, and the PI of the striatal complex is 16.4 in humans (compared to 9.0 in chimpanzees and 4.7 in prosimians), which could be indicative of the increasing importance of motivated behaviour and reward-prediction and anticipation (Knutson et al. 2001), whereby connections of the striatum to the orbitofrontal cortex (OFC) contribute to the processing of hedonic experiences (Schultz et al. 2000; Kringelbach 2005).

Of specific interest is the cingulate gyrus, which belongs cytoarchitectonically to the limbic system. The most anterior part has undergone significant evolutionary changes (see section 2.9) and contributes to the differentiation of salient from non-salient stimuli and decision-making (Allman et al. 2001; Paus 2001). Finally, the cerebellum is also larger in humans than expected for a primate of equivalent body size, but tends to be smaller compared to other apes (Rilling and Insel 1998; MacLeod et al. 2003). Thus it would seem that the increase in size of the cerebellum could not keep pace with neocortical expansion during hominid evolution. However, the neocerebellum, in particular, has greatly increased in size in apes and humans relative to monkeys, and this might have to do with its involvement in visuospatial skills, planning of complex movements, procedural learning, and attention shifting between different modalities, and with the role these functions had during hominoid evolution, perhaps in developing more sophisticated foraging techniques (MacLeod et al. 2003).

The human cerebellum has increased in size relative to other primates, but not relative to other apes. The frontal cortex—though not larger than expected for an ape of human body size—is significantly more convoluted compared to other ape brains.

At first sight, a perplexing finding is that the human frontal lobes—relative to neocortex size—are not bigger than expected for an ape of our body size (Semendeferi et al. 1997, 2002). However, the human PFC is significantly more convoluted or gyrified than expected for a primate of the same brain size, and the same is probably true for the posterior temporal and parietal lobes, whereas the motor, premotor, and primary visual areas are the least convoluted (Rilling and Insel 1999a, 1999b; Rilling and Seligman 2002). Interestingly, the PFC and the temporoparietal junction are the last to myelinate during ontogeny. Due to complex reorganizations, some areas located in the OFC such as Brodmann area (BA) 13 are even smaller in humans, relative to other ape species (Semendeferi et al. 1998). BA 10, by contrast, has undergone an evolutionary shift in location by moving from the orbital frontal cortex to cover the entire frontal pole in apes (Semendeferi et al. 2001). In terms of function, the frontal poles are engaged in future action planning and initiation of action, whereas the OFC is involved in evaluating the emotional significance of social stimuli (Bechara et al. 2000a, 2000b). Damage to the medial part of the OFC produces a profound impairment of empathy, and dysfunction of the dorsolateral part of the OFC leads to lack of drive and motivation (Bechara et al. 2000a). Moreover, the medial part of the PFC is specifically involved in social cognitive processes including the representation of one's own and others' thoughts and intentions (Frith and Frith 1999, 2001). Of particular importance is the paracingulate sulcus, which can be found in only 50 percent of individuals and is thought to be under ongoing adaptive modification (Paus et al. 1996; Walter et al. 2004).

The prefrontal and parietal cortices myelinate last in humans. The paracingulate sulcus as part of the limbic system is present in only 50 percent of humans and is believed to undergo ongoing adaptive modification.

Within the frontal cortex the frontal poles are engaged in future action planning and initiation of action; the OFC is involved in evaluating the emotional significance of social stimuli; the medial part of the orbitofrontal controls social emotions such as empathy; the dorsolateral part of the OFC regulates drive and motivation; and the medial part of the PFC is specifically involved in social cognitive processes including the representation of one's own and others' thoughts and intentions.

The temporal lobes have also disproportionally increased in the human lineage relative to other apes, particularly with respect to white matter volume, possibly reflecting its functional significance in speech comprehension and production, face processing, and recognition of intentional movements (Rilling and Seligman 2002). The temporal poles contribute to the storage of autobiographical memory. The fusiform gyrus at the lower surface of the temporal lobe is critical for recognizing invariant aspects of faces such that individuals can be identified irrespective of the angle from which their faces are visible.

The temporal lobe is functionally important for speech comprehension and production, face processing, and recognition of intentional movements. The temporal poles contribute to the storage of autobiographical memory.
The infraparietal lobule contributes to complex cognitive functions such as self-recognition and attribution of agency.

For some reason, the evolutionary history of the parietal lobes has remained, to some extent, obscure. However, the infraparietal lobule, which comprises the supramarginal gyrus and the adjacent angular gyrus, has probably also undergone recent evolutionary reorganization. It has rich connections to the prefrontal and temporal cortices and plays an important role in multimodal sensory integration, self-perception, and differentiation of self from others (Torrey 2007). Thus, damage to this brain area may lead to bodily neglect (e.g. anosognosia after damage to the right parietal lobe), lack of insight and self-reflection, and misattribution of thoughts and behaviours as alien-made (called passivity symptoms; Torrey 2007). In contrast to the more anterior parts of the neocortex, the primary visual cortex has been displaced posteriorly and its relative size is reduced in humans relative to other primates, yet with large interindividual differences (Aboitiz et al. 2003).

Notably, the relative brain weight in primates is also closely associated with relative longevity of individuals of different species. This can be explained by the fact that species that enjoy a long lifespan experience—statistically—more adverse events, such as food shortages and other unpredictable environmental variations, than short-lived species, and therefore require more computational resources to cope with such adversities. The maximum human lifespan as predicted from brain weight is about 101.5 years, which comes close to the actual maximum. In humans, relative longevity has been found to correlate with different parts of the brain in similar ways, notably the size of the neocortex, amygdala, hypothalamus, and cerebellum (Allman 1999).

2.5 **Cytoarchitecture of the human neocortex**

The total number of neurons of the PFC has increased over evolutionary time. Humans possess approximately four times more neurons compared with other apes, comprising 14 cm^3 in humans compared with 2.8 cm^3 in chimpanzees. By contrast, the density of neurons reveals an inverse relationship: humans have the lowest density per centimetre cubed due to an increase in connecting tissue; thus, an increasing number of neurons constrains the density of white matter. In humans grey matter is about 50 percent of total brain volume and the human neocortex contains 40 percent white matter. Thus, although brain size matters, patterns of brain reorganization in terms of function are at least equally important (Hofman 2001; Jerison 2001). For example, further growth of cortical surface would require such an increase in size of the skull that the passage through the birth canal would become impossible (or require timing of birth to be even more displaced preterm). Moreover, if the cortex expanded along the horizontal axis only, the length of connecting fibres would inevitably increase such that the flow of information from one cell or cell assembly to another would be slowed.

Thus, one reason why cortical folding (gyrification) occurred in brain evolution was to facilitate neural transmission by reducing the number and length of connecting axons. The number of connecting fibres was reduced by compartmentalization of neurons into modular circuits, whereas the length of connecting tissue was diminished by cortical folding (Hofman 2001). In other words, gyrification represents a solution for large brains to pack a maximum of surface into a minimal volume. Thus, in the adult human brain, about two-thirds of cortical surface is buried in the sulci and only one-third is superficially exposed. All gyri and sulci are already visible at birth, but it takes two decades of growth to conceal two-thirds of the cortex surface in the sulci (Allman 1999; Roth and Wullimann 2001). The modular organization at the neuronal level probably matches, in part, the organization according to function as proposed by evolutionary psychology (see Chapter 1).

Cortical folding (gyrification) emerged in brain evolution as a way to facilitate neural transmission by a reduction in number and length of connecting axons.

For more than 100 years scientist have tried to develop brain atlases on the basis of cytoarchitectonic details, such as the number of cortical layers, cell packing densities, and shape of neurons, or based on the degree of myelination. The most influential cartography of the neocortex—to date—was put forth by Korbinian Brodmann. It turned out that Brodmann's map of the cortex surface was in many respects consistent with functional specializations of cytoarchitectonically defined brain areas. Studies using functional brain imaging still use Brodmann's cartography as a reference system, even though it is perhaps too schematic.

Novel approaches now combine the traditional parcellation procedures with brain imaging techniques such as magnetic resonance imaging (MRI), diffusion tensor imaging (DTI), positron emission tomography (PET), and receptor autoradiography (Toga et al. 2006). The latter technology could demonstrate that receptors for acetylcholine, norepinephrine, dopamine, serotonin, glutamate, and gamma-aminobutyric acid (GABA) are heterogeneously distributed across the human neocortex and archicortex. The patterns of distribution of different receptors in anatomically defined areas of the cortex can be graphically overlain in two-dimensional coordinates such that receptor fingerprints for individual regions of the brain can be visualized. This kind of molecular architectonic brain mapping seems more accurate than conventional atlases and may be used in the near future to define more precisely the functional representation of cognitive and emotional processes in healthy subjects and patients with psychiatric disorders (Toga et al. 2006).

Traditional cartography of the brain is now being combined with novel techniques such as MRI, DTI, PET, and receptor autoradiography, showing that receptors for acetylcholine, norepinephrine, dopamine, serotonin, glutamate, and GABA are heterogeneously distributed across the human neocortex and archicortex.

2.6 **Evolutionary ontogeny of the human brain**

The study of evolutionary ontogeny, or heterochrony, refers to the observation that changes in timing or rate of developmental events, relative to the homologous patterns in the ancestor, are the key mechanisms of how evolutionary modifications are translated into ontogeny (McKinney and McNamara 1991). Scientists have long believed in the idea developed by Ernst Haeckel that ontogeny recapitulates phylogeny. This is now conceived to be imprecise, though, superficially, embryonic stages of different species resemble each other more closely than later stages of development. Ontogenetic development is highly conservative, but organisms do not pass through the adult stages of their ancestors; rather changes in developmental genes influence both early and late ontogeny (Deacon 1990a, 1990b). Thus, developmental processes can be accelerated and terminated earlier, or delayed and set off later during ontogeny (Figure 2.4).

Heterochrony describes changes in timing or rate of developmental events, relative to the homologous patterns in the ancestor, as the key mechanism of how evolutionary modifications are translated into ontogeny.

The idea that the adult human skull resembles the skull of juvenile apes in shape and form was put forth by anthropologists many decades ago. Indeed, several human body features including hairlessness and the anterior position of the vagina have been interpreted as the result of a retention of juvenile characteristics of the ancestral species into adulthood of the extant human species, known as paedomorphosis (McKinney and McNamara 1991). Moreover, persistent playfulness and curiosity into adulthood have been likened to behaviours found in juvenile apes (and other animals), hence giving rise to the hypothesis of behavioural paedomorphosis (Montagu 1989). Put slightly differently, the hypothesis suggests that paedomorphic organisms reach sexual maturity while retaining features of a juvenile body. Paedomorphosis is one of several developmental timing processes, which are embraced under the term 'heterochrony'. Heterochrony

Many anatomical and behavioural features, including findings from dentition and myelination, suggest that humans are paedomorphic, that is, that juvenile characteristics are retained in adulthood. In addition, hypermorphosis—the delay of growth offset—may have produced additional computational brain capacity.

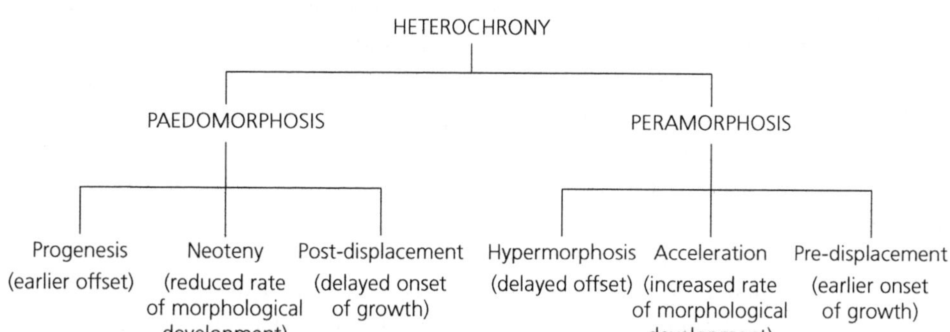

Fig. 2.4 Hierarchical classification of heterochronic processes. (Reproduced from Michael L. McKinney, 'Classifying and Analyzing Heterochrony', in Heterochrony: The Evolution of Ontogeny, pp. 17, Figure 2–3, Copyright © 1991, Springer Science + Business Media.)

explains why during ontogeny the growth of different parts of the body (including the brain) diverges. Some tissues grow faster (and longer) than others (McKinney and McNamara 1991).

Whether or not some aspects of brain enlargement and organization are associated with paedomorphic timing of maturation is a matter of controversy. There are, however, several facts that point in this direction. Sexual maturity in primates is a function of brain weight relative to body weight. For a primate with a human-sized brain, sexual maturity should be reached by age 44. The actual time point at which humans become sexually mature is, however, much earlier (with differences between men and women; see Chapter 3). Similarly, the eruption of wisdom teeth correlates with brain weight. The projection of the regression line would predict the eruption of the third molars to occur at about 38 years of age, where the wisdom teeth actually erupt in humans on average around age 20. Comparisons of growth processes in teeth between fossil human species and anatomical modern humans suggest that the typical human-like growth pattern emerged relatively late in human evolution. Taken together, these human characteristics indicate that humans become sexually mature earlier than predicted from their relative brain weight, whereas development in general is delayed (Allman 1999).

In further support of the paedomorphosis hypothesis, it is noteworthy that the PFC is the brain region that matures latest during ontogeny, and myelination and synaptogenesis may continue to develop well into the third decade. Grey matter volume increases postnatally until 4–5 years of age and declines gradually through the third decade. In contrast, white matter and corpus callosum thickness increase from birth through the third decade, and possibly through the fifth decade, in frontal and temporal areas. These effects are more pronounced in boys compared with girls. A 40 percent synapse overproduction primarily takes place from the 30th gestational week through the first to the second year postnatally, with a peak rate of 40,000 synapses per second (Rakic et al. 1986). Within the neocortex, synapse production peaks in the occipital cortex by 6 months of age, and in the PFC by 2 years. This extension of synaptogenesis is considerably longer than in other primates. In essence, brain growth is considerably expanded in humans compared to other primates, and the extension of the human juvenile period may in part be mediated by regulatory genes producing a shift towards greater paedomorphosis. Although not exactly known, it is conceivable that selection pressures from the social environment have contributed to this shift in developmental timing, possibly including the need for a reduction in intraspecies aggression (Leach et al. 2003).

In any event, paedomorphosis was certainly not the only mechanism in timing the growth of the human brain. The human brain does not resemble any juvenile ape brain, and the complex addition of new traits has probably been regulated by another developmental timing process referred to as hypermorphosis. Hypermorphosis involves a delay of growth offset. Accordingly, hypermorphic structures grow for an extended period of time, and this may be another important mechanism that produced additional computational brain capacity (besides other physical features in humans, such as longer legs compared to other apes). Thus, the best heterochronic model for the human brain is probably a combination of paedomorphosis and (subsequent) hypermorphosis (McKinney and McNamara 1991). Interestingly, heterochronic processes are linked with a species' life history. Neoteny and hypermorphosis typically occur in K-selected species with extended life histories. K-selection is more likely to develop in stable or predictable seasonal environmental conditions. Among primates, human life history represents the extreme of K-selection, with far-reaching consequences for cognitive, emotional, and behavioural systems (for further details see Chapter 3).

2.7 Lateralization and connectivity in the human brain

The human brain comprises many functions that are carried out by neural networks, most of which are differentially represented in the left or right cerebral hemisphere. This division of labour by the two hemispheres is referred to as lateralization (Saugstad 1998). Language has been considered the prime example of functional lateralization. However, whereas 'linear' functions such as speech production and grammar as well as auditory processing of spoken language are lateralized to the left (in right-handed individuals), the 'holistic' comprehension of content of speech such as intonation, metaphor, and emotional prosody, that is, the ability to recognize the affective overtone of spoken language, is lateralized to the right (Mitchell and Crow 2005). In addition, spatial orientation is usually localized in the right hemisphere. Recent research has revealed that even the capacity to distinguish self from others is to some degree lateralized. The first-person perspective is represented in the left inferior parietal cortex, whereas the third-person perspective is localized in the corresponding region on the right side of the human brain. For example, the imitation of another person's action activates the left inferior parietal cortex; conversely, the opposite side is involved when subjects view their actions being imitated (Decety and Chaminade 2005).

Many brain functions are lateralized to the right or left hemisphere. With regard to language, 'linear' functions such as speech production and grammar, as well as auditory processing of spoken language, are lateralized to the left (in right-handed individuals), whereas the 'holistic' comprehension of content of speech, such as intonation, metaphor, and emotional prosody, is lateralized to the right.

Anatomically, there is a leftward occipital and rightward frontal lobe asymmetry, known as the cerebral torque, and perhaps a mild leftward planum temporale asymmetry (Crow 1997a-c). Asymmetry of the planum temporale, a portion of Wernicke's speech area, however, is not human-specific (Gannon et al. 1998; Hopkins et al. 1998). Rather it has been shown to be already present in great apes, a finding suggesting that apes may have some functional specialization located in the temporal lobe indicative of gestural proto-language. However, handedness is much less pronounced in

Self and other representation is also lateralized to left and right, respectively.

apes compared to humans, such that there is still uncertainty about how to interpret these results.

In any event, increasing functional and anatomical specialization of the cerebral hemispheres of a large brain causes some problems regarding the connectivity of anatomically distributed neural networks. In mammals the size and thickness of the corpus callosum has increased with neocortex size and is also related to the strength of cerebral dominance. However, the callosal fibre diameter and fibre packing density has remained fairly constant, such that an increase in size of both hemispheres constrains the proportional growth of connecting fibre tracts. In humans, the interhemispheric connectivity is indeed reduced relative to other primates, whereas intrahemispheric connectivity is augmented, as indicated by a greater white matter volume relative to neocortical grey matter volume. This, in turn, may have been important for the evolution of brain lateralization.

Functional specialization of the hemispheres constrains the proportional growth of interhemispheric connectivity. Accordingly, corpus callosum size has decreased in humans relative to other primates. In contrast, intrahemispheric connectivity, which is maintained by four large fibre tracts, has increased during human evolution.

The ratio of the corpus callosum volume to neocortex surface size decreases in primate species as hemispheric asymmetry and handedness (cerebral dominance) increase, suggesting a relationship between directional asymmetry and interhemispheric connectivity (Hopkins and Rilling 2000). Intrahemispheric connectivity in the human brain is maintained by white matter bundles. There are four major tracts, called the arcuate fasciculus, the inferior longitudinal fasciculus, the fronto-occipital fasciculus, and the uncinate fasciculus. The arcuate fasciculus connects the dorsolateral PFC with cortical areas in the temporal, parietal, and occipital lobes. It also links Broca's and Wernicke's speech areas. The anterior cingulum bundle connects the anterior part of the anterior cingulate cortex and the dorsolateral PFC with the parahippocampal gyrus and with the medial parts of the parietal cortex. The uncinate fasciculus connects the OFC and the anterior cingulate cortex with the medial and anterior temporal lobe, the superior temporal gyrus, the entorhinal cortex, and the amygdala (Zilles 1987). These structures are thought to contribute to the evaluation and processing of social information and fear responses, in part by using autobiographical material. The term 'inferior longitudinal fasciculus' is probably somewhat misleading, because this bundle primarily connects the occipital with the temporal lobe. It is believed to be important for visual recognition, including face recognition.

The reasons why cerebral lateralization evolved are probably manifold. It could be that hemispheric specialization emerged as a consequence of reduced interhemispheric connectivity, which in turn arose as a result of increasing brain size. But why does functional asymmetry prevail in humans and other vertebrates in the same direction, instead of random lateralization of functions within populations? From an evolutionary point of view the preferential use of the right or left visual hemifield during activities such as searching for food, agonistic responses, or escape from predators may be disadvantageous because relevant stimuli may occur randomly in both hemifields, and predators may exploit the predictability of behaviour arising from lateral biases at population level. In many species, predator escape reactions and associated fear are controlled by the right brain, because individuals are more reactive when predators occur in their left visual hemifield (processed by the right hemisphere). Similarly, control of intraspecies aggression seems to be lateralized to the right brain. By contrast, there seems to be a rightward bias for feeding, including catching prey (which could have predisposed to right-handedness). In humans there is a clear asymmetry regarding face processing. For example, emotions are more evidently expressed on the left side of the face as a function of emotion control via the right hemisphere, such that humans expose more often the left side of their faces, at least if the emotional expression is meant to be honest (interestingly, the examination of portraits of males shows no leftward bias, suggesting an intention to conceal the real emotion, that is, to show the right side of the face when lying). Thus, a possible explanation could be that the direction of behavioural asymmetries may be selected for by social pressures to coordinate behaviour with other asymmetrical individuals of the same species (Vallortigara and Rogers 2005).

The direction of behavioural asymmetries may be selected for by social pressures to coordinate behaviour with other asymmetrical individuals of the same species, despite disadvantages regarding escape from predators. In humans, emotional expression is lateralized to the right brain such that the left side of the face is preferentially exposed if emotions are honest: interestingly, the left side of the face is often concealed if the emotional expression is dishonest.

2.8 Brain sexual dimorphism

Males have slightly larger brains in terms of cortical volume by about 11–18 percent, and overall brain weight differs between men and women by about 110 g, even when body weight is covaried out. The total number of cortical neurons seems to be slightly lower in women compared with men, with a difference of about 15.5 percent. The density of cortical neurons is by contrast the same in both sexes. The overall ratio of cortex to the whole brain volume is about 46 percent in both men and women, and the ratio of cortical to subcortical brain mass is identical in both sexes. The right hemisphere is usually slightly larger than the left hemisphere, with differences of about 3.5 g for both sexes. The thickness of the corpus callosum is similar for men and women. However, in light of the smaller brain size of women, the commissural connectivity is about 10 percent larger, which may support the assumption of a lesser hemispheric lateralization in women (Gur et al. 2002).

Sex differences in brain weight and number of cortical neurons in favour of men, and differences in interhemispheric connectivity in favour of females, are measurable, but the functional significance of these findings remains elusive. Behaviourally, women have superior verbal fluency and are more skilled than men in object location, whereas men are better at visuospatial orientation. Women's larger ratio of the OFC volume relative to amygdala volume may explain the greater significance of empathetic behaviour in women.

The functional significance of these differences is fairly obscure. It is well known that women have superior verbal fluency compared with men, whereas men, on average, are better at visuospatial orientation. However, women are more skilled than men in object location. These functions have been associated with divergent selection pressures for men and women in ancestral times, where early humans lived as hunter-gatherers and women with infants and juveniles formed the core of the community (as 'cooperative breeders'; see Chapter 3), whereas men were engaged in travelling large distances in order to hunt large game. In line with this, research has revealed that women tend to have greater orbitofrontal cortices (involved in emotion regulation and empathy) compared with men, whereas no sex differences have been found regarding the size of the amygdalae, hippocampi, and dorsolateral prefrontal cortices. However, the ratio of OFC volume and amygdala volume has been found to be greater in women, which may explain sex differences in emotion processing and affect-driven behaviour (Gur et al. 2002).

2.9 **Evolutionary novelties in primate and ape brains**

In the context of human brain evolution it is noteworthy to highlight those neuronal adaptations that are perhaps somewhat unique to primates. Some of these adaptations occurred because primates are essentially gregarious animals, their ontogenetic development is slow, and their maximum lifespans are long, such that social learning became increasingly important. Moreover, inhibitory control of behaviour as well as novel ways of communication became a crucial factor in apes and humans.

Single cell recordings in macaque monkeys have revealed that neurons in the middle portion of the temporal lobe, particularly in the superior temporal sulcus (STS), selectively fire when monkeys observe the gaze direction of other monkeys. These neurons are also active when animals observe goal-directed behaviour. In humans a homologous area of the temporal lobe is activated by observation of seemingly purposeful movements of inanimate objects (as opposed to random movements), even when still photographs depict 'implied' motion (Kourtzi and Kanwisher 2000). Activity in parts of the STS, therefore, is linked to the observation of intentional movements. Although this does not imply conscious awareness, the representation of 'intentions' is certainly a critical aspect of complex social interactions.

Primates possess unique types of neurons that are selectively activated by movements that imply intention. Mirror neurons discharge during both the execution of a certain hand or mouth action and the mere observation of the same behaviour carried out by another individual. These neurons are believed to be involved in imitation and learning, as well as in human language. Spindle-shaped cells in the anterior cingulate cortex and the anterior insula, known as 'von Economo neurons' (VENs), have increased in density and size during human evolution. The density of VENs is inversely correlated with the phylogenetic distance of apes to humans. VENs may play a role in self-awareness (interoception), empathy, and emotion processing, including disgust and more complex emotions such as guilt and shame.

The temporal and the frontal lobes of primates also contain a specific type of cells called 'mirror neurons' due to their unique quality to discharge during both the execution of a certain hand or mouth action and the mere observation of the same behaviour carried out by another individual, even if the terminal part of the movement is hidden from observation (Umiltà et al. 2001; Rizzolatti and Craighero 2004). This suggests that mirror neurons provide a basic mechanism for predicting behaviour and imitating the actions of others (Gallese and Goldman 1998). Mirror neurons have also been found in great density in the ventral premotor cortex (area F5) of monkeys, an area that is probably homologous to Broca's speech area in humans (Rizzolatti et al. 2002). Human language might therefore have evolved from the ability to use gestures for communication (Corballis 2003). Interestingly, the mirror neuron system is elegantly accessible by measuring the suppression of alpha and beta bands of the electroencephalogram, referred to as 'mu rhythm' suppression (due to similarities of the alpha waves with the Greek letter 'mu'; Pineda 2005), which may open new avenues for the study of such basic social cognitive processes in neuropsychiatric conditions, including the role of reward mechanisms (Brown et al. 2013; Brown and Brüne 2014).

Another brain area that has undergone recent evolutionary modification is the anterior cingulate cortex (ACC). The ACC receives input from the motor cortex and the spinal cord, from the ipsilateral PFC, and from the thalamus and brainstem nuclei. It is highly heterogeneous in terms of its cytoarchitecture and functional organization. The ACC is believed to serve as an important mediator of motor control, cognition, and arousal, as well as an inhibitory control device to suppress impulsive reactions in favour of 'rational' decisions (Devinsky et al. 1995; Allman et al. 2001). Bilateral damage to the ACC may produce akinetic mutism and other complex abnormalities including disinhibition of primitive behaviours. The anterior human ACC inconsistently forms a paracingulate sulcus that is present in only 30–50 percent of individuals and is perhaps still under selection pressure (Paus et al. 1996).

Moreover, the ACC contains a spindle-shaped cell type (thus somewhat misleadingly termed 'spindle cells', also known as 'von Economo neurons', VENs) unique to apes and humans. VENs, named after their discoverer, Constantin von Economo (1926), have apparently been selected during the evolution of hominins (there is now growing evidence that VENs also exist in other mammalian species, including whales (Butti and Hof 2010), macaques (Evrard et al. 2012), and other, mostly social species). When comparing the extant great apes and humans, the size and density of VENs has steadily increased in an inverse correlative fashion. That is, their size and density is most advanced in humans, somewhat smaller in chimpanzees and bonobos, and even more reduced in gorillas and orangutans (Nimchinsky et al. 1999). VENs are also densely located in the anterior part of the insular cortex (AI) (Nieuwenhuys 2012), and in more scattered distribution in the dorsolateral PFC (Fajardo et al. 2008). They mature fully after birth and seem to be more abundant in the right hemisphere (Allman et al. 2011).

Although the exact function of VENs is as yet unknown, there is some evidence to suggest that they play an important role in self-awareness (interoception), empathy, and emotion processing, including disgust and more complex emotions such as guilt and shame (Craig 2003; Allman et al. 2011). Both ACC and AI are also sensitive to social exclusion (Eisenberger 2012; Powers and Heatherton 2012). Interestingly, the density of VENs in the ACC has been found to be reduced in several neuropsychiatric conditions (Allman et al. 2010), including schizophrenia (Brüne et al. 2010), frontotemporal dementia (Santillo et al. 2013), and possibly autism (Santos et al. 2011). Conversely, the density is apparently increased in the ACC of psychiatric patients who committed suicide, which may justify speculations about the functional role of VENs in regard to complex emotions (Brüne et al. 2011).

2.10 Neurotransmitter systems in the brain

Neurotransmitters are ancient molecules that have long existed before nervous systems evolved. They may, therefore, be better termed 'biomodulators', as many of these agents evolved to promote bacterial growth, to which plants evolved counter-strategies, utilized by animals through pharmacophagy (Roshchina 2010; St John-Smith et al. 2013; see Chapter 23). Acetylcholine, the biogenic amines (epinephrine, norepinephrine, dopamine, and serotonin), amino acid transmitters (e.g. glycine and adenosine), enzymatically modified amino acids such as glutamate and GABA, and various neuropeptides have already been found in protozoa (Roshchina 2010). Over evolutionary time, many of these molecules were 'co-opted' as neurotransmitters to serve the communication between neurons (Allman 1999).

Neurotransmitters comprise different classes of molecules. Many of these agents evolved to promote bacterial growth, to which plants evolved counter-strategies, utilized by animals through pharmacophagy The activity of acetylcholine, the biogenic amines (epinephrine, norepinephrine, dopamine, and serotonin), amino acid transmitters (e.g. glycine, and adenosine), glutamate, and GABA, and neuropeptides is best known, even though interactions of different neurotransmitters are yet to be scrutinized.

Neurotransmitters are stored in vesicles in the presynaptic endings of neurons from where they are usually released into the synaptic cleft upon arrival of an electric impulse. They bind to postsynaptic and presynaptic receptors and modify the electrical excitability of the receiving neuron. As a rule of thumb, it can be said that axosomatic synapses are largely inhibitory, whereas the majority of axodendritic synapses are excitatory, and axo-axonal synapses are double inhibitory, and thus disinhibitory (Zilles 1987). The action of neurotransmitters is terminated by reuptake mechanisms, enzymatic degradation, or diffusion. Reuptake is the most important mechanism for many neurotransmitters, because their synthesis is metabolically expensive. Thus, it is in the organism's interest not to waste such precious molecules. Some neurotransmitters produce rather short, sharply peaking action potentials at ionotropic receptors, whereas others produce much slower alterations at metabotropic receptors that last much longer (Panksepp 1998).

Synthesis of these molecules in the vertebrate brain mainly takes place in nuclei that are located in phylogenetically old parts of the brain, the 'reptilian brain' (see section 2.3). Ontogenetically, neurotransmitter receptors emerge before birth. Postnatally, they are overexpressed, with a peak at around 2–4 months of age, and receptor density subsequently declines to adult levels at age 3 years, which is similar across all cortical areas. The major (known) neurotransmitters are briefly described in sections 2.10.1 to 2.10.6. It has to be kept in mind, however, that this overview is a simplification of the real picture. There are many more substances that

Neurotransmitters are stored in vesicles and released into the synaptic cleft by electric stimulation of the neuron. Reuptake of neurotransmitters is the most important mechanism for terminating neurotransmitter activity.

may act as neurotransmitters, many of which are probably yet to be discovered. The same applies to the number of different receptor types to which neurotransmitters are able to bind. Moreover, neurotransmitters interact in many ways, and individual neurons usually express receptor binding sites in close proximity on the same dendrite (Panksepp 1998).

2.10.1 **Acetylcholine**

The largest nuclei that produce acetylcholine are found in the basal forebrain controlling hippocampal and cortical functions, and in the midbrain controlling thalamic and hypothalamic functions. During ontogeny, cholinergic projections from the basal forebrain reach the cortex in the early prenatal period. Acetylcholine is synthesized from the nutrient choline and acetyl coenzyme A in the presence of choline acetyltransferase, and degraded enzymatically by acetylcholine esterase. Acetylcholine binds to two types of receptors, called nicotinic and muscarinic, the functions of which are influenced by cholesterol. Cholesterol contributes to the stabilization of the cell membrane, and nicotinic receptors are found in skeletal muscle cells, whereas muscarinic receptors modify visceral parasympathic activity (Panksepp 1998).

Acetylcholine is synthesized from the nutrient choline and acetyl coenzyme A in the basal forebrain. Degeneration of the nucleus basalis of Meynert causes Alzheimer's disease.

Clinically, the acetylcholinergic system is relevant in the context of cognitive dysfunction. For example, the nucleus basalis of Meynert degenerates early in the course of Alzheimer's disease, leading to hippocampal dysfunction (memory loss) and other cognitive impairments, including attention and arousal.

2.10.2 **Catecholamines**

The catecholamines are synthesized from the amino acid tyrosine by hydroxylation, leading to L-DOPA, which can cross the blood–brain barrier. In the brain L-DOPA is transformed into dopamine by decarboxylation and can further be processed into norepinephrine by hydroxylation. Epinephrine results from methylation of norepinephrine, but this metabolic step is more important in the periphery than in the brain. Ontogenetically, monoamine neuron groups in the brainstem are generated in the first trimester of embryogenesis.

Catecholamines have rather widespread functions in the human brain. They bind to several receptors that are differentially distributed across the brain. Norepinephrine binds to alpha 1 and 2 receptors, as well as to beta 1 to 3 receptors. Dopamine binds to five different dopamine receptor types that convey different functions. The action of the catecholamines is mainly terminated by reuptake into the presynaptic ending, and they are degraded by an enzyme called COMT, as well as by an enzyme called monoamino-oxidase (MAO-A and MAO-B), both of which are encoded by polymorphic genes. Either allelic variant conveys advantages and disadvantages such that they are balanced in

Catecholamines (dopamine, norepinephrine, and epinephrine) are synthesized from the amino acid tyrosine. They are degraded by two enzymes called COMT and MAO. The catecholamines are involved in regulating cognitive and motor processes. Depletion of dopamine causes Parkinson's disease. Mesolimbic overactivity of dopamine is presumably involved in positive symptoms associated with schizophrenia. Norepinephrine deficiency is involved in ADHD.

prevalence (see also Chapter 1). In essence, the allelic variations determine the speed at which the catecholamines are degraded.

Norepinephrine synthesizing cells are abundant in the locus coeruleus, from which pathways connect with the neocortex, hypothalamus, cerebellum, brainstem, and spinal cord. Norepinephrine is a crucial regulator of sensory arousal and attention. It increases the signal-to-noise ratio such that sensory input is filtered according to its biological relevance to the organism. In human psychiatric disorders, deficiency of norepinephrine is, for example, suggested to be involved in ADHD, somatization, lowered pain threshold, and impulsivity.

Dopaminergic neurons are concentrated in the pars compacta of the substantia nigra from which projections are sent to the caudate nuclei. Dopamine deficiency in this circuit causes Parkinson's disease. Dopaminergic neurons are also abundant in the ventral tegmental area connecting to the nucleus accumbens in the ventral striatum and the cortex via mesolimbic and mesocortical pathways. The former circuit is crucial for motivated behaviour. Dopamine turnover increases in the ventral striatum when a reward is expected, whereas it decreases upon receiving the reward. Projections to the cortex are involved in motor arousal. A reduced dopaminergic activity in the frontal cortex may produce avolition and apathy. Excessive dopamine in the frontal cortex, by contrast, may lead to stereotyped behaviours that are carried out repetitively and purposeless, which may be part of drug-induced states (Panksepp 1998). Mesolimbic overactivity of dopamine is thought to be involved in the causation of positive symptoms associated with schizophrenia, whereas a prefrontal deficit in dopamine causes negative symptoms.

2.10.3 **Serotonin**

In contrast to the catecholamines, serotonin is synthesized from the amino acid tryptophane via 5-hydroxytryptophane, which can cross the blood—brain barrier and is transformed into serotonin by decarboxylation. Serotonin is produced in the raphe nuclei of the brainstem, which have maintained the same location in the vertebrate brain perhaps for 500 my. In primates, serotonergic neurons emerge in clusters, and ascending, often myelinated axons project to the lower brainstem and spinal cord, and to the striatum, the hypothalamus, the amygdala, the hippocampus, and the cortex. Serotonin is abundant in plants, but as the ability to synthesize tryptophane was lost in animal evolution, organisms had to develop (through natural selection) other means to secure this amino acid (Azmitia 2010). Serotonin is synthesized in two enzymatic steps (another important derivative of tryptophane is melatonin, which in plants acts as an antioxidant; Azmitia 2010).

Serotonin is synthesized from the amino acid tryptophane. It modulates the response of neurons to other neurotransmitters rather than exerting an excitatory function itself. Serotonin controls many functions including feeding and digestion, sexual behaviour, aggression, and explorative behaviour. Serotonin deficiency is associated with pathological anxiety, OCD, depression, and eating disorders.

Serotonin controls many body functions including feeding and digestion, sexual behaviour, aggression, and explorative behaviour. Serotonin modulates the response of neurons to other neurotransmitters rather than exerting an excitatory function itself, except in pyramidal neurons in the cerebral cortex. Generally, serotonin has dampening effects on neuronal activity. At least 16 types of serotonin receptors have evolved, by a series of gene duplications. The different serotonin receptors are distributed across different brain regions in different densities. The reuptake of serotonin from the synaptic cleft into the terminal axon is under control of a serotonin transporter gene. The transporter gene is influenced by a DNA promoter sequence, which apparently evolved in primates some 40 mya. Variations of this promoter gene in humans are associated with differences in personality traits such as anxiousness, impulsivity, hostility, and depression-proneness. Serotonin deficiency is found in a broad spectrum of emotional disorders including pathological anxiety, OCD, depression, and eating disorders.

Interestingly, serotonergic activity in primate brains is associated with social status as well as with explorative and aggressive behaviour (Suomi 2003). Experimental evidence suggests that individuals with low social status have lower serotonin concentrations, as measured using its main metabolite, 5-hydroxyindole-acetic acetate (5-HIAA). Moreover, individuals with low serotonin turnover show a greater sensitivity towards reward and risk-taking, and it is well established that humans with low levels of serotonin are also more likely to behave aggressively towards self and others. On the other hand, aggression, impulsivity, and antisocial behaviour have been linked to low-activity variants of both MAO-A and COMT, which also contribute to the enzymatic degradation of serotonin. Thus, high levels of dopamine, norepinephrine, and serotonin put individuals at risk of behaving aggressively, particularly if the genetic disposition is associated with adverse experiences during early childhood, such as abuse or neglect (see Chapter 19). Of note, the indole structure of tryptophane has light-absorbing properties. It is therefore straightforward to speculate about the interaction between serotonergic (and melatonergic) action and exposure to sunlight with regard to mood regulation and sleep (Azmitia 2010).

2.10.4 Glutamate and GABA

Glutamate is synthesized from the amino acid glutamine. Glutamate is the major excitatory transmitter and globally distributed across the brain. It binds to three major receptors, N-methyl-D-aspartic acid (NMDA), kainate, and alpha-amino-3-hydroxy-5-methyl-isoxazole-4-proprionic acid (AMPA). Glutamate is involved in the control of thalamic input to the cortex and probably contributes to learning processes and consciousness. It has been experimentally shown that the administration of glutamate antagonists such as ketamine may produce psychotic symptoms, and that agonists at the NMDA receptor such as glycine may reduce psychotic symptoms (Panksepp 1998).

Glutamate is synthesized from glutamine. Glutamate is involved in the control of thalamic input to the cortex and contributes to learning processes and consciousness. Administration of glutamate antagonists such as ketamine may produce psychotic symptoms, whereas agonists at the NMDA receptor such as glycine may reduce psychotic symptoms.

GABA is the most abundant inhibitory neurotransmitter in the brain. It is synthesized from glutamate in a single step through decarboxylation. GABA binds to

$GABA_{A-C}$ receptors that are preferentially localized at the soma and proximate axon of GABAergic interneurons, which makes inhibitory control most efficient. In the human brain, GABA receptors are particularly abundant in the primary sensory cortex, Heschl's gyrus (temporal cortex), and the ACC, and it can be said that the human brain contains an exceptionally large number of GABAergic neurons. Both glutamatergic projection neurons and GABAergic interneurons are largely generated before birth. GABAergic substances effectively control cortical and subcortical excitation. Thus, benzodiazepines, which bind to $GABA_A$ receptors are able to reduce anxiety and aggression and are indispensable for treating potentially life-threatening catatonic syndromes and epileptic seizures (Panksepp 1998).

GABA is the most abundant inhibitory neurotransmitter in the brain. It is synthesized from glutamate in a single step through decarboxylation. GABA is the most abundant inhibitory neurotransmitter in the brain. GABAergic substances such as benzodiazepine receptors reduce anxiety and aggression.

2.10.5 **Neuropeptides**

Another group of neurotransmitters comprise the neuropeptides which are synthesized in the hypothalamus and the pituitary gland and other areas of the brain. Neuropeptides are even more expensive in energetic terms than the classical neurotransmitters. The synthesis of neuropeptides is regulated by many different genes. Neuropeptides act as modulators of neurotransmitter activities rather than exerting direct excitatory or inhibitory effects. Beta-endorphin, for example, has a calming effect and induces a feeling of pleasure. It binds to opioid receptors in the brain and reduces separation distress in young animals. It is therefore conceivable that the artificial stimulation of endogenous opioid receptors by illicit drugs help overcome negative feelings resembling separation distress (Panksepp 1998).

Neuropeptides are modulators of neurotransmitter activities rather than exerting direct excitatory or inhibitory effects. Beta-endorphin has calming effects. Oxytocin and vasopressin modulate female and male sexuality. Oxytocin is also crucial for parental bonding and impacts on social cognition.

Similarly, oxytocin, which is produced under the control of oestrogen in the nucleus paraventricularis and nucleus supraopticus and stored in the pituitary gland, has profound effects on social behaviour. It reduces aggressive tendencies, and it promotes both parental bonding and partner bonding (Donaldson and Young 2008). Moreover, oxytocin improves 'mindreading', empathy, and trust, although such 'prosocial' effects very likely depend on the quality of early attachment experiences (Domes et al. 2007; Bartz et al. 2011; Ebert et al. 2013). Oxytocin is released during orgasm in large quantities and has also been found to facilitate (at physiological doses) social memories and empathy. Oxytocin is more abundant in female brains, and is also released upon infant suckling, a process that strengthens the mother–child dyad (Feldman 2012). Oxytocin receptors are highly expressed in the nucleus basalis (Meynert), in the pons, amygdala, and nucleus accumbens (Hammock and Young 2006; Ross et al. 2009), and it interacts with dopamine, serotonin, and the opioidergic system in manifold ways (Walker and Glone 2013), whereby the interaction of oxytocin and serotonin seems to be crucial for the experience of social reward (Dölen et al. 2013).

Vasopressin, which differs from oxytocin in only one (out of nine) amino acid, is more prevalent in the male brain and its synthesis is facilitated by testosterone. Vasopressin promotes male sexuality and aggression. In contrast to oxytocin, vasopressin peaks during sexual arousal (Panksepp 1998). The role of these peptides in psychopathology is only emerging, but it is most likely that disruptions of early infant attachment have profound effects on the expression of these social affiliation-promoting neuropeptides (Meyer-Lindenberg et al. 2011; Hammock 2015).

Another class of neuropeptides called neurotrophins controls the proliferation, migration, and replacement of damaged neurons by regulating neural stem cell proliferation. Neurotrophins bind to tyrosine kinase receptors. The first neurotrophin that was discovered is called nerve growth factor (NGF). NGF is involved in differentiation and protection of nerve cells. Similarly, the brain-derived neurotrophic factor (BDNF) is a peptide that is active in the hippocampus, basal forebrain, and cortex. It exerts protective effects and is perhaps the most important neurotrophin for neurogenesis from neural stem cells. It is therefore crucially involved in cell migration during ontogeny. Of note, stress has been shown to reduce BDNF levels in the brain, such that BDNF deficiency has been suggested to play a role in several psychiatric disorders, including depression, OCD, autism, and Alzheimer's disease. Neuregulins are proteins that contribute to the development of Schwann cells involved in myelination of neurons, and to the survival of oligodendrozytes (Panksepp 1998). Neuregulin 1 is perhaps involved in the pathogenesis of schizophrenia by downregulating glutamatergic NMDA receptor activity in the PFC (Sei et al. 2007).

Neurotrophins are peptides involved in the differentiation and protection of nerve cells. The role of neurotrophins in the pathogenesis of affective disorders, schizophrenia, autism, and Alzheimer's disease has only begun to be uncovered.

2.10.6 **Endocannabinoids**

It has long been known that ingestion or inhalation of the plant cannabis sativa exerts psychotropic effects. As late as the 1990s, researchers discovered G-protein-coupled cannabinoid receptors, CB1 and CB2. The CB1 receptor is stimulated by endogenously produced anandamide and 2-arachidonoylglycerol (2-AG), which acts as a retrograde messenger and downregulates the activity of other neurotransmitters. Endocannabinoid receptors are widely distributed in the nervous system of vertebrates. CB1 receptors are mainly located on GABAergic neurons in the basal ganglia, hippocampus, neocortex, spinal cord, and in the periphery (including the heart), which may account for the dampening effect of cannabinoids on movement (catalepsy), memory (impairment), nociception (analgesia), and the cardiovascular system (bradycardia and hypotension via blockade of noradrenaline release; Elphick and Egertová

Endocannabinoid receptors are widely distributed in the nervous system of vertebrates. CB1 receptors are mainly located on GABAergic neurons in the basal ganglia, hippocampus, neocortex, spinal cord, and in the periphery (including the heart), which may account for the dampening effect of cannabinoids on movement (catalepsy), memory (impairment), nociception (analgesia), and the cardiovascular system.

2001). A smaller proportion of CB1 receptors is also located on glutamatergic terminals. Activation of these receptors seems to be associated with neuroprotective effects (Chiarlone et al. 2014). Animal studies suggest that experimental upregulation of CB1 receptors in the medial PFC of the rat induces marked changes in social behaviour, and impairs cognitive flexibility (Klugmann et al. 2011). In addition, anandamide has been shown to be involved in the reward processing of social play in rats (Trezza et al. 2012), which is consistent with findings from imaging studies in humans showing that genetic variation of the CB1 receptor modulates physiological responses to happy faces (Chakrabarti and Baron-Cohen 2011).

From a clinical perspective, it is important that delta-9-tetrahydrocannabinol (THC) is the main psychoactive component of *Cannabis sativa*, which binds to CB1 receptors. The widespread abuse of THC may be linked to its calming effect, and perhaps its influence on the polyvagal system, although it has been suggested that chronic THC abuse can increase the risk for psychosis.

This brief overview of the major neurotransmitter systems may illustrate how economical Nature has designed novel substances by often adding simple chemical steps. For example, the catecholamines can be understood as successive evolutionary refinement of neurotransmission, and the same is true for glutamate and GABA, which can fine-tune the balance between excitatory and inhibitory control of neuronal activity. Similarly, vasopressin and oxytocin are so similar in amino acid structure that it seems parsimonious to conclude that these substances emerged from a single mutation in the coding gene.

In general, the action of neurotransmitters is not only limited be their availability. Several complex mechanisms control the susceptibility and number of pre- and postsynaptic receptors, known as up- and downregulation. Thus, receptors can be hyper- or hyposensitive to transmitter exposure, and this can have profound effects on the progression of disease processes and response to pharmacological treatment. For example, chronic administration of antipsychotic substances may induce an upregulation of dopamine-sensitive receptors, and this may be mediated by modulation of gene expression in the brain. Why is this so important?

2.11 Gene expression in the human brain

Roughly half of all coding genes (55 percent) of the human genome are expressed in the brain. This is remarkable, because it renders the brain the prime target for mutations and evolutionary changes (Caceres et al. 2003; Myers et al. 2007). In fact, a comparison of the genome of our closest relative, the chimpanzee, with the human genome has revealed that both species share about 98 percent of DNA sequence. Thus, the human genome differs from the chimpanzee DNA by only about 35 million bases. About 5 million bases are inserted or deleted in humans or chimpanzees, and an additional 3 million differences may lie in protein-coding genes or

More than half of all coding genes are expressed in the human brain. This renders the brain a prime target for evolutionary changes. In humans, gene expression is greatly accelerated compared to other primates.

other functional areas of the genome (Khaitovich et al. 2005). At the protein level, however, only 29 percent of amino sequences in chimps and humans are identical. For example, the amino acid sequence for haemoglobin is virtually the same in both. Genetic differences between humans and chimpanzees are therefore about ten times smaller than between mice and rats. So why are humans and chimpanzees so different in terms of cognitive functioning and behaviour?

Recent research into the evolution of the human and the chimpanzee's genomes has shown that the gene expression pattern in the brain differs less between the two species compared to other tissues such as liver, kidney, heart, or testes. However, when comparing upregulation and downregulation of genes in both species it would seem that more rapid changes occurred on the lineage leading to humans than on the chimpanzee lineage since the two split from a common ancestor, whereby these rapidly evolving regions do not pertain to coding regions directly, but parts of the genome concerned with gene regulation (Pollard et al. 2006). This acceleration of gene expression was found to be largest in brain tissue, and this evolutionary trend could also be demonstrated for human-specific amino acid changes compared to chimpanzee-specific changes. It is plausible to assume that these changes occurred due to positive selection of functions associated with changes in gene expression in the human brain (Khaitovich et al. 2005; Somel et al. 2013). Two recent discoveries of genes associated with brain size and language may illustrate that this story could indeed be true.

The abnormal spindle-like microcephaly associated gene (ASPM) is probably involved in the regulation of neural stem cell proliferation. The strange name of this gene comes from a mutation found in humans that is associated with microcephaly. The gene is, however, of ancient origin, but has undergone several changes during human evolution that were probably positively selected. One such change occurred quite recently about 5,800 years ago, perhaps in populations in the Middle East. Regardless of whether or not the coincidence with the domestication of animals (except wolves, which happened much earlier) or with the emergence of written language occurred just by chance, this example shows that anatomically modern humans have substantially changed in their genetic makeup, and probably still undergo further selection (Mekel-Brobov et al. 2005), although the targets of selection may be different from ancestral ones (Stearns et al. 2010a).

The ASPM gene is an ancient gene that underwent recent positive selection in humans. The most recent change occurred in coincidence with the domestication of animals and with written language.

The second example deals with the genetic foundation of human language. Language is perhaps the faculty that sets humans apart from other animals in that human language has complex syntactical, semantic, and pragmatic qualities. The forkhead box P2 (FOXP2) is an ancient gene that regulates the activity of other genes. It has changed very little during mammalian evolution. In fact, in roughly 130 million years separating the mouse from the common human–chimpanzee ancestor's lineage, only a single amino acid change took place. Since then, however, two additional changes have occurred in the human lineage, whereas none took place in

In the FOXP2 gene three amino acid changes occurred in the last 130 my, two of which emerged after humans split from the last common ancestor of chimps and humans. The FOXP2 gene has been functionally associated with the evolution of human language.

the chimpanzee lineage, and it has been estimated that the change in the human lineage became genetically fixed some 200,000 years ago (Enard et al. 2002). A rare mutation in the FOXP2 gene on chromosome 7 that is autosomal dominantly transmitted in a three-generation pedigree causing problems with articulated speech ('verbal dyspraxia') suggests that the gene could have been involved in the evolution of language. Recently, a SNP of the FOXP2 gene has been associated with auditory hallucinations and incoherent speech in schizophrenia, but this finding needs replication in independent samples (Sanjuan et al. 2006).

In any event, the human genome has undergone genetic modifications, and mutations at single loci (SNP) occur frequently. Perhaps only a minority of allelic variations exert positive effects. The majority are probably selectively neutral or convey disadvantages in concert with additive or epistatic effects. According to conservative estimates, each individual human genome contains 500–2,000 potentially harmful SNPs in coding regions, and perhaps twice that number in non-coding regions of the DNA, 50 percent of which may affect brain functioning. Most likely, this astonishingly large number of alterations of the human genome is one of the main research obstacles for detecting allelic variations with large effect sizes in human psychiatric disorders (Keller and Miller 2006).

Afterthought: the 'social brain' hypothesis—an integrative perspective

The fact that the human brain comprises about 2 percent of adult body weight but consumes between 15 and 20 percent of total energy requires an evolutionary explanation, because such 'expensive tissue' would not have been selected had its benefits not outweighed its costs (Aiello and Wheeler 1995). A compelling hypothesis first put forth in the 1960s suggests that it was foremost the social environment that led to an increase in brain size during primate evolution, eventually culminating in the evolution of human psychological mechanisms that are specialized on the processing of social information (Jolly 1966; Humphrey 1976). The 'social brain' hypothesis (Brothers 1990b; Dunbar 2003a, 2003b) is probably complementary rather than incompatible with the assumption that the evolution of technical intelligence and cultural transmission of knowledge has also been a driving force in human brain evolution (Tomasello and Call 1997). The idea of a 'social brain', however, nicely integrates an evolutionary scenario of human brain development, comparative research into non-human primates, and recent findings from neuroscience, including functional brain imaging and genetics of social behaviour (Ebstein et al. 2010).

Evolutionary psychology suggests that the human brain's enormous capacity to store information, to flexibly interact with the environment, and to quickly affiliate with others is rooted in the fact that selection favoured the formation of larger social groups in which social interactions became increasingly complex (Chance 1988). The increase in size of ancestral hominin groups was adaptive, probably because—as the climate in East Africa became cooler—trees were more sparsely dispersed in the open savannah such that larger social groups yielded better protection from large predators (Jones et al. 1992; Cerling et al. 2011). On the other hand, this situation posed greater pressure on the individual to successfully compete for food and sexual partners. The dilemma between the need for growing gregariousness and social competition may have led to a runaway selection of higher cognitive functions, increasing social competence, and emotional systems of attachment and bonding, all of which ultimately increased the chance of survival and reproduction of those who had such capacities over others who were less well endowed with these abilities. Accordingly, selection pressures may have increased the demands of greater computational resources and thus bigger brains.

Two independent predictors strongly support the social brain hypotheses. In primates, average group size correlates with the ratio of the neocortex volume (excluding the visual cortex) to the rest of the brain (Dunbar 1995). In other words, the larger the neocortex ratio, the larger the average group size in different primate species. Similarly, the maximum lifespan of different primate species is highly correlated with the relative size of the neocortex, but not with group size, suggesting that group size and longevity are independent factors predicting the relative size of the neocortex in primates (Allman 1999). In addition, neocortex size seems to correlate with the length of childhood and adolescence (Joffe 1997).

Interestingly, the neocortex ratio does not predict group size in apes, because apes usually live in much smaller groups than do many other primate species, but have larger brains relative to body size. However, when looking at strategic social interactions, including what has been called 'tactical deception', that is, the ability to intentionally manipulate the behaviour of other individuals to one's own advantage, relative neocortex size correlates with the number of deceptive acts in apes (Byrne and Whiten 1992). As predicted from these approaches, humans are expected to live in groups of 150 people on average, a number that has been found to strikingly match contemporary hunter-gatherer groups (Dunbar 1998).

A recent reformulation of the 'social brain' hypothesis posits that the driving force behind increased brain size might be social complexity, rather than group size alone, whereby social complexity is reflected in the ability to form coalitions and maintain cooperative relationships (Dunbar and Shultz 2007a, 2007b). In fact, human societies, compared with chimpanzees, for example, are characterized by much more cooperative behaviour (Tomasello and Vaish 2013), which is essentially linked to a sophisticated emotional repertoire, including trust, sympathy, liking, love, but also shame, guilt, envy, and schadenfreude (Trivers 1971; Dvash et al. 2010; Damasio and Carvalho 2013). In fact, fairness behaviour is associated with the activation of the reward system, which may serve as a proxy to maintain altruistic behaviour in social groups (Tabibnia et al. 2008). However, in order to maintain cooperation, individuals must be able to detect non-cooperative behavioural strategies of others. Due to the need for group cohesion and cooperation between genetically unrelated or distantly related individuals, it probably paid off not only to cooperate to a high degree, but also to develop rules of collective punishment of individuals who disobeyed the rules of cooperation (Trivers 1971). Collective punishment and the evolution of morality must have been important landmarks of human cognitive and emotional evolution, because, most remarkably, people tend to punish others for their misdemeanour even if the punishment incurs costs to the punisher (Camerer 2003a, 2003b). On the other hand, selection has also operated on mechanisms involved in reparative altruism, for example, forgiveness, because restoration of mutual cooperation in social groups can be advantageous, depending on the estimated risk of further exploitation by a defector (McCullough et al. 2013). Accordingly, many rules of moral punishment do not follow any mathematical logic; on the contrary, they often appear highly irrational at first sight, which underscores their value for early and contemporary human societies—otherwise such rules would not have evolved.

The brain comprises, therefore, neural representations of cognitive and emotional capacities that make humans experts in reflecting own and others' mental states and feelings, which, together contribute to the ability to maintain complex social relationships. There are two domains that can theoretically be separated from one another, although they broadly overlap, behaviourally and neurally: empathy and 'theory of mind' or 'mentalizing'. Empathy concerns the ability to intuitively feel what others are feeling and to understand cause and effect. Phylo- and ontogenetically, empathy is predated by emotional contagion, where the understanding of a causal relationship between the contextual factors that elicited a specific emotion is not required (Gonzalez-Liencres et al. 2013). Empathy-related processes probably evolved early during mammalian evolution as a consequence of intensive maternal care and nurturance (Preston 2013). Empathy is therefore not specific to primates, let alone humans. Generally, empathy can be elicited by every emotion, which includes not only the 'classic' basic emotions such as happiness, sadness, fear, surprise, anger, and disgust (as well as contempt), but also complex emotions such as shame, guilt, envy, and schadenfreude. As a prerequisite, it is essential to be able to decipher observable social signals such as facial expressions of emotions, body posture, and gestures. Emotion processing networks develop slowly during human infancy, childhood, and adolescence, whereby amygdala and orbitofrontal function seems to emerge at around 5–7 months of age (Leppänen and Nelson 2009).

A large body of research has examined empathic concern elicited by the observation of others who are exposed to physical or emotional pain. This research has shown that the neural representations of physical and emotional pain broadly overlap (Eisenberger 2012), and similar brain activation can be measured when one is observing another person in a painful situation (Singer et al. 2004). Key structures involved in empathy for pain include the ACC, the anterior insula, and the somatosensory cortex. Empathic responses to another person's sickness behaviour and suffering vary widely in intensity, however, and such responses are also greatly influenced by the way the sufferer actually expresses his or her way of coping with illness (Preston et al. 2013).

The other domain, 'theory of mind', concerns the ability to reflect upon one's own and other persons' mental states in terms of beliefs, knowledge, intentions, feelings, and so forth (Premack and Woodruff 1978; the terms 'mentalizing', 'mental state attribution', and 'reflexive functioning' are used more or less interchangeably). Theory of mind seems to be quite human-specific (as compared to empathy). Comparative research suggests that this is achieved in similar ways in every known culture (Avis and Harris 1991), though culture modulates the speed and timing of social competence development (Greenfield et al. 2003). Neurally, theory of mind is associated with activation of the medial PFC, the precuneus, and regions containing mirror neurons (Frith and Frith 2001).

The cognitive development of a 'theory of mind' is inseparably linked with the close affectional bond between mother and child (von Klitzing et al. 1999; Hughes and Ensor 2006; for details see Chapter 3), but also the child's closeness with siblings and peers. There seem to be slightly different neural signatures for the representation of emotional ('affective' theory of mind) as opposed to the representation of thoughts and intentions ('cognitive' theory of mind). Notably, affective and cognitive theory of mind can functionally dissociate in a variety of psychiatric conditions such as schizophrenia and borderline personality disorder (Harari et al. 2010).

In a very general sense, the developmental trajectories of 'theory of mind' follow quite distinct steps. As early as around the age of 6 months, human infants are able to distinguish between the motion of inanimate and animate objects. At about 12 months the infant develops the ability of what has been called joint attention. Joint attention refers to the cognitive capacity to form a triadic representation involving the infant's own perception, the perception of an agent, often its mother, and an object. At the age of about 14–18 months the human infant is able to turn its head into the direction the gaze of an agent suggests an object to be, and the infant begins to understand the mental states of desire and intention, and the causal relation between a person's emotions and goals. Between 18 and 24 months of age toddlers discover the difference between the representation of a real event and the representation of a hypothetical state (such as a thought) and start to engage in 'pretend play' (Leslie 1987). At about the same time infants learn to recognize themselves in a mirror (a cognitive capacity that some human-raised apes, foremost chimpanzees, are also able to achieve). Not until the age of 3–4 years, however, is a child able to distinguish between his or her own and others' beliefs and knowledge about the world, including the differentiation between one's own true and others' false beliefs (Perner and Wimmer 1985; Baron-Cohen 1997). Five to six year olds understand that someone can hold beliefs about another person's beliefs. However, children do not understand metaphor or irony before the age of 6–7, and they cannot reliably distinguish jokes from lies at the same age. Even more complex is the comprehension of a 'faux pas' situation. A faux pas happens when a person says something she should not have said, not grasping her mistake. Understanding faux pas requires a developmentally advanced theory of mind ability because it requires simultaneous representation of two mental states: the perspective of the person who commits the faux pas, and the representation of the second person involved who may feel hurt or irritated. 'Faux pas' may not be reliably understood before the age of 9–11 years (Baron-Cohen et al. 1999).

'Theory of mind' development is accelerated if parents frequently use expressions referring to mental states when talking to their infants, compared with children whose parents use such terms less often. In addition, the presence of older siblings speeds up young children's appreciation of other minds. Research has also shown that theory of mind abilities predict social competence in preadolescence and in school-age children at large (Bosacki and Astington 1999; Liddle and Nettle 2006). Taken together, it is therefore parsimonious to suggest an adaptive role for the general extension of all stages of human development. The extraordinary complexity of human social interaction requires an extended juvenile period to attain all the social rules and norms necessary to stand one's ground in social competition later in life. In support of the assumption that social learning plays an outstanding role in primates including humans, it has been shown that the length of the juvenile period correlates with both the size of the non-visual cortex and average group size. In turn, the extended care for immature offspring has selected for longevity, a life-history pattern that has been driven to an extreme in humans with a *post*reproductive lifespan of several decades (see Chapter 3).

The representation of own and others' minds is a prerequisite for mutual cooperation, but also for cheating and the detection of deceptive intentions (Trivers 1971). Moreover, the ability to deceive others may even require the capacity for deceiving the self. Self-deception may increase individual fitness, because it may improve one's success in deceiving others; in other words, an individual that is unaware of his or her (perhaps morally unacceptable) wishes may appear more sincere and trustworthy to others (Trivers 2000; von Hippel and Trivers 2011). There is probably a delicate balance between trust and mistrust (see Chapter 1, section 1.2.2.1 on 'reciprocal altruism'). However, transitory errors in 'mind reading' are probably part of the evolutionary costs of the 'mind reading' system, whereby persistent or incorrigible erroneous beliefs about the intentions of others may emerge into habitual suspiciousness or paranoia (Green and Phillips 2004). Likewise, whereas self-deception including concealing selfish wishes before the self (through a mechanism commonly termed 'repression') may to some extent be adaptive, complete inaccessibility of one's own wishes and intentions may turn problematic in terms of maintaining complex social relationships. Furthermore, (unconscious) intrapsychic conflict may arise from selfish desires that may increase short-term individual fitness and moral demands, which benefit the social group and perhaps only secondarily the self, problems that have long been recognized in analytic psychotherapy (Nesse and Lloyd 1992; see also Chapter 22).

There is now increasing evidence suggesting that early experiences with caregivers and significant others impact on the developmental structuring of the mind-reading system and the mechanisms negotiating selfish and altruistic behaviour. Moreover, social decision-making, including the ability to maintain reciprocal and trustful relationships, is mediated, in part, by 'bonding hormones' such as oxytocin and genetics. These ideas are further developed in Chapter 3.

Chapter 3

Human life history

Abstract

Human life-history patterns are characterized by slow maturation, long parental dependency, longevity, and low number of offspring. These developmental peculiarities determine the amount of parental investment in offspring and mating effort, and assign an adaptive role to postmenopausal women. Hence evolution has produced specific adaptations pertaining to the relationship of human infants with their primary caregivers, subsumed under the term 'attachment'. The way attachment patterns or 'styles' develop during early infancy coin the child's view of the world in terms of the emotional availability and trustworthiness of others. Harsh environmental conditions during infancy promote insecure attachment styles and a 'faster' life-history strategy, including earlier sexual maturation and sexual activity and less parental investment in own offspring. The opposite is more likely to emerge when children grow up in secure conditions with responsive and emotionally available caregivers. These developmental trajectories have profound implications for social interaction and stress-regulation abilities.

Keywords

attachment, life-history strategies, mating effort, parental investment, stress regulation, sexual maturation

3.1 Introductory remarks to human life history

Life-history theory deals with species-typical solutions for problems associated with survival and reproduction that change over an individual's lifespan. Accordingly, life-history strategies involve a trade-off between the allocation of energy to body growth or reproduction. Life-history strategies, therefore, determine important biological developments, including the timing of sexual maturation, number of offspring, mating effort, parental investment, and length of lifespan (Stearns 1992; Roff 2007).

Life-history theory deals with species-typical solutions for problems associated with survival and reproduction that change over an individual's lifespan. Accordingly, life-history strategies involve a trade-off between the allocation of energy to body growth or reproduction. Life-history strategies, therefore, determine important biological developments, including the timing of sexual maturation, number of offspring, mating effort, parental investment, and length of lifespan.

The concept was originally applied to between-species comparison with regard to life-history traits, based on observations of considerable variation between species in the organization and timing of characteristic life courses. K-selection and r-selection are strategies reflecting diametrically opposite solutions to survival and reproductive problems. K-selected species develop slowly, they reproduce repetitively (iteroparity), the number of offspring per litter is small with long-lasting intensive parental investment including a long gestation period, and death rates in infancy and childhood are low. The onset of reproductive activity is delayed, and K-selected species enjoy long lives. Typically, K-selected species grow large bodies, and competition between adults of K-selected species is high, because—due to prolonged lifespans—competition determines survival and reproductive success. K-selected species usually live in conditions with little random environmental variation. Conversely, r-selection involves the opposite pattern; r-selected species develop fast, they often reproduce only once in their life-time (semelparity), the number of offspring is large (to vast), but only a small fraction lives to reach adult stages. Parental investment after birth (or hatching) is low or absent in r-selected species, sexual maturity sets in early, and individuals die at an early age. R-selected species usually grow small bodies, and random environmental variation is high in r-selected species (MacArthur and Wilson 1967). Offspring of K-selected species is relatively mature at birth (precocial), whereas in r-selected species offspring is often much more immature (altricial).

Secure attachment develops if the attachment-figure is able to positively respond to the infant's signals such that the infant perceives the mother as available and responsive when needed.

Among mammals, many rodent species typically follow an r-selected life-history pattern, whereas primates are highly K-selected species. Apes and humans in particular stand out for their extreme K-selected life histories, and this developmental pattern has profound impact on the species' psychological make-up, with changing demands over an individual's lifespan. Interestingly, the extreme K-selection of humans is probably intimately tied to the heterochronic processes of paedomorphosis and subsequent hypermorphosis. Hypermorphosis is perhaps the most important mechanism through which *Homo sapiens* has attained K-selected traits, including the large human brain (McKinney and McNamara 1991).

The most outstanding feature of human life history is that the typical primate pattern is extended in all stages of development. However, as we will see later in this chapter, there is within-species variation in life-history patterns, such that some human life histories appear to be slightly more pushed to an r-selection-like pattern, others more to an extreme K-selected pattern (although the terms r- and K-selection are usually not used for within-species variation). To put it another way, there is variation among humans with regard to the timing of biological maturation, age at onset of sexual activity and reproduction, choice of partners, number of offspring, and amount of care provided for offspring, which can be subsumed under the terms 'faster' as opposed to 'slower' life-history strategies (Ellis et al. 2011b). Differences in life-history strategies are partly under genetic control;

There is variation among humans with regard to the timing of biological maturation, age at onset of sexual activity and reproduction, choice of partners, number of offspring, and amount of care provided for offspring, which can be subsumed under the terms 'faster' as opposed to 'slower' life-history strategies.

however, the more critical factor in determining an individual's life-history strategy seems to be the quality of the early family environment (Belsky et al. 1991; Ellis et al. 2011a, 2011b). This renders life-history theory one of the most important concepts for the understanding of psychiatric conditions (Del Giudice 2014; Ellis and Del Giudice 2014).

3.2 **Infancy and childhood**

Biologically speaking, the most crucial task for all newborn offspring is to manage to survive infancy and childhood in order to reach sexual maturity. Human babies are no exception in this respect. However, they face the problem of being extremely immature at birth. Compared with other apes, for example, human newborns are physiologically preterm by about 13 months (Jones et al. 1992). In other words, if human babies were at birth as mature as chimpanzee babies the human gestation period would last approximately 22 months. Human preterm parturition represents an evolved design compromise, which is ultimately linked to the evolution of bipedalism. Upright walking was accompanied by a change in the human pelvis anatomy, which consequently led to a narrowing of the birth canal. This was not a problem as long as ancestral hominoid species had relatively small chimpanzee-like brains of about 350 cm^3 in size and, hence, small skulls. However, as the brain (and body) started to grow larger over evolutionary time, the problem of a narrow birth canal became more vital (Bradshaw 1997).

Human babies are preterm at birth by about 13 months compared to other apes. Immaturity at birth represents a design compromise associated with changes in pelvis anatomy due to bipedalism. Brain enlargement during human evolution increased the pressure towards early parturition.

Brain enlargement in human ancestral species probably happened discontinuously. A first growth spurt of the brain set in roughly 1.8 mya, most likely fostered by a dietary change towards greater amounts of protein, leading to doubling in brain size from 350 to 800 cm^3 in *Homo habilis*. Note that ancestral hominoid species had walked upright long before; thus bipedalism and brain enlargement are not that intimately linked as was previously thought (Jones et al. 1992). A second 'leap' in brain size occurred around 400,000 years ago when archaic *Homo sapiens* evolved, leading to an average brain size of 1,300 cm^3. This second increase in brain size was probably linked to changes in social structure giving rise to the human social brain (see Afterthought to Chapter 2).

These successive increases in brain size selected for antedating parturition, which came at the expense of greater immaturity of offspring at birth (Bjorklund 1997). Nevertheless, in spite of this evolved design compromise the human birth process has become an extremely perilous enterprise for both mother and baby. In order to pass the birth canal, human babies have to perform two torsion movements with their heads, bodies, and extremities (see Figure 3.1), such that birth places both the baby and the mother at great risk of dying from a broad spectrum of possible complications (Bradshaw 1997). Midwifery was perhaps the first 'profession' in early humans in that experienced females helped other females to give birth. This was part of a cooperative breeding strategy that evolved in humans to decrease interbirth intervals to approximately 3 years, which is considerably shorter than in other

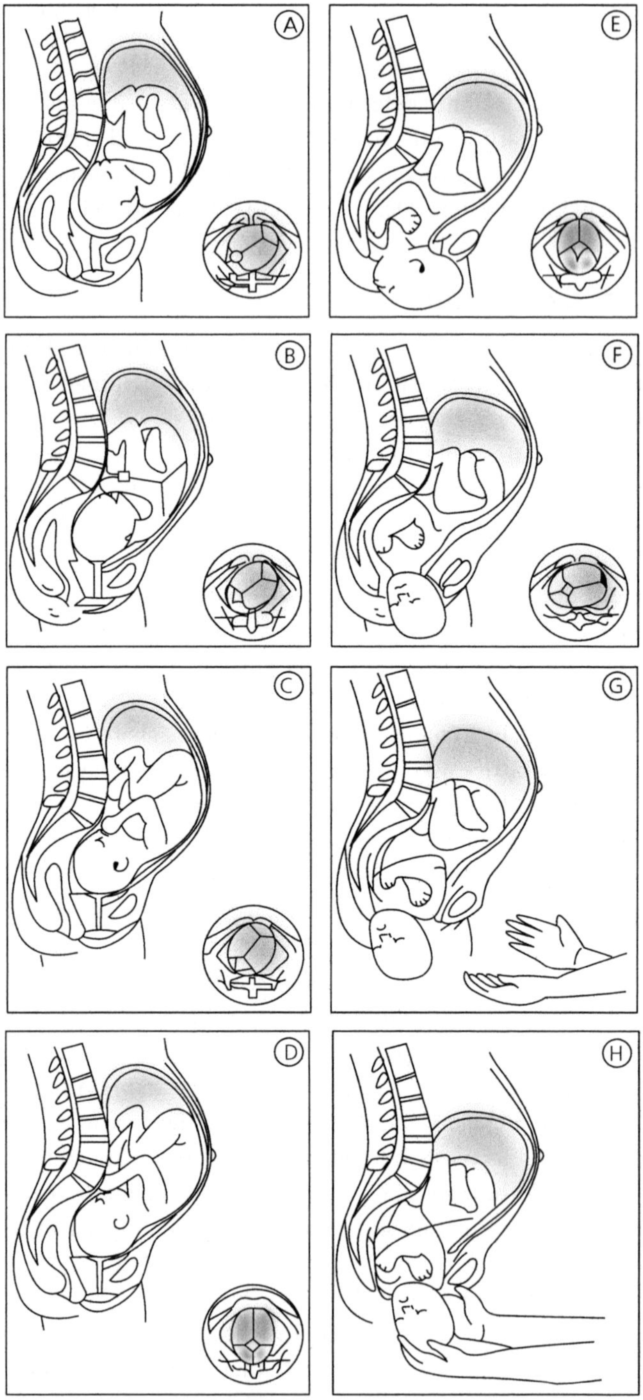

Fig. 3.1 The stages of human childbirth. Each box depicts a sagittal section through the maternal body during labour. The maternal pubic bone and vertebral column are shown in black. The inserted images show the cranial sutures and fontanels of the foetus from a midwife's perspective, illustrating the complicated rotations of the foetus's head and body during its passage through the narrow human birth canal. (Reproduced from The evolution of modern human childbirth, Karen R. Rosenberg, American Journal of Physical Anthropology, 35 (S15), pp. 89–124, DOI: 10.1002/ajpa.1330350605, Copyright © 2005, John Wiley and Sons.)

apes (Hrdy 2000). This shortening of birth intervals may have contributed to the great reproductive advantage of the human species over any other primate.

Due to preterm birth, human newborns are less precocial compared to young apes, and therefore have secondarily retained some altricial features. Precociality refers to the ability of offspring to move on their own legs soon after birth. The eyes and ears of precocial animals are open at birth or soon afterwards. Precocial features of newborn human babies include open eyes at birth, the ability to soon interact with their mothers, and to cling to the carrying person. Altriciality, by contrast, embraces signs of immaturity such as sealed eyes and ears at birth, immobility, and nakedness, which necessitate a period of development in a nest, burrow, or den. The inability to move on their own and to actively seek comfort and shelter are altricial features of human newborns (Jones et al. 1992). Because there is no fur to cling to, human babies need to be actively carried by their mothers. In German the biological term introduced for human newborns is 'Tragling' (Eibl-Eibesfeldt 1995) to which there is no comparable English expression ('one who is carried'). This could only become possible, of course, in conjunction with bipedalism, which freed the mother's hands for carrying offspring (and food).

Human babies display precocial features, such as open eyes and ears at birth, and an ability to interact with the primary caregiver; at the same time, however, altricial features such as immobility and nakedness necessitate intense parental care.

This special situation of human newborns implies that the formation of the dyad between mother and offspring became one of the most crucial psychological adaptations in early humans. Successful attachment on the baby's side and bonding on the mother's side have remained vital for psychological well-being throughout human evolution to the present day in every known culture (Bowlby 1969). In addition, the dependence of the mother on helpers increased proportionally, such that close cooperation between women, between mother and father of the child, and kinship alliances were positively selected (Hrdy 2000). Bogin (2009) suggests that childhood evolved as a novel developmental stage in humans to shorten infancy (terminated by weaning), such that mothers could have another baby considerably faster than any one of our closest extant relatives (apes). All the more important became the role of attachment in human development that helped human offspring survive, even if the mother's attention had to be shared with one or more siblings.

The formation of the dyad between mother and offspring by infant attachment behaviour became one of the most crucial psychological adaptations in early humans. Childhood evolved as a novel developmental stage in humans to shorten infancy (terminated by weaning), such that mothers could have another baby considerably faster than any one of our closest extant relatives (apes).

The biological function of attachment was first recognized by John Bowlby and developed by himself and his followers into a theory of universal human behaviour with far-reaching consequences for the understanding of close relationships throughout the entire lifespan (Bowlby 1991; van Ijzendoorn and Sagi 1999). Attachment theory has proven to be entirely consistent with an evolutionary framework (Simpson 1999). It integrates empirical studies in non-human primates (Kraemer 1997), normal attachment and bonding in humans, and pathological conditions such as foster care, and other adverse events during infancy and early childhood, including physical, emotional, and sexual abuse (Cassidy and Shaver 1999; Dozier et al. 1999). Attachment theory represents a powerful tool that can be used to make predictions about the psychological, physiological, and behavioural consequences of secure and insecure attachment (Belsky et al. 1996; Carter et al. 2001). These predictions are open to empirical testing, and complex gene–environment interactions in relation to attachment research have only begun to become unravelled.

Initially, Bowlby was struck by the fact that many young boys who grew up in foster homes displayed delinquent and antisocial behaviour, and were emotionally inept, despite being regularly provided with basic care and food. These boys were, however, deprived of a close relationship with a mother-figure, and Bowlby concluded that this could be at the core of their behavioural problems (Bowlby 1944). Research into non-human primates later confirmed the outstanding importance of closeness of young monkeys with their biological or surrogate mothers. Newborn monkeys, when separated from their mothers at an early age and raised in social isolation, prefer clinging to a fur-covered dummy mother rather than to a mesh-wired dummy providing milk (Harlow and Zimmerman 1959; Harlow et al. 1965). Depending on the duration of isolation, young monkeys develop severe forms of depression that does not lift even upon reunion with mothers or peers. Moreover, as adults these monkeys are socially incompetent and unable to raise their own offspring (Troisi 2003). These—in many respects merciless—experiments clearly confirmed the importance of social closeness with a mother-figure early in life for psychological well-being and social competence throughout successive life-history stages.

The importance of attachment has experimentally been shown in many studies with non-human primates. Depending on the duration of isolation from caregivers, young monkeys develop severe forms of depression. As adults, these monkeys are socially incompetent and unable to raise their own offspring.

In light of the great similarities in life history and evolved psychological attachment mechanisms, represented in homologous—foremost limbic—brain structures, it is evident that healthy human development critically depends on proximity and emotional warmth from very early on, probably even before birth (Kofman 2002; see Afterthought, this chapter). Young primates including humans are indeed biologically preprogrammed to seek proximity. Attachment behaviours were selected to increase the likelihood of the infant's survival, and to facilitate social learning. For example, human newborns' regulatory system for body temperature is still immature and they may also easily suffer from dehydration. This is so, in part, due to the lack of insulation by fur (although to a certain degree compensated by a subcutaneous layer of brown fat) and the fact that the developing brain consumes almost two-thirds of the total energy intake (Levitt 2003; Williams 2008). Of note, due to the physiological antedate of the human birth, the brain continues to grow after birth at the same pace as prebirth for more than a year (Jones et al. 1992). Only then does the brain's energy consumption slowly decline relative to the body's energy demand. This growth pattern deviates from that of other primates in which soon after birth the brain starts to grow more slowly relative to body growth (compare Figure 2.3). However, as already pointed out, attachment formation is not primarily associated with the need or drive for being fed, even though a strong affectional bond between mother and baby may best protect against malnutrition; the primary goal of young infants is to seek proximity and security (Bowlby 1969). This has arguably selected for intense empathy-related emotions (Preston 2013). As a side note, the outcome of human premature infants significantly improves if close skin-to-skin contact ('kangarooing') with the mother is provided, compared to standard incubator treatment. That is, kangaroo care increases autonomic function, stress regulation, sleep patterns, and maturation of the prefrontal cortex (Feldman et al. 2014).

Human infants have several means to form strong attachment relationships with caregivers. At the age of 4 weeks human infants have already a strong preference for human face contours. They are responsive to human voices, particularly the mother's voice, and actively seek contact by crying or smiling. Interestingly, in contrast to the delay in development of locomotion compared with other primates, the baby's smile and play-face occurs ontogenetically much earlier than in other primates. After 3–4 months human infants learn to distinguish between familiar and unfamiliar individuals. Xenophobia—the fear of strangers—emerges from 6 months on, a behaviour that probably represents an adaptive response to the potential dangerousness of other (particularly male) humans (Eibl-Eibesfeldt 1995). At the age of 6–9 months infants can control proximity to their attachment figures through crawling within a limited range (Marvin and Britner 1999).

Human infants have several means to accomplish proximity with caregivers. At the age of 4 weeks, human infants have already a strong preference for human face contours. They are responsive to human voices and actively seek contact by crying or smiling. Moreover, the baby's smile and play-face occurs ontogenetically much earlier than in other primates.

Parental care is, however, not only elicited by behavioural means. In addition, human infants, like all mammalian young and bird hatchlings, display features such as large eyes, round faces and skulls, and short extremities, which normally reduce aggression and are perceived as 'cute' (referred to as 'Kindchen schema'; Lorenz 1943). Although the reaction to these babyish features are deeply biologically rooted, the mother's responsiveness to her child's signals is much less preprogrammed than the proximity-seeking behaviours on the infant's side (Hrdy 2000). Thus, in contrast to 'attachment', the term 'bonding' has been chosen to describe maternal behaviours that support the development of a stable mother–infant dyad. Mothers are usually highly responsive to their babies' needs, and suckling strengthens the affectional bond between mother and child via psychological and physiological processes including oxytocin secretion, which is stimulated by breastfeeding (Insel 1997, 2003; Feldman et al. 2010). However, the availability of resources, including supportive resources from the partner and kin, has considerable impact on the mother's ability to accept and bond to her baby (Hrdy 2000).

Human infants display features such as large eyes, round faces and skulls, and short extremities, which normally reduce aggression and are perceived as 'cute'. However, the mother's responsiveness to her child's signals is much less preprogrammed than the proximity-seeking behaviours on the infant's side. Thus, in contrast to 'attachment', the term 'bonding' has been chosen to describe maternal behaviours that support the development of a stable mother–infant dyad.

The first 24 hours or so after birth have been critical throughout human evolution in regard of whether or not bonding develops, and a newborn's risk of dying from maternal neonaticide or abandonment is largest within this critical period, even in modern societies (Hrdy et al. 1994). By contrast, the risk of infanticide (after the neonatal period) is greatest in children who grow up with a stepfather (who is biologically unrelated to the child). Here, persistent crying and the lack of an affectional bond between (step-)father and child may create a vicious circle, which may lead to violent behaviour and victimization of the child (Daly and Wilson 1988; Weekes-Shackelford and Shackelford 2004; for a divergent view see Temrin et al. 2000). Infanticide carried out by mothers is much more often associated with maternal psychopathology, foremost depression. Severely depressed mothers may even intend to 'rescue' the infant from growing up under adverse conditions, sometimes as attempted homicide-suicide (Spinelli 2004; Stone et al. 2005). This is fundamentally different from neonaticide or abandonment of the newborn, which is rarely associated with maternal psychopathology in the strict sense, but often enough pursued by desperate single teenage mothers (for more details see Chapter 16).

Neonaticide may occur if attachment and bonding fail to establish.

The mother–child dyad and the affectional bond between them is, once established, enduring and practically irreversible. Attachment is specifically oriented towards a particular person that is not interchangeable. Attachments can also be formed with more than one person, for example, the mother and the father, but usually in a hierarchical fashion. Paternal investment (and emotional engagement) is probably highest in human fathers compared with other mammals, and one attachment figure can be important in some areas, whereas another attachment figure can be important in other areas. Interestingly, well-functioning individuals often have two secure relationships with both mother and father (Hrdy 2000).

Attachments can also be formed with more than one person, for example, the mother and the father, but usually in a hierarchical fashion.

Once attachment has been established, infants and toddlers develop emotional and cognitive representations of their attachment figures and their selves. These 'internal working models' essentially foster the child's ability to explore the environment, because children make predictions about future events on the basis of their internal working models. This happens largely outside conscious awareness. If a child perceives the world as a safe place, a feeling that is most consistently supported by a secure attachment, it starts exploring the environment, including the social environment. In such a situation the attachment system is 'offline', and the child may seek proximity to peers and be encouraged to socialize. Conversely, experiencing the environment as dangerous activates attachment behaviours, which can be elicited by darkness, sudden movements, loud noises, height, or feelings of loneliness. Positive emotions such as joy and love are brought about in infants by closeness and security, whereas negative emotions such as anxiety and grief emerge upon perceived or actual separation from the

The developing emotional and cognitive representations of attachment-figures and the self are called 'internal working models'. They determine the way a child explores the environment, as children make predictions about future events on the basis of their internal working models.

mother-figure (Bowlby 1973). A child's negative reaction depends, however, on the quality or nature of the affectional bond and the duration of separation.

The initial phase after separation is usually dominated by protest. The display of fear, anger, crying, or tantrums has probably served as an adaptive response to real threat during the human evolutionary past. An infant left unattended was at great risk of predation or injury. Thus, protest aims at forcing the attachment-figure to immediately return (Bowlby 1973; Belsky 1999). The protest phase may last from a few hours to days, but eventually gives way to a phase of despair, if the primary caregiver fails to return. The phase of despair is characterized by increasing signs of hopelessness, withdrawal, and disengagement. Motor activity is reduced and the infant remains silent, perhaps as adaptation not to attract predators. In many respects this phase resembles deep mourning or depression. The final phase is characterized by detachment, where the child actively turns his or her attention towards the environment and may eventually accept other caregivers. However, if the primary attachment figure returns unexpectedly, the child typically turns away, ignoring the attachment-figure, which may be followed by alternating clinging and fear of recurrent loss of the attachment-figure (Bowlby 1973). In evolutionary perspective, detachment can be seen as the *ultima ratio* to secure survival and possibly pave the way for a new affectional bond.

Separation from the attachment-figure produces protest, despair, and eventually detachment behaviour in the child.

Attachment theorists distinguish between four attachment styles, which have been studied in an experimentally created separation scenario, referred to as 'strange situation', through which separation distress and coping styles of infants can be systematically examined (Ainsworth and Bell 1970). Infants at the age of 12–18 months respond differently when separated from their mothers for a short period of time, and this is strongly related to the quality of the infant's attachment. The different attachment styles may reflect differences in the amount and quality of parental investment, which interact with differences in biological predispositions of infants regarding personality and temperament traits such as harm avoidance, novelty-seeking, extraversion, and agreeableness (Noftle and Shaver 2006).

Attachment theory distinguishes four types of attachment, which depend on the amount of emotional availability and responsiveness of the primary caregiver.

Secure attachment develops most easily if the mother or other attachment-figure is able to positively respond to the infant's signals, such that the infant perceives the mother as available and responsive when needed. Secure attachment reflects the parents' willingness and ability to provide emotional (and financial) resources, thus showing a high amount of parental investment. Typically, securely attached children approach their mothers upon reunion and seek proximity, but may resume playing in the presence of their mothers. Securely attached children use their mothers as a secure base or safe haven from which the environment can be explored with a sense of curiosity. In adulthood, secure attachment is reflected by coherent description of attachment-related experiences, which is referred to as 'autonomous state of mind' (Fonagy 1999). Secure attachment is the most prevalent attachment style across cultures and has probably been positively selected in the evolutionary past (Simpson 1999).

However, in line with parental investment theory (see Chapter 1), there may be conflict between the child and caregiver over the amount of nurture and emotional availability. In strange situation scenarios it has been observed, for example, that some infants avoid or ignore their mothers upon reunion. Attachment-figures of avoidantly attached infants have been found to often respond in a rejecting and cold manner to their infants' needs. They seem to invest less and to urge their children to become independent early, compared to care-givers of securely attached children. The avoidant reaction of infants can be interpreted as an attempt to maintain proximity to some extent while reducing the risk of being abandoned. As adults, avoidantly attached individuals often idealize attachment-related experiences and play down negative experiences, which may reflect an attempt to minimize the impact of early attachment on present-day life. This state of mind is referred to as 'dismissing' (Belsky 1999).

Another attachment style referred to as 'ambivalent' or 'resistant' is characterized by a mix of contact-seeking and angry reactions of the infant shown upon reunion. Many caregivers of ambivalently attached children are inconsistent in their behaviours. In contrast to caregivers of avoidantly attached children, who are often unwilling to invest, caregivers of ambivalently attached children are more often *unable* to invest, perhaps as a function of emotional instability. The attachment-figure may be in principle accessible to the infant but unable to provide comforting behaviour when the child is stressed. Temper tantrums may therefore be an adaptive response to maximize parental effort. In adulthood, ambivalent attachment is reflected in 'preoccupied states of mind', which can manifest as vagueness in describing attachment-associated experiences (Kobak 1999).

Insecurely attached children show different behaviours that aim at securing proximity and avoidance of being abandoned. Insecure attachment can be divided into avoidant, ambivalent (resistant), and disorganized patterns of behaviour.

Finally, disorganized or disoriented attachment style is coined by a pattern of contradictory behaviours in children upon reunion. Avoidance may follow strong contact-seeking behaviour or be displayed simultaneously. 'Freezing' is another form of behaviour that may occur as a consequence of disorganized attachment. Expressions of distress may arise in conjunction with movements directed away from the caregiver. As adults, disorganizedly attached individuals display an 'unresolved' or 'disorganized state of mind', which becomes evident in loosening of associations or other reasoning lapses when describing attachment relationships. Attachment-figures of disorganizedly attached children are often experienced as frightening, or they may feel frightened by their own infants (Kobak 1999). Abusive behaviour is most prevalent in caregivers of infants with disorganized attachment, which renders those children particularly vulnerable to developing a variety of psychopathologies, including abnormally high levels of aggression, dissociative symptoms, depression, anxiety, or redirected aggression towards peers or objects. Such behaviours can be explained as responses to perceived threats to the availability of an attachment-figure, such that the negative emotions of fear, anger, and sadness may become more pervasive (Kobak 1999).

The latter three attachment styles can be subsumed under the term 'insecure attachment' as opposed to secure attachment. Insecurely attached children may display strong attachment behaviours—they may struggle for emotional warmth and availability of an attachment-figure, that is, frantic efforts to avoid abandonment. That is, the intensity of the attachment behaviour must not be confused with the strength of the affective bond between infant and caregiver. Insecurely attached children develop expectations about how their social environment reacts that are different from those of securely attached children. These differences in anticipation of social interactions are causally linked to differences in internal working models. A child, for example, that anticipates rejection will approach her mother cautiously upon reunion compared to a child who is confident that the mother will comfort her. In the worst case, problems for young infants can arise from the need to seek proximity to an abusive caregiver, that is, infants might be caught in the ambivalent situation of attaching to caregivers who, in fact, are a source of threat and danger. Such a situation can create an emotional state of intense fear of abandonment, which further increases the infant's efforts to attach, thus causing great uncertainty and unpredictability, which precludes the development of a stable internal working model (Kobak 1999).

Unstable internal working models also have a profound impact on how insecurely attached individuals think about other people's thoughts and intentions, referred to as 'mentalizing' (an alternative expression used in the psychoanalytic literature is 'reflective functioning'; for details see Afterthought to Chapter 2 on the 'social brain'). Research suggests that securely attached individuals learn faster to think about other people's mental states, because caregivers of securely attached children may be likely to use 'mentalistic' expressions more often than rejecting caregivers of insecurely attached children. In contrast, insecure attachment may be coupled with developmentally delayed or even defective mentalizing, which is activated much more frequently in situations associated with negative affect. This may give rise to psychopathological signs and symptoms including suspiciousness and paranoid reactions (compare Chapter 17). Likewise, verbal communication between children and caregivers may open new possibilities for both maintaining open communication and creating threats to the availability of attachment-figures.

Unstable internal working models—as a result of insecure attachment—have a profound impact on how individuals think about other people's thoughts and intentions, referred to as 'mentalizing'. Securely attached individuals learn faster to think about other people's mental states. On the other hand, a feeling of security and emotional warmth may actually turn off the mentalizing system.

Differences between children in attachment and communication skills and caregivers interact in many ways, and attachment styles can be 'inherited' over successive generations (Kobak 1999). This research is consistent with the view that attachment security is intimately linked to stress regulation abilities in measurable ways. For example, studies have shown that people with fearful attachment styles (and those with preoccupied attachment) report higher levels of perceived stress, but have attenuated cortisol responses to a laboratory stress test compared to people with secure attachment and dismissive attachment styles (Kidd et al. 2011). Even though behavioural and neurophysiological differences among different attachment styles are largely triggered by environmental conditions, there is considerable evidence for important gene–environment interactions. For example, carriers of a certain polymorphism of the MAO-A and MAO-B coding gene that leads to a reduced activity of MAO-A are at greater risk of developing personality disorder or antisocial behaviour only if they are exposed to adverse conditions early in life such as violence, abuse, or neglect, whereas the risk of antisocial behaviour is even reduced in children who grow up under favourable early life conditions. In other words, MAO-A activity alone does not explain individual differences in behaviour, but findings strongly suggest that genetic variation accounts for differential sensitivity to social experiences during early stages of development (see Chapter 1, section 1.4.2 on 'differential susceptibility'). These interactions exert a profound influence on personality development, as shown in section 3.3.

Attachment security is intimately linked to stress regulation abilities.

Genetic variation accounts for differential sensitivity to social experiences during early stages of development, and these gene–environment interactions exert a profound influence on personality development.

3.3 Adolescence and early adulthood

From a biological perspective, adolescence and adulthood bring about major physiological and social changes, which prepare an individual to form cooperative alliances and to seek romantic relationships. During the extremely prolonged period of childhood and youth, humans acquire social skills and refine their internal working models about the social and physical world, which enable individuals to attain independence of their caregivers. Importantly, sensitive responding of a caregiver to an infant's needs fosters independence later in life, rather than promoting dependence; a fact that is often misconceived (Bowlby 1991). Thus, the importance of childhood experience, particularly the quality of early relationships, for peer and intimate relationships, relationships with own children, and even developmental timing of puberty, sexual activity, and amount of parental investment in own children can hardly be overestimated (Ellis et al. 2011b).

A caregiver's emotional availability fosters independence of offspring later in life, rather than reinforcing dependence.

Of note, from a biological point of view, is that there are striking differences between adolescent boys and girls. In fact, evidence suggests that adolescence emerged in hominin evolution, while it is absent in great apes. Boys, for example, become sexually fertile approximately 2 years prior to the final growth spurt. Phenotypically, they remain juvenile in stature, body hair, and pitch. Accordingly, they may learn adult social role models while sexually fertile, without being recognized as sexually mature, which helps them avoid intrasexual competition (Bogin 1999; Hochberg and Belsky 2013). Adolescent girls, in contrast, complete half of their breast development and growth of pubic hair during their final growth peak. However, while looking sexually mature, they remain infertile, as they reach adult frequency of ovulation and size of the birth canal at around 18 years of age (with significant differences between ethnic groups in relation to environmental contingencies; Kramer 2008). So, they learn adult social role models while looking feminine but still being infertile (Bogin 1999; Hochberg and Belsky 2013).

Differences between boys and girls developing during adolescence pertain to the dissimilarity in biological maturation and social role learning.

In any event, an individual's early rearing conditions shape his or her developing internal working model, which in turn guides the individual's expectations in terms of availability and predictability of resources, including trustworthiness and stability of interpersonal relationships (Bowlby 1969; Cassidy 1999; Cohen and Belsky 2008). Bowlby originally believed that only secure attachment and the development of a trustful internal working model were adaptive in an evolutionary frame of reference, and that other (insecure) forms of attachment were deviations from the norm. From an evolutionary point of view, however, it is plausible to assume that fluctuations in environmental conditions—although probably limited—have selected for a set of flexible adaptive behavioural responses to environmental contingencies.

Behavioural flexibility ultimately emerged to promote reproductive fitness by enabling an individual to choose among different strategies to accomplish important biosocial goals. For example, an individual growing up in harsh physical or emotional environmental conditions—regardless whether real or perceived—is more likely to aim at immediate resource extraction, which included the exploitation of others' resources, early mating and reproduction, and little care for own offspring (Belsky et al. 1991). The logic behind this is that the individual's internal working model suggests unpredictability of future availability of resources, both in terms of the reliability of social relationships and the prospects of the physical environment (i.e. social safeness; Kelly et al. 2012). In contrast, emotional warmth and availability of caregivers are more likely to induce an internal working model suggesting that others are trustworthy and that the world is a safe place, which makes individuals predict future resource abundance. In other words, despite being extreme K-strategists at the species level, there is interindividual variation in human life-history strategies depending on environmental contingencies. Unfavourable rearing conditions (from the perspective of the child) may cause psychological and biological preparedness such that behaviour later in life is shifted, however moderate, towards r-selection (or faster life history), whereas abundant resources and emotional availability of caregivers may enhance K-selected orientation (or slower life history) (Ellis et al. 2011a, 2011b). Viewed this way, avoidant and ambivalent attachment may, to some extent, reflect adaptive strategies that evolved to ensure survival and to maximize reproductive success under unpredictable environmental conditions (Belsky et al. 1991).

Children who grow up under unfavourable conditions such as high familial stress, parental unavailability and rejection, and perhaps scarcity of financial resources may develop mistrustful internal working models suggesting that others are untrustworthy and that future opportunities to achieve biosocial goals are dim. These children may as adolescents act in more opportunistic ways in order to extract maximum resources and to achieve short-term goals at the expense of engaging in high-risk behaviour. Thus, children with a background of insecure attachment are less tolerant to frustration or to reward delay. They also show, on average, less empathy for distressed peers and are often less liked by their peers (Allen et al. 1998).

Unfavourable rearing conditions (from the perspective of the child) may cause psychological and biological preparedness that is shifted towards 'faster' life-history strategies, whereas abundant resources and emotional availability of caregivers may enhance 'slower' life-history strategies within species-specific boundaries.

Notably, the quality of the family environment also impacts biological maturation. That is, early adversity is associated with antedated puberty, earlier engagement in sexual activity, and larger number of intimate partners compared to individuals who grow up in more favourable conditions (Ellis et al. 2011b). For example, a girl who experiences that her single mother has intimate relationships with multiple partners may internalize her mother's behaviour as a model for her own future behaviour, because the prospects of attaining a stable relationship may be perceived to be poor. Along similar lines, adolescent girls with a history of sexual abuse are more likely than their peers to engage in risky sexual behaviour (Houck et al. 2010). At the biological level, father absence accelerates menarche. Early adversity may also explain girls' greater propensity to 'internalize' problems, which may not only cause sadness, depression, and social withdrawal, but also lower metabolism and increase fat storage as proximate causation of early menarche. As adults, women who grew up under unfavourable conditions may be more likely to engage in multiple short-term relationships, to be sexually less faithful, and to give birth to children in which they are less willing to invest, compared to women whose internal working model is more trust-oriented and predict good access to future resources. Today's explosion in the number of teenage pregnancies may serve as an example for this scenario (Nettle et al. 2011). A similar development may occur in boys who, in contrast to girls, are more likely to 'externalize' problems, as evidenced by high levels of aggression, non-compliance, and impulsivity (Belsky et al. 1991). Like their female counterparts, however, young men who have experienced early adversity are more likely to engage in indiscriminate and opportunistic sexual relationships. Due to non-random (assortative) mating, depressed women are more likely to marry men with antisocial traits such that low levels of parental investment seemingly become 'heritable' (Marmorstein et al. 2004).

Unlike other primates, father absence or stressful family environment accelerate menarche and promote earlier sexual activity. This could be related to girls' greater propensity to 'internalize' problems, which may not only generate sadness, depression, and social withdrawal, but also lower metabolism and increase fat storage as a proximate cause for inducing menarche.

In contrast, children who grow up in families with spousal harmony, low levels of familial stress, and adequate financial resources are more likely to experience emotional warmth and availability of their caregivers. These children more often develop trusting internal working models, predicting sufficient future resource availability. Accordingly, their interpersonal attitudes are oriented towards greater reciprocality and cooperation. They, therefore, depend much less on immediate resource acquisition and are better able to tolerate reward delay. As juveniles, securely attached individuals tend to mature late, they reach puberty at a later age, and are less likely to have premature sexual intercourse. As adults, securely attached individuals engage more often in long-term relationships and tend to invest more in their own children (Figure 3.2).

Securely attached individuals tend to mature later, they reach puberty at a later age, and are less likely to have premature sexual intercourse. As adults, securely attached individuals engage more often in long-term relationships and tend to invest more in their own children.

These diametrically opposite life-history strategies can be seen as extremes on a within-species scale between r-selection (faster life history) and K-selection (slower life history), with all possible variations in between.

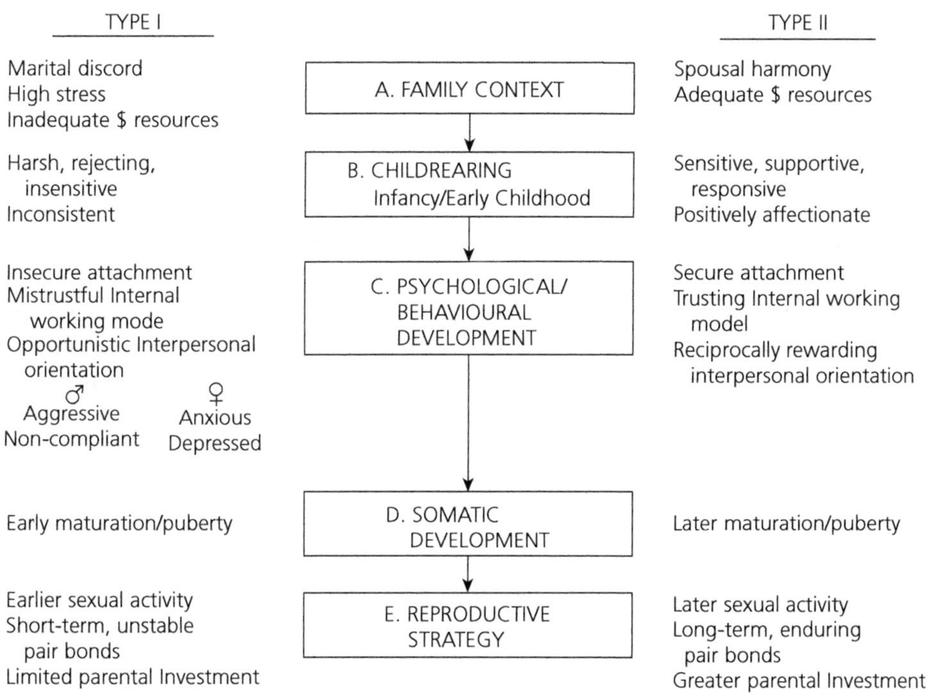

Fig. 3.2 Evolutionary developmental pathways of divergent reproductive strategies depending on resource availability. (Reproduced from Childhood Experience, Interpersonal Development, and Reproductive Strategy: An Evolutionary Theory of Socialization, Jay Belsky, Laurence Steinberg, and Patricia Draper, Child Development, 62 (4), pp. 647–70, DOI: 10.1111/j.1467-8624.1991.tb01558.x, Copyright © 1991, John Wiley and Sons.)

Approximately two-thirds of children are securely attached across populations, 20 percent are avoidantly attached, and roughly 10 percent ambivalently attached, with some variations depending on the cultural background (van Ijzendoorn and Sagi 1999). No cross-cultural data are available for disorganized attachment. In any event, insecure attachment styles represent (non-specific) risk factors for a broad spectrum of psychopathologies, but critically interact with the individual genetic make-up.

In a cross-cultural comparison approximately two-thirds of children are securely attached, 20 percent are avoidantly attached, and roughly 10 percent ambivalently attached. No cross-cultural data are available for disorganized attachment.

As already indicated, parenting styles may be 'inherited' over successive generations according to anticipated or actually available resources for both mother (or family) and child. Unconscious prediction of future environmental resource availability based on one's early life experiences is not a by-product of modern life. On the contrary, behavioural plasticity in relation to life-history strategies has been prevalent throughout human evolutionary history. As already mentioned, human mothers carry the burden of having more than one dependent child at the same time, which became possible by early weaning, by evolving mechanisms to strengthen partnership with men, among which concealed ovulation, and by strong emotional ties which contributed most to the formation of the 'nuclear family' (Konner 1977). In addition, human women were selected to assume a particular role beyond their own reproductive life-time, which is dealt with in section 3.4.

3.4 The postreproductive period

One of the great mysteries in human biology concerns the evolutionary puzzle that women survive menopause by two to three decades. At first sight, this does not seem to be plausible in terms of reproductive fitness. Menopause is not unusual in the animal kingdom per se; however, the long postreproductive lifespan of human women is. Fertility in humans increases gradually from menarche and peaks around age 30, before it steadily declines and eventually ceases. Similar to other apes, human women stop ovulating around age 50. This is adaptive because the risk of miscarriage or genetic birth defects increases with age. Unlike other primates, however, only humen women live another 20–30 years, and this life-history pattern is not a by-product of our modern life circumstances—women in hunter-gatherer societies who reach age 60 have a good chance of living another 10–20 years (Hrdy 2000).

The long postmenopausal human lifespan is probably closely related to the overall extended life history at all stages (Finch 2007; Bogin 2009), and possibly also to shifting energy budgets from direct to indirect reproduction (Reiches et al. 2009). It usually takes humans about two decades to start reproducing, and an offspring's dependence on the parental generation is accordingly long. From this perspective, it would not make sense to reproduce beyond age 50, because chances of survival of mothers until their last offspring has achieved full independence might be unpredictable. Instead, it has been argued that selection has favoured altruism directed towards close kin, such that the provision of additional resources by postmenopausal women especially helped offspring of their own children to survive, a scenario known as the 'grandmother hypothesis' (Voland 1998). Indeed, postreproductive women in hunter-gatherer societies supply much more edible resources to their tribe than they can consume themselves, and some spend more time gathering and processing food than women in their reproductive age. In most hunter-gatherer societies (as a model of the human ancestral condition) this surplus foremost benefits the offspring of own kin, particularly grandchildren (Voland 1998). This makes evolutionary sense, because in ancestral environments children just weaned were at risk of starvation, such that additional provision of calories by grandmothers increased their chances of surviving (Hrdy 2000). Thus, delaying senescence and selection for longevity might in the first place have been associated with the extremely decelerated human lifecycle and the need to increase the likelihood of survival of highly dependent, though already weaned, offspring by providing additional high-caloric diet (Hrdy 2000). Indeed, many postmenopausal women in contemporary hunter-gatherer societies are physically remarkably fit (Hrdy 2000).

The long postreproductive (postmenopausal) lifespan of women may have evolutionarily been selected because postmenopausal women have contributed to the survival of grandchildren ('grandmother hypothesis').

In western societies, members of families with disproportionally high numbers of individuals with long lifespans delay age-related diseases such as cancer, cardiovascular disease, and diabetes by a decade compared to members of families without a history of longevity (Sebastiani et al. 2013), whereby longevity is often inversely related to fertility and number of offspring (Jasienska 2009). Consistent with this discovery, there are apparently several genetic components involved in individual differences in longevity, some of which seem to be remarkably evolutionarily conserved (Lopez et al. 2012). However, human aging patterns do not seem to be qualitatively different from that of other primates (Bronikowski et al. 2011). In any event, grandmothers (and grandfathers?) have evolved significant roles in helping close kin to survive. A recent example of the importance of grandmothers that we currently witness concerns the tragedy of millions of HIV orphans in Africa whose parents deceased from acquired immune deficiency syndrome (AIDS), and who now grow up under the auspices of their grandmothers.

Longevity in humans is often inversely related to fertility and number of offspring.

Postreproductive women were probably also valued for their knowledge about locations and seasonal variations of valuable resources and for their advanced social skills, including conflict resolution. Likewise, older men might have been valued for similar reasons in terms of hunting skills and negotiation of social matters within their tribal societies. In line with these considerations it is worth mentioning that the crystalline intelligence necessary for the storage of semantic knowledge remains stable throughout higher ages, whereas fluid intelligence and cognitive flexibility declines as a function of age.

However, reverence of elderly women was much lower in human cultures less dependent on foraging. Until quite recently, tribal societies with a high amount of meat in their diet even practised euthanasia (carried out by socially sanctioned men) of elderly women, because women were unable to contribute much to the provision of food (Hrdy 2000). This negative side of the coin was perhaps counter-balanced by the special affectional bond between mother and child, and the great importance of altruism and kinship in humans. Attachment to a caregiver may in turn even predispose to role reversal through which an aging parent seeks proximity to a younger adult, usually their own adult son or daughter. However, devaluation of the elderly is certainly not specific to hunter-gatherer societies. Our modern culture has led to a break-up of the multigenerational family, and the consequent lack of involvement of the elderly in family life is perhaps one of the reasons for the exceptionally high rates of depression in the aged population.

The contemporary devaluation of the elderly may be one of the reasons for the exceptionally high rates of depression in the aged population.

Afterthought: prenatal environment and biopsychosocial preparedness

A growing literature on prenatal stress in mothers suggests that psychological problems of offspring later in life may be related to the intensity and timing of antenatal stressors. The concept of 'foetal programming' implies that the intrauterine environment prepares the foetal organism for postnatal conditions. Depression or anxiety of the mother during pregnancy, for example, is associated with lower birth weight and earlier delivery, as well as with elevated cortisol levels in children and with childhood behavioural problems at school age (Andersson et al. 2004; van den Bergh and Marcoen 2004; Brennan et al. 2008). Along similar lines, high levels of negative effect of the mother during the 12th–22nd week of gestation predict impulsivity and hyperactivity in children (boys more than girls) at age 8–9 and 14–15 years (Talge et al. 2007). Moreover, antenatal stress in the mother may predict anxiety symptoms, externalizing problems, and attention deficits in children. Interestingly, prenatal stress also predicts reduced laterality, which has been associated with autism and schizophrenia. This possible pathophysiological mechanism of schizophrenia has recently been corroborated by the observation that maternal stress due to loss of a close relative in the first trimester of pregnancy significantly increases the risk for schizophrenia in the offspring (Spauwen et al. 2004; Khashan et al. 2008).

Although it is clear that stressful experiences of the mother may have profound effects on the offspring's behaviour, there is little consensus over the questions of specificity, nature, and timing of stressors. It is plausible to assume that chronic stress over extended periods of time exerts greater effects on the foetus than single stressful events (Fontenot et al. 1995; Kofman 2002). Marital discord or separation seems to be particularly critical. It has been shown that plasma cortisol levels correlate highly in mother and foetus, and animal models point to the fact that epigenetic factors (methylation) associated with prenatal stress may reduce the expression of glucocorticoid receptors in the hippocampus, which may impair feedback control of the stress-induced cortisol response via the HPA axis

(Brennan et al. 2008). In line with these findings, prenatal stress leads to a smaller volume and decreased neurogenesis in the hippocampus, altered HPA functioning, and chronic elevated stress responses to novel stimuli or social isolation in non-human primates (Lee et al. 2002a). Moreover, prenatal stress may also impair the development of inhibitory control executed by prefrontal cortex function (Fine et al. 2014). These effects seem to be pronounced in primates if stress exposure happens early in gestation (Coplan et al. 1996).

However, in light of the expanded period of brain growth in humans and the physiologically preterm birth, it is conceivable that the brains of human foetuses and infants are vulnerable to maternal stress for a considerably longer period of time (Graham et al. 1999). In fact, abundant evidence suggests that postnatal stress may also exert lasting effects on stress responsivity. For example, continuous exposure to socio-economic stress increases an individual's 'allostatic load', that is, the way the organism can cope with stress through increased activation of the sympathetic nervous system, HPA axis, lipid metabolism and fat deposition, and immune function (McEwen 2002). In other words, under heightened stress the body is able to mobilize resources effectively, yet in times of lower stress it is unable to downregulate these processes, which in turn may promote the development of hypertension, diabetes, and cardiovascular disease (Brody et al. 2013), as well as psychiatric conditions such as depression and post-traumatic stress disorder (PTSD).

These scenarios seem to be a logical extension of the model of fast versus slow life-history strategies. Human mothers in the environment of EEA, who for social reasons or in times of increased danger were more distressed, anxious, and vigilant, might have prepared their unborn offspring for unpredictable environmental conditions and, hence, push their offspring's behaviour slightly more into the faster life-history direction of immediate resource extraction and early reproduction.

Another example—although perhaps speculative to some extent—may illustrate the plausibility of biological principles in explaining the relation of human psychology and behaviour: foetal death rates disproportionally increased for males compared with females 2 months after the terrorist attacks in New York City (Bruckner et al. 2010), a finding reminiscent of the Trivers–Willard hypothesis outlined in Chapter 1. Did women (unconsciously, of course) selectively abort male foetuses because the perceived prospects for postnatal reproductive fitness were greater for female offspring? These hypothetical causal relationships need to be prospectively studied in the future.

Chapter 4

Causes of psychopathology

Abstract

The causes of psychiatric and psychosomatic conditions can be categorized into two groups: proximate and ultimate (evolutionary) causes. Proximate causes comprise genetic factors, epigenetic modulation, childhood trauma and other life events, and senescence. Ultimate or evolutionary causes concern mismatch between adaptation and current environment, suboptimal design, and design compromises. Examples of evolutionary causes of dysfunction include cognitive and emotional adaptations to small-scale societies (mismatch), anxiety (suboptimal design), premature birth (design compromise), and other features associated with human life history. Furthermore, many 'diseases of civilization' fall under the category of mismatch, as well as immunological diseases that may arise from a lack of exposure to pathogens early in life. Prevention of psychopathology, though desirable, may not always be possible due to the fact that evolution does not select for emotional well-being. However, reducing the impact of early adversity and helping people develop alternative life-history strategies may be an attainable goal.

Keywords

proximate causes, ultimate causes, mismatch, design compromise, diseases of civilization, prevention

4.1 Introductory remarks to causes of psychopathology

The question why psychopathology exists can be approached from various, in general complementary, scientific angles. The traditional view is limited in explanatory power to the focus on proximate causations or mechanisms of signs, symptoms, or disorders (see also Chapter 1). Proximate causes comprise genetic factors (inherited risks), adverse experiences in early childhood associated with potential epigenetic modulation of gene function (see Chapter 3), or other psychologically traumatizing events that may occur at any time during an individual's life-time, brain injury, or senescence. There is nothing fundamentally wrong with this approach. Knowledge about the different mechanisms involved in the causation of psychopathology has greatly increased over the last decades, mainly due to advances in psychiatric genetics, gene–environment interaction, brain imaging, and other non-invasive techniques. Moreover, understanding the relationship between adverse early childhood experiences and the development of psychopathology later in life has improved, even though controversy remains as to whether inadequate environmental input (neglect and deprivation) may be associated with neurobiological consequences different from that following harmful environmental input (abuse and trauma; Humphreys and Zeanah 2015).

However, a modern conceptual framework that is useful for both clinical psychiatry and experimental neuroscience has to tackle additional, to date barely resolved, problems. One relates to the fact that subspecialties within psychiatry tend to drift apart and to lead separate lives with limited mutual exchange. In other words, there is apparently little common ground between the fields of genetics, neuroscience, and animal models of psychiatric disorders on the one hand, and the various disciplines of psychotherapy, social psychiatry, and cross-cultural psychiatry on the other. The former are often recognized as 'biological' and the latter as 'psychological'. Only quite recently has a dialogue commenced between the biological and the psychological 'schools' within psychiatry.

Nevertheless, the scientific exploration of the proximate causations (i.e. mechanisms) of psychopathological conditions alone is insufficient, because convergence of findings from psychiatric genetics, neuroscience, and the behavioural clinical perspective falls short of integrating the questions 'what' causes dysfunction (mechanism), 'when' does dysfunction set in (ontogeny), why is the original function of the mechanism designed the way it is (adaptive function), and how did it evolve (phylogeny). These four questions, originally proposed by Nikolaas Tinbergen (see Chapter 1), form the basis of a metatheoretical framework that embraces both the proximate and the ultimate causation of function and dysfunction (Nesse 2013; Brüne 2014b). This is not to say that any psychopathological sign or symptom has adaptive value in its own right. Per definition, they are maladaptive in both current (proximate) perspective and ultimate perspective, because they cause harm to the individual and are dysfunctional by their abnormal intensity (hypofunctioning, hyperfunctioning, or dysregulation), appearance in inappropriate context, and/or abnormal duration (Wakefield 1999).

However, every single dysfunctional sign or symptom has its functional counterpart as part of a set of evolved psychological mechanisms. Accordingly, dysfunctions (or psychopathological signs and symptoms as we call them) can be described as extremes of variation of normal adaptive mechanisms, of which the evolved function can be explored. Yet what is perceived as abnormal is not simply a matter of objective evaluation that is free of cultural norms and values. On the

Psychiatric genetics, neuroscience, and animal models of psychiatric disorders on the one hand, and psychotherapy, social psychiatry, or cross-cultural psychiatry on the other are conceptually disintegrated. A new framework needs to address the questions: (1) 'what' causes dysfunction (mechanism); (2) 'when' does dysfunction set in (ontogeny); (3) why is the original function of the mechanism designed the way it is (adaptive function); and (4) how did it evolve (phylogeny).

Per definition, psychopathological signs and symptoms are maladaptive in both current (proximate) perspective and ultimate perspective, because they cause harm to the individual and are dysfunctional by their abnormal intensity (hypofunctioning, hyperfunctioning, or dysregulation), appearance in inappropriate context, and/or abnormal duration. However, every single sign or symptom has its functional counterpart as part of a set of evolved psychological mechanisms. Accordingly, dysfunctions (or psychopathological signs and symptoms) can be described as extremes of variation of normal adaptive mechanisms, of which the evolved function can be explored.

contrary, there may be quite large differences of what is considered abnormal depending on the cultural background (Fabrega 2002). This must not be overlooked, in spite of the fact, or perhaps due to the fact, that current knowledge is mainly based on research in high-income countries, and that current diagnostic manuals (the Diagnostic and Statistical Manual of Mental Disorders (DSM) and International Classification of Diseases (ICD)) have been compiled in European and North American populations that share, to a large amount, a common cultural heritage. Accordingly, the nosological systems of DSM and ICD may be inadequate to capture psychopathology in non-western cultures (Burton-Bradley 1979). Our culture-chauvinistic perspective suggests that the way we conceptualize psychopathology is the only scientifically justified one, and that 'culture-bound syndromes' are to be dealt with as exotic exceptions to the system. In a broader view, however, ADHD, eating disorders, or the epidemic of drug and alcohol dependence may be similarly 'culture-bound' as 'amok', 'latah', or 'koro' are. In any event, diagnosing psychopathological conditions is perhaps to some degree culture-independent (Pfeiffer 1994), but at least equally depending on values and diagnostic conventions. The latter may wax and wane even within cultures, sometimes perhaps to the point at which a discipline like psychiatry creates its own market by altering diagnostic thresholds: not every state of sadness evolves into depression, restless and curious children do not necessarily have ADHD, and so forth. People working in the field may keep this self-criticism in mind to avoid over-diagnosing psychiatric conditions (Frances 2013).

Psychiatric diagnoses are—to some degree—not independent of culture; current conceptualizations have been generated in a small geographical area of western Europe. Thus, ADHD, eating disorders, or the epidemic of drug and alcohol dependence may be similarly 'culture-bound' as 'amok', 'latah', or 'koro' are. Diagnostic conventions may even vary within cultures. The threshold at which a certain condition becomes a 'disorder' is flexible rather than fixed. This must not be confused with early recognition of psychiatric disorders.

Figure 4.1 depicts the possible problems arising from changing diagnostic thresholds.

However, the threshold problem must not be confused with any endeavour to make an accurate diagnosis as early as possible. Whether or not primary prevention of psychiatric disorders is a realistic goal is hotly debated; in any event, the outcome and prognosis of psychiatric disorders can certainly be improved if early signs and symptoms do not go undetected for months or even years, as is currently still the case in most disorders (e.g. Häfner and Maurer 2006).

Current psychiatric conceptualizations also insufficiently account for sex differences in presentation of psychopathological signs and symptoms. Emphasizing the (proximate) role of sex hormones, for instance, does not explain at all *why* differences in cognition, emotion, and behaviour between the sexes exist, and *how* this translates into the diagnostic schemes of psychiatric disorders. For example, BPD is much more prevalent (or diagnosed) in young women, whereas the opposite is true for antisocial personality disorder. Erotomania, the delusion of being loved by a socially high-ranking person, is more common in women. By contrast, delusional jealousy occurs

Sex differences in presentation of psychopathological signs and symptoms are insufficiently reflected in current diagnostic systems.

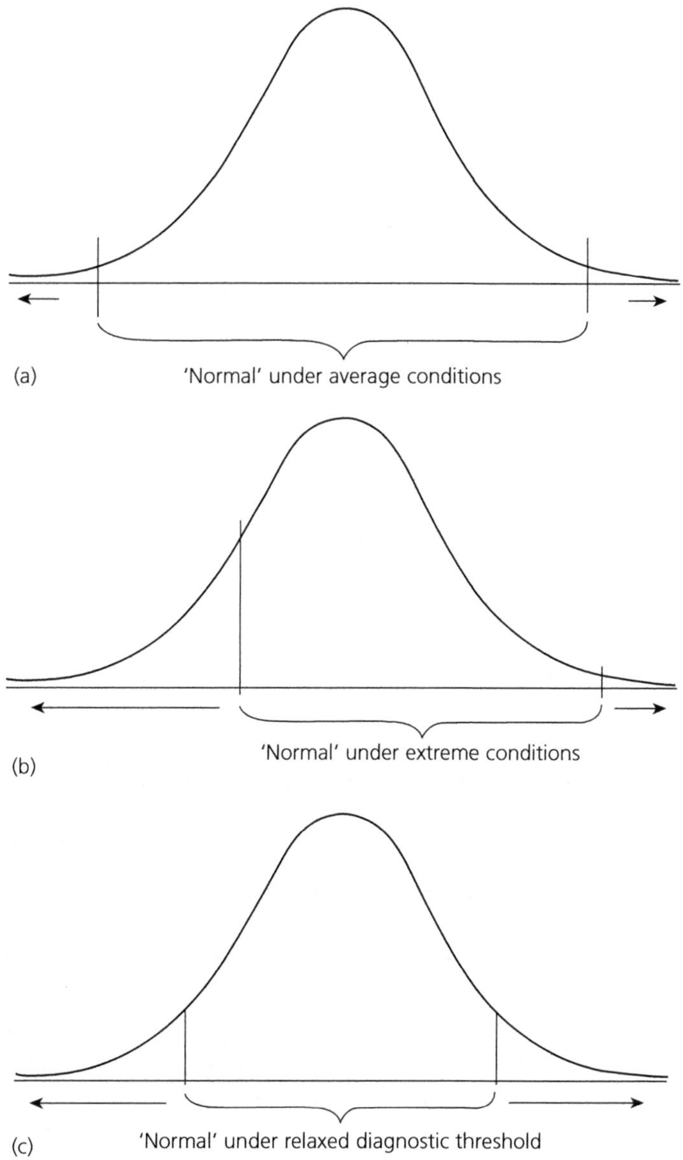

Fig. 4.1 (a) Psychopathological signs and symptoms as extremes of variation. Only significant hypo- or hyperfunction of an adaptive trait is considered pathological. (b) Under extreme environmental conditions, the diagnostic threshold may move along the X-axis, such that extreme trait variation at one end may still be rendered 'normal' (right-hand side of the graph), whereas at the other end, variation may be considered pathological, which under average conditions would be 'normal' (left). For example, in times of impending threat or danger (such as warfare) extreme suspiciousness on the edge of paranoia may be regarded as 'normal', whereas trust at the border of credulousness may be deemed 'abnormal'. Similarly, under extreme conditions, heightened alertness and anxiety may be regarded as 'normal', whereas low levels of alertness and anxiety are already outside the normal range. (c) Relaxed diagnostic thresholds for psychopathological signs and symptoms, perhaps as the result of changing diagnostic criteria or the desire of the medical industry to open new arenas for 'treatment' of mild, non-specific ailments.

almost exclusively in men (Brüne 2003a). No explanation for these discrepancies has been given by standard psychiatric nosology.

In addition, differences between the sexes in terms of vulnerability to stress have largely been disregarded. For example, men may be more vulnerable to develop psychological distress upon experiencing negative events relating to social status, whereas women are perhaps more vulnerable to developing psychological problems due to negative interpersonal events (Troisi 2001). By no means does this suggest that men are impervious to interpersonal distress and women to professional failure. There is quite good empirical evidence, however, that there is a tendency in men and women that points in this direction.

Moreover, contemporary conceptualizations struggle with the growing evidence that categorically distinct disease entities do not exist. For example, there are continua not only between schizophrenia and bipolar affective disorder (a fact that has been recognized since the days of Kraepelin), but also between 'normalcy' and psychosis, depression, and anxiety disorders, and between OCD and delusional disorder, to name just a few.

Psychiatric disorders broadly overlap, and there is also continuity between disordered states and 'normalcy'.

A related problem pertains to the diagnosis of comorbidity. The atheoretical diagnostic manuals of DSM and ICD allow for making diagnoses of an infinite number of comorbid psychiatric disorders, but certainly some disorders go together more often than others. This is so because comorbid disorders may reflect problems associated with the same or similar life-history strategies (Del Giudice 2014). For example, recurrent depression, social phobia, and avoidant personality disorder may plausibly be diagnosed, whereas it is much more difficult to diagnose anxiety disorder in a patient with schizophrenia or bipolar disorder. Finally, in a psychotherapeutic perspective, some concepts from the beginnings of psychoanalysis and behaviour therapy have surprisingly long half-lives and are still being taught in (some) medical schools, although there is little empirical evidence for the validity of the Oedipus complex (Erickson 2000), or the assumption that all behaviour is learned and can thus be unlearned.

It is at the core of this book to promote the endeavour to integrate the subspecialties within psychiatry, because it is in the patients' interest that diagnosis and therapy is individually tailored, taking into account age, gender, biological predisposition, adverse (early) experiences, and socio-economic background. This necessitates acknowledging the biological history of our species, particularly if we want to understand the worldwide increasing prevalence of psychiatric disorders and the individual circumstances that render a person vulnerable to developing psychological problems.

Another important aspect of integrating proximate and ultimate causation of psychiatric disorders is that knowledge of how and why psychological mechanisms evolved in our species and how genes interact with environmental contingencies may strengthen

Table 4.1 Risk and protective factors for mental disorders. (Reproduced from World Health Organization, *Prevention of Mental Disorders: Effective interventions and policy options, Summary Report*, page 23, box 5, © 2004, World Health Organization, <http://www.who.int/mental_health/publications/prevention_mh_2004/en/>.)

Risk factors	Protective factors
Academic failure and scholastic demoralization	Ability to cope with stress
Attention deficits	Ability to face adversity
Caring for chronically ill or dementia patients	Adaptability
Child abuse and neglect	Autonomy
Chronic insomnia	Early cognitive stimulation
Chronic pain	Exercise
Communication deviance	Feelings of security
Early pregnancies	Feelings of mastery and control
Elder abuse	Good parenting
Emotional immaturity and dyscontrol	Literacy
Excessive substance use	Positive attachment and early bonding
Exposure to aggression, violence, and trauma	Positive parent–child interaction
Family conflict or family disorganization	Problem-solving skills
Loneliness	Pro-social behaviour
Low birth weight	Self-esteem
Low social class	Skills for life
Medical illness	Social and conflict management skills
Neurochemical imbalance	Socioemotional growth
Parental mental illness	Stress management
Parental substance abuse	Social support of family and friends
Perinatal complications	
Personal loss—bereavement	
Poor word skills and habits	
Reading disabilities	
Sensory disabilities or organic handicaps	
Social incompetence	
Stressful life events	
Substance use during pregnancy	

research into the prevention of psychopathological conditions. The World Health Organization (WHO) has identified several risk factors as well as protective factors for psychopathology, many of which reflect adverse or favourable circumstances that meet built-in vulnerabilities (or plasticity) and evolved psychological needs of our species, respectively (Table 4.1).

Research into psychopathology including an evolutionary perspective may not only help explain the worldwide increase in prevalence of psychiatric disorders, but also inform studies of resilience and vulnerability factors of mental disorders.

As we will see in section 4.2, one of the most important reasons for psychopathology is that some individuals are more likely than others to suffer from a mismatch of their behavioural biological heritage and modern environmental living conditions (for an overview of psychiatric genetics and evolutionary explanations of the paradox that genes causing psychiatric disorders persist in the gene pool of populations see Chapter 1).

4.2 **Evolutionary constraints of psychological adaptedness**

Clinicians take for granted that any body part can go wrong at some point in life, as much as a faulty gadget that is poorly adapted to the burden of life. But why? From an evolutionary point of view it is all but straightforward to assume that the human body is fraught with design flaws that cause vulnerability to disease or disorder (Nesse and Williams 1994). Common understanding of evolutionary processes suggests that pathologies—regardless of whether physical, cognitive, emotional, or behavioural—convey fitness disadvantages in terms of survival and reproduction, and should therefore be eliminated by selection over generations. This assumption, however, disregards at least two readily overlooked facts.

First, the majority of adaptations are not optimal by design. Evolution by selection is usually a 'thrifty' process, such that evolved physical or psychological traits are just sufficiently well designed to fulfil their function proper, and only as long as needed (Nesse and Williams 1994). Second, evolution cannot create physical or mental traits de novo. New adaptations derive from pre-existing structures. The evolutionary process of acquiring new function by modification of pre-existing traits is sometimes misleadingly referred to as 'co-optation' (Brüne and Mulcahy 2003). It must, however, not be mistaken as goal-directed (teleological) or progressive development. By definition, evolution through selection is neither purposeful nor progressive (Mayr 2001).

The majority of adaptations are not optimal by design. Evolution by selection is a 'thrifty' process, such that evolved physical or psychological traits are just sufficiently well designed to fulfil their function proper. Moreover, evolution cannot create physical or mental traits de novo.

To understand the problem of design optimality, consider the example of the evolution of bipedalism in hominoids. Upright walking evolved in human ancestral species probably due to a slow but dramatic climate change in southern Africa (Cerling et al. 2011). About 2.5 mya rainforests receded and gave way to a savannah-like environment, with trees being more scattered such that bipedalism evolved to traverse larger distances between trees and to survey the surroundings for the presence of predators (National Research Council (US) Committee on the Earth System Context for Hominin Evolution 2010). Upright walking required a complex reorganization of the pelvis and vertebral column anatomy. In anatomically modern humans, the vertebral column forms a double 'S' curve, which allows travelling large distances at relatively low energetic costs. However, the vertical alignment of the inner organs and the elevated centre of mass of the human body slightly above the hip joints may cause vulnerability to degenerative problems, because the vertebral discs are squeezed between the vertebrae and can slip to compress the cauda equina or the spinal cord (Bradshaw 1997). Thus, lumbar or cervical disc prolapses are built-in design compromises of bipedalism, because the solution to the adaptive problem was sufficient but not optimal. Slipping discs are, however, certainly not adaptive, but an inevitable vulnerability factor for lower back pain.

Similarly, brain function is replete with design compromises. As brain size and cortical folding increased in ancestral human species, a number of energetic problems arose, as well as the problem of passing a narrow birth canal (for details see Chapters 2 and 3). Two obvious solutions to these problems were to increase the amount of high-protein diet, which was accompanied by decreasing gut size (Aiello and Wheeler 1995), and to antedate parturition towards greater immaturity (Jones et al. 1992). Moreover, the large human brain needed a well-developed cooling device maintained by an extended system of venous sinuses, which is susceptible to head trauma and exsiccosis (Allman 1999). Many design compromises within the brain pertain to the large distances for information to travel in extended neural networks, as well as the problem that all top-down information from the neocortex has to pass the midbrain and brainstem. Damage to the lowest layer of the triune brain (see also Chapter 2) therefore has a profound impact on the function of the other two.

Brain function is replete with design compromises. Increasing brain size and cortical folding have caused energetic problems, as well as the problem of passing through a narrow birth canal.

A problem relating to design suboptimality of psychological mechanisms lies in the variation of threshold at which a stimulus can elicit a response. This problem particularly pertains to defence mechanisms signalling threat or danger to the individual. Evolution by selection has equipped defence mechanisms with low and perhaps labile stimulus thresholds. Fear and anxiety, for example, are helpful internal signals of impending danger or actual threat. The threshold of eliciting anxious reactions is usually low (with interindividual differences), because the cost of being injured or killed as a consequence of not reacting to a threat is much higher than responding to false alarms (Nesse 2001). On the other hand, it is not useful to be permanently anxious, because the proximate mechanisms associated with anxiety such as epinephrine and cortisol secretion (through activation of the HPA axis), hypertension, and tachycardia may cause tissue damage in the long run (which is actually the case in PTSD). Fear reactions can be elicited much easier by stimuli that played a significant adaptive role in the past—snakes, spiders, height, strange people, open space—but much less so by modern threats such as automobiles, radioactivity, and so forth.

Defence mechanisms such as fear and anxiety have labile triggering thresholds. Unfavourable environmental conditions and/or individual predisposition may cause abnormally frequent release of fear reactions, which, in turn, may lead to tissue damage due to hyperactivity of the HPA axis.

The mechanism of eliciting fear reactions has been likened to a 'smoke detector principle' (Nesse 2001), which operates at low thresholds sensitive enough to detect small concentrations of smoke. However, in contrast to a smoke detector, the threshold of anxious reactions can vary within an individual. For example, a person walking alone in the dark almost certainly has a lower threshold for fear reactions than the same individual has if he or she is in good company with trustworthy people. Thus, an individual's sense of safety and security critically depends on environmental circumstances, of which the experience of closeness with others is perhaps most important.

Second, modern environments have little in common with ancestral living conditions. For example, for most of our evolutionary history, probably for several hundred thousand years or so, ancestral humans lived in close-knit communities in which everyone knew everybody else personally; the smallest functional unit within ancestral human societies was the nuclear family consisting of father, mother, and children. Anatomical features including testes size and sexual dimorphism suggest that mild polygyny was perhaps common in ancestral humans, yet critically depending on whether or not a male could 'afford' more than one spouse, including offspring he sired, in terms of provision of sufficient resources. Individual families were surrounded by extended kinship, and communities critically depended on mutual aid and cooperation (Hrdy 2000). Anonymity was virtually absent, and every-day confrontation with thousands of strangers was not an adaptive problem in the past. Thus, although humans in modern times try to create social conditions that resemble ancestral ones—for example, the average number of an individual's personal acquaintances has been estimated to be around 150 (Dunbar 1995), which is strikingly similar to what has been predicted from neocortex ratio (see Chapters 1 and 2)—competition for resources, social status, and intimate partners is probably much higher than it ever was in our evolutionary past (Gilbert 1998), such that urban unbringing alone can be considered a 'risk factor' for psychiatric conditions (Lederbogen et al. 2011).

Modern environmental conditions are dissimilar to ancestral ones ('mismatch hypothesis'). The likelihood that modern environmental conditions including accentuated social competition potentiate the risk that an individual's biosocial goals such as care-seeking, caregiving, mate attraction, cooperation with others, and attaining an acceptable social status are thwarted has increased by magnitudes compared to the EEA.

Moreover, due to the high degree of mutual dependence among all members of ancestral communities, child neglect or abuse might have virtually been absent in the EEAs. In contemporary societies such dramatic adversities are quite easily hidden from public awareness, sometimes for an appallingly long time. Thus it seems reasonable to argue that modern environmental conditions, including intensified social competition or child neglect and abuse, have potentiated the risk that an individual's biosocial goals such as care-seeking, caregiving, mate attraction, cooperation with others, and attaining an acceptable social status are thwarted compared to the EEAs in which our species' psychological make-up evolved (Gilbert 1998). In fact, there is evidence to suggest that early adversity can leave permanent marks on brain mechanisms and structures dealing with threat evaluation (Teicher et al. 2003; Dannlowski et al. 2012), as well as on physical health in ways that lead to an acceleration of somatic damage (Nettle 2014).

Mismatch of psychological mechanisms that evolved in the past and current environmental stressors is perhaps one of the most important evolutionary causes of psychopathology (Nesse and Williams 1994). Another parsimonious explanation for the mismatch between adaptations to past conditions and present-day environments is that human cultural evolution has overtaken biological evolution, such that biology could not keep pace with cultural changes. The mismatch problem does not only affect psychological mechanisms, however. Many 'diseases of civilization', including the risk for hypertension, stroke, myocardial infarction, and type-II diabetes, can be interpreted in line with a mismatch scenario (Brüne and Hochberg 2013). Chronic activation of the HPA axis due to environmental, (foremost) social, stressors may be the prime causal factor for disorders affecting the cardiovascular system. Moreover, harsh environmental living conditions in terms of episodic food shortages were probably prevalent throughout human evolutionary history, such that selection favoured individuals who were carriers of 'thrifty genes'. The 'thrifty gene hypothesis' (Neel 1962) posits that genes for maximum calorie extraction were selected in ancestral conditions, which now in times of oversupply and abundance of high-caloric diet cause harm. Thrifty genes, for example, may account for our preference for sweets and food rich in cholesterol, and contemporary human populations such as the indigenous peoples of North and South America, which until recently lived under environmental restrictions on the availability of such food, now suffer from enormous prevalence rates of type-II diabetes and coronary heart disease causing premature death (Brüne and Hochberg 2013). Whether or not thrifty genes are also linked to psychological problems is currently unknown.

Early adversity can leave permanent marks on brain mechanisms and structures dealing with threat evaluation, as well as on physical health in ways that lead to an acceleration of somatic damage.

Many 'diseases of civilization', including the risk for hypertension, stroke, myocardial infarction, and type-II diabetes, can be interpreted in line with a mismatch scenario. 'Thrifty genes' that were selected for maximum calorie extraction may now—in times of abundance of calorie-rich diets—play a causal factor in these disorders.

Another example of mismatch between ancestral adaptations and modern environments concerns the exposure to pathogens early in life and its impact on immune function later in life. When comparing ancestral with modern environmental conditions, it is quite obvious that the exposure to pathogenic agents has substantially changed. Even contemporary rural areas differ from urban residential quarters with regard to the prevalence of micro-organisms (Ege et al. 2011). In any event, over the course of human evolution several infectious diseases have been highly prevalent, including malaria, tuberculosis, and leprosy, thus creating significant selection pressures on the immune system. Some of the positively selected genes that convey immunity to such infectious diseases may now increase our vulnerability to autoimmune disease (Karlsson et al. 2014).

According to the 'hygiene hypothesis', a lack of exposure to pathogens early in life deprives the immune system of fighting infectious diseases, leading to increased risk for autoimmunological attacks on one's own tissue (Rook 2009). Beyond classic autoimmune diseases such as atopy, asthma, and type-I diabetes, there is some evidence to suggest that a dysregulated immune system may play a role in psychiatric disorders, including depression (Raison and Miller 2013), based on observations that assign several genetic risk alleles a role in pathogen host defence. A novel line of research suggests that the gut microbiota exerts considerable impact on brain function, whereby animal studies have revealed far-reaching consequences of the action of micro-organisms for behaviour and cognition, possibly via neuroendocrine, neuroimmune, and vagal pathways (Cryan and Dinan 2012). It can be expected that insights from immunological research will substantially improve our understanding of (psycho-)somatic and psychiatric disorders.

The 'hygiene hypothesis' posits that a lack of exposure to pathogens early in life deprives the immune system of fighting infectious diseases, leading to increased risk for autoimmunological attacks on own tissue.

A further case of mismatch is intimately linked with human immaturity at birth and the extremely expanded period of dependence of infants and children from their caregivers. In 'modern' societies it is still common practice to separate human newborns from their mothers (at least temporarily) after birth, and to separate young mothers from their supporting social environment (Sharma 2007). It has long been propagated that infants should sleep separate from mothers, because accidental overlaying may be a cause of sudden infant death syndrome (SIDS) (the risk for which is indeed increased if the mother or father are intoxicated with drugs or alcohol, or if one of them smokes tobacco; occasionally, however, infanticide is hidden behind the label). Physical separation of infants from their mothers, at least during the earliest stages of the postnatal period (Morgan et al. 2011), is now known to be a threat to the developing affectionate bond between the two (see Chapter 3), and insecure attachment can be seen as one important risk factor for psychopathology later in life.

As outlined in Chapter 3, avoidant and resistant attachment styles can be seen as adaptive responses to unpredictable environmental conditions and immediate resource extraction (Simpson 1999). Disorganized attachment, by contrast, is perhaps a particular style that cannot be interpreted as adaptive morph. Disorganized attachment is more prevalent in infants of parents with psychiatric disorders, including affective disorders and substance dependence, compared to healthy parents, and the child's contradictory behaviours oriented towards his or her caregiver reflect the ambivalence between being attracted to a caregiver who at the same time is a source of threat or maltreatment. Such a constellation produces persistent fear in the child without the possibility to escape. A parent, for example, who expresses threats of suicide not only induces fear of loss and abandonment in the child, but also confounds attachment-related fears with feelings of guilt. Similarly, parents who are chronically anxious or constantly fear that something dreadful may happen to the child may induce a role-reversal such that the child feels compelled to comfort a distressed caregiver (Liotti 2000).

Human immaturity at birth has created the necessity to form close attachment with primary caregivers. Insufficient parental responsiveness to infants' needs poses a risk factor for psychopathology later in life.

These kinds of physical or emotional abuse may lead to negative perception of the self as worthless or overburdened, which may be transferred to adult attachment figures later in life, for example, spouses, and to the role as a parent. Insecurity in partnerships, for instance, may lead to accusation of the partner that he or she has been unfaithful and, in the long term, disengagement of the partner (Del Giudice 2014). This, in turn, may paradoxically increase the individual's effort to engage the withdrawing partner, because threat to the availability of the partner may cause intense fear. As parents, individuals with severe attachment problems, particularly disorganized attachment styles, may display more frightened and frightening behaviours than securely attached individuals. Insecurely attached individuals are less well able to sense their infants' needs or to accurately reflect upon their infants' mental states in terms of desires, feelings, and intentions, and hence act in a less responsive way or even abusive ways (Shaver and Miculincer 2005).

The ability to appreciate one's own and others' mental states is perhaps one of the most critical evolved psychological mechanisms involved in regulating social interaction among individuals and within social groups. Mentalizing develops during childhood and adolescence with considerable impact of the specific social context. Although humans inherit the biological basis for mentalizing, it is probably one of the most 'open programmes' which, on the one hand, produces enormous flexibility, but, on the other, almost certainly at the cost of potentially dysfunctional development (see Chapter 2).

The ability to appreciate own and others' mental states ('mentalizing') is perhaps one of the most critical evolved psychological mechanisms involved in regulating social interaction between individuals and within social groups. Dysfunction of mentalizing may cause a broad array of psychopathological signs and symptoms.

Other potential risk factors for psychopathology are more generally related to immaturity and prolonged dependence. The period of greatest vulnerability to infectious pathogens, toxins, and malnutrition is probably the prenatal and perinatal period of development. In a broader sense, these risk factors may be seen as the result of a mismatch, because the higher population density in modern compared to ancestral human societies is associated with an increased likelihood that infectious diseases spread in the population. Likewise, accumulation of toxic substances in the mother's body and milk is an even more pressing problem of modern times. Moreover, infant malnutrition has exploded in underdeveloped countries, the causality of which is multifactorial. These factors may affect brain development in rather unspecific ways. The adaptively decelerated paedomorphic brain maturation, particularly the late myelination of the prefrontal temporal and parietal cortices, and the evolution of greater openness of brain circuits that allow for increased behavioural flexibility may come at the cost of greater vulnerability to harmful events, regardless whether emotional, infectious, or toxic in nature. However, the role of timing of adverse events and its specific effects on brain development and neural circuits is insufficiently understood.

The adaptively decelerated paedomorphic brain maturation, particularly the late myelination of the prefrontal temporal and parietal cortices, and the evolution of greater openness of brain circuits that allows for increased behavioural flexibility may come at the cost of greater vulnerability to harmful events, regardless of whether emotional, infectious, or toxic in nature.

Abnormal birth spacing may be another mechanism that causes vulnerability to psychological problems. In humans, cooperative breeding and grandmothering has already contributed to the shrinkage of ape-typical birth intervals by several years (Jones 1986; Galdikas and Woods 1990). If birth intervals are further shortened, particularly in the absence of adequate social support, which may particularly be problematic in undereducated and socio-economically impoverished people, the risk of maltreatment, neglect, and abuse may dramatically increase (e.g. El-Kamary et al. 2004).

Abnormal shortening of interbirth intervals associated with poor education and poverty increases the risk for child maltreatment, neglect, and abuse.

Design suboptimality and environmental mismatch, in conjunction with genetic susceptibility through variation, are probably the most powerful causal mechanisms to explain psychopathology from an ultimate evolutionary point of view, with which proximate causes such as allelic variation and experience-dependent factors interact. For example, anxiety disorders may emerge from an alteration of the threshold at which perceived threatening stimuli elicit a response, and this altered threshold may be triggered by insecure attachment (Dozier et al. 1999). At the genetic level, this may be paralleled by an allelic variation at the serotonin transporter gene locus, leading to a reduced availability of serotonin, which may eventually impede the pursuit of significant biosocial goals. Similarly, attachment styles may be mediated by genetic variation, for example, dopamine, serotonin, or oxytocin receptor polymorphisms, such that insecure attachment may be more likely to occur under circumstances associated with both insensitive parenting and a specific allelic variant (Bennett et al. 2002; van Ijzendoorn et al. 2008; Ellis et al. 2011b; Bakermans-Kranenburg and van Ijzendoorn 2013). These variants may selectively be favoured in unpredictable environmental conditions in which immediate resource extraction could be advantageous over more long-term-oriented behavioural strategies. In other words, suboptimal design and mismatch of evolved behavioural propensities with modern environmental conditions are by no means mutually exclusive, but rather complementary explanations of how psychopathology can be understood in proximate and ultimate perspective.

Since biosocial demands change with life-history stages, the likelihood and nature of dysfunction varies with age (and brain maturation). Those periods of life during which the need for adjustment of adaptive strategies is greatest may be associated with greater susceptibility or dysfunctional solutions to specific adaptive problems. Early infancy is foremost characterized by the need (from the infant's perspective) to secure sufficient resources both emotionally (parental care) and physically (food) to survive. Childhood and youth are life-history stages during which the acquisition of knowledge, social rules, and interaction with peers is critical. Adolescence and early adulthood are predominated by cementing peer relations, finding a suitable mate, and perhaps having children (Bogin 2009).

Those periods of life during which the need for adjustment of adaptive strategies is greatest may be associated with greater susceptibility of dysfunctional solutions to specific adaptive problems. Incidence rates of psychiatric disorders may peak around those life-history stages that bring about the greatest developmental changes, because the impact of thwarted biosocial goals during stages of developmental transition is greatest when people acquire new social roles.

Late adulthood, particularly the postmenopausal period, brings about the need for continuing investment in own kin, especially adult children and their dependent (weaned) grandchildren, as well as transferring essential knowledge to the next generation. Senescence and old age are perhaps somewhat special because natural and sexual selection have little impact on these life-history stages (Nesse 1988). However, the genetic underpinnings of traits that are advantageous early in life may have deleterious effects later on, a possibility referred to as 'balanced polymorphism'. Thwarting of biosocial goals during any one of these periods may increase the risk for developing psychiatric disorders, and peaks of prevalence rates are consequently to be expected during those life-history stages that bring about the greatest changes in terms of reorganization of the brain and behaviour (Paus et al. 2008).

4.3 Conceptualization of individual psychopathological signs, symptoms, and syndromes: an overview

An important question is whether or not the proximate and ultimate explanations (discussed in sections 4.1 and 4.2) at the macro level can be boiled down to individual signs and symptoms. A more detailed description of classic psychiatric phenomenology is given in Chapter 5. Here, a brief outline may exemplify the need to additionally get at least a rough understanding of the meaning of individual signs and symptoms or syndromes. Traditional conceptualizations and classifications of psychiatric disorders barely reflect evidence from modern (evolutionary) neuroscience as to their corresponding normal neuropsychology and representation in the brain. Moreover, they are limited in expressing coherence between signs and symptoms and in explaining the functional significance of cognitive–emotional–behavioural units (Geerts and Brüne 2009).

Traditional classifications of psychiatric disorders are limited in expressing coherence between signs and symptoms and in explaining the functional significance of cognitive–emotional–behavioural units.

In classic psychopathology the term 'consciousness' has multiple meanings, including states of wakefulness, vigilance, and reflexive awareness of the self as a person. These different aspects of consciousness are supported by different and largely unrelated brain systems.

To begin with, the term 'consciousness' as used in psychiatry has multiple meanings, embracing the states of wakefulness, vigilance, and reflexive awareness of the self as a person. These different aspects of consciousness—as used in classic psychopathological terminology—are supported by different and largely unrelated brain systems. It is easily comprehensible that the basic states of vigilance and wakefulness confer fitness advantages in terms of survival, for example, through improved ability to escape predators. These functions are maintained by evolutionary ancient structures located in the brainstem, notably the ascending reticular system (Roth 2001). Lesions to this system produce deep coma.

The more 'advanced' capacity to consciously reflect upon the self, that is, the ability to have representations about representations of somatic states, emotions, and thoughts (Damasio 1996), and the ability to experience 'agency' (Frith et al. 2000), is fundamentally different with regard to both its evolutionary history and representation in the brain. Conscious self-reflection can be found—to some extent—in our closest relatives, the great apes, but is clearly much more sophisticated in humans. Apes can recognize themselves in mirrors and they may be able to cognitively represent that other individuals may have plans, goals, and desires (Suddendorf 2013). But probably only humans can entertain multiple mental representations at a time, own and others' (Suddendorf and Whiten 2001). Moreover, the ability to reflect upon one's 'agency' is intimately linked with conscious awareness of the self (Synofzik et al. 2008).

Many pathological symptoms of impaired thought disorder may be conceptualized along these lines, which classic psychopathology has disregarded so far. For example, an impaired ability to represent one's own and others' mental states in terms of thoughts, feelings, and intentions may lead to signs typically conceived of as formal thought disorder if a patient erroneously assumes that his interlocutor may have knowledge about the patient's mental states, though the interlocutor actually has no access to such knowledge (Abu-Akel 1999). This may, therefore, appear as incoherence or derailment (Frith 1992). Moreover, if a patient is unable to accurately ponder others' intentions and to consider alternative explanations, the patient may hold incorrigible fixed beliefs that others are after him and plan to harm him.

Finally, the inaccurate perception of one's own 'inner speech' may be experienced as external voices giving advice or commenting on one's behaviour (Frith 1992). As described in Chapter 2, a parsimonious explanation why self-reflexive abilities evolved is that they convey an adaptive advantage in response to selection pressures from the social environment (Dunbar 2003a, 2003b).

Orientation in space and time is certainly phylogenetically old and may have evolved independently several times. In birds, for example, seasonal migration is exclusively instinct-bound, as is the ability to store and retrieve food in hibernators. In primates, spatial and chronological orientation represent adaptive properties, because they are similarly indispensable for retrieving valuable food resources that may only seasonally be available (Allman 1999). In contrast to hibernators, however, primates have to learn how to find the most resourceful spots (Suddendorf and Corballis 1997). Here, imitation of the most experienced individuals may be particularly useful to recover energy-rich nutrients.

Orientation in space and time has lead to the evolution of memory systems, among which episodic or autonoetic memory is most advanced in humans.

In addition, it is necessary to have semantic storage capacity for this kind of information. Episodic memory has greatly advanced in primates including humans over evolutionary time (Schwartz and Evans 2001). The adaptive advantage of episodic memory certainly lies in its contribution to future survival. Episodic memory, that is, the cognitive representation of past events as subjective experiences (the term 'autonoetic consciousness' has been used synonymously), is perhaps unique to humans. It may have coevolved with the capacity to represent the mental states of self and others. Loss of orientation and memory has devastating effects, as can be seen in the various forms of dementia. In particular, loss of episodic memory deprives affected individuals of making sense of current and future events in relation to their unique past and they may not be able to lead independent lives.

From a functional point of view, it is also fruitful to classify psychomotor signs according to the evolutionary meaning of their 'normal' equivalents. For example, proskinetic behaviours and echophenomena may be understood as pathological variants of behaviours (in ethological terms called 'vacuum behaviours') normally promoting imitation and learning. On the contrary, negativism and cataleptic signs can be conceptualized as pathologies of assertive behaviour. Motor restlessness and perhaps akathisia represent another class of behaviours that typically occur during motivational conflict (e.g. fight–flight). Such movements indicating ambivalence are called 'displacement activities' (Troisi 2002). A great step forward in this direction has been made by the introduction of coding systems of non-verbal behaviours based on ethological observation (see Afterthought to Chapter 5).

Catatonic signs can be differentiated according to their meaning in social interaction.

At the syndromal level, mood disorders and associated behaviours can be understood as exaggerated (and therefore maladaptive) defence mechanisms. Depression, for example, often occurs in situations associated with intense social stress or conflict, in which the affected individual feels entrapped with no escape (Gilbert et al. 2002). Rumination of negative thoughts and self-devaluation, as well as non-verbal behaviours that signal admission of defeat (submission), can be interpreted as (pathological) variants of strategies of coping with interpersonal stress (Rohde 2001). For example, in the most severe forms of depression, a patient may display catatonic stupor, strongly resembling phylogenetically old behavioural patterns of 'playing dead' or 'freezing' (Moskowitz 2004), which has been found in many animals threatened by predation when flight is impossible (Bracha 2004). Interestingly, in retrospect many patients report states of intense anxiety during catatonic stupor, and a similar mechanism may account for many dissociative signs and symptoms, including altered states of consciousness.

Mood disorders can be understood as dysfunctional (exaggerated) defence mechanisms.

These examples may illustrate the importance of attributing biological (evolved) meaning to cognitive, emotional, and behavioural processes of which signs and symptoms reflect anomalous variants. The multidimensional analysis of psychopathology along these lines may eventually improve our understanding of patients' subjective feelings, complaints, and behaviour, and the significance of categorizing cognition, emotion, and behaviour in the context of humans as essentially social animals.

Afterthought: on the possibility to prevent mental illness

There is no doubt that the best way to ameliorate the impact of psychopathology on subjective well-being and quality of life is to prevent its manifestation. Alleles that contribute to phenotypic variation are so prevalent in any human population that eugenics is not even a theoretical option to reduce the prevalence of psychiatric disorders, let alone a moral one (see also Afterthought to Chapter 1). Fortunately, environmental conditions are much more readily malleable than genetics (even though genetic drift can change population genetics in just a few generations), and are thus a legitimate target for prevention measures. Consequently, the 2004 WHO report identifies primary prevention as the main task for ameliorating the impact of psychiatric disorders on disability-adjusted life years (DALY).

Current knowledge about the causes of psychopathology, however, is mainly based on research in developed countries, and much less is known about the prevalence of psychiatric disorders in developing countries. That the problem is pressing, though, is illustrated by the figure of approximately 450 million people worldwide who currently suffer from psychiatric disorders. It is estimated that by the year 2020 about one-third of a billion people will be affected by depression alone. Currently, five of the ten leading causes of disability and premature death concern psychiatric disorders, and depression will rank number two in 2020. Moreover, it has been shown that psychological distress increases the risk for physical illness, including cardiovascular diseases (World Health Organization 2004).

Two related strategies have been shown effective in improving mental health. Promotion of mental health and prevention of psychiatric disorders are complementary means, in that the former aims to increase psychological well-being, resilience against mental health risks, and improve living and environmental conditions, whereas the latter focuses on the reduction of symptoms, often by using mental health promotion. Ideally, primary prevention reduces the risk of mental health problems at the population level, which is, as a unit, not at a specifically increased risk. By contrast, selective prevention aims to prevent the development of psychiatric disorders in populations at risk, defined by biological, psychological, or social risk factors. Indicated prevention targets individuals at high-risk who have already minimal signs or symptoms of a disorder, or are carriers of biological markers, but who do not meet the criteria for disorder. Thus, to some degree, indicated prevention overlaps with secondary prevention, which aims to reduce prevalence rates of disorders by early detection and treatment of established or diagnosable disorders. Tertiary prevention seeks to reduce disability, relapse, or recurrence of illness and to enhance rehabilitation (World Health Organization 2004).

Any means of prevention of mental disorders or promotion of mental health critically depends on the identification of risk factors and protective factors. Risk factors are defined as those factors that increase the probability of manifestation and the severity or duration of a disorder. By contrast, protective factors of psychopathology are those that increase resilience. These factors often overlap with factors promoting mental health such as self-esteem, positive thinking, problem-solving, and social competence. In a general vein, psychological well-being is mainly threatened by a combination of multiple risk factors and the lack of protective factors. Risk factors for the manifestation of psychopathology can be distinguished on the basis of their specificity. Generic risk factors are non-specific and common to several mental health problems. Disease-specific risks are related to the development of a particular disorder.

Aside from socio-economic risk factors, such as poverty and poor nutrition, or exposure to between-group aggression, including war, displacement, or racial discrimination, individual and family-related risk factors have the greatest impact on psychological well-being. Child neglect and abuse and parental mental illness figure most prominently as non-specific or generic risk factors for psychiatric disorders. Among preventive factors, secure attachment, parental emotional responsivity, and social support represent important mechanisms improving resistance against risk factors. In any event, from an evolutionary point of view, vulnerability to disorder and disease depends on complex interactions between developmental exposures to stress, stress responsivity, and behavioural strategies. From a life-history perspective, stress-related psychological and somatic disorders are trade-offs of biological goals (i.e. survival and reproduction), whereby a reduction in adverse experiences would need to be complemented by the development of alternative life-history strategies that help cope with stress (Ellis and Del Giudice 2014).

For example, studies have shown that adolescent teenage mothers are at high risk of preterm delivery of underweight infants, and also of abusing or maltreating their children. The evolutionary background for this situation has been outlined in detail in Chapter 3. It is at face value that such rearing conditions are probably causally associated with the unpredictability of future prospects from the teenage mother's point of view.

Home-visiting programmes for socially disadvantaged young mothers during pregnancy and infancy of newborns, however, could demonstrate a reduction in emotional and physical abuse of infants, and a reduction in maladaptive behavioural consequences in childhood and adolescence (Olds 2002). Moreover, reduced birth weight could be ameliorated. There was also a reduction in preterm delivery and a significant delay of birth of a second child by 12 months. At follow-up, children of mothers in home-visiting programmes had higher IQ scores compared to controls, fewer drug and alcohol problems, and fewer conflicts with legal authorities, and there was a reduction in number of sexual partners in adolescence, as well as increased employment of mothers (Olds et al. 1997). These encouraging results once again demonstrate that evolutionary propensities are not at all impervious to modification. Rather, these studies convincingly show that young mothers who previously had little expectations about the future may change their strategy towards intensified parental care and emotional availability.

An additional group of individuals that is particularly at enhanced risk of developing mental health problems is children of depressed mothers, facing a 50 percent (non-genetic) risk of developing a depressive disorder before age 20. Moreover, it has been revealed that depressed women, more often than non-depressed women, have relationships with antisocial men (Marmorstein et al. 2004). This reflects a (non-conscious) strategy that is intuitively consistent with the evolutionary developmental scenario that emerges from poor parenting and harsh rearing styles, leading to opportunistic resource extraction in both sexes, and, hence, poor parental care provided for offspring (see Chapter 3). Family disruption or divorce of parents is also associated with an increased risk of teenage pregnancy, early marriage, school drop-out, delinquency, substance use, externalizing and internalizing problems, reduced academic success and social competence, unhappy relationships, divorce, and premature mortality (Del Giudice 2014). Although the risk for a transgenerational non-genetic transfer of psychiatric disorders through shared, or better, recreated environments is high, home-visiting programmes for children of depressed mothers were able to reduce the risk for depression down to 8 percent versus 25 percent in control children after 1 year, and to 21 percent versus 31 percent at 2-year follow-up (Olds 2002).

These promising findings may underscore the need for adapting environmental conditions to the needs of both parents and children to facilitate the emotional availability of caregivers and to promote secure attachment in infants, which, in turn, is one of the strongest protective factors against the risks for psychopathology.

Chapter 5

Psychiatric assessment

Abstract

Clinical assessment of patients and therapeutic interaction relies on the clinician's interpersonal skills. The psychiatric interview serves the purposes to understand signs and symptoms in terms of their (maladaptive) meaning, to ascertain a (preliminary) diagnosis, and to initiate therapy. The clinician's task, therefore, is to simultaneously listen to the patient's subjective report, observe the patient's non-verbal and paraverbal behaviour, and be attentive to his or her own emotional reactions (self-reflection). Specifically, sometimes the non-verbal expressions of behaviour tell more about a patient's inner state than his or her verbal report, simply because the former is less under conscious control. The traditional psychiatric terminology distinguished between cognitive, emotional, and behavioural manifestations of psychopathology. An ethology-based description of non-verbal behaviours according to the meaning of the behavioural unit (eye contact, affiliation, assertiveness, flight, ambivalence, relaxation) is suitable to complement the traditional examination.

Keywords

assessment, therapeutic interaction, non-verbal behaviour, paraverbal behaviour, ethology

5.1 Introductory remarks to psychiatric assessment

The clinical assessment of psychiatric patients is complicated by the fact that, in comparison to other medical disciplines, it almost exclusively relies on the clinician's interpersonal skills. A complete psychiatric assessment is usually a mix of a structured or semistructured interview, an exploration, where the clinician makes use of a more directing approach, and anamnesis, which mostly relies on the patient's subjective report. Generally speaking, the psychiatric interview serves several purposes: to understand signs and symptoms in terms of their (maladaptive) meaning, to ascertain a (preliminary) diagnosis, which includes differential diagnostic

The clinical assessment of psychiatric patients is complicated by the fact that, in comparison with other medical disciplines, it almost exclusively relies on the clinician's interpersonal skills. The psychiatric interview serves to understand the symptoms in terms of their maladaptive meaning, to ascertain a (preliminary) diagnosis, which includes differential diagnostic considerations, and to initiate therapy.

considerations, and to initiate therapy. It is therefore essential to not only focus on the patient's subjective report. Careful observation of the patient's non-verbal ('what is expressed') and paraverbal behaviour ('how something is expressed'), as well as meticulous perception and reflection of one's own responses (both psychological and somatic) to patients' utterances and behaviour are of equal importance. Accordingly, the interviewer has to constantly switch between the role of an empathetic listener and that of a more distant observer. In a sense, the clinician's situation is somewhat similar to an anthropologist's approach when exploring foreign cultures. Anthropologists distinguish between the *emic* and the *etic* view. The *emic* perspective is intrinsic and therefore similar to the clinician's empathizing attitude and role-taking of the patient, whereas the *etic* perspective is analogous to 'objective' (extrinsic) behavioural observation (Calogeras 1973).

With regard to the subjective patient report, it is mandatory to establish good rapport (at least as good as possible) by listening to the patient's complaints with empathy and compassion. The patient should feel accepted in his or her needs, such that a trustful clinician–patient relationship can develop. Even though this is not always easy to achieve, insights from ethology may help to achieve this goal (Grant 1968, 1969). For one, humans are sensitive to dominance hierarchies, such that the interviewer's body language ought not to force the patient into an inappropriately submissive position or provoke increasing hostility in tense patients. Along similar lines, folding one's arms is usually perceived as a sign of rejection and should therefore be avoided. The setting in the consultation office ideally seats both patient and interviewer on a par, without barriers like large desks between them. Chairs should be arranged in an open angle to allow for eye contact, but also to permit gaze diversion in order to prevent situations in which persistent eye contact may be perceived as a threat signal (Ellsworth et al. 1972; McGuire et al. 1981; Schelde and Hertz 1994).

Simultaneous empathetic listening and distanced observation of patients' non-verbal behaviour is one of the most difficult tasks for clinicians. It is essential to pick up discrepancies between a patient's verbal and non-verbal report, which are often indicated by signs of motivational ambivalence.

Non-verbal and paraverbal behaviour comprise facial expression of emotions, gesture, body posture, and prosody. Common elements of non-verbal behaviour include frequency and duration of eye contact, affiliative signals, submission, flight, assertiveness, ambivalence, and relaxation (Grant 1968; Troisi 1999). 'Eye contact' is a significant aspect of social interactions. Usually the frequency of eye contact indicates attention and interpersonal involvement. 'Affiliation' concerns behavioural signals that invite and positively reassure social interaction. Pacifying signals are included in the category of 'submissive behaviour', while 'flight' items indicate cut-off reactions signalling social adversity. 'Assertion' refers to behaviours akin to low levels of aggression and hostility. 'Gestures' are used to emphasize or embody the meaning of

Common elements of non-verbal behaviour include frequency and duration of eye contact, affiliative signals, submission, flight, assertiveness, ambivalence, and relaxation.

spoken language. Motivational ambivalence is often expressed by 'displacement activities' (Tinbergen 1952), which comprise self-oriented behaviours such as fumbling and scratching or locomotion. 'Relaxation' includes behaviours that suggest low levels of emotional arousal (Troisi 1999).

Careful observation of these non-verbal cues may sometimes help identify discrepancies between a patient's verbally given information and his or her non-verbal behaviour (Schelde et al. 1988; Schelde 1998). For example, a patient who after a suicide attempt affirms that he is distanced from any further suicidal ideas may display subtle signs of motivational ambivalence (i.e. 'displacement activities') (Troisi 2002). Because non-verbal behaviour is under less conscious control than verbal report, it is considered more reliable with regard to an individual's emotional state, and subtle non-verbal cues may even help distinguish between deception and truth telling (Troisi 1999; Yu et al. 2014).

Because non-verbal behaviour is under less conscious control than verbal report, it is considered more reliable with regard to an individual's emotional state, and subtle non-verbal cues may even help distinguish between deception and truth telling.

In addition to careful listening and behavioural observation during the psychiatric assessment, it is essential for clinicians to control and monitor their own non-verbal behaviour. Unconsciously expressed negative emotions, such as fear or anger, or other forms of unconscious rejection must be contained. This necessitates continuous monitoring of one's own feelings and attitudes during the assessment, particularly when confronted with hostile or aggressive patients. Anger or rejection on the clinician's side may, however, also arise from patients' (unconscious) deceptive behaviour, which may be part of disorders involving somatization, that is, psychiatric conditions associated with somatic complaints for which no organic cause can be identified (Troisi and McGuire 1990; see Chapter 14).

Clinicians ought to be able to control and monitor their own non-verbal behaviour.

At the end of the assessment, the patient should be given the opportunity to ask questions or express his expectations. Occasionally, patients say something important just before leaving the consultation office, particularly if interpersonal conflicts play a role; this should not escape the clinician's attention.

5.2 **Contents of psychiatric assessment**

The psychiatric examination should start with the identification of patient and informants. This includes the patient's age, sex, marital status, and occupation. The patient should then get the opportunity to state his or her chief complaints. Here it is advisable to use open-ended questions first and to let the patient talk freely, before focusing the talk on the history of the present problem or episode. This comprises onset (acute or insidious) of the most recent episode, presence (or absence) of particular life events, and course of the illness until the day of presentation. The history of past episodes comprises the first life-time signs and symptoms, the number and duration of past illness episodes, the number of hospitalizations, symptom severity, treatment, and response to treatment.

The history of a patient's present illness comprises onset (acute or insidious) of the most recent episode, presence (or absence) of particular life events, and course of the illness until the day of presentation. The personal history provides information about the patient's place of birth, where the patient grew up, and the perceived quality of early relationships with parents or other significant attachment figures.

The personal history provides information about the patient's life history, including place of birth, where the patient grew up, and under what circumstances. Emphasis should be given to the quality of early relationships with parents or other significant attachment figures, and problems with emotion regulation like temper tantrums, anxiety, depression, or delinquency during childhood or adolescence. Information should be obtained regarding important developmental steps, for example, when did the patient learn to walk, to talk, and gain control over excretory functions. In addition, the number of siblings, birth order position, relation with peers during adolescence, first sexual experiences, experiences with illicit drugs, and educational history should be recorded.

The family history concerns information on parents' and siblings' age and occupation, their illness history, particularly psychiatric illnesses in first- and second-degree relatives, and premature deaths of family members, especially suicides or suicide attempts.

The social history contains a summary of the patient's marital status, marital satisfaction, number of children, occupation, income situation, hobbies, and other leisure activities. Note that individual differences in early childhood attachment style are often 'transferred' to significant relationships later in life, including relationships with romantic partners, peer group, and own children (for details see Chapter 3).

Finally, the general medical history should list past surgeries, traumatic injuries, and other serious health problems, including past and present medication, allergic reactions, or other idiosyncrasies. It must never be overlooked that 'organic' medical problems may cause all kinds of psychopathological signs and symptoms.

5.3 Description of psychopathological signs and symptoms

One of the most difficult tasks for psychiatrists is to mould both their observations and the patient's subjective report into a detailed description of psychopathology. The term 'sign' usually refers to observable phenomena, whereas 'symptom' denotes a patient's subjective experience. Many psychiatric conditions can be described as syndromes, that is, groups of signs and symptoms (e.g. a depressive syndrome). Signs and symptoms do not cluster randomly. Rather they group together in a meaningful way, usually expressing extremes of variation of normal cognitions, emotions, and behaviours. For example, panic attacks, phobias, or depressive reactions may be understood as exaggerated defence mechanisms, and craving in substance use disorders may express a dysregulation of the brain's phylogenetically old built-in reward system.

A detailed description of psychopathological signs and symptoms is essential and should at least comprise a preliminary diagnostic evaluation at the syndromal level, suggestions of further diagnostic steps, and treatment recommendations.

A comprehensive psychiatric report is essential to enable the uninformed colleague to get an idea of a patient's cognitive functioning, mood and emotions, and behaviour. It should at least comprise a preliminary diagnostic evaluation at the syndromal level, suggestions of further diagnostic steps, and treatment recommendations. Although not ideal in many respects, a systematic description can be accomplished by using one of the classification schemes such as the Diagnostic and Statistical Manual of Mental Disorders in its current version (DSM-5) and the International Classification of Diseases (ICD-11, in development). Both have been conceptualized as largely atheoretical frameworks to facilitate communication between clinicians from different backgrounds. However, this comes at the cost of saying very little about the causes of mental disorders and functional significance of individual symptoms or syndromes. For example, the distinction between 'reactive' and 'endogenous' depression has been abandoned, and psychodynamic aspects including possible adverse childhood experiences for the development of a particular disorder cannot be coded. Moreover, DSM and ICD seem to suggest clear boundaries between different disorders where in fact continua exist (e.g. between schizophrenia and bipolar disorders). Furthermore, in support of a dimensional view on psychiatric disorders, there is increasing evidence that psychopathological conditions reflect extremes of variation of traits, rather than being categorically distinct from 'normalcy'.

Although not ideal, the classification systems currently in use (DSM-5 and ICD-10) help structure the clinical description of psychiatric disorders.

5.4 Clinical signs and symptoms and psychiatric terminology

The following sections give an overview of the major signs and symptoms of psychiatric conditions. This overview is partly based on the Manual for the Assessment and Documentation of Psychopathology (AMDP) (Guy et al. 1982) and has been reorganized and expanded in the present chapter. The psychopathological categories are traditionally arranged roughly following the (somewhat arbitrary) distinction between cognition, emotion, and behaviour.

5.4.1 Outer appearance

Usually, people dress more or less according to their cultural fashion. They are able to look after their personal appearance and hygiene in an appropriate way.

Bizarre appearance and neglect of personal hygiene: the patient dresses in an unusual or bizarre manner, for example, wearing fantastic costumes or an unkempt hairstyle. Sometimes, patients shave off their hair or parts of their hair. They may grossly neglect personal hygiene and grooming, or clothing may be inappropriate for the present climate conditions.

5.4.2 Consciousness and vigilance

Normal: the patient is awake with sensory functions (cognitive functioning of senses) intact.

Lowered vigilance: a rise in the threshold for all incoming stimuli, decreased responsiveness to environmental contingencies, or reduction of vigilance. Lowered vigilance ranges from decreased clarity—scored 'mild'—through somnolence (moderate), to sopor, pre-coma, and coma (severe and extremely severe). The patient is apathetic, slowed down, and drowsy, and easily awakened in somnolence, but only with great difficulty in sopor.

Clouded consciousness (oneiroid): dream-like state of consciousness characterized by the inability to distinguish between inner and outer experiences. These states can be constant or intermittent (fragmented consciousness).

Narrowed consciousness: constriction of what enters into awareness. Seen with fixation on or fascination with certain experiences. A characteristic of narrowed consciousness is diminished reactivity to external events, that is, shutting oneself off from stimuli.

Expanded consciousness: heightened or intensified awareness of inner and outer events. An experience of expanded awareness is distinct from the usual level of consciousness. Heightened consciousness may occur spontaneously or in endogenous psychoses, for example, in early schizophrenia and mania, but can also be induced by drugs or meditation. States of ecstasy are included here.

5.4.3 **Orientation**

Normal: the patient is oriented in time, place, situation, and person.

Disorientation refers to the inability to differentiate or accurately evaluate the reality of temporal, spatial, and/or personal situations.

Time: lack of awareness of day, month, year, or season. It is not uncommon for patients—or non-patients for that matter—to be imprecise in stating the numerical date, that is, to be 'off' 1 or 2 days from the actual date. Such deviations should be judged leniently.

Place: lack of awareness of one's present location. The patient does not know where he is.

Situation: inability to assess correctly the surroundings and one's place in it, for example, a patient being examined by the doctor.

Self: lack of awareness of one's identity. The patient does not know his name and/or misconstrues his personal history.

5.4.4 **Attention and memory**

Normal: the patient is able to concentrate and pay sustained attention to a focus or activity over an extended period of time.

Attention and memory disturbances are to be rated as objectifiable manifestations—not subjective feelings—of impaired apperception, concentration, and memory.

Impaired apperception: the inability to grasp the meaning and significance of experience or to see the meaningful connections between them; in a broader sense, the inability to integrate new experiences with one's own past experience. Apperception may be inappropriate, slow, or absent.

Poor concentration: the inability to focus on a topic and remain focused; failure to keep one's attention on a specific matter or objective for a reasonable period of time.

Memorization: disturbed immediate memory; the partial or total inability to retain *newly acquired* material for more than 10 min. It may be tested by asking the patient to repeat a series of numbers or sentences, remember objects, etc. after a 10-min delay. Immediate memory impairment may vary from one sense modality to another and is dependent upon the emotional state of the patient or the emotional loading of the material presented.

Retention: reduction or loss of ability to retain or recall previously *learned* material for longer than 10 min, for example, hypomnesia, amnesia. Amnesias are memory gaps limited in content (systematized) or more often in time (localized). They are subdivided into lacunar or global on the basis of completeness, into congrade (simple), retrograde, or anterograde on the basis of their relationship to time, and into transitory or persistent on the basis of their course.

Confabulation: the filling of memory gaps with reports of imagined or supposedly experienced events which the patient regards as real. The content of confabulation for the same memory gap can change continually. This last point is important for differentiation from *pseudologia fantastica*.

Paramnesias: four types of pathological recall are evaluated under this item:

- *Delusional memories*: falsification of memories by delusional thinking. Also includes erroneous memories.
- *False recognitions*: never-experienced recognitions (*déjà-vu*) or unrecognized previous experiences (*jamais-vu*) are rated here. In *déjà-vu* the patient reacts as though everything seen has been seen and experienced before in exactly the same way—down to the last detail. Conversely, *jamais-vu* consists of reacting to everything as though it is seen for the first time; everything is unfamiliar, fresh, or incomprehensible.
- *Ecmnesia*: disturbance of time sense, that is, temporal sequence, in which the past is experienced as present.
- *Hypermnesia*: increased or heightened recall of the details of events.

5.4.5 Form of thought

Normal: the patient's thinking reflects a goal-directed flow of ideas in logical sequence. The patient is able to use and understand the meaning of non-literal or metaphorical speech during conversation.

Formal thought disorders are characterized by a lack of normal flow of ideas or misrepresentation of the actual meaning of spoken language.

Inhibited thinking: experienced by the patient as a slowing-down, irregularity, or cessation in the processing of ideas. The inhibition in speed, content, or goal-directedness cannot be removed, however hard the patient tries. Inhibited thinking is subjectively experienced.

Retarded thinking: slow, laborious flow of thought processes. Continuous delay in expressing thoughts, with almost no progress. The viscosity and torpidity in speech and reactions are observable to the examiner. Retardation must be differentiated from inhibited thinking and perseveration.

Circumstantial thinking: inability to differentiate the essential from the unessential, getting lost in insignificant details without losing track of the question. Circumstantiality may be the result of loss of abstract thinking ability or the result of an inability to omit insignificant details, for example, pedantry.

Perseveration: poverty of ideas. Characterized by shrinking of the thought content and fixation on one or a few themes. The patient has difficulties in switching from one topic to another or returns to a given topic again and again. Constant repetition of a specific content (theme) is the most severe form of restricted thinking.

Stereotyped thinking: persistent repetition of words, phrases, or sentences to the point they become meaningless. Verbigeration, the senseless reiteration of words, is a severe form of verbal stereotypies.

Rumination: endless preoccupation or incessant concern with sometimes unpleasant thoughts not experienced as alien and usually related to a real situation in the patient's life. Do not rate obsessional thinking here.

Pressured thinking: driven or kaleidoscopic thinking. The patient feels himself under great stress from disruptive or constantly recurring thoughts—sometimes sensible, sometimes senseless—which seem to tumble over one another.

Flight of ideas: increased number of ideas with a loosening of internal direction or goal. Ideas flow so rapidly that sentences or thoughts are not completed, because thinking is continuously interrupted by diverse associations, often in the form of clang associations. In contrast to incoherence, the examiner can usually follow the flight of ideas. The acceleration in the flight of ideas is sometimes subjectively perceived as pressured thinking.

Accelerated thinking: abnormally rapid flow of ideas and verbal output; often but not necessarily associated with flight of ideas and logorrhoea.

Tangential thinking: talking past or around the point. Although appearing to understand the question, the patient does not answer directly but brings up another topic or something different in context. Do not rate deliberately misconstrued answers.

Blocking: sudden blocks or interruptions in the flow of the thought process without obvious reason. The patient stops in the middle of a sentence, is silent, and then resumes conversation on another theme. Blocking occurs in states of clear consciousness and must not be confused with interruptions of thinking due to *petit mal*. The blocking is experienced by the patient, who is, however, unaware of any motive(s) behind the breaks or blocks.

Incoherence: thought and consequently speech no longer have understandable connections. What remain are fragmented incomprehensible thoughts, phrases, and sentences arbitrarily thrown together. Thoughts jump from one topic to another. This differs from flight of ideas in that there are no connections whatsoever among the ideas. In the mild form, paralogia, the sentence structure can still remain intact, while in the severe form (paragrammatism), words and syllables are a senseless mixture, as in schizophasia.

Knight's move thinking: largely synonymously used with 'derailment of thought' or 'loosening of associations', which is characterized by a disrupted train of thought without blocking.

Other symptoms of formal thought disorder that may occur in association with incoherence are:

- *Contamination*: fusion of two or more unrelated items.
- *Condensation*: combination of more or less unrelated widely diverse ideas into one.
- *Substitution*: replacement of familiar concepts with unusual but nearly similar ones.

Neologisms: new word- or phrase-building in which the usual language conventions are not observed and which usually cannot be easily understood. Includes paralogisms, that is, semantically unusual use of words.

Concretism: inability to grasp the metaphorical meaning of utterances with a tendency to interpret words or expressions literally.

5.4.6 **Content of thought**

Normal: the patient is able to reflect upon thoughts and ideas and to critically evaluate their plausibility.

Delusions can be defined as a disease-induced failure in reality testing which is maintained on the basis of subjective belief and a priori evidence. A delusion is a contradiction of reality which is not supported by collective beliefs and concepts. The patient feels no need to prove the reality of his delusion since, to him, its correctness (reality) is unequivocally certain. Delusions can be bizarre, that is, implausible, absurd false beliefs, or systematized, that is, assembled into a coherent—albeit irrational—interconnected construct. New delusional perceptions or ideas as well as secondary delusions (delusional elaborations) may be used to produce the system.

Delusional ideas: isolated, irrational, or delusional thoughts which emerge singly or in combination; may be persistent but are unsystematized.

Delusional dynamics: the force or intensity of the affective drive which accompanies the delusion. It is possible to estimate the dynamics by the way in which the delusion is reported. There are many variations, ranging from vivid delusions forcefully narrated and intensely described to monotonous, stiff recitations of usually old delusions reported without affective resonance or productivity. The dynamics are strong when delusional experiences appear on a vivid or intense affective (sometimes parathymic) background with psychomotor activity and increased drive and when the delusional ideas are flowing rapidly and are marked by intense reactions.

Delusion of control (disorders of ego boundary or integrity): these ego disturbances can be fleeting or persistent. A disturbance of ego-identity over the course of time is present when the patient perceives himself as somebody different than he was at an earlier time and questions whether it was him or someone else.

Thought broadcasting: the experience that one's thoughts are not exclusively one's own but are shared by others.

Thought sonorization: hearing one's own thoughts spoken aloud; distinguish from thought broadcasting where one's thoughts can be heard by others.

Thought withdrawal: the experience that thoughts are being removed or pulled out of one's mind. Thought withdrawal should be differentiated from blocking.

Thought insertion: thoughts are externally introduced into one's mind and influence, direct, or impel behaviour.

Other feelings of alien influence: similar to the feeling that one's thoughts are directed by outside forces, the patient believes that other aspects of his being (feelings, strivings, will, behaviour) are being influenced from outside. As a consequence, the patient must say something peculiar, scream, roar, behave in a peculiar way, attack someone, bluster, etc.

Delusions of reference: the conviction that environmental events or objects have a special meaning for the patient. The patient is convinced that events in the surroundings—which, in fact, have nothing to do with him—have a definite significance for him, for example, conversation between others has some reference to him, or a casual eye blink from a passer-by conveys an important message. The patient feels himself to be the focus of observation and attention, and even the most insignificant events are sources of extremely important signals for him. Delusions of reference may occur in an isolated form or as the basis or background for other types of delusions, for example, persecution, grandeur, etc.

A special subtype of delusions of reference comprises the delusional conviction of being loved by a certain person (*erotomania; de Clérambault syndrome*). The patient is convinced that a person of high social status loves him. The patient often harasses this person to make him confess his devotion.

Delusions of jealousy (Othello syndrome): conviction of being deceived or sexually betrayed by a loved one.

Delusions of persecution: conviction that persons or organizations are attempting to do harm to the patient. The patient sees himself as the focus of animosity and feels threatened, offended, insulted, mocked, or derided by others who are striving to take his money, property, health, or even his life. Querulous (litigious) delusions are a special type of persecutory delusion in which the patient struggles for justice because of some supposed judicial injury.

Delusions of grandeur: expansive or fantastic claims of one's abilities or position. The patient is convinced that he is superior to all other people by virtue of his talents, power, abilities, wealth, etc. He believes himself to be most powerful, the ruler of the world, God, or an envoy of God. There may be delusions of distinguished birth or having made great inventions. Religious delusions are included here. The patient may believe he has been sent by or has some special relation with God or has been given a sacred mission to perform in the world.

Delusions of guilt: conviction of having failed in one's duty or having discredited others. The patient believes he has failed in his duty to God or to some higher moral code, or has broken the law or a trust. It can be either an imagined guilt or an extreme exaggeration—due to pathological guilt—of actual errors or failures. The patient feels he is evil, inferior, rejected, or unpardonably damned. The guilt may be related to acts of omission, for example, not taking care of his children, not returning for the doctor's appointment. Frequently, self-accusations are seen, for example, masturbation, perversion, abortion.

Delusions of impoverishment: conviction of having lost one's fortune or livelihood. The themes of these delusions focus on material loss, for example, money, clothes, home, sustenance, job.

Somatic (hypochondriac) delusions: conviction of improbable or impossible physical illness. The patient is convinced that his health is threatened, that he is chronically ill, or that he is about to die. The delusion can also be concerned with specific illnesses, for example, cancer, syphilis, multiple sclerosis, brain tumour or injury, or mental illness.

Nihilistic delusions (Cotard syndrome): conviction that parts of the body or the entire body are dead or that the world is non-existent.

Capgras syndrome: the patient holds the delusional conviction that a person familiar to him, usually a family member, has been replaced by an identical-looking impostor.

Fregoli syndrome: the patient is convinced that a specific person appears in different disguises to persecute or harm him (named after an Italian actor).

Reduplicative paramnesia: the patient is convinced that his environment exists in more than one physical location. Capgras syndrome and Fregoli syndrome together with reduplicative paramnesia are subsumed under the term 'delusional misidentification syndromes'.

Folie à deux (induced psychosis): delusional disorder shared by two or more persons who are emotionally closely related. One has real psychosis (the inducer), while the false belief is shared by another person or persons due to close attachment to the inducer.

5.4.7 **Perception**

Normal: the patient is able to integrate incoming sensory information into psychologically meaningful concepts and to bring them to conscious awareness.

Disorders of perception comprise perceptual experiences in the absence of internal or external stimuli, the misinterpretation of stimuli, or unawareness of missing perceptual input.

Derealization: the experience of one's environment being unreal, strange, or otherwise changed. To the patient, the world appears unfamiliar, peculiar, ghostly, or somehow changed. These feelings of estrangement can be part of a delusional mood. Changes in time perception are included here, as is the loss of vividness of sensory experiences, for example, in depression.

Depersonalization: disturbances of the unity (oneness) of the self in the present or in one's identity in the present period of life. The experience of oneself being unreal, detached, strange, changed, or unidentifiable.

Illusions: distortion or misinterpretation of a real perception or falsified actual perceptions; the presence of a real object (percept) differentiates an illusion from a hallucination.

Pareidolia: a special type of illusion where a random stimulus is mistakenly perceived as having a distinct form, for example, perceiving the image of sheep in clouds.

Hallucinations are perceptual experiences without a corresponding stimulus in the environment. One can hallucinate in all sense modalities and frequently in more than one. The judgement of reality is more or less narrowed or suspended. If the patient is aware of the wrongness of his experiences, these phenomena are called pseudo-hallucinations.

Verbal (phonemic) hallucinations: perception of human voices in the absence of external stimuli. Voices of humanoids are also included, for example, God, Satan, spacemen, leprechauns. There are different degrees of clarity and substance to the voices. The voices may speak directly to the patient or may be experienced (overheard) as conversations between third persons. It is sometimes difficult to differentiate phonemes from thought insertion.

Other auditory hallucinations: these include all non-verbal, non-human auditory hallucinations, for example, animals, birds, trees, and inanimate objects.

Visual hallucinations: visual perceptions without corresponding external stimuli. These range from simple optical phenomena (photomes) to elaborate scenes.

Somatic hallucinations (coenaesthetic): unfounded tactile and somatic perceptions including touch, kinaesthesic, pain, pressure, and thermic phenomena. Many such hallucinations have the character of being produced by external forces, for example, the patient has the feeling of being abused sexually or by electricity or 'rays'. It is not always easy to differentiate bodily hallucinations from other delusional experiences, especially when perceptions of space and motion as well as of internal organs are involved.

Olfactory or gustatory hallucinations: hallucinations of smell or taste often occur together, alternately, or merge with one another.

Delusional perception: a normally perceived event (stimulus) is endowed with abnormal significance—usually related to the self—which it does not objectively possess. A delusional perception is actually a delusional misinterpretation of a real perception.

Delusional perception must be distinguished from illusions. Delusional memories should be rated as paramnesia.

Anosognosia: the patient is unaware of his own illness or denies being ill.

Anton's syndrome: the patient is unaware of his blindness and may attempt to walk, bumping into objects and injuring himself. Anton's syndrome is caused by damage to the visual association cortex.

Synaesthesia: a condition in which two or more bodily senses are coupled: sounds may be perceived as colours, etc.

Palinacousis: persistent perception of an auditory stimulus after the stimulus has ceased to exist.

Palinopsia: persistent visual image after the stimulus has gone.

5.4.8 **Emotion**

Emotions can be defined as complex spontaneously arising mental states that are associated with physiological changes. The term 'affect' refers to the observable expression of emotion, which, in contrast to 'mood', is relatively short lasting. 'Mood' denotes a pervasive and sustained emotional state that is subjectively experienced and expressed in facial movements, body language (posture, gait), or prosody.

Normal: the patient's mood is euthymic or appropriate in the context of important life events and can adapt to environmental stimuli. Affective responsiveness is within normal range.

Depressed mood: a negatively tinged affective state characterized by lowered mood and experienced as sadness. It must be present during the evaluation or within the prescribed rating period. Depression covers a wide spectrum of feelings, from sadness, uneasiness, being downcast, loss of pleasure, dullness, dejectedness, and loss of interest to feelings of grief, sorrow, despair, helplessness, and extreme, indescribable inner torment. The expressions of depressive symptomatology vary: crying, looking sad, downcast, or in despair, and looking as though in pain or torment are all expressions of depression.

Hopelessness: pessimistic mood with lack of positive expectations in the future.

Feeling of loss of feeling: feeling that one has lost the ability for emotional resonance; loss or absence of feeling, feeling of emotional emptiness, feeling that one's emotions are 'dead'.

Felt loss of vitality: depression of general bodily feelings subjectively experienced by the patient. Disturbance in the underlying feeling of being alive. Loss or reduction in energy, liveliness, and vigour. Also included are the general feelings of fatigue, weakness, bodily discomfort, and lack of 'pep' or animation.

Complaintiveness: expressions of pain and grief through words, mimicry, and gesture. Wailing, weeping, sighing, groaning, and other similar phenomena are seen.

Lamentation—loud and repetitive complaints expressed in a morose way—is also included here.

Feelings of inadequacy: imagined lessened capacity. Non-delusional feeling that one is incompetent, incapable, clumsy, awkward, indecisive, dumb, ignorant, dowdy, etc.

Feelings of guilt: exaggerated remorse for past behaviour, thoughts, or wishes, which, in the patient's eyes, goes against moral or religious tenets.

Feelings of impoverishment: a non-delusional feeling that one does not have the means to sustain one's livelihood.

Inner restlessness: complaints or feelings of psychic unrest. The patient complains spontaneously—or in answer to questions—that he is stirred by and suffers from agitation and tension. Inner restlessness is frequently associated with depressive, fearful, hopeless, and despondent feelings and with manic states, delusional mood, and delusional states with various content.

Euphoria: heightened mood or elevated sense of well-being. Excessive cheerfulness or serenity, reaching to feelings of elation and ecstasy.

Moria (Witzelsucht): flat euphoric mood, characterized by frivolity and the inability to act seriously. Often associated with a lack of foresight and a general indifference.

Dysphoria: a morose, sullen, dissatisfied mood. An ill-humoured, crabby, discordant attitude.

Irritability: undercurrent of anger or aggressiveness. The examiner can sense the imminence of aggressively tinged, affective outbursts even when the patient exhibits a seemingly calm exterior (tense calm).

Exaggerated self-esteem: heightened self-confidence. The patient has a high opinion of one's abilities. Although non-delusional, the patient believes himself to be very unusual, for example, very smart, very strong, very competent, very talented, very powerful, very rich.

Perplexity: mood of uncertainty or puzzlement. The patient is no longer sure of himself, his situation, his surroundings, or his future. He cannot understand what is happening to him, what he is supposed to think, plan, or do. He is unable to come to grips with events or provide himself an overview of them. Objective manifestations of perplexity are a puzzled, strange, or anxiously uncertain facial expression, sometimes restlessness or hesitant immobility, indecisiveness, or searching behaviour.

Blunted affect: observed decrease in emotional responsiveness, for example, emotional indifference, lack of concern, loss of interest.

Ambivalence: coexisting, contradictory conscious feelings which the patient experiences simultaneously and most often as harassing.

Parathymia: paradoxical affect. Inappropriate emotional expression or response to a situation.

Affective lability: rapid changes in affect. Increases in affective variability in which an affect persists for only a very short period and shows many ups and downs. Take into consideration temperament and cultural tradition.

Affective incontinence: lack or loss of emotional control. Rash outbursts of affect, which are uncontrolled and often of great intensity.

Affective rigidity: reduction or loss of emotional modulation. The patient persists, without modulation or oscillation, in certain moods or affects regardless of the external situation.

Anxiety: fearfulness or apprehensive feelings without specification or objective basis. The symptom should be explored explicitly with the patient and the rating should be based on the subjective experience of and expression by the patient.

Phobias: overwhelming fear, which repeatedly occurs in certain situations or in the presence of certain objects—more often than not resulting in the avoidance of the stimulus. Phobias differ from ordinary anxiety in that the compulsive inevitability of the fear is combined with intellectual insight (full, partial, or transient) of its unreasonableness and with the experience of inner resistance against the fear.

Somatic concerns (hypochondriasis): anxious, fearful perception of one's body. Misgivings of a non-delusional type about the 'reality' of the illness. Objectively unfounded fear of falling ill or being ill. Somatic sensations are perceived fearfully and are given undue attention. Somatic delusions (delusional hypochondriasis) are differentiated by the strength of the conviction of illness. There is some doubt in the non-delusional type despite the fear. Intermediate forms of hypochondriasis range from fear of cancer, syphilis, or heart disease to mortal dread, for example, carcinophobia, syphilophobia, cardiophobia, in which a delusional conviction is present. Non-delusional hypochondriasis can become delusional over time.

Obsessive thoughts: preoccupation with thoughts, which persist against one's will. While obsessive thoughts are not necessarily senseless, their persistence must be regarded as senseless and meaningless. Include obsessive ideas, thoughts, questions, and fears under this category.

Compulsive impulses: persistent drive (urge) to carry out actions against one's will, for example, the urge to control something, to jump out the window, to attack somebody, to curse or utter obscene words, to count or calculate.

Compulsive actions: actions persistently carried out against one's will—usually based on thoughts or impulses. Frequently a ritual or ceremony is carried out, for example, hand washing in a precise, uniform, and repetitive manner. When the ritual has been performed there is often a '*folie de doute*', that is, doubt that the ritual has been performed correctly—thus requiring repetition of the ritual. Repetitiveness, however, can also be seen without such doubt. Pathological laughing or weeping—as release phenomena of inborn expressive movements seen in cerebral disease processes—is not included here.

Alexithymia: the patient is unaware of or unable to describe his emotions or mood.

Anhedonia: the patient withdraws from or is entirely uninterested in any kind of pleasurable activity. He may be unable to savour anything.

Suspiciousness: non-delusional propensity to view the world with anxious uncertainty and mistrust. Disinclination to engage in the usual positive social interactions. A special form is non-delusional jealousy.

Delusional mood: the affect, which forms the background of the delusional experience. An atmosphere of perplexity and involvement in which the world or the self is experienced as strangely changed. The patient very often cannot give details of the content of the changes. The mood consists of unsubstantiated guesses, suppositions, and expectations, which, to the healthy person, have no meaning or relationship. There are a variety of moods associated with the subjective belief in the delusional experience. Most often, it is a sense of awe or mystery about the changes in one's self or in the environment. Other common moods are: apprehension, terror, foreboding, fear, suspiciousness, perplexity, and occasionally elation and self-confidence. Delusions can be mood-congruent or mood-incongruent.

5.4.9 **Motivation and drive**

The terms 'drive' and 'motivation' are often used interchangeably. They refer to the initiation, direction, intensity, and persistence of behaviour. Drive and motivation are usually temporal and dynamic states that are goal-directed and temporarily decrease upon consummatory behaviour.

Normal: short and long-term goals can be pursued with sufficient persistence and energy.

Lack of drive: deficient energy or initiative. Subjectively reported by the patient or observed by the interviewer as sparse motor behaviour and/or decreased initiation of conversation. An example is the quiet, passive patient who cannot be prompted into conversation and who seems to be submerged within himself.

Inhibition of drive: in contrast to lack of drive, inhibition does not refer to the diminution of energy and initiative of the patient but rather to a slowing down of drive. The patient's efforts to overcome the inhibition can be seen in psychomotor activity, perceptual experience, and thought processing.

Abulia: lack of initiative. The patient is unable to act or make decisions independently. It may range from subtle to overwhelming in severity.

Increased drive: increase in activity and initiative as compared to the usual activity level. The behaviour usually remains organized and purposeful.

5.4.10 **Psychomotor activity and expression**

'Psychomotor activity' embraces patterns of behaviour, which are, in part, influenced by psychological processes including impulses, drives, instincts, and cravings. Psychomotor activity is different from 'motility', which is under control of the autonomic nervous system.

Normal: movements carried out by the striated musculature can be brought under voluntary control, are concerted and coordinated, and harmoniously integrated with involuntary or accessory movements. This includes the fluent production of speech.

Movement disorders (including speech production) may be quantitatively or qualitatively different from normalcy. They can either be performed excessively or be diminished, or appear snatchy and irregular. Many symptoms listed below are subsumed under the term 'catatonia', although there is little agreement over what shall be labelled catatonic.

Alogia: poverty of speech, as expressed by monosyllabic replies or use of simple phrases.

Mutism: parsimonious speech or the absence of speech on a psychological basis. The patient generally no longer speaks or, at the most, utters only very few words or syllables. Mutism can be the result of drive deficiency, inhibition, or blocking. It may also be an active, negativistic refusal to make verbal contact.

Logorrhoea: voluble speech; speaking with unquenchable pressure and too excessively for understanding. Depending on its tempo, clarity, internal cohesiveness, logical or meaningful connections, logorrhoea can be quite comprehensible or not at all comprehensible to the interviewer.

Coprolalia: involuntary utterance of socially inappropriate or obscene phrases.

Verbigeration: see also stereotyped thinking. Purposeless repetition of words, phrases, or sentences.

Palilalia: purposeless repetition of the last word or syllable of a sentence or phrase.

Echolalia: the patient repeats word or sentences spoken to him, sometimes in a robotic or mechanical intonation.

Stupor: the patient lacks voluntary movements or movements are extremely slowed down in clear consciousness. He may follow what is going on around him with his gaze.

Negativism: the patient does not respond to instructions of the examiner (passive negativism) or resists attempts to move him and does the opposite to what is asked (active negativism).

Gegenhalten: a special type of negativistic behaviour where the patient opposes passive movements with the same degree of force as applied by the examiner.

Catalepsy: rigidity of the limbs, which often results in abnormal posturing for long periods of time.

Flexibilitas cerea ('waxy flexibility'): a specific kind of resistance felt by the examiner when moving the patient's limbs as if the person were made of wax.

Parakinesia: qualitatively abnormal movements, characterized by a loss of harmony and smoothness.

Stereotypic behaviours: persistent and repetitive purposeless movements or postures, or visiting a certain location without being able to suppress the behaviour. The patient does not show signs of distress (unlike akathisia).

Mannerisms: natural movements and behaviour (gestures, facial expressions, speech) become exaggerated, distorted, posed, and baroque—often in a pronounced playful fashion. Manneristic behaviour also refers to unnatural, pompous, boastful (in the sense of bombastic), studied, affected and artificial, cramped, stylistic, showy, and bizarre behaviour. A manneristic patient behaves in an extraordinarily conspicuous fashion in speech, movement, or dress—compared with his group standards.

Schnauzkrampf: stereotyped grimacing resembling pouting.

Staring: prolonged fixation on a point or gazing at the examiner with eyes wide open, which may be perceived as threatening.

Proskinetic behaviours are characterized by an abnormal tendency to cooperate with the examiner or other persons.

Automatic obedience: the patient cooperates with the examiner in an exaggerated manner. For example, if repeatedly asked to shake hands, the patient is unable to suppress the urge to stretch out his hand again, even if explicitly told not to do so.

Mitgehen, mitmachen: weaker expressions of abnormal cooperation; the patient may perform any movement or be put in any posture on very slight pressure.

Echopraxia, echomimia: the patient imitates movements or facial expression in an automatic way.

Motor restlessness: aimless and purposeless motor activity, which can increase to frenzy (catatonic excitement). The patient is continually in motion, running around (motor restlessness with locomotion), or moving his limbs while remaining in place. Restlessness can also be circumscribed, for example, scratching, hand wringing, tic-like movements.

Conversion or dissociative disturbances: the patient may present with anaesthesia (loss of sensory modalities), blindness, fugue (taking on a new identity with amnesia for the old identity), or paralysis of the limbs (e.g. astasia–abasia). These disturbances are usually conceived of as somatization of repressed conflicts and are not under voluntary control. In striking contrast to the severity of symptoms, the patient is often indifferent about the disability and does not show any signs of serious concern ('*la belle indifference*').

Theatricality: the patient gives the impression that he is exaggerating his situation, difficulties, and disturbances. His behaviour often appears markedly demonstrative.

Vorbeireden: the patient responds to a question by giving obviously and grotesque incorrect answers. For example, 'How many legs does a cow have?'—'Five'. This symptom is typical of Ganser syndrome and was first described in prisoners awaiting trial in order to escape punishment.

Pseudologia fantastica: the patient grossly exaggerates his symptoms or even tells a lie about his symptoms in order to get medical attention. Seen in malingering and Münchhausen's syndrome.

Akathisia: literally the 'inability to sit'. Patients usually describe a feeling of 'inner restlessness' and urge to move, most often affecting the legs, which they try to overcome by constantly moving the legs or walking around.

Rabbit syndrome: rapid rhythmic movements of the upper lip or lips, resembling a rabbit chewing.

5.4.11 **Intellectual functioning**

A deficit in intellectual functioning refers to retardation and/or deterioration of intellectual functions and not to impaired judgement secondary to an acute exogenous reaction or functional psychosis.

5.4.12 **Circadian rhythm**

Oscillations in the patient's condition or behaviour during a 24-hour period should be assessed.

Worse in the morning: condition is worse between 12 midnight and 12 noon.

Worse in the evening: condition is worse between 12 noon and 12 midnight.

Better in the evening: distinct improvement of condition in the evening. Do not score if improvement is only relative when compared to morning low.

5.4.13 **Other terms used in psychiatric assessment**

Social withdrawal: decreased social contact. Judge by the accessibility of the patient in conversation or by the ability to communicate on the ward and/or with people outside the clinic.

Excessive social contact: markedly increased social contact in comparison with earlier behaviour. The patient turns towards many people with an almost total loss of psychological distance, for example, behaviour, which is sticky, clinging, superficial, machinating, stifling, querulous.

Aggressiveness: aggressive tendencies; this refers to the inclination for violence (verbal or physical) either in attacking others or in defending self. Aggressive acts refer to physical assault on persons or surroundings. Both tendency and behaviour must be rated according to severity.

Suicidal tendencies: suicidal intentions, plans, death wishes, preparations, or attempts. Each of these can be rated—from mild to extremely severe.

Loss of desire to live: expression of a desire to discontinue living but without suicidal intent. A positive desire for non-existence. 'I don't want to live, but I don't want to kill myself.' 'I'm trapped in life, but I can't end it.'

Self-mutilation: non-life-threatening, self-inflicted damage, for example, banging the head against the wall, scratching the skin, pricking with a needle, plucking out hair.

Asthenia: the experience of fatigue or debility. The physical draining, which precedes the effort and tends to increase during the course of action. Asthenia is often more marked in the morning and tends to dissipate as the day progresses. The sleep pattern is either unchanged or aggravated. All these attributes distinguish asthenia from physiological fatigue.

Tension: the tonic neuromuscular expression of affect or arousal which the patient seemingly cannot control, that is, relax. Seen objectively by furrowed brow, clenched fists, taut musculature, and 'uptight' appearance.

Increased libido: the subjective state of sexual excitement as reported by the patient as well as observable genital excitement. Imagination may be the only outlet for gratification if actual consummation is impossible.

Sexual dysfunction: habitual dissatisfaction, impairment, or absence of genital gratification as reported by the patient, for example, ejaculatory or orgiastic dysfunction.

Altered sexuality: include all deviant sexual behaviour, for example, transvestitism, fetishism, zoophilia.

5.4.14 **Insight and judgement**

Lack of feeling ill: the patient denies, spontaneously or upon questioning, that he feels ill. The differentiation between feeling ill psychologically or physically is not relevant.

Lack of insight: the patient is unable to recognize as morbid those experiences or behaviour that his doctor has judged to be due to disease.

Uncooperativeness: negative or oppositional behaviour. Resistance against or refusal of various therapeutic measures and/or against admission to the hospital.

Lack of self-care: the patient is not able to eat or drink by himself, to attend to personal hygiene, or is bedridden. Incontinence of bowels and/or bladder is rated here.

5.4.15 **Culture-bound syndromes**

Amok or mata galap: sudden violent behaviour (first described in Malaysian people) directed towards objects and persons, followed by sleep or stupor. The patient may be amnesic for the state of amok.

Koro: fear or delusional conviction of retraction of the penis into the abdomen with the belief that this will lead to death (mostly prevalent in people of Chinese origin).

Latah, imu: startle-induced disorganized behaviour, hypersuggestibility, automatic obedience, echopraxia, and aggressive behaviour. Latah is mostly seen in women in South-East Asia, whereas the similar syndrome of imu was first described in the indigenous Japanese Ainu people.

Afterthought: what non-verbal behaviour can tell—on the necessity of ethological research in psychiatry

A clinically prevalent problem during taking patients' anamnesis is that their verbal reports can differ in manifold ways from what they express non-verbally. This may be so either due to attempts of patients to consciously withhold important information, for example, about suicidal intents ('I do not want to tell you what is really going on in my mind'), or due to the unavailability of information to the patient's conscious awareness, that is, the patient is unaware of his or her own states of mind in terms of affect and mood, intentions and dispositions, a problem that is also ubiquitous in psychopathological conditions. In such situations the clinician may have only a vague feeling of incongruity of verbal and non-verbal information (referred to as 'praecox feeling'; Rümke 1941; Grube 2006).

For example, patients who intentionally try to hide their real emotions or intentions may be unable to show a genuine smile (the genuine one referred to as 'Duchenne smile'). The Duchenne smile is characterized by the activation of the muscles surrounding the eyes (m. orbicularis oculi), which are not under voluntary control. Thus, an individual trying to mimic a smile (consciously or unconsciously) is less well able to activate the m. orbicularis oculi, and hence displays a 'false' smile (Ekman 2003). It requires a lot of training, however, to uncover such subtleties of non-verbal expressions. As a matter of fact, in psychiatric practice the patients' non-verbal behaviour is utilized too little to confirm a diagnosis or to uncover discrepancies between verbal and non-verbal information, and formal training to recognize subtle non-verbal cues to predict future behaviour has received little attention.

It has been convincingly shown, however, that ethological studies into non-verbal behaviour can reveal crucial additional information about a patient's 'real' state of mind. The ethology of psychiatric populations has been described as a systematic and quantitative study of patients' behaviour in natural or seminatural settings, such as interviews, or behaviour on the ward, for instance, in interactions with other patients or staff. Pathological behaviour is defined as being structurally, temporally, or contextually abnormal and, hence, expressing functional impairment (Geerts and Brüne 2009).

Alterations of non-verbal behaviour in timing, duration, or context have been systematically described in a variety of psychiatric disorders, foremost depression and schizophrenia (fewer ethological studies have been carried out in psychiatric patients with personality disorders). Depression is usually characterized by a low diversity of behaviour and low activity, a paucity of affiliative or socializing behaviour, reduced facial expressions of emotions, yet abundant behavioural elements indicating submission or flight (Pedersen et al. 1988). In agitated depressed patients, there may also be a substantial amount of observable displacement activity.

One of the great advantages of ethological observation of patients' behaviour is its predictive superiority over standard evaluations of the severity of psychopathology by use of rating scales. For example, a subtle increase of behavioural activity in depression at week two has been shown to predict subsequent improvement better than self-ratings of depression, and case reports have illustrated that a decrease of behavioural diversity in depression may indicate relapse at a time at which standard ratings are unable to determine a deterioration of the condition (Schelde et al. 1988). Moreover, depressed patients have been shown to fail to attune or converge with interviewers on expressive behaviours. Usually, interlocutors show an increasing degree of behavioural similarity over the course of social interaction (referred to as convergence or attunement). The more similar the behaviour, the more is social interaction perceived as gratifying. The failure in patients to become more similar in non-verbal behaviour with their interviewers not only predicts short-term outcome of depression, but also has proved to be an indicator for the recurrence of depression in clinically remitted patients (Geerts et al. 2006). Lack of interpersonal convergence in depressed patients also predicts negative personal life events during a 2-year follow-up (Bos et al. 2007). Overall, it has been demonstrated that the analysis of non-verbal behaviour has greater predictive value in terms of response to treatment and relapse than standard rating scales for psychopathology (Bos et al. 2006).

Studies into schizophrenia have similarly shown an overall reduction of facial expressivity, particularly a paucity of upper face movements expressing positive emotions. Patients with schizophrenia also tend to avoid physical proximity to others in 'natural' settings on the ward (McGuire and Polsky 1979, 1983). Paranoid schizophrenia patients may be distinguished from non-paranoid patients by their amount of abnormally persistent gaze (staring) in social interactions, which is usually perceived as a threatening signal. Such effects are largely independent of antipsychotic medication. Unmedicated schizophrenia patients and patients on second-generation antipsychotics can be distinguished from normal controls on the basis of their behavioural repertoire during interviews. Patients use behaviours that invite social interaction less often compared with controls (Troisi 1999; Brüne et al. 2008). By contrast, they display behavioural elements suggestive of flight or motivation conflict more often during interviews.

When comparing patients with depression and patients with schizophrenia directly, it has turned out that depressed patients avoided eye contact with the interviewer more often and displayed more self-touching behaviours than patients with schizophrenia, which disappeared with clinical improvement (Jones and Pansa 1979). Dimic and colleagues (2010) showed that patients with schizophrenia displayed more flight behaviour compared to depressed patients, which was associated with greater symptom severity. A comparison of patients with schizophrenia, depression, and mania revealed distinguishable patterns of behaviour during clinical interviews, however subtle. Patients with mania significantly more often showed gesturing than patients with schizophrenia or depression. Moreover, patients with mania more often showed 'thrust' compared to the other two clinical groups, whereas both manic and depressed patients more often displayed a 'small mouth' compared to schizophrenia patients ('thrust' has been defined as a sharp forward movement of the head towards the interviewer, while 'small mouth' refers to a lip movement, by which the lip corners are brought towards each other so that the mouth looks small, indicating a subtle sign of suppressed aggression) (Troisi, 1999). This finding could underscore the view that depression is associated with issues relating to social rank (Price et al. 2007) and the expression of anger (Fava and Rosenbaum 1999).

As expected, patients' non-verbal behaviour influences the way clinicians rate the severity of psychopathology on standard rating scales. For example, in schizophrenia, affiliation and gesturing correlated inversely with the anergia subscore of the Brief Psychiatric Rating Scale (BPRS). Likewise, the inverse correlation of submission with the total BPRS score, as well as gesturing with the total BPRS score in manic patients suggests that the amount of assertive behaviour is linked with the severity of psychopathological signs and symptoms such as thought disorder, agitation, and hostility (Annen et al. 2012). Patients with BPD have been found to frequently show the facial expression of disgust when talking about themselves (Benecke and Dammann 2004). They also display less affiliative behaviour during clinical interviews, especially when experimentally triggered by the intranasal administration of oxytocin (Brüne et al. 2015). From a psychotherapeutic perspective, non-verbal synchrony of client and therapist's head and body movements during therapeutic sessions has predictive value with regard to (short-term) session outcome as well as (long-term) therapy outcome, which may be exploited in the future with regard to therapy success on a broader scale (Ramseyer and Tschacher 2014).

In summary, ethological studies of patients' non-verbal behaviour can help predict treatment response and relapse. Ethological methodology is therefore perhaps more suitable for treatment studies than clinical standard ratings based on subjective experience. A major disadvantage of ethological observation of non-verbal behaviour is that it is a time-consuming method, usually based on videotaped behaviours that are evaluated in small timeframes. Thus, computer-based ethological analysis of non-verbal behaviour is of little use in everyday clinical practice, but the ability to recognize non-verbal behavioural elements during interactions can be achieved through training, and a standardized scale for rating patients' non-verbal behaviour is direly needed.

Part II

Psychiatric and psychosomatic disorders

Chapter 6

Autism spectrum disorder

Abstract

Autism spectrum disorder (ASD) is characterized by social communication deficits, impaired social interaction, and restricted and stereotyped behaviours and interests. The typical onset is during early childhood. Behaviourally, people with ASD have difficulties in tolerating proximity. Insecure attachment is frequently observed. At the cognitive level, people with ASD have selective difficulties in mentalizing or 'theory of mind', possibly related to a dysfunctional mirror neuron system and alterations of the oxytocin system. Conversely, many with ASD (particularly those formerly diagnosed with Asperger's syndrome) have superior technical skills. It has been hypothesized that the brains of individuals with ASD are skewed to maleness, possibly linked to genomic imprinting of paternal genes. The preservation of genes that predispose to ASD may have undergone sexual selection fostering 'slow' life-history strategies. None of the evolutionary hypotheses on ASD is conclusive so far, but open to empirical testing.

Keywords

autism, communication, mentalizing, mirror neuron system, oxytocin, maleness, genomic imprinting, slow life-history strategy

6.1 Symptomatology and diagnostic criteria

Autism spectrum disorder (ASD) is one of several syndromes that are subsumed under the term 'neurodevelopmental disorders'. Neurodevelopmental disorders typically involve impaired interpersonal, social, academic, or occupational dysfunction and manifest early in development (American Psychiatric Association 2013).

ASD is characterized by a symptom triad comprising communication deficits, impaired social interaction, and restricted and stereotyped behaviours. Onset of the disorder is in early infancy.

ASD is clinically characterized by a symptom triad comprising social communication deficits, impaired social interaction, and restricted and stereotyped behaviours and interests, with onset in early infancy. Social and communicative impairments include a lack of exploration of faces and appreciation of other communicative signals, avoidance of eye contact, inability to monitor other people's gaze direction (Pelphrey et al. 2005) or to form joint attention with others, as well as a profound deficit or developmental delay of the ability to appreciate other persons' mental states in terms of beliefs, desires, knowledge, intentions, and dispositions (Baron-Cohen 1995; Critchley et al. 2000). Individuals with ASD also show a marked lack of empathy and social reciprocity and—in severe cases—even ignore the presence of others. In addition, children with ASD are impaired in their ability to imitate (emulate) observed behaviours and to make use of symbolic play. On the other hand, an obligatory diagnostic feature is that individuals with ASD engage in stereotyped behaviours, sometimes in the form of meaningless mimicking behaviour (echopraxia) or speech (echolalia) of others, where in the case of echolalia even the intonation may be retained.

Deficits in recognizing and processing social signals and in imitation can be profound.

The severity of ASD can vary, from mild forms such as Asperger's syndrome or 'high-functioning autism' (the boundaries of which are vaguely defined) with preserved verbal communication to severe forms (formerly known as Kanner autism) associated with mental retardation (in approximately two-thirds of cases with Kanner autism) or epilepsy (one-third). Intellectual functioning is normal in about 20 percent of ASD subjects. In stark contrast to the severity of social cognitive deficits, people with ASD and normal intellectual functioning may have superior technical intelligence and visual discrimination abilities, and relatives with technical professions may be more prevalent in the families of autistic individuals than in control families. Moreover, some individuals with autism have extraordinary skills in divergent domains such as calendar calculation, music, or drawing. These so-called savants are often intellectually severely impaired.

The severity of autistic symptoms can vary considerably. In Asperger's syndrome verbal communication is preserved, whereas Kanner autism is associated with mental retardation and epilepsy. Autistic individuals with preserved intellectual abilities often have superior technical intelligence or even savant-like skills, which is in stark contrast to their impairments in the social realm.

Even though the symptom triad is considered typical for autism, population-based studies have shown that the three core areas correlate only moderately, and isolated difficulties in one of these areas may occur in children, who, then, do not meet the diagnostic criteria for autism, but may better be diagnosed with one of the other communication disorders (e.g. social (pragmatic) communication disorder).

Behavioural abnormalities in ASD may be recognizable shortly after birth; however, a diagnosis is usually made at age 15–24 months, for example, when a delay in language development becomes evident.

6.2 **Epidemiology**

Autism, narrowly defined, is a rare disorder affecting on average 5.2 per 10,000 population with a relative increase to 7.2/10,000 since 1990 due to changes in case definition and diagnostic sensitivity (Fombonne 1999). ASD is now believed to affect around 1 percent of the population (American Psychiatric Association 2013). Although the worldwide

The prevalence of ASD in the general population is believed to be 1 in 100. The male to female ratio is about 3–4:1.

prevalence rates differ to some extent, cases have been reported from a broad variety of cultural backgrounds. The male to female ratio is about 3–4:1.

6.3 Genetic risk factors

Autism is highly heritable such that the risk of developing the disorder is 30–120 times higher for siblings of autistic children compared to the general population. The concordance rate for monozygotic (MZ) twins is between 40 and 90 percent (around 60 percent if narrow definitional criteria are applied), and for dizygotic (DZ) twins it is between 0 and 10 percent.

Autism is highly heritable. The concordance rate for MZ twins is between 40 and 90 percent. Inheritance is polygenetic, but the exact contribution of individual genes is unknown. Epigenetic factors such as genomic imprinting may also be involved.

Autism is not a disease entity but a syndrome in which 10–20 different alleles are involved (Muhle et al. 2004). There is evidence that genes located on chromosomes 1q, 2q, 3p, 4, 7q, 15q, and 17q and on the sex chromosomes play a role in ASD. The functional significance of these gene loci is only partially known. Of particular interest are alleles on chromosome 7q (Schnellenberg et al. 2006), which are located close to a putative speech and language area (FOXP2), allelic variants of the oxytocin receptor on chromosome 3p (Jacob et al. 2007), cytogenetic abnormalities including duplications of chromosome 15q, and serotonin transporter gene variations on chromosome 17q. In addition, DISC1 ('Disrupted In SChizophrenia'), a gene on chromosome 1q presumably involved in neurogenesis, has been assigned a role in ASD (Kilpinen et al. 2008).

It is as yet unclear whether or not epigenetic factors such as genomic imprinting are involved in the pathogenesis of autism, but theoretical models suggest that paternal or maternal imprinting could lead to an overexpression of male characteristics in the brain (Skuse 2000) and social cognitive impairments, respectively. However, it should be emphasized that twin studies suggest that the three areas of the symptom triad, though highly heritable, at best partially overlap genetically, such that characterizing endophenotypes using biological markers may help clarify the contribution of genes to different symptomatic aspects.

6.4 Environmental risk factors

Specific environmental risk factors for ASD are unknown. The relative risk for developing ASD is increased in individuals with tuberous sclerosis, fragile X syndrome, prenatal rubella, cytomegalovirus infection, or prenatal exposure to toxins or teratogens. However, these factors account for less that 10–15 percent of cases. There is some evidence that higher parental age, low birth weight, and foetal exposure to valproic acid may be associated with a greater prevalence of ASD.

Specific environmental risk factors for autism are unknown.

6.5 Pathophysiological mechanisms

The pathophysiological mechanisms of ASD are only partially understood. There is some evidence that levels of endorphins and BDNF are elevated in individuals with autism, whereas contradictory findings pertaining to serotonin have shown elevated blood levels but reduced availability in the central nervous system. Oxytocin, an important mediator of social cognition, bonding, and sexuality, is downregulated in autism. Apoptosis (programmed and selective cell death) is apparently reduced, which may account for the increased number of small, densely packed neurons in some parts of the autistic brain, which are, however, poorly connected with the rest of the brain. There has been some speculation that some alterations at the neurotransmitter level may be mediated by elevated foetal testosterone or an increased number of androgen receptors in the developing brain, but, as yet, this has not been empirically demonstrated. Similarly, reduced serotonin levels in mothers of autistic children have been related to alterations of brain development and maturation. However, in light of the heterogeneity of autistic disorders, findings are overall inconclusive (Lam et al. 2006).

The pathophysiology of autism is poorly understood. BDNF may be upregulated in the autistic brain, whereas apoptosis is reduced. Oxytocin is downregulated.

Due to the difficulties in imitation and in inferring mental states, it has been hypothesized that the mirror neuron system, which is considered critical for imitation learning and probably contributes to the simulation of other people's states of mind, may be functionally impaired in individuals with autism.

6.6 **Evolutionary synthesis**

Even though ASD are highly heterogeneous in nature (Happé et al. 2006), they seem to selectively affect psychological mechanisms associated with social brain function at the behavioural, cognitive, and emotional level. Ethological observation of autistic children suggests, at least in some milder forms of the disorder, a motivational conflict between approaching a caregiver and avoidance, perhaps due to enhanced timidity and fear (Tinbergen and Tinbergen 1972; Macintosh and Dissanayake 2006). Avoidance of close contact is evident from very early on and makes it difficult for both child and caregiver to establish an affectional bond. Accordingly, insecure attachment styles are found to be more prevalent in autistic children compared to healthy controls (Van Ijzendoorn et al. 2007). At the proximate level, this could be related to alterations of oxytocin and serotonin turnover in the autistic child (Hammock and Young 2006). The response of caregivers to the child's shyness may either facilitate bonding by not forcing the infant into social interaction, or aggravate the situation by repeated attempts to make eye-to-eye contact or to establish physical proximity too forcefully. Parents of autistic children, however, are on average no less sensitive than parents of normally developing children. The problem of forming a stable mother–child dyad may, therefore, be more prominent on the side of the autistic child, and in severe cases of autism an affectionate bond between child and caregiver may perhaps never be established.

Ethological observation of autistic children suggests a motivational conflict between approaching a caregiver and avoidance. Avoidance of close contact makes it difficult for both child and caregiver to establish an affectional bond. Accordingly, insecure attachment styles are more prevalent in autistic children compared to healthy controls.

Autistic school-age children, including those with high-functioning autism and Asperger's syndrome, engage less in social play with their peers and experience more often social isolation. As adults, autistic individuals, even those with high-functioning autism or Asperger's syndrome, still have profound difficulties in establishing close social relationships or intimacy (Asperger 1944). Conversely, it has been reported that people with ASD may have an advantage in threat detection in facial expressions (Krysko and Rutherford 2009) and superior visual search abilities (O'Riordan 2004).

Since the 1980s many studies have consistently shown that autistic individuals have severe problems in understanding thoughts, intentions, feelings, desires, and dispositions of others by making inferences about their mental states (Baron-Cohen et al. 1986; Baron-Cohen 1988; Perner et al. 1989). This deficit in 'theory of mind' or 'mentalizing' is not a direct consequence of other cognitive dysfunction (although accompanied by executive planning deficits and poor reconstruction of autobiographic events), but may reflect a selective impairment of social information-processing including mentalizing, emotion recognition, and face processing (Baron-Cohen 1991, 1997; Baron-Cohen et al. 2001; Buitelaar and van der Wees 1997; Buitelaar, et al. 1999a, 1999b). In line with this, autistic individuals have been found to display difficulties in appreciating social rules and norms such as fairness and reciprocity (Brent et al. 2004; Sally and Hill 2006).

Autism is associated with a selective deficit in social information processing, including deficits in appreciating the mental states of others. Imitation and other developmental steps preceding mentalizing, such as gaze monitoring and shared attention, are dysfunctional in autism, which could be linked to a defective mirror neuron system.

Mentalizing deficits in autism are, however, not directly linked to intelligence. Rather, even in autistic individuals with above-average intelligence and perhaps superior technical and mathematical skills (Wheelwright and Baron-Cohen 2001), the developmental delay in social cognition is profound (Baron-Cohen et al. 1997). Even in mild forms of autism where some basic understanding of other people's minds may develop with increasing developmental age (Ponnet et al. 2004), autism is not a disorder that is simply grown out (Holroyd and Baron-Cohen 1993).

Social cognitive functioning involved in mentalizing emerges in children in distinct developmental steps (see Afterthought to Chapter 2). Impaired mentalizing is, however, not sufficient to explain social aloofness in autism, since the onset of behavioural abnormalities in autism clearly precedes the age at which normally developing children acquire mentalizing abilities. A failure of the mirror neuron system may plausibly link early behavioural abnormalities with a defective mentalizing system in autism (Obermann et al. 2005; Cattaneo et al. 2007).

Abundant evidence from cross-species comparison and research in non-human primates suggests that learning by imitation is linked to the activity of specific neuronal cell populations called mirror neurons. These neurons are named after their conspicuous firing during both observation of a hand movement and performance of the very same movement. Mirror neurons are even active when the outcome of a movement is hidden from observation. They therefore connect complex visual perception with the cognitive process of anticipation. Imitation of behaviour and establishing an association between observed behaviour and performance of the behaviour is not only important for early learning experiences; the capacity for imitation also represents a precursor of mentalizing abilities. Imitating behaviour and simulating mental states have in common the ability to imaginatively take the perspective of another individual. Mentalizing, however, requires additional mechanisms including self–other discrimination and differentiation of reality and appearance. In any event, imitation and other developmental steps preceding mentalizing, such as gaze monitoring and shared attention, are already underdeveloped in autism. Dysfunction of the mirror neuron system may explain both the difficulties in mentalizing or perspective-taking through inhibition and the existence of pathological imitation in the form of echopraxia or echolalia through disinhibition of neuronal activity (Williams et al. 2001).

The assumption of a defective mirror neuron system in autism is further supported by the observation that in autism cortical thickness is reduced in those prefrontal and temporal areas, which putatively contain mirror neurons, which contrasts with the otherwise increased cortical thickness in autism (Hardan et al. 2006). Other brain areas consistently involved in mentalizing are underactive during functional brain imaging, and such abnormal activation patterns include the ACC and paracingulate cortex, which are densely serotonergically innervated, and, given a serotonergic deficit in the prefrontal cortex, perhaps dysfunctionally inhibited in autism (Boddaert and Zilbovicius 2002).

Empathetic perspective-taking and mentalizing, as well as social sensitivity and verbal fluency are probably more advanced in women compared with men, perhaps due to the greater amount of female parental investment. In contrast, mental rotation, spatial orientation, and physical problem solving are, on average, superior in men. The marked (and selective) social cognitive deficit in autism, in contrast to the often preserved or even superior technical understanding, has therefore led to the hypothesis that the autistic brain could be an extreme variation of 'male brain' traits (Skuse 2000; Baron-Cohen et al. 2005), which may develop under control of excessive foetal testosterone, perhaps as a consequence of paternally imprinted genes (Badcock and Crespi 2006).

The observation that the autistic brain could be an extreme of variation of the 'male brain' has led to the hypothesis that the exposure to foetal testosterone is involved in the pathogenesis of autism.

Indirect evidence in support of this hypothesis comes from observations that girls with congenital adrenal hyperplasia display more boyish behaviour and more autism-like traits compared with their unaffected sisters. Foetal testosterone is inversely correlated with the ratio of the second-to-fourth digit length, and such a low ratio is found in autism. Moreover, there is some evidence that onset of puberty is precocious in autistic boys. In normally developing children, the level of foetal testosterone inversely correlates with the amount of eye-to-eye contact, shared attention, speech development, social functioning, and restricted range of interests, which in extreme form would resemble autistic symptoms. It is unclear whether autism is associated with elevated foetal testosterone levels or increased number of androgen receptors in sexually dimorphic brain areas. In any event, anatomical data suggest that autism is associated with brain enlargement, larger size of the amygdalae at birth with relative size declining to subnormal volumes after puberty, increased neuronal density (though poorly connected), and increased white matter volume in the first years of life (Keller et al. 2007).

Conversely, data on intra- and interhemispheric connectivity in autism are contradictory, with findings showing decreased interhemispheric connectivity and reduced intrahemispheric connectivity (Villalobos et al. 2005; Mizuno et al. 2006; Just et al. 2007). Reduced interhemispheric connectivity could, however, explain dysfunction of cognitive processes such as a lack of 'central coherence', that is, the ability to recognize the whole (gestalt) rather than its parts (Happé 1993; Hoy et al. 2004). Consistent with this finding, autistic savants have been proposed to see the world literally, because they lack the normal acquisition of concepts or mental templates, and therefore rely on the perception of details, rather than the gestalt (Snyder and Thomas 1997). This could also partly explain autistic persons' literalness in interpreting spoken language. Such differences also exist—albeit to a much lesser degree—between normal males and females. It is therefore conceivable that differential inheritance or expression of male and female traits is involved in the pathogenesis of autism.

Evolutionary inclusive fitness theory suggests that intragenomic conflict may arise between maternally and paternally inherited genes. Genes from the father are designed to extract more resources from the mother than maternally inherited genes. If, as is the case in genomic imprinting, genes from the other parent are silenced, paternally or maternally derived genes may be overly expressed in the offspring. At this stage, it is speculative that genomic imprinting has a major role in autism. However, the overexpression of male traits, both behaviourally and anatomically, as well as greater size of the placenta, with signs of increased proliferative growth and higher birth weight of children with autism, strongly support the assumption that paternal imprinting is involved at least in a subset of ASD (Crespi and Badcock 2008). Moreover, Angelman syndrome, a disorder caused by overexpression of paternal genes on chromosome 15 (see Chapter 1), is characterized by high prevalence of autistic symptoms, including impaired language acquisition, poor eye contact, and stereotypic behaviours, which may be interpreted as further evidence for a imbalance of gene expression towards paternal inheritance.

Another hypothesis—based on the assumption of genomic imprinting—suggests that genes imprinted from the father or the mother contribute to the phenotypic characteristics of autism.

A somewhat competing hypothesis regarding genomic imprinting in autism comes from studies into Turner's syndrome, which is characterized by a partial or complete deletion of one X chromosome (Skuse et al. 1997). Females with only one X chromosome differ in their social cognitive abilities and executive functioning depending on whether they inherit the X chromosome from their father or mother. If the X chromosome stems from the mother (70 percent of cases), social cognitive impairments and autistic-like features are more prevalent, compared to individuals with Turner's syndrome whose X chromosome is paternally derived. This suggests that there could be a genetic locus on the X chromosome involved in social cognition, which in normal females (46, XX) is expressed only from the paternal X chromosome, whereas the maternally inherited locus is silenced (Donnelly et al. 2000). This could explain not only why females are better at social cognition compared with males in general (because males always inherit their X chromosome from their mothers, such that inactivation of the maternal X chromosome does not take place), but also why males are much more vulnerable to developmental disorders including ASD, and why individuals with Turner's syndrome (45, X0) have more autistic symptoms if carrying a maternally derived X chromosome compared to X0 females with a paternal X chromosome.

Both imprinting hypotheses have received partial empirical support, but neither is probably sufficient to explain all features of the autistic spectrum. It is likely that imprinted genes, be they expressed from maternal or paternal chromosomes, interact with susceptibility loci elsewhere on the genome to produce the actual phenotype. It is therefore conceivable that both imprinting scenarios apply to different subtypes of the autism spectrum, a speculation that may be a target for future research.

Whatever the contribution of genomic imprinting and other genetic factors to ASD might be, there is no conclusive theoretical framework that explains why genes that predispose to ASD are maintained in the gene pool. One possibility is that autism is the extreme of variation of sexually selected genes involved in long-term mating strategies in males. That is, some autistic-like traits are compatible with the idea that individuals with ASD display reduced effort to engage in short-term mating and tend to retain valuable resources akin to a 'slow' life-history strategy (Del Giudice et al. 2010). Another plausible scenario views autistic-like phenotypes as the low-fitness variant of behaviour that evolved to force parents to provide attention, protection, and nurturance. Such 'charming' behaviours could serve as fitness indicators of offspring signalled to parents (Shaner et al. 2008b). Finally, ASD may occur as a trade-off of selection for general (or perhaps technical) intelligence (Ploeger and Galis 2011).

There is no conclusive theoretical framework that explains why genes that predispose to ASD are maintained in the gene pool. One possibility is that autism is the extreme of variation of sexually selected genes involved in long-term mating strategies in males. Another plausible scenario views autistic-like phenotypes as the low-fitness variant of behaviour that evolved to force parents to provide attention, protection, and nurturance.

In light of the heterogeneity of autistic phenotypes (Happé et al. 2006), these hypotheses need not be mutually exclusive and may be open to empirical testing.

6.7 **Differential diagnosis and comorbidity**

The most important differential diagnoses of ASD entail other syndromes in which social communication deficits are diagnostically mandatory, such as Rett syndrome, selective mutism, and language disorders. In addition, ASD may share features with ADHD, stereotypic movement disorder, and schizophrenia. Childhood schizophrenia is rare before age 12 and usually involves delusions and hallucinations, which rarely occur in ASD (Abell and Hare 2005). Mental retardation with behavioural symptoms differs from autism in that subjects are less often socially withdrawn and usually interact with family and peers. Cases of psychosocial deprivation may

The most important differential diagnoses of ASD are childhood schizophrenia and mental retardation. Comorbidity exists with ADHD, GTS, and catatonia. Intellectual disability and structural language disorder are the most frequent comorbidities.

be confused with autism, but these children often rapidly improve in enriched environments, depending on the duration of deprivation and developmental age.

About 70 percent of individuals with ASD have a comorbid psychiatric disorder and 40 percent meet the criteria of two or more comorbid conditions. Intellectual disability and structural language disorder are the most frequent comorbidities (American Psychiatric Association 2013). Other comorbid disorders of ASD comprise ADHD, Gilles-de-la-Tourette syndrome (GTS), and occasionally catatonia. In terms of comorbidity it should be kept in mind that psychiatric disorders are dimensional expressions of traits rather than discrete disease entities. Hence, symptomatic overlap with other disorders can be frequently observed.

6.8 **Course and outcome**

ASD is a chronic disorder with no known spontaneous remission. However, with increasing chronological and developmental age, the severity and nature of social deficits may change. As infants, autistic individuals often show a social aloofness, sometimes completely disregarding other people. This pattern of behaviour may emerge into a passive receptive style of social interaction, with little initiative on the side of the child to make contact. As adolescents and adults, people with ASD may eventually adopt a more active role in social interaction, which, however, appears odd or bizarre. Older individuals, particularly those with milder forms of ASD, may reach a developmental stage at which they acquire a basic understanding of other minds. However, they may still have difficulties in comprehending more subtle states of mind, such as sarcasm or faux-pas situations, in which somebody has said something he or she should not have expressed before a particular person (Baron-Cohen et al. 1999). Even individuals with high-functioning autism or Asperger's syndrome usually retain a self-centred perspective, and in some cases paranoid ideation may occur. IQ above 70 and the presence of language skills are associated with a relatively good prognosis. However, only a minority of subjects with ASD reach a developmental status that enables them to lead independent or at least semi-independent lives.

ASD are chronic with no known spontaneous remission. With increasing chronological and developmental age, the social deficits observed in autism may change. Even in high-functioning autism, difficulties remain in comprehending subtle states of mind, such as sarcasm and faux-pas situations.

6.9 **Treatment**

There is no causal therapy for ASD. Psychoeducational interventions include fostering social interaction and behaviour interventions tailored to the child's individual needs. In addition, social and communication skills training and vocational therapy are important non-pharmacological intervention strategies. Forcing autistic subjects to engage in social interaction has not proven useful, because this rather increases stress responses and social withdrawal. Thus, avoiding overstimulation may be appropriate for children with autism, particularly in light of

There is no causal therapy for autism. Social and communication skills training and vocational therapy are important non-pharmacological intervention strategies. Pharmacological treatment is generally not recommended and reserved for severe behavioural problems.

their problems with sustained attention. Moreover, because of the difficulties of autistic people to make sense of other people's minds, it might be useful to avoid conversation with double meaning, but perhaps also to cautiously educate them that other people have expectations, knowledge, and intentions different from their own.

Family interventions and support should be an integral part of assessment and treatment procedures. Psychotherapy of autism has proven unsuccessful, except for comorbid disorders including depression and anxiety in high-functioning autism and Asperger's syndrome.

Pharmacological treatment is generally not recommended and reserved for severe behavioural problems. There is some evidence that serotonin reuptake inhibitors (SSRI) may be effective in reducing stereotyped and self-injurious behaviours. Hyperaggression and impulsivity may also respond to second-generation antipsychotics or naltrexone (McCracken et al. 2002). Experimental administration of oxytocin has revealed improved affect recognition from speech (prosody) in patients with autism and Asperger's syndrome (Hollander et al. 2007).

Treatment recommendations and other helpful information are provided by the American Academy of Child and Adolescence Psychiatry (AACAP).

Chapter 7

Attention deficit/hyperactivity disorder

Abstract

Attention deficit-/hyperactivity disorder (ADHD) is characterized by inattention, impulsivity, and hyperactivity. It features among the neurodevelopmental disorders with childhood onset. Behaviourally, individuals with ADHD show increased novelty-seeking and risk-taking, suggesting that ADHD reflects a 'fast' life-history strategy. Poor sustained attention and inhibitory control, as well as sensitivity to social reward are typical for ADHD. Accordingly, ADHD people are at risk of consuming illicit drugs, suffering from physical injuries, or engaging in teenage pregnancy. Genes involved in catecholamine turnover that confer risk for ADHD seem to have undergone positive selection, at least in some populations. For example, it is plausible to assume that novelty-seeking and impulsivity may have been associated with reproductive success in migrating hunter-gatherers, whereby these traits may turn out as a disadvantage in 'modern' environments (i.e. evolutionary mismatch).

Keywords

attention deficit, hyperactivity, impulsivity, novelty-seeking, risk-taking, positive selection, evolutionary mismatch

7.1 Symptomatology and diagnostic criteria

Attention deficit/hyperactivity disorder (ADHD) features among the neurodevelopmental disorders. ADHD is a disorder of childhood onset whereby inattention, hyperactivity, and impulsivity clearly exceed the degree that is typical for the child's developmental age (Sagvolden et al. 2005). Inattention involves failure to give close attention to details, to keep attention in tasks over longer periods of time, difficulties in organizing tasks, losing things, forgetfulness, and increased distractibility (Aase and Sagvolden 2006). Children with ADHD often do not seem to listen or follow instructions. Hyperactivity and impulsivity comprise fidgetiness, leaving one's seat in

ADHD is a common disorder of childhood onset, with inattentiveness, hyperactivity, and impulsivity clearly exceeding the degree of typical child development.

inappropriate ways, running about, inability to engage in silent play, talking excessively, and interrupting or intruding on others (American Psychiatric Association 2013). Depending on the leading symptom constellation, a hyperactive/impulsive type can be distinguished from a predominantly inattentive subtype or combined type of ADHD. Individuals with ADHD have usually problems in organizing and planning of behaviour. Inhibitory control of behavioural impulses is often reduced, in many cases associated with the inability to tolerate delay of being rewarded (Ströhle et al. 2008).

ADHD has received increasing clinical attention in recent years, and a diagnosis is usually made at preschool or primary school age, but in some cases a diagnosis is made as late as in adulthood. DSM-5 has relaxed the criterion regarding age at onset, now allowing the emergence of first symptoms prior to age 12 (rather than 7), which may lead to a growing rate of false positives. In any event, as hyperactivity and impulsivity tend to decline over time, and secondary features including personality disorders and other comorbid conditions may obscure the clinical picture, a diagnosis is more difficult to establish in adulthood and essentially requires the verification of continuity of symptoms since childhood in retrospect. A de-novo diagnosis of adult ADHD is not possible.

A diagnosis of ADHD is usually made at preschool or primary school age, but sometimes as late as adulthood. A diagnosis of ADHD in adulthood requires the verification of continuity of symptoms since childhood.

7.2 **Epidemiology**

Recent epidemiological studies suggest that ADHD is present in up to 10 percent of primary school children. More conservative estimates figure around 5 percent, with regional differences and pockets of higher prevalence rates. Differences in prevalence estimates are due, in part, to the choice of informant, clinical awareness, and diagnostic threshold. Self-report figures are usually lower than parent or teacher reports (Scahill and Schwab-Stone 2000; Rowland et al. 2002).

Although the typical symptoms associated with ADHD decrease in severity over time, approximately 60–85 percent of ADHD children still meet diagnostic criteria for the disorder in their teenage years. Moreover, young adults who as children were diagnosed with ADHD have the full syndrome in 2–8 percent of cases; however, subthreshold criteria are present in up to 90 percent, with figures of about 3 percent and 16 percent, if narrow criteria are applied. In adults aged 19–44 years the prevalence of ADHD is about 4 percent of the population. It is therefore clear that the condition does not spontaneously remit after puberty and persists well into adulthood.

ADHD is present in up to 10 percent of primary school children. The typical symptoms associated with ADHD decrease in severity over time. The male to female ratio is estimated at around 2–9:1 in favour of males. However, ADHD, inattentive type, may be at least equally prevalent in girls, but it is more difficult to diagnose.

The male to female ratio is estimated around 2–9:1 in favour of males. However, ADHD, inattentive type, may be at least equally prevalent in girls, but it is more difficult to diagnose (Biedermann et al. 2002, 2004).

7.3 Genetic risk factors

ADHD is a highly heritable polygenetic disorder. The concordance between MZ twins is 60–88 percent according to parent ratings and 39–72 percent according to teacher ratings. By contrast, the concordance rate for DZ twins has been estimated at zero or even negative. Genome scan studies suggest susceptibility markers on chromosomes 4, 5, 6, 8, 11, 16, and 17. Of particular interest—though inconsistently linked to ADHD—are the 10-repeat allelic variant of the dopamine transporter allele (DAT1) on chromosome 5p, the dopamine D4 receptor (DRD4), serotonin transporter and serotonin receptor polymorphisms, and allelic variants of the dopamine-beta-hydroxylase, which converts dopamine into norepinephrine (Laucht et al. 2007).

ADHD is a highly heritable polygenetic disorder with fairly high concordance rates between MZ twins. Allelic variations of genes involved in regulating the dopamine and serotonin turnover in the brain have been proposed to be associated with ADHD.

The dopamine receptor DRD4 is coded by a gene on chromosome 11p and has several polymorphic variants, with a single to up to 11 repeats of a coding section in exon 3, of which the 7-repeat allele has been associated with ADHD susceptibility, but also with the personality trait 'novelty-seeking', OCD, and GTS. The DRD4 receptor also shows high affinity for norepinephrine. However, 50 percent of ADHD children do not have a 7-repeat variant, whereas 20 percent of unaffected individuals do. Polymorphisms of the serotonin transporter gene HTR2A and the serotonin receptor 5-HT1B have (inconsistently) been associated with ADHD, as well as several alpha-adrenergic receptors. Variation of the synaptosomal-associated protein-coding gene (SNAP-25) has also been linked to increased ADHD risk, based on the observation that mouse mutants lacking the gene display marked overactivity. Overall, ADHD is associated with multiple genetic polymorphisms, each of which has a rather small effect size, but with possible additive or epistatic effects.

7.4 Environmental risk factors

Several environmental risk factors such as maternal smoking and alcohol abuse during pregnancy seem to increase the risk for developing ADHD. In addition, perinatal stress, preterm delivery, low birth weight, and traumatic brain injury are associated with increased risk for ADHD. Maternal anxiety during the first half of pregnancy (particularly between the 12th and 22nd week of gestation), which is a sensitive period for brain development (differentiation of the limbic cortex including the anterior cingulate cortex starts around week 12), severe early deprivation, institutional rearing, child maltreatment, family conflict, and maternal psychopathology including parental ADHD (a genetic risk factor as well) are associated with a heightened risk for ADHD (van den Berg and Marcoen 2004; Rucklidge et al. 2006).

Pre- and postnatal stressors including maternal smoking or drinking during pregnancy, negative affect during the first trimester, institutional rearing, child maltreatment, and parental ADHD increase the risk for ADHD.

7.5 Pathophysiological mechanisms

ADHD is a syndrome in which dopamine and norepinephrine deficiency contributes most to the cognitive and behavioural phenotype of the syndrome. A lack of dopamine in mesolimbic, mesocortical, and nigrostriatal pathways produces behavioural disinhibition, reduced tolerance for delayed reward, attention deficits, poor executive planning skills, and motor clumsiness (Sagvolden et al. 2005). Reduced availability of dopamine in the synaptic cleft can be in part explained by increased dopamine reuptake in individuals who carry the 10-repeat DAT1 haplotype. However, due to gene–environment interaction, inattention, hyperactivity, and impulsivity are more pronounced in individuals with ADHD carrying the 10-repeat variant if this particular polymorphism is associated with adverse psychosocial circumstances early in life.

Dopamine and norepinephrine deficiency contributes most to the cognitive and behavioural phenotype of the syndrome. Due to gene–environment interaction, inattention, hyperactivity, and impulsivity are more pronounced in individuals with ADHD carrying the 10-repeat variant if this particular polymorphism is associated with adverse psychosocial circumstances early in life. Moreover, the DRD4 7-repeat allele of the dopamine receptor family producing decreased postsynaptic sensitivity to dopamine has been associated with antisocial behaviour and ADHD.

Notably, the risk for ADHD conveyed by the DRD4 7-repeat variant is reduced when parenting is more sensitive to the child's needs.

Season of birth may have an impact on the expression of traits associated with ADHD.

In support of this finding, the phenotypic effect of this variation is pronounced if the mother had consumed alcohol or smoked during pregnancy. Moreover, the DRD4 7-repeat allele of the dopamine receptor family producing decreased postsynaptic sensitivity to dopamine has been associated with antisocial behaviour and ADHD. DRD4 receptors are most abundant in cortical and limbic brain areas, which are critical for cognitive functioning and emotional processes. Notably, the risk for ADHD conveyed by the DRD4 7-repeat variant is reduced when parenting is more sensitive to the child's needs (Bakermans-Kranenburg and van Ijzendoorn 2006; see Chapter 1, section 1.4.2 on 'differential susceptibility').

Curiously, the risk for ADHD is apparently contingent on the season of birth. Children with one copy of the DRD4 7-repeat variant who are born in autumn have a significantly decreased risk for developing ADHD and conduct disorder relative to controls, whereas children with the same genetic make-up who are born in spring have an increased risk for ADHD and conduct disorder (Seeger et al. 2004). This finding could relate to differences in light exposure during pregnancy and mutually inhibitory effects of the melatonin and dopamine systems.

In contrast to the behavioural symptoms of the ADHD spectrum, attention deficits may be more strongly linked with reduced norepinephrine availability in the prefrontal cortex, perhaps as a result of decreased dopamine-beta-hydroxylase enzyme activity. Norepinephrine increases the signal-to-noise ratio and thus improves cognitive functioning. Reduced serotonin levels may also play a role in ADHD, because low serotonergic activity has been linked with poor impulse control and emotional lability, both of which are part of the ADHD phenotype.

Aside from multiple variations at the neurotransmitter level, various anatomical brain abnormalities have been described in ADHD. Treatment-naïve children with ADHD, for example, have reduced cortical grey and white matter volumes, particularly in the frontal and temporal lobes. The caudate nucleus volume is also reduced and normal asymmetry is lacking (in ADHD boys). Cerebellar abnormalities and smaller thickness of the rostral part of the corpus callosum, the latter associated with hyperactivity and impulsivity, have also been found. In addition, functional brain imaging has revealed reduced brain activation in the caudate, frontal lobes, and ACC during task performance requiring inhibitory control.

Children with ADHD have a greater number of anatomical brain abnormalities compared to healthy controls.

7.6 **Evolutionary synthesis**

ADHD is a highly heritable syndrome that involves multiple epistatic genetic effects and important gene–environment correlations (Thapar et al. 2007; see Chapter 1). In many respects, the ADHD phenotype reflects the extreme of variation associated with increased risk-oriented behaviour indicative of a fast life-history strategy (see Chapter 3). Children with ADHD, for example, are at greater risk of serious injuries and accidents than their unaffected counterparts; as adolescents they are more vulnerable to start smoking and to use alcohol or illicit substances. Teenage pregnancy is also increased in individuals with ADHD. Adults with a history of ADHD or persistent ADHD have higher than average rates of antisocial and criminal behaviour compared to healthy control subjects. They are more likely to have employment problems and marital difficulties, as well as extramarital children (McGough et al. 2005).

The ADHD phenotype reflects the extreme of variation of adaptive risk-oriented behaviour. Gene–environment correlations suggest that people with ADHD are more opportunistic with regard to interpersonal relationships, indicative of a fast life-history strategy.

These behavioural tendencies, in conjunction with problems in tolerating delay of rewarding, enhanced impulsivity, impaired sustained attention, and increased distractibility, suggest that people with ADHD seek immediate resource extraction and may be prone to adopt an opportunistic stance in interpersonal relationships. Although this would suggest insecure attachment styles in children with ADHD, there is no unequivocal evidence that attachment patterns in general differ from that of controls.

One possible explanation could be that early infant attachment develops before the ADHD behaviour manifests, and that attachment styles tend to remain stable despite (mildly) adverse home conditions. However, ADHD children recall harsh and punitive parenting styles and lack of emotional availability of the primary caregiver more often compared with non-ADHD subjects. In particular, mothers of ADHD children tend to show more punitive behaviour if their children display guilt or anxiety. Such parental restrictions may in some cases lead to avoidant attachment in children with high temperamental activity, and perhaps perceptual blindness for negative emotions in individuals with ADHD (Finzi-Dottan et al. 2006).

Taking prenatal risk factors such as maternal smoking, substance abuse, and elevated levels of anxiety into account, suggestive of 'foetal programming' (see Afterthought to Chapter 3), patterns of parental behaviour associated with pronounced negative affect support the assumption that children with ADHD are at greater risk of seeing the world as a dangerous and unpredictable place, in which it is adaptive—from a biological point of view—to strive for immediate reward extraction in order to maximize reproductive success, with relatively little parental investment in potential own offspring (i.e. to pursue a 'fast' life-history strategy; see Chapter 3).

In addition, due to the high heritability of ADHD, it is likely that parents of ADHD children—as each shares 50 percent of genes with children—fall within the broader ADHD phenotype. Thus, elevated levels of motor activity and impulsivity in the child may provoke harsh emotional reactions in emotionally labile parents, which, in extreme cases, may create a vicious circle. Moreover, assortative mating (non-random selection of partner; see also Chapter 1) may lead to a constellation in which an emotionally unstable woman is more likely to choose a partner with antisocial personality traits, such that the familial milieu is characterized by highly expressed emotions and antisocial tendencies.

As ADHD children grow older, increased impulsivity and aggression may lead to rejection and ostracism by peers. This may contribute to the persistence of the vicious circle, and, in the long run, induce additional and enduring neurobiological alterations, for example, in the serotonergic system, the function of which is closely linked to an individual's social status. For example, serotonin decreases as a function of status loss and leads to an increase in aggressiveness and solitary behaviour. Interestingly, problems with peers seem to increase in pubertal girls more than in boys, perhaps because aggressiveness and competitive behaviour is generally more accepted among pubescent boys compared to girls.

From an evolutionary point of view, it is easily conceivable that increased motor activity and explorative behaviour, heightened vigilance, and rapid attention shifting can be adaptive behavioural traits, especially in unpredictable environmental conditions (Shelley-Tremblay and Rosen 1996; Baird et al. 2000). However, such behaviours may become maladaptive in more secure conditions, requiring sustained attention and enduring problem-solving behaviour (Jensen et al. 1997). There is evidence that 'novelty-seeking' as a temperamental trait was positively selected at some point during human evolution.

Increased motor activity and explorative behaviour, heightened vigilance, and rapid attention shifting can be adaptive behavioural traits, especially in unpredictable environmental conditions.

Specifically, research into the genetics of dopamine receptors has revealed that the 7-repeat variant of the DRD4 receptor gene evolved quite recently (Wang et al. 2004). The pattern of linkage disequilibrium associated with the 7-repeat allele suggests that this variant occurred about 40,000–50,000 years ago, probably as a rare mutational sequence of at least six events from the ancestral highly conservative 4-repeat allele (Ding et al. 2002).

The 7-repeat variant has been found worldwide, whereas the 2-repeat variant, which is comparably young in origin, is much more prevalent in Asian populations, and may have filled the functional gap of the absent 7-repeat variant. The 2-repeat allele has similar properties at the synaptic membrane as the 7-repeat allele, leading to a reduced postsynaptic dopamine receptor sensitivity, and is assumed to be a recombination product of the 7-repeat and the 4-repeat allele. Overall, the 4-repeat variant is most prevalent worldwide at a rate of 65 percent, the 7-repeat variant is present in about 19 percent, and the 2-repeat allele in roughly 9 percent across populations, which suggests that these allelic variations represent a balanced polymorphism.

Two polymorphisms of the DRD4 receptor gene evolved recently in humans and may have been positively selected, presumably because 'novelty-seeking' has been an adaptive personality trait in ancestral environments.

The large differences in evolutionary age of the different alleles suggest that both the 7-repeat and the 2-repeat variants underwent strong positive selection (Ding et al. 2002; Wang et al. 2004). It is tempting to speculate that the 7-repeat variant coincided with the dispersal of anatomically modern humans out of Africa. The association of the 7-repeat allele with the personality trait 'novelty-seeking' may support the assumption that increased exploration and risk-taking were selected at a time of increased environmental variability and unpredictability, which paid off through enhanced reproductive success, perhaps because these traits were also exposed to positive sexual selection. Sexual selection may be the key mechanism through which both the 7-repeat and 2-repeat may be maintained in populations at relatively low frequencies. Indirect support comes from a study in which the frequency of the 7-repeat variant was higher in nomadic compared to sedentary ethnic groups in Kenya, suggesting a particularly beneficial effect in nomads (Eisenberg et al. 2008).

If this scenario were true, ADHD—as the extreme of variation of 'novelty-seeking' and enhanced risk-taking—would be a prime example for a gene–environment mismatch (see Chapter 4). Contemporary environments, at least in the western world, require improved sustained attention and problem-solving abilities, with impulsivity and enhanced motor activity being less advantageous compared to ancestral times (Barkley et al. 2001). Moreover, rough and tumble play and exploration of novel situations are part of the normal ontogenetic development of children and essential for brain maturation, including prefrontal cortex functioning. Social play has been shown to increase dopamine utilization in animals. Thus it is conceivable that diminished opportunities to act-out basic needs for play in modern environments may contribute to the increase in prevalence of ADHD (Panksepp 1998).

ADHD can be seen as the extreme of variation of 'novelty-seeking' behaviour. Traits associated with ADHD are perhaps no longer adaptively advantageous, because modern environments require sustained attention and reduced impulsivity.

It is important to emphasize that the variations of the DRD4 receptor gene contribute only a minor portion to the genetic vulnerability for ADHD, and deleterious effects may only emerge in combination with other genetic variations, as well as gene–environment correlations. For example, allelic variations of the dopamine-beta-hydroxylase gene that converts dopamine to norepinephrine, which have been found to be involved in the aetiology of ADHD, may only exert deleterious effects in conjunction with neglect or abuse during early infancy.

Typically developing children show sex differences in impulsivity, motor activity, and attention, with boys being more impulsive, aggressive, and overactive, yet performing less well in tasks requiring sustained attention or verbal fluency. These sex differences are most likely the result of sexual selection and differences in parental investment. Good self-regulation abilities, sublimation of own interests and feelings relative to children's interests, and inhibition of immediate responses to environmental stimuli may have been selected in females as a consequence of their greater parental investment in offspring (Bjorklund and Kipp 1996; Stevenson and Williams 2000). Improved inhibitory control in females may, in turn, protect girls, relative to boys, from developing ADHD.

Sex differences in impulsivity, motor activity, and attention may explain why boys are more susceptible to developing ADHD than girls. However, if girls are affected, they may have a greater genetic load or experienced more often adverse early rearing conditions.

Consistent with this assumption is the observation that externalizing behaviours directed against others are more common in males (with and without ADHD), whereas internalizing behaviours (oriented towards oneself) are more prevalent in females. These behavioural tendencies may also reflect sex differences in comorbidity, as well as the syndromal overlap of ADHD with hypomania (Brody 2001). If true that females are better protected from developing ADHD due to differences in evolved cognitive and emotional design, it could follow that *if* girls and women are affected, they may either carry a higher genetic load (i.e. a larger number of 'unfavourable' alleles) and/or be exposed to more adverse environmental conditions during early childhood. In line with this hypothesis, females with ADHD report higher rates of childhood abuse compared to males, whereas to date there is insufficient evidence for a differential genetic load between males and females.

From a therapeutic perspective it is worth noting that ADHD children seem to be particularly susceptible to social reward. While there is a heightened sensitivity to reinforcement contingencies in ADHD in general, inhibitory control has been found to selectively respond better when coupled with a social (as compared to a monetary) incentive (Kohls et al. 2009). This finding may open new non-pharmacological therapeutic avenues for the treatment of ADHD.

In summary, ADHD seems to emerge from complex gene–environment interactions. Evidence suggests that positive selection of genes involved in dopamine turnover occurred in recent human history. These genes promote novelty-seeking, but may also, in conjunction with early adversity (perhaps even prenatal), increase the risk for ADHD. Modern environmental conditions such has high demands on sustained attention and lack of physical exercise also seem to foster the development of ADHD symptoms in vulnerable individuals. Preventive action may therefore focus on the amelioration of environmental factors contributing to ADHD.

7.7 **Differential diagnosis and comorbidity**

Children and adults with ADHD have high rates of comorbid disorders. About 40–80 percent of children and adolescents with ADHD meet the criteria for oppositional defiant disorder (ODD) or conduct disorder (CD), with males being more frequently affected than females (McGough et al. 2005).

ADHD has high comorbidity rates with conduct disorder or oppositional defiant disorder during childhood. In adults with ADHD, the inattentive type is more often associated with depression and anxiety disorders (more common in women), whereas the hyperactive or mixed type is typically associated with bipolar affective disorder or substance abuse (in men).

Twenty-five to thirty-five percent of ADHD patients have learning or language problems. Tic disorder or GTS are often associated with ADHD. Anxiety disorders may occur in up to one-third of ADHD patients, with figures for depressive disorders ranging between 0 and 33 percent. In adult ADHD a substantial number of patients meet the criteria for bipolar affective disorder, substance abuse, or antisocial personality disorder. Comorbidity with BPD may also be found, particularly in women. BPD is, at the same time, an important differential diagnosis, because of a considerable overlap of symptoms, foremost emotional instability and irritability (but not inattention; Philipsen 2006). It may sometimes be a matter of diagnostic convention to diagnose ADHD, BPD, or both in adults, particularly if childhood history is obscure.

The nature of comorbid disorders may vary depending on the ADHD subtype (Miller et al. 2007). The inattentive subtype is more often associated with internalizing problems like social withdrawal or academic difficulties. Thus, comorbidity with anxiety or depression is more common. In contrast, the impulsive-hyperactive type is more often associated with externalizing problems such as aggression, delinquency, and substance abuse, and therefore occurs more often in association with bipolar disorder or antisocial personality disorder. As a rule, externalizing behaviours are more prevalent in males, whereas internalizing problems occur more frequently in females with ADHD.

7.8 **Course and outcome**

Hyperactivity and impulsivity have the tendency to decrease with developmental age. However, only quite recently have clinicians become more aware of the fact that ADHD may persist into adulthood in up to 60 percent of cases, either in the form of subclinical manifestation (such that criteria for the full syndrome are no longer met) or in the disguise of personality disorders, substance abuse, or mood or anxiety disorder secondary to persistent ADHD. These comorbid disorders may even be more relevant for functioning and outcome than the core ADHD symptoms (Rasmussen and Gillberg 2000). It is therefore essential to routinely screen for ADHD in these disorders, because a history or diagnosis of current ADHD may have an impact on treatment regimes and counselling.

ADHD may persist into adulthood in up to 60 percent of cases, either in the form of subclinical manifestation or in the disguise of personality disorders, substance abuse, or mood or anxiety disorder.

7.9 **Treatment**

Treatment with dopamine-releasing stimulants such as methylphenidate is most effective for ADHD (Arnsten 2006). Stimulation of dopamine receptors in the prefrontal cortex follows an inverted U-shaped dose response. Modest levels of dopamine are essential for proper functioning, and the administration of low-dose stimulants can improve attention, inhibitory control, and working memory in both patients with ADHD and healthy subjects. At higher doses, however, task performance declines, similar to excessive stress-related dopamine release. The risk of abuse is apparently low in the normal (low) dose range. In fact, patients with ADHD and comorbid abuse of dopamine-releasing substances such as cocaine can often be stabilized when properly medicated. Overdosing of stimulants, however, can induce stereotyped behaviour, and even proper administration of methylphenidate may be associated with undesirable side-effects (see Chapter 23). Norepinephrine reuptake inhibitors such as atomoxetine are less efficacious compared to classic stimulants, but have been proven useful as an alternative to methylphenidate or amphetamines, particularly in cases with comorbid depression.

Pharmacological treatment with stimulants may ameliorate the symptoms of ADHD and improve attention. The risk of stimulant abuse is considered to be low. Norepinephrine reuptake inhibitors are efficacious particularly in cases with comorbid depression. Non-pharmacological treatment may include psychoeducation, behaviour therapy, or dialectic behaviour therapy.

Non-pharmacological treatments include psychoeducation, self-regulation training, and behaviour therapy. Due to altered reinforcement gradients and perhaps abnormal extinction of learned behaviour, it could be advisable to frequently and immediately reinforce desirable behaviours in ADHD children, whereas the occurrence of undesirable behaviour should be prevented (Gibbins and Weiss 2007). For adults with comorbid personality disorder, dialectic behaviour therapy has been proven useful.

On a critical note, the diagnosis of ADHD has become—to some extent—fashionable. The recent increase in prevalence may thus reflect a change of diagnostic convention. At present, an alarming number (up to 7 percent) of primary school children in the USA receive medication for ADHD. Whether or not this has to do with a genuine increase of the disorder or perhaps with changing expectations of child behaviour remains a contentious issue. In a world with decreasing opportunities for social play (which is fundamentally different from computer games), not only may children be precluded from exercising their motor system, but also they are at risk of experiencing deleterious effects on cognitive functioning, including sustained attention and inhibitory control through insufficient synaptic pruning. This should be considered with regard to programmes to improve preschool and primary school curricula, as well as the education of parents.

Promotion of social play in children may help prevent the development or reduce severity of ADHD.

Useful practice parameters and treatment recommendations for children and adolescents with ADHD have recently been updated by the AACAP.

Chapter 8

Schizophrenia spectrum and other psychotic disorders

Abstract

Schizophrenia spectrum disorders are characterized by the presence of delusions, hallucination, disorganized thinking, motor abnormalities, and/or negative symptoms. Behaviourally, schizophrenia patients have profound difficulties in regulating approach and avoidance, causing social withdrawal or aggressive behaviour. Evolutionary hypotheses of schizophrenia abound, but none covers all phenotypic aspects of the syndrome(s). Genetic risk for schizophrenia is partly conferred by genes that have undergone positive selection, whereby the reproductive advantage compensating for the reduced fecundity is as yet unknown. Environmental risk factors for schizophrenia comprise poverty, migration, and urbanicity, which has given rise to the hypothesis that individuals with schizophrenia are particularly sensitive to the exposure of strangers. In a more general vein, many signs and symptoms associated with schizophrenia can be interpreted from an evolutionary point of view. They pertain to diverse aspects of social life, including cooperation and trust (paranoia), mating (delusional jealousy, erotomania), and social rank (catatonic stupor, mutism).

Keywords

schizophrenia, approach-avoidance behaviour, fecundity, positive selection, cooperation, trust

8.1 Symptomatology and diagnostic criteria

This chapter discusses schizophrenia and other psychotic disorders as well as schizotypal disorder. These disorders are characterized by (1) the presence of delusions, (2) hallucinations, (3) disorganized thinking, (4) disorganized or abnormal motor behaviour, including catatonic features, and (5) negative symptoms such as affective flattening and inappropriate affect. Schizophrenia involves at least two of these five main domains, of which one must be (1), (2), or (3). Schizophrenia is associated with marked occupational or social dysfunction. The symptoms must

The term schizophrenia refers to a group of clinically heterogeneous psychotic disorders characterized by the presence of delusion, hallucinations, disorganized thinking, disorganized or abnormal motor behaviour, including catatonic symptoms and negative symptoms such as affective flattening or inappropriate affect.

have been present for at least 6 months, including a 1-month active phase during which delusions, hallucinations, or disorganization must have been prominent. The Swiss psychiatrist Eugen Bleuler who coined the term 'schizophrenia' described ambivalence, autism, affective flattening, and disordered thinking (loosening of associations) as the core symptoms of this 'group of disorders' (Bleuler 1911).

Depending on the prevailing symptomatology, schizophrenia was divided into several subtypes. The most frequently observed type has been paranoid schizophrenia, with disorganized and catatonic subtypes being less common. If none of these subtypes can be diagnosed, but symptoms of schizophrenia are clearly present, the category 'undifferentiated type' applied. DSM-5 has now dropped this distinction and has instead introduced a dimensional rating of the primary symptoms (American Psychiatric Association 2013).

Traditional subtypes of schizophrenia comprise paranoid schizophrenia, disorganized schizophrenia, catatonic schizophrenia, undifferentiated schizophrenia, and residual schizophrenia.

Schizophreniform disorder pertains to psychotic states that do not fulfil the time criterion for schizophrenia, but which is otherwise identical to schizophrenia, except that a diagnosis of schizophreniform disorder does not require impaired social and occupational functioning (prodromal states may fall into this category). The relationship of schizoaffective disorder and delusional disorder to schizophrenia is a matter of debate. Both belong to the broader phenotypic spectrum of schizophrenia. It is debated whether or not schizophrenia forms a continuum with bipolar disorder, with schizoaffective disorder lying in-between.

Delusional disorder is rare (at least in clinical settings) and has some commonalities with schizophrenia (abnormal content of thought), but also overlaps to some extent with OCD (preoccupation with improbable beliefs). Finally, cycloid psychoses (brief psychotic disorder) are associated with symptoms of the schizophrenia spectrum, but differ in terms of their strictly episodic course and good prognosis. The nosological place of these clinically quite well-defined disorders within the schizophrenia–bipolar disorder spectrum has been controversially discussed.

It should be emphasized that none of the symptoms is pathognomonic or specific to schizophrenia. Disorders within the schizophrenia spectrum are associated with widespread cognitive deficits in different domains. Executive control and social cognition, including the ability to reflect upon one's own and others' states of mind, are most severely, perhaps selectively, compromised (Frith 1992; Langdon et al. 1997; Sarfati and Hardy-Baylé 1999; Brüne 2003b). One hallmark of schizophrenia is impaired social competence, and such deficits are, by and large, best predicted by deficits in social cognition. Moreover, many people with schizophrenia lack insight into the disorder, which is associated with poorer adherence to treatment, higher rates of relapse, and poorer prognosis. Hostility and aggression can also be associated with schizophrenia, particularly in cases with comorbid substance abuse.

Schizophrenia is frequently associated with deficits in executive functioning and social cognition. Attenuated psychotic symptoms can precede the manifestation of the first episode by months or years.

Many symptoms associated with schizophrenia can already be found in preclinical or prodromal stages of the disorder in the form of attenuated psychotic features. Moreover, social withdrawal and other symptoms reminiscent of depression may precede the onset of psychosis.

There is some evidence for a neurodevelopmental subtype of schizophrenia that is characterized by motor abnormalities, such as clumsy movements and other neurological soft-signs since early childhood, by early-onset behavioural problems with peers, and by poor educational performance, which precede manifestation of the first psychotic episode (Murray 1994). This subtype possibly represents one of several endophenotypes that are associated with different biological or behavioural markers (Jablensky 2006).

A neurodevelopmental subtype of schizophrenia is characterized by motor abnormalities, neurological soft-signs, behavioural problems with peers, and poor educational performance since early childhood, which precede the manifestation of the disorder.

8.2 **Epidemiology**

Schizophrenia is thought to have a life-time prevalence of about 1 percent worldwide across populations, with some regional differences, partly depending on diagnostic conventions and the presence or absence of environmental risk factors. This dogma has, however, been challenged, and it now seems more accurate to acknowledge differences in prevalence between populations (McGrath 2006). The average incidence is 0.2–0.6 percent in 1,000. Onset of schizophrenia is typically in late adolescence or young adulthood (Jennen-Steinmetz et al. 1997), whereby the onset in women is, on average, several years later than in men (DeLisi 1997; Leung and Chue 2000; Ruiz et al. 2000), but perhaps not in all populations (Jablensky and Cole 1997; Gangadhar et al. 2002). However, prodromal states with attenuated psychotic symptoms or social withdrawal often precede the manifestation of the first episode by several years. Onset after the fourth decade is unusual and more common among women (Leung and Chue 2000). The male to female ratio is about 1.2:1.

Schizophrenia is thought to have a life-time prevalence of about 1 percent worldwide, though differences in prevalence between populations have been demonstrated. Onset of schizophrenia is typically in late adolescence or young adulthood.

8.3 **Genetic risk factors**

Schizophrenia is a highly heritable polygenetic disorder with concordance rates in MZ twins of about 48 percent. If both parents have schizophrenia the risk for offspring is roughly 46 percent. The concordance rate for DZ twins is 17 percent, and the relative risk for siblings of schizophrenia patients is 9 percent, with further decline of risk for schizophrenia with increasing genetic distance (Owen et al. 2007). Adoption studies point to a greater importance of shared genetic background compared with shared environment (Karlsson 1968; Kety et al. 1994; Tienari et al. 2000), with differences between narrowly

Schizophrenia is a complex polygenetic disorder. Twin and adoption studies have revealed a considerable heritable component. The risk for MZ twins to develop schizophrenia is about 48 percent.

defined phenotypes and broadly defined 'schizophrenia spectrum' disorders (Tienari et al. 2003), whereby those with a high genetic risk are also more susceptible to adverse rearing conditions (Tienari et al. 2004).

Genetic linkage studies have found susceptibility loci for schizophrenia on chromosomes 1p, 1q, 5q, 6p, 6q, 8p, 10p, 11p, 13q, and 22q and a homologous region of the X and Y chromosome, but findings are inconclusive, because replication in different populations has proven difficult (Laval et al. 1998; Kim et al. 1999; Hung et al. 2001; Badner and Gershon 2002; Bailer et al. 2002; Sanders et al. 2008). Moreover, research shows that the genetics of schizophrenia overlap with genetic risk factors for bipolar affective disorder (Berrettini 2000a; Lewis et al. 2003; Craddock et al. 2006; Laursen et al. 2007) and with the genetics of schizotypy (Fanous et al. 2007). A recent large genome-wide association study (GWAS) identified 108 independent loci putatively conveying genetic risk for schizophrenia (Schizophrenia Working Group of the Psychiatric Genomics Consortium 2014).

Linkage studies have revealed multiple susceptibility loci. Genes involved in the regulation of dopamine and serotonin turnover seem to be pathogenetically critical. Moreover, polymorphisms of several neurotrophins have recently received increasing attention, because schizophrenia is now seen as a progressive degenerative disorder. DISC1, TCF4, MBP, and a heat-shock protein (HSPA1B) are important candidate genes involved in schizophrenia.

Candidate genes involved in the pathogenesis of schizophrenia comprise a gene encoding the dopamine D3 receptor (DRD3) and a gene encoding the serotonergic 5-HT2a receptor, but effect sizes are small. However, some polymorphisms of the DRD3 coding gene may be associated with a particularly strong affinity for endogenous dopamine, and, hence, earlier onset of the disorder (Garver et al. 2001; Renou et al. 2007). In addition, there is evidence for genes coding for the DRD2 receptor and genes involved in glutamatergic transmission contributing to the genetic risk for schizophrenia (Schizophrenia Working Group of the Psychiatric Genomics Consortium 2014).

Moreover, polymorphisms of genes encoding neurotrophins, such as NGF and BDNF, as well as neuregulin, dysbindin (dystrobrevin-binding protein 1), and DISC1 (disrupted in schizophrenia) have received increasing attention, particularly because schizophrenia is now seen as a progressive degenerative disorder to which disrupted pathways of the neurotrophins may contribute. Polymorphisms at these gene loci may be involved in abnormal synaptogenesis and pruning, reduced plasticity, compromised neural repair mechanisms, and abnormal cell migration (Feinberg 1983; McGlashan and Hoffman 2000; Sei et al. 2007). Furthermore, allelic variation of the COMT gene has been associated with increased vulnerability of psychosis, particularly in cannabis abusers (see Chapter 1). Finally, the cannabinoid receptor coding gene (CNR1) has been hypothesized to be involved in the pathogenesis of schizophrenia, perhaps via its modulatory effects on dopaminergic and glutamatergic neurotransmission.

Recent research has begun to unravel the epistatic effects of several of these polymorphisms. For example, the COMT genotype seems to interact with neuregulin in complex ways, such that carriers of the val/val allele of the COMT gene showed reduced cell migration in lymphocyte cultures compared to met/met allele carriers with schizophrenia. Moreover, there is evidence that the COMT genotype interacts with other genes with effects on prefrontal cortex function, such as the regulator of G-protein signalling gene (RGS4) (Buckholtz et al. 2007). However, the latest GWAS failed to confirm a role of the COMT gene in schizophrenia (Schizophrenia Working Group of the Psychiatric Genomics Consortium 2014).

In addition, a novel convergent functional genomics approach has identified genes and corroborated previous findings, suggesting that DISC1, transcription factor 4 (TCF4), myelin basic protein (MBP), and a heat-shock protein (HSPA1B) are important candidate genes involved in schizophrenia (Ayalew et al. 2012). While DISC1 has a role in neurodevelopment, and MBP in myelination, TCF4 is expressed in the immune system as well as in neurons, and HSPA1B is involved in stress-response mechanisms. The most significant association found in the latest GWAS concerns a locus on chromosome 6 near a region coding for the major histocompatibility complex (MHC), yet the idea that schizophrenia may be linked to immune function awaits further exploration (Flint and Munafò 2014).

8.4 **Environmental risk factors**

There are a variety of environmental risk factors for schizophrenia, among which maternal influenza during the second trimester of pregnancy and exposure to other viruses is being discussed (Fatemi et al. 2008). In addition, higher paternal age, birth complications, low intelligence, and developmental delay seem to predispose for schizophrenia. Furthermore, schizophrenia occurs apparently more often in urban environments compared with rural, and especially migration markedly increases the risk for schizophrenia in at least the first and second generation. This has strikingly been shown in the indigenous population of Papua New Guinea, where the incidence of schizophrenia sharply increased with greater intensity of contact with western civilization (Torrey et al. 1974). Another risk factor seems to be the widespread use of illicit drugs, particularly cannabis. In recent years the influence of adverse events during early childhood, including physical and emotional abuse, as risk factors for schizophrenia has been shown to be significant, though not specific for schizophrenia (Wahlbeck et al. 2001; Khashan et al. 2008). No evidence exists for a specific rearing style of mothers of individuals who later develop schizophrenia ('schizophrenogenic mother'; Parker 1982).

Maternal influenza during the second trimester of pregnancy, birth complications, urbanicity, migration, use of illicit drugs, and adverse events during early childhood comprise environmental risk factors for schizophrenia.

8.5 **Pathophysiological mechanisms**

Many aspects of the pathophysiology of schizophrenia are still unknown, and the diversity of findings is probably due to the heterogeneity of the schizophrenia spectrum.

The most plausible neurodevelopmental model of schizophrenia, called the 'two-hit hypothesis', posits that, based on a genetic or exogenously acquired vulnerability, neuronal migration is disrupted in the early phase of the second trimester of pregnancy (Lewis and Levitt 2002). Influenza infection of the mother during the late first or early second trimenon, for example, leads to a sevenfold increase in the risk for schizophrenia in offspring. Consistent with the assumption of early maturational disruption of the nervous system, schizophrenia patients have enlarged lateral ventricles (on average), reduced grey matter and neuropil volumes, increased microglial activity indicating inflammatory processes, and multiple alterations at the neurotransmitter levels, among which abnormal levels of dopamine, glutamate, and serotonin (and partly acetylcholine) are thought to produce the manifold symptoms of schizophrenia (Hanson and Gottesman 2005). Reductions of grey matter and connecting tissue seem to selectively (or at least predominantly) affect those brain circuits involved in executive functioning and social cognition, including cortical midline structures of the prefrontal lobe, the ACC, the dorsolateral prefrontal cortex, medial and superior temporal areas, and regions of the temporoparietal junction and infraparietal lobule (Ritter et al. 2004).

The 'two-hit' hypothesis of schizophrenia posits that early neuronal disruption, perhaps caused by intrauterine infection, is followed by a second hit during adolescence, when brain maturation and reorganization start slowing down.

Grey and white matter reduction seems to selectively (or at least predominantly) affect brain circuits involved in executive functioning and social cognition.

Subtle deviations at the neuronal level may also be responsible for a delay of psychomotor development, delayed speech acquisition, and communication problems in childhood (Cannon et al. 2002). Social stressors in adolescence, both positive, such as first romantic love, and negative, among which the use of cannabis is critical, are believed to contribute to the development of prodromal symptoms. This 'second hit' strikes at a critical developmental stage where maturation and reorganization of the nervous system begin to slow down. Emotional overengagement of the family and highly expressed emotions may further contribute to continuously heightened stress levels. Manifestation of first episode usually occurs in early adulthood (earlier in males compared to females). It is assumed that each further episode may exert 'neurotoxic' effects. Insufficient repair mechanisms and reduced plasticity, mediated by alterations of neurotrophins, may induce a neurodegenerative cascade via increased apoptosis that could account for increasing negative symptoms over the course of the illness (Jarskog 2006).

Insufficient repair mechanisms and reduced plasticity, mediated by alterations of neurotrophins, may induce a neurodegenerative cascade in schizophrenia.

At the neurotransmitter level, the most widely acknowledged model suggests a reduced prefrontal inhibition of subcortical dopamine release. Stress normally induces a release of dopamine and norepinephrine in the prefrontal cortex; in schizophrenia, however, prefrontal dopamine is reduced, whereas dopamine is excessively produced in the ventral striatum. Prefrontal reduction of dopamine is thought to be linked to negative symptoms, whereas the overshoot of striatal dopamine is believed to produce positive symptoms, especially under conditions associated with stress-induced phasic dopamine release, which causes aberrant attribution of salience to irrelevant stimuli (Kapur 2003).

The complex regulation of prefrontal and striatal dopamine is probably under neuromodulatory control of GABA and glutamate. Neuregulin and dysbindin are believed to influence the expression of glutamate receptors.

The complex regulation of prefrontal and striatal dopamine is probably under neuromodulatory control of GABAergic and glutamatergic neurotransmission. The excitatory neurotransmitter glutamate is assumed to be reduced in the prefrontal cortex in schizophrenia, and thus cannot exert dampening effects on striatal dopaminergic neurons via GABAergic interneurons in schizophrenia. It is believed that neuregulin and dysbindin influence the expression of glutamate receptors. Substances with antagonistic effects at the glutamatergic NMDA receptor, such as ketamine and memantine, are known to produce psychotic symptoms in healthy subjects. Glutamate is the most widespread excitatory transmitter in the mammalian brain. In the human cortex it is released from cortical pyramidal cells and hippocampal neurons, with extensive projections to the limbic system and basal ganglia. In physiological concentrations, glutamate facilitates cognition and memory formation; non-physiologically high concentrations of glutamate are, however, neurotoxic.

It is likely that many other neurotransmitter substances are, in one way or the other, involved in the pathophysiology of schizophrenia and related disorders. Current research focuses on neurotrophins and their regulatory power of repair mechanisms, and apoptosis via expression of glutamate receptors, which may also open new therapeutic avenues in the future (Schizophrenia Working Group of the Psychiatric Genomics Consortium 2014). Moreover, it seems that the oxytocin system plays a role in schizophrenia, indicated by alterations of basal serum oxytocin levels in schizophrenia (Rubin et al. 2010), and there is a differential role of oxytocin in social approach and avoidance (Brown et al. 2014) and kinship recognition in schizophrenia (Fischer-Shofty et al. 2013).

8.6 **Evolutionary synthesis**

Schizophrenia spectrum disorders comprise so many divergent findings at the clinical–behavioural, neuroanatomical, physiological, and genetic levels that a unifying theory covering all facets of these disorders cannot be expected (Brüne 2004).

One of the hallmarks of schizophrenia is, however, that patients have profound difficulties in social interaction, which often precede the manifestation of the first psychotic episode. Children who as adults develop schizophrenia present not only with neurological soft-signs, but also with increased prevalence of socially abnormal behaviour, including extreme shyness, withdrawal, and aggression towards peers (Crow et al. 1995a-c). These behavioural abnormalities may be paralleled by children's difficulties in understanding other people's behaviour in terms of their mental states.

Ethological research into non-verbal behaviour of schizophrenic patients has revealed that such patients are impaired in their ability to promote social interaction.

Ethological research into non-verbal behaviour of schizophrenic patients has revealed that they are reduced in their ability to promote social interaction (McGuire and Polsky 1979; Pitman et al. 1987a, 1987b; Gaebel 1989; Krause et al. 1989; Troisi et al. 1998, 2007; Gaebel and Wölwer 2004). Schizophrenia patients with pronounced negative symptoms more often display behavioural patterns suggestive of avoidance or 'cutting-off' social contact altogether, whereas others, particularly those with paranoid ideation, may be more likely to show subtle cues signalling threat, such as 'staring' (see also Afterthought to Chapter 5). Interestingly, the non-verbal behaviour of patients with schizophrenia may sometimes appear indistinguishable from behavioural patterns found in depression, which, in a general vein, can be interpreted as correlates of submissive behaviour (Jones and Pansa 1979; Schelde 2000; Brüne et al. 2008; see Chapter 10; see paragraph on catatonia).

Whether or not children who later develop psychosis are more frequently insecurely attached to caregivers is a matter of debate; as adults, the majority of schizophrenia patients report early attachment bonds in a dismissive or unresolved style, which correspond to insecure–avoidant or disorganized attachment (Dozier et al. 1999; Berry et al. 2007). It is, however, conceivable, similar to the case of autism, that disruptive neurodevelopment in the child exerts negative effects on early social interaction, including the formation of an affectional bond between infant and primary caregiver. If such gene–environment correlations play a role early in childhood development of individuals who later become psychotic, additional aversive events to the point of physical or emotional abuse may be more likely to occur in problematic familial environments, and, in turn, may increase vulnerability for psychosis via chronic activation of the hormonal stress axis.

Evolutionary hypotheses regarding schizophrenia have revolved around the apparent paradox of why such devastating disorders exist at all, despite the marked reproductive disadvantage of affected individuals by 30–70 percent, particularly males. Similar to other disorders, it has been proposed that a selective advantage of traits may exist, of which only the extremes of variation are disadvantageous. The number and diversity of evolutionary hypotheses of schizophrenia, however, are unparalleled in other major psychiatric disorders (Brüne 2004; Burns 2004, 2007). These hypotheses suggest some advantages of schizotypal traits in relation to group selection, schizophrenia as a trade-off of human language acquisition or creativity, reduced risk of cancer in relatives of schizophrenic patients, schizophrenia as an extreme negative variation of sexually selected traits, and effects of maternally imprinted genes (Kuttner and Lorincz 1966; Kuttner et al. 1967; Erlenmeyer-Kimling 1968; Carter and Watts 1971; Crow 1988, 1990, 1991, 1995a-c, 1997a-c; Feierman 1994; Price 1998b; Yovel et al. 2000; Boin et al. 2001; Polimeni and Reiss 2002, 2003; Levav et al. 2007; Crespi and Badcock 2008; Kéri 2009; Preti and Wilson 2011). Many of these explanatory approaches are implausible because they implicitly assume that schizophrenia is a homogenous

Evolutionary hypotheses regarding schizophrenia have revolved around the paradox of why such devastating disorders exist despite the marked reproductive disadvantage of affected individuals by 30–70 percent.

'disease entity', or that the risk for schizophrenia is conveyed by a single gene or several genetic polymorphisms with large effect size (Keller and Miller 2006). Both assumptions are currently not supported by empirical evidence.

For example, schizophrenia is probably not the result of a single balanced polymorphism, as was suggested by Huxley et al. (1964), where the risk for schizophrenia (and reduced fecundity of affected individuals) is compensated by advantageous effects within the brain (e.g. benefit for the social group conveyed by schizotypal personality traits in relatives of affected individuals) or outside the brain (e.g. reduced cancer risk, immunological advantages, and increased survival rates in relatives of schizophrenia patients; Jarvik and Deckard 1977; Horrobin 1999; Chiavetto et al. 2002), although genes involved in immune function may play a role (Ayalew et al. 2012). However, there is some evidence for a recent positive selection in the human lineage at several loci, including those coding for DISC1, dysbindin, and neuregulin, of which the exact functional significance is as yet unknown (Bord et al. 2006; Crespi et al. 2007), whereby creativity could be one possible trait that has undergone positive selection (Kéri 2009). Along similar lines, Khaitovich et al. (2008) reported that brain metabolic processes involved in schizophrenia have undergone more recent positive selection compared to brain metabolism that is unaltered in schizophrenia, suggesting that schizophrenia could be a costly 'by-product' of human brain evolution.

Even though evolutionary models suggesting a balanced polymorphism involved in schizophrenia have not been confirmed, a recent study found evidence for positive selection in the human lineage at several loci, including those coding for DISC1, dysbindin, and neuregulin, of which the exact functional significance is as yet unknown, whereby creativity could be one possible trait that has undergone positive selection.

An intensely discussed evolutionary hypothesis of schizophrenia has linked the disorder to a failure to establish functional dominance and language in one or the other hemisphere of the brain. It has been proposed that cerebral dominance is under the control of only a few regulatory genes, and that polymorphisms at one or several of these loci would not only reduce cerebral dominance but also convey a risk for schizophrenia (Crow, 1991, 1995a-c, 1997a-c, 1999; DeLisi 2001). In support of this hypothesis it has been found that children who later develop psychotic disorders are more often ambidextrous and have more language disorders and behavioural disturbances than children who as adults do not become psychotic (Crow et al. 1995a-c, 1996). Moreover, some studies have revealed a reduced cerebral asymmetry in schizophrenic adults compared with healthy subjects, and sex differences in normal asymmetry have been found disrupted in schizophrenia (Crow 1999).

'First rank' symptoms of schizophrenia can be explained by a failure to establish cerebral dominance in schizophrenia.

With regard to the representation of language, it is assumed that under normal conditions the organization of language is segregated such that the spatial or 'logical' component is represented in the non-dominant hemisphere and the temporal or 'phonetic' aspect in the dominant hemisphere, both of which normally interact via the corpus callosum. Accordingly, schizophrenia 'first rank symptoms' could reflect a disruption of the normal transcallosal connection of the two hemispheres (Crow 1998a, 1998b; Mitchell and Crow 2005).

Imprecise coordination of the logical and the phonetic aspect of language could produce symptoms such that an individual perceives his or her own thoughts as alien.

However, there is no unequivocal link of handedness and language, nor has cerebral dominance been successfully linked to oligogenetic effects (DeLisi et al. 2000). Furthermore, this hypothesis does not explain symptoms other than formal thought disorder or delusional beliefs.

In any event, the hypothesis points to the interesting observation that sexual selection could be involved in the pathogenesis of schizophrenia, since age at onset and symptom severity differ between the sexes (DeLisi et al. 1997). Age at onset is usually earlier and symptom severity is greater in men, and both features may be associated with the normally greater asymmetry between the cerebral hemispheres in men, which fails to be established in schizophrenia (Saugstad 1989, 1998, 1999).

Several studies have shown that developmental instability is pronounced in patients with schizophrenia. Normally, genes involved in neurodevelopment help to 'buffer' against the negative effects of multiple mutations, pathogens, and toxins. Variation at these loci may lead to increased 'fluctuating asymmetry' (FA), that is, a near-normally distributed asymmetry of bilateral characters that are on average symmetrical in the population. In schizophrenia, FA is greater in twin pairs concordant for schizophrenia than in discordant pairs, which suggests that greater FA may indicate an imprecise expression of the developmental design due to genetically or environmentally caused developmental disruption. This could explain, for example, why patients with schizophrenia have a greater number of minor physical abnormalities, such as hypertelorism, that could be indicative of an incomplete early cell migration.

Findings of increased fluctuating asymmetry in schizophrenia, cross-cultural differences in age at onset associated with environmental contingencies, as well as deficits in intelligence and social cognition suggest that the schizophrenia phenotype represents the unattractive extreme of variation of sexually selected traits.

Other characteristics putatively associated with a developmental instability in schizophrenia are greater homozygosity of blood alleles, lower premorbid intelligence, reduced cortical volume, and a relative instability of functional and anatomical lateralization of brain functions in schizophrenia. FA is under partial control of sexual selection, as small FA is usually perceived to be more attractive than large FA (Yeo et al. 1999). It could therefore be that, in a very general vein, the broad spectrum of schizophrenia represents the unattractive extreme of variation of sexually selected traits, including FA, language, intelligence, and social cognitive capacities, which may be important for successful courtship behaviour. In fact, many behavioural signs and symptoms and epidemiological findings seem to support this assumption, including the onset of the disorder at a life-time when mating and courtship behaviour normally peaks. Competition for potential mates is pronounced for males compared with females, and the peak of mating effort is at a younger age for males, which could explain the earlier onset of schizophrenia and the more severe course and outcome in men. By contrast, the need to attract suitable mates reaches a second peak in women near the end of their reproductive cycle, which may account for the higher prevalence of erotomanic delusions in women.

If the schizophrenia phenotype represents the low-fitness extreme of sexually selected traits (Shaner et al. 2004), it is also plausible to ask why patients with schizophrenia have lower than average reproduction rates. In line with this hypothesis, it has recently been discovered that age at onset of schizophrenia varies with latitude, in the direction that onset is earlier the closer people live to the equator (Saha et al. 2006; Shaner et al. 2007). One possibility for this finding could be that factors such as increased exposure to pathogens and higher levels of polygyny create pressure towards mating at a younger age. This, in turn, may lead to earlier expression of schizophrenia-associated signs and symptoms produced by a stress-induced dopamine overshoot in the ventral striatum, where the need for intensified (premature) courtship behaviour serves as a non-specific stressor. Such a scenario may also explain why the search for replicable allelic variation involved in the pathogenesis of schizophrenia has been unsuccessful. Since stabilizing selection tends to reduce deleterious mutations, it could be that an individual's higher than average number of fitness-reducing alleles leads to the expression of the schizophrenia phenotype, but that many of these alleles are evolutionarily transient. However, the emergence of new fitness-decreasing mutations may contribute to an equilibrium through which the average prevalence of schizophrenia in a population is maintained. Taken together, the polygenetic inheritance of schizophrenia and the heterogeneity of the disorder can be understood as the negative side of sexually selected fitness-enhancing additive genetic variance (Shaner et al. 2004; Shaner et al. 2008a).

Consistent though not identical with the hypothesis of schizophrenia as a maladaptive extreme of variation of sexually selected traits, some physical and behavioural characteristics indicate that genomic imprinting may play a role in the expression of schizophrenia-associated features. Generally speaking, several characteristics seem to support the assumption that maternal imprinting leads to a pattern of general undergrowth and 'femaleness' of the brain in schizophrenia. This could include reduction of grey matter, reduced lateralization, and overactive mechanisms involved in social cognition—quasi, the opposite of what is found in autism (Crespi and Badcock 2008).

It is as yet unclear whether genomic imprinting is involved in schizophrenia.

These general evolutionary hypotheses of schizophrenia are, in part, flawed by the fact that they hardly cover all clinical aspects of schizophrenia. Thus, in addition to these broad approaches to understanding the heterogeneous nature of the schizophrenia spectrum phenotype, it is useful to analyse individual symptoms based on evolutionary theory as pathological exaggerations of adaptive mechanisms: symptoms that may be attributed to a disturbed interplay between one or more levels of the triune brain (see Chapter 2).

The distinct deficit in social competence in schizophrenia, which often precedes the manifestation of the first psychotic episode, is paralleled by deficits in social cognition, including the recognition of facial emotions, mentalizing, and interpersonal processes involving an understanding of fairness, reciprocity, and trust (Cutting and Murphy 1990; Frith 1992; Langdon et al. 2001; Brüne 2003b, 2005; Brekke et al. 2005; Addington et al. 2006a, 2006b; Agay et al. 2008). This deficit is perhaps triggered by a dopaminergic overstimulation of mesolimbic circuits, which one-sidedly influences the emotional evaluation of social situations. Patients with marked positive symptoms of schizophrenia, for example, tend to be hypervigilant, in particular regarding gaze monitoring of others, and to interpret social cues as threat. They may also overattribute the mental states of others, often in a way that they falsely infer malicious intents of others, clinically expressed as persecutory delusion or delusion of reference.

At symptom level, hypervigilance and overattribution of (malicious) intentions to others (i.e. persecutory delusions) suggest that in schizophrenia mechanisms involved in the evaluation of social threats are overactive.

Excessive mental state attribution may also contribute to some aspects of formal thought disorder. For example, a patient who incorrectly assumes that his or her interlocutor shares his or her knowledge—perhaps due to the patient's fragile ego-boundaries associated with thought transference—may present with loose associations or derailment. Moreover, the tendency in some patients to form too many hypotheses about the mental states of others, while at the same time being unable to choose the most plausible one among these hypotheses, may lead to secondary negative symptoms, perhaps as self-protection from overstimulation and arousal (Salvatore et al. 2007). Consistent with this assumption, patients with schizophrenia fail to correctly attribute mental states 'on the spot', despite their tendency to over-infer mental states. Over the course of the illness, negative symptoms often increase (whereas positive symptoms are still present, but less emotionally salient), accompanied by a decreased potential of the prefrontal cortex to be activated by dopamine. Thus, in chronic schizophrenia, patients evaluate social situations less, and have even more difficulties in inferring mental states of self and others.

It is at present unclear whether this 'mentalizing' deficit in schizophrenia is as selective as it seems to be in autism. There is at least convincing evidence that patients with schizophrenia also have difficulties in integrating contextual and autobiographical information when judging mental states on the basis of observed behaviour.

Another frequent clinical finding in schizophrenia is the striking lack of awareness of illness and insight (Mysore et al. 2007; Tirupati et al. 2007). It would seem that impaired insight is related to patients' difficulties to reflect upon their own states of mind. Patients also frequently experience so-called passivity symptoms, for example, that a patient's own action is perceived as being influenced by an external agent (Frith et al. 2000). Thus it is conceivable that disturbances in the neural network underlying the representation of self and others may be central to many 'core' symptoms associated with schizophrenia.

Lack of awareness and insight reflect abnormalities of recently evolved neuronal circuits involved in the cognitive representation of the self.

The neural basis for the ability of mental state attribution or 'mentalizing' and self-representation is now well known (for details see Afterthought to Chapter 2). It comprises several interconnected regions of the frontal, temporal, and parietal lobes, among which adaptations, perhaps unique to primates, such as the mirror neuron system plays a crucial role in simulating actions and behavioural dispositions of significant others (Torrey 2007). In addition, it has been speculated that the paracingulate sulcus, which separates the ACC from the medial wall of the prefrontal cortex and is inconsistently present in humans, represents an evolutionary novelty involved in social cognitive processes. Furthermore, the infraparietal lobule, which consists of the angular gyrus and the supramarginal gyrus, is probably involved in self–other distinction and representation of the self as acting agent (Torrey 2007). Similar to prefrontal cortical midline structures, the infraparietal lobule myelinates late during ontogeny and is only rudimentary in great apes, suggesting that selection has operated on these particular brain areas involved in self-reflexivity and mental state attribution. These brain regions have been found to be functionally and/or structurally damaged in patients with schizophrenia.

Apart from formal thought disorder, many aspects pertaining to the content of delusional beliefs appear to be tightly linked to scenarios that were selectively important in the evolutionary past of humans. This does certainly not preclude influences on delusion formation from an individual's personal background, but the uniformity of delusional content across cultures suggests that universal patterns relating to survival and reproduction are mirrored in delusions.

For example, Abed and Abbas (2011, 2014) have advanced the hypothesis that schizophrenia may arise from a mismatch between ancestral and current environments, whereby schizophrenia (at least the paranoid type) could be the extreme of variation concerning the intolerance of outgroup membership. In fact, humans have lived, for most of their existence, in small-scale communities based on kin relationships (see Chapter 1), and departure from these conditions may produce heightened vigilance, fear of being assaulted by others, and suspiciousness with regard to others' malicious intentions. Individual vulnerability (conditions of upbringing, genes) may, in combination with recent changes of environmental contingencies (changing roles in society, migration, urbanicity, poverty, and ostracism), produce a psychotic phenotype (Abed and Abbas 2011, 2014). Predictions from this model include higher rates of schizophrenia in males, in people who migrated to other countries or social systems (extending to the second generation), in those who have experienced exclusion from the community (or social defeat; Selten and Cantor-Graee 2005; Taylor et al. 2010), in young people during transition from juvenility to adulthood (i.e. during adolescence), and in those whose social environment has departed most from ancestral conditions. Conversely, social environments that are more kinship-oriented may confer a lower risk for schizophrenia.

Schizophrenia (paranoid type) could be the extreme of variation concerning the intolerance of outgroup membership, which is consistent with environmental risk factors such as migration, urbanicity, poverty, and ostracism.

In support of the outgroup intolerance hypothesis, the content of persecutory delusions has been found to differ between men and women regarding the number and sex of persecutors, as well as regarding the degree of familiarity with the perceived persecutor. Whereas men usually feel more often threatened by groups of strange males, women more often feel persecuted by individuals from their personal environment. Both deluded men and women primarily report fears of being physically injured or assaulted. The rationale for these sex differences in persecutory delusional content could be that the main source of ancestral threats

The contents of delusional beliefs (persecutory, erotomanic, jealous) reflect scenarios that were selectively important in the evolutionary past of humans.

for men in the EEA were indeed strange males from other tribes; by contrast, women, under ancestral conditions, formed the core of the kin-based highly cooperative social group, such that expulsion from the community was a real threat for women living in the EEA (Zolotova and Brüne 2006). This assumption is further supported by data from chimpanzees, our closest living relatives, in which territorial competition and warfare between troops of rivalling males has been reported to be high, perhaps similar to what happened in ancestral human conditions (Wrangham 1999). Moreover, until quite recently, similar scenarios were described in extant hunter-gatherer and horticultural societies, where a substantial number of men (up to 25 percent) and women (up to 13 percent) die premature violent deaths.

Similarly, delusions relating to mating effort and reproduction differ markedly between men and women, and, again, these patterns are highly uniform across cultures. Since parental investment differs between men and women (see Chapter 1), with women investing more than men in potential offspring, the former were selected to be choosier in terms of mate choice. In other words, women are, on average, more likely to seek as potential partners socially high-ranking men who are willing to invest in offspring. In contrast, in established pair-bonds, paternity is less certain than maternity, such that strategies to ensure sexual fidelity were more strongly selected in males.

These divergent selection pressures for males and females are strikingly mirrored in erotomania, the delusional conviction of being loved by another person, and delusional jealousy (Brüne 2003a). Erotomania is much more common in women, who usually choose socially high-standing men (politicians, physicians, actors, sportsmen, etc.) as 'love objects'. Women with erotomania often try to 'convince' their love objects of their own mate value and tend to harass them. This form of following is, however, different from what is found in stalking behaviour. Stalkers are much more often men who pursue their victims, sometimes using violent means (Kienlen et al. 1997). Erotomania is uncommon among stalkers; however, jealousy (both delusional and non-delusional) is frequently involved in stalking (Mullen et al. 1999; Mullen et al. 2001). There is probably some phenomenological overlap between stalking behaviour and delusional jealousy. Delusional jealousy is much more frequently observed in men compared with women. It can be seen as the counterpart to erotomania, aimed at partner retention and securing sexual fidelity (see Chapter 16).

Finally, many signs and symptoms commonly subsumed under the term 'catatonia' can be interpreted as contextually abnormal and exaggerated fear response, fight–flight ambivalence, or behavioural patterns relating to submission or assertive behaviour. Catatonic stupor, for example, strongly resembles a primitive fear reaction, which markedly resembles tonic immobility, seen in many animal species (Moskowitz 2004; Abrams et al. 2009). In tonic immobility, which is most likely elicited by impeding predatory threat where flight is impossible, the animal stops moving to avoid detection. At the same time, it shows heightened alertness, reduced

Catatonic signs and symptoms can be interpreted as contextually abnormal and exaggerated fear response, fight–flight ambivalence, or behavioural patterns relating to submission or assertive behaviour.

vocalization, unfocused gaze, analgesia, and abrupt onset and offset of the behaviour, followed by a ferocious struggle to escape.

Further similarities are found regarding autonomic instability. In tonic immobility, heart rate initially rises and then drops below baseline, which can also be observed in catatonic stupor. The parallels between catatonic stupor and tonic immobility as (primitive) fear responses—represented in the most ancient parts of the triune brain—are also supported by the fact that catatonia responds well to anxiolytic treatment with benzodiazepines and can be worsened by dopamine-depleting drugs. Autonomic instability seems to be a trait marker of schizophrenia, however (Ostermann et al. 2013), possibly caused by a dysfunction of the myelinated vagus (Porges 2007; see also Chapter 2). In addition, patients with catatonic stupor often report in retrospect extreme feelings of overwhelming anxiety during the catatonic state (Northoff 2002a). Catatonic stupor may be preceded or followed by states of extreme hyperactivity or excitement, sometimes associated with assaultive behaviour. However, catatonic excitement is usually poorly coordinated, which may reflect a primitive behavioural escape response in situations in which the source of the perceived danger is hard to recognize.

Other behavioural symptoms labelled as catatonic, such as waxy flexibility, abnormal imitation, and echoing movements, including automatic obedience, can be interpreted as contextually abnormal submissive behaviours, the counterpart of which are represented by behaviours suggestive of exaggerated resistance to requests, such as negativism.

The pathophysiological underpinnings of these inappropriate expressions of fear, fight–flight ambivalence, and communicative behaviours are incompletely understood. Dysfunction of the prefrontal cortex is probably involved, as bilateral lesions to the anterior cingulate cortex produce akinetic mutism (Northoff 2002b). Inhibition of imitative behaviour also implicate the distinction from self and other, such that it is conceivable that dysfunction of the infraparietal lobule contributes to catatonic behaviours. There is also limited evidence to suggest that the mirror neuron system is dysfunctional in schizophrenia, so disinhibition of mirror neurons may plausibly contribute to the occurrence of echo phenomena (Pridmore et al. 2008).

Moreover, there is possibly a lack of inhibitory control of the amygdala via the orbitofrontal cortex, which is reciprocally connected with the limbic system. Little is currently known about the role of the amygdala in catatonia, but given its impact on fear and aggression-related behaviour, and the response of catatonic symptoms to anxiolytic treatment, it can be presumed that this structure is central to the aetiology of catatonia. In addition to the assumption of an inhibitory deficit, it could be that catatonic behaviours can be elicited in individuals who are vulnerable to overstimulation of these brain areas. In this context, it is important to note that many catatonic symptoms are indistinguishable from dissociative symptoms, and that a terminological distinction is more due to convention rather than neurophysiological differences. This notion is essential, because it throws light on the possibility that patients with early traumatization are perhaps more susceptible to develop dissociative/

catatonic states if experiencing retraumatization or other situations associated with unbearably intense fear (Shilo et al. 1995).

Catatonic symptoms are phenomenologically indistinguishable from dissociative symptoms. Accordingly, patients with early traumatization are perhaps more susceptible to developing dissociative/catatonic states if experiencing retraumatization or other situations associated with unbearably intense fear.

Finally, catatonic behaviours (like all symptoms found in schizophrenia) can frequently be observed in other psychiatric disorders, foremost depression and bipolar affective disorder, which is, from an evolutionary point of view, not surprising, given the importance of these behaviours for submission and appeasement strategies.

In summary, evolutionary hypotheses about schizophrenia are abundant, but many are difficult to test. Problems relate to the heterogeneity of the phenotypic picture (Pearlson and Folley 2008), vague boundaries between psychosis and 'normalcy' (van Os et al. 1999, 2000; Verdoux and van Os 2002) which have provoked claims to abandon the concept altogether (Bentall et al. 1988), and uncertain diagnostic validity of 'core' symptoms, as reflected in recent changes from DSM-IV to DSM-5.

It could therefore be more appropriate to study individual symptoms, symptom clusters, or endophenotypes, rather than choosing a broad phenotypic concept for evolutionary enquiries (Brüne 2004). A number of testable hypotheses arise when focusing on paranoia (Abed and Abbas 2011, 2014), which makes perfect sense with regard to epidemiological data and to recent findings concerning the action of neuropeptides in schizophrenia.

Resolving the puzzle of high heritability, high prevalence, and low reproductive fitness necessitates evolutionarily informed research on gene–environment interaction, as well as clarifying the role of immune function in psychosis.

In addition, there is a need for addressing open genetic questions, that is, to resolve the 'Devil's triangle' (Doi et al. 2009) comprising high heritability, high prevalence, and low reproductive fitness; this may include answers to the question why genes conferring increased vulnerability to psychosis have apparently been positively selected during human evolution (Crespi et al. 2007; Kéri 2009), and what the role of immune function might be (Flint and Munafò 2014).

8.7 **Differential diagnosis and comorbidity**

The most significant differential diagnoses of schizophrenia comprise 'organic' psychotic disorders and substance-induced psychosis. The term 'organic' is unfortunate because it suggests that 'endogenous' psychosis is non-organic in origin; however, such a view is obsolete to date. It is probably better to speak of *known* organic causes of psychotic syndromes, among which encephalitis is most important.

'Organic' psychotic disorders such as encephalitis and substance-induced psychosis are important differential diagnoses of schizophrenia. Bipolar affective disorder with psychotic symptoms may be difficult to differentiate from schizophrenia. Depression can comorbidly occur in patients with schizophrenia, and overlaps with negative syndrome schizophrenia. Alcohol and cannabis abuse are frequent in patients with schizophrenia.

Within the psychosis spectrum, bipolar affective disorder with psychotic features (especially mood-incongruent) is sometimes difficult to differentiate from schizophrenia, and in some cases a definite diagnosis can only be made on the basis of longitudinal observation.

A substantial number of patients with schizophrenia have comorbid depression and/or substance abuse. These conditions deserve special attention because they may complicate treatment and outcome. Depression is sometimes difficult to distinguish from negative syndrome, with which it may coincide. Substance abuse has been interpreted as an attempt by patients to self-treat the side-effects of antipsychotic medication or negative syndrome. Alcohol abuse or dependence is present in up to 50 percent of schizophrenia patients. Cannabis is consumed by 15–25 percent of patients.

8.8 **Course and outcome**

Schizophrenia is a severe disorder, which often takes a chronic course (Jablensky 2000). Only 20–30 percent of patients have a benign course and outcome, with a fraction reaching full recovery. Another 30 percent experience recurrent episodes, with remission or partial remission. About 50 percent of patients are impaired in terms of social and occupational functioning. In one-third of patients the disorder takes a persistent or chronic course, with increasing severity of negative symptoms requiring special housing or assertive community treatment. Ten to fifteen percent of patients with schizophrenia die by suicide, particularly if comorbid depression is present.

Only 20–30 percent of patients with schizophrenia have a benign course and good outcome with remission. Another 30 percent have recurrent episodes with remission of partial remission. About 50 percent of patients are impaired in terms of social and occupational functioning. Cognitive dysfunction, poor premorbid adjustment, schizotypal personality traits, and psychosocial stressors negatively influence course and outcome of the disorder.

Outcome critically depends on patient and environmental variables (Owens et al. 2010). Cognitive dysfunction, poor premorbid adjustment, schizotypal personality traits, and psychosocial stressors, including emotional overstimulation or high levels of expressed emotions in the family, negatively influence course and outcome. By contrast, adherence to antipsychotic treatment, good coping strategies, self-management, and supportive family functioning are associated with improved outcome. Relapse after the first psychotic episode is 70–80 percent in the first 3–7 months after discontinuation of antipsychotic medication, compared with 20–30 percent under continuous drug treatment.

Outcome parameters are determined not only by reduction of positive and negative symptoms, but also by factors such as quality of life, psychosocial functioning, treatment, and caregiver burden.

Outcome parameters are, however, determined not only by a reduction of positive and negative symptoms, but also by factors such as quality of life, psychosocial functioning, treatment, and caregiver burden. For example, interpersonal functioning and affect regulation are influenced by attachment styles, and it has been shown that patients with schizophrenia, who as children were securely attached, have better outcome predictors and fewer relapses compared to insecurely attached individuals (Ringer et al. 2014).

Whether or not schizophrenia is, on average, less severe than it was 100 years or so ago is a contentious issue (McGlashan 2006). The evidence seems to be robust, however, to suggest that the course and outcome are more benign in developing countries compared to most parts of Europe and the USA (Jablensky 2000).

8.9 Treatment

The introduction of antipsychotic medication has revolutionized the treatment of psychotic disorders (Lieberman et al. 2005). Since antipsychotic drugs became available in the 1950s, however, treatment goals have changed dramatically. Whereas prevention of harmful behaviour and reduction of positive symptoms were initially at the core, the focus has somewhat shifted to the need to control negative symptoms, which are prognostically at least equally relevant compared to positive symptoms, and to improve patients' quality of life. It is now widely acknowledged that second-generation antipsychotic drugs (still misleadingly referred to as 'atypical neuroleptics') are more effective in reducing negative symptoms, with fewer extrapyramidal side-effects such as parkinsonism, dystonia and akathisia. Treatment-resistant patients may benefit from electroconvulsive therapy (ECT). Individual tailoring of treatment is, however, still in its infancy, but characterization of endophenotypes within the schizophrenia spectrum may help to achieve this goal in the near future (Braff et al. 2007). In any event, despite promising improvements, one should keep in mind that antipsychotic drug treatment seems to exert only limited effects on patients' conviction of delusional beliefs and social competence (Mizrahi et al. 2006). Novel approaches may include the administration of neuropeptides such as oxytocin or agonists acting via the oxytocinergic system (Feifel et al. 2010).

Whereas prevention of harmful behaviour and reduction of positive symptoms were primary targets after antipsychotic drugs became available, the focus has somewhat shifted to the need to control negative symptoms, and to improve patients' quality of life.

In addition to pharmacological treatment, it has proven fruitful to educate patients in recognizing early signs of impending relapse and avoiding extensive psychosocial stress. Moreover, the evolutionary cognitive perspective may add the recommendation that training in social cognitive abilities, including understanding others' minds and emotions, as well as psychotherapeutic interventions focusing on interpersonal relationships may help reduce the risk of relapse and deterioration of the illness (Pilling et al. 2002). Given the tendency of many patients with schizophrenia to overmentalize, it is essential for clinicians to use unambiguous expressions, and to avoid the use of ironic or otherwise (too) metaphorical speech.

Educating patients in recognizing early signs of impending relapse and avoiding extensive psychosocial stress has proven effective.

Useful treatment recommendations are provided online by the American Psychiatric Association (APA). Guidelines have also been published by the Royal Australian and New Zealand College of Psychiatrists (RANZCP). Information for lay persons and carers is provided by the Royal College of Psychiatrists (RCP) and by RANZCP.

Chapter 9

Bipolar and related disorders

Abstract

Bipolar disorder concerns a syndrome in which both manic and depressive episodes occur, or states where manic and depressive symptoms co-occur. Mania is characterized by elevated mood, drive, and accelerated cognition. Behaviourally, mania reflects an extreme phenotypic variation of cognitive, emotional, and behavioural traits involved in competitiveness and dominance. Evolutionary explanations of mania suggest that dilute versions of the syndrome may confer increased reproductive success, which could partly account for the preservation of genes that predispose to bipolar disorder. Life-history perspectives suggest that mania reflects a 'fast' life-history strategy. Why such a strategy can switch—sometimes rapidly—to the extreme of a 'slow' strategy (i.e. depression) remains unclear.

Keywords

bipolar disorder, mania, competitiveness, dominance, reproductive success

9.1 Symptomatology and diagnostic criteria

DSM-5 has placed Bipolar and Related Disorders between the diagnostic classes of Schizophrenia and Depressive Disorders to emphasize the view that bipolar disorders (BD) overlap with both in terms of symptomatology, family history, and genetics (American Psychiatric Association 2013). Like all affective disorders, BD is characterized by abnormalities of mood, drive, and cognition. The new category of Bipolar and Related Disorders comprises the 'classic' bipolar I disorder, bipolar II disorder, cyclothymic disorder, and bipolar syndromes caused or induced by substances, medication, or other medical conditions.

Bipolar and Related Disorders have been placed between the diagnostic classes of Schizophrenia and Depressive Disorders to emphasize the view that BD overlap with both in terms of symptomatology, family history and genetics.

Bipolar I disorder requires the experience of at least one manic episode, but not necessarily the experience of depressive episodes. Bipolar II disorder requires the occurrence of a major depressive episode and a hypomanic episode. Cyclothymia is a somewhat dilute form of BD, whereby the criteria for a manic, a hypomanic, or a depressive episode are not fully met (Akiskal and Akiskal 2005).

A classic manic episode is characterized by elevated or irritable mood, increased drive, and accelerated cognition to the point of flight of ideas and a sense of inflated self-esteem or grandiosity. The full picture of mania is also usually associated with a decreased need for sleep, inattentiveness or distractibility, an increase in goal-directed or senseless behaviour (i.e. agitation), and excessive involvement in activities that may cause harm to the affected individual or others (e.g. promiscuity, inappropriate financial investments). Mania is always accompanied by marked impairment in social or occupational functioning.

A manic episode is characterized by elevated or irritable mood, increased drive, and accelerated cognition to the point of flight of ideas and a sense of inflated self-esteem or grandiosity. The full picture of mania is also usually associated with a decreased need for sleep, inattentiveness or distractibility, an increase in goal-directed or senseless behaviour (i.e. agitation), and excessive involvement in activities that may cause harm to the affected individual or others.

Hypomania is similar to mania, whereby the observed changes in behaviour, mood, and cognition do not compromise functioning. DSM-5 provides specifiers for BD that allow for coding specific features regarding course (e.g. rapid cycling), symptomatology (mixed episodes with both manic and depressive symptoms present at the same time, or presence of melancholic features such as loss of pleasure, somatic symptoms, and disturbances of the circadian rhythm), presence or absence of psychotic symptoms that can be mood-congruent (delusions of grandeur) or mood-incongruent (persecutory delusions), and presence of catatonic symptoms (American Psychiatric Association 2013). The presence of psychotic or catatonic symptoms makes it sometimes difficult to distinguish BD from schizophrenia spectrum disorders, and longitudinal follow-up assessment may be mandatory for a distinction.

Mixed episodes comprise features of both depression and mania, where 'mood', 'drive', and 'thought' dissociate. Thus, theoretically, there are 2×2×2 possibilities (already noticed by Kraepelin), among which the most frequently observed mixed state is agitated depression (whereby DSM-5 does not classify agitated depression as a mixed state). However, mania associated with psychomotor retardation, depression with flight of ideas, and so forth can also be found.

Mixed episodes comprise features of both depression and mania, where 'mood', 'drive', and 'thought' dissociate.

9.2 **Epidemiology**

The population risk for bipolar affective disorder is estimated between 0.5 and 1.5 percent. Males and females differ marginally with respect to life-time risk for bipolar affective disorder. Age at onset of bipolar and related disorders peaks at around 18 years. Mixed states and rapid cycling seem to be more frequent in women (Angst 1995; Bauer and Pfennig 2005).

The population risk for bipolar affective disorder is estimated between 0.5 and 1.5 percent. Males and females differ marginally with respect to life-time risk.

9.3 Genetic risk factors

The risk for BD is about sevenfold increased for first-degree relatives of patients with BD. Twin studies suggest a 60 percent concordance rate for BD in MZ twins, in contrast to only 25 percent in DZ twins (Potash et al. 2001). A greater genetic risk for BD is possibly associated with early age of onset, the number of affected relatives, and when the disorder is triggered by puerperium.

Linkage studies into BD suggest allelic variations of genes located on chromosomes 4p, 12q, 15q, 16p, 18q, 21q, and Xq (Berrettini 2001; Badner and Gershon 2002). Several susceptibility loci overlap with those found in schizophrenia, which supports the assumption of a continuum between the two (Berrettini 2000a, 2000b; Craddock and Jones 2001; Bailer et al. 2002; Craddock et al. 2006). No gene of major effect has been determined. Candidate genes include the gene coding tyrosine hydroxylase, an enzyme involved in the synthesis of catecholamines, the serotonin transporter gene, and the gene encoding COMT. The latter is probably not associated with an elevated risk for BD in general, but perhaps plays a role in rapid cycling (defined as four or more mood episodes in 12 months).

The risk for BD is about sevenfold increased for first-degree relatives of patients with BD. Twin studies suggest a 60 percent concordance rate for BD in MZ twins in contrast to only 25 percent in DZ twins.

Several susceptibility loci for BD overlap with those found in schizophrenia, which supports the assumption of a continuum between the two. However, no gene of major effect has been determined.

9.4 Environmental risk factors

Loss of the primary caregiver prior to puberty increases the risk for BD. In addition, spousal separation, divorce, and widowhood are associated with higher rates of BD than in individuals who are married or single (Laursen et al. 2007).

Environmental risk factors for BD comprise loss of the primary caregiver prior to puberty, spousal separation, divorce, and widowhood.

9.5 Pathophysiological mechanisms

Affective disorders are thought to arise from complex dysregulations of neurotransmitter systems, among which the catecholamines and serotonin are considered to be most important. In contrast to depression, where dopamine availability appears to be diminished, dopamine is temporarily increased in mania.

Early traumatization and other causes of chronic stress may in addition lead to lability of the HPA axis via overactivation of limbic structures, which in turn induces excessive glucocorticoid activity. Exposure of the developing brain to chronic stress has neurotoxic effects especially on the vulnerable hippocampal region, which then is diminished in its ability to control the HPA system via negative feedback mechanisms. Grey matter and neuropil are diminished in the OFC, PFC, and ACC in patients with BD (Blumberg et al. 1999; López-Larson et al. 2002). However, the

Early traumatization and chronic stress may cause lability of the HPA axis via overactivation of limbic structures, which in turn induces excessive glucocorticoid activity. Grey matter and neuropil are diminished in the OFC, PFC, and ACC in patients with BD.

majority of patients with bipolar affective disorders experience more depressive episodes than manic episodes, such that the specificity of alterations at the transmitter or anatomical level is less clear. At the anatomical level, bipolar affective disorder is associated with ventricular enlargement and smaller left dorsolateral PFC volume and volume reductions of inferior and middle PFC regions on the right (Soares et al. 2005).

9.6 **Evolutionary synthesis**

In contrast to depression, mania represents the pathologically extreme of variation of dominance behaviour and competition-enhancing strategy at the behavioural, emotional, and cognitive level. Behaviourally, manic patients seek social contact, often interact with people of the opposite sex in salacious ways, and escalate contest with same-sex individuals. This is ethologically measurable by increased eye-to-eye contact, gestures and facial expressivity, and dominance-suggesting body postures (Polsky and McGuire 1979; Annen et al. 2012). Asymmetries in social status are perceived reversed compared to depression, and the constantly challenging behaviour of manic patients may be quite demanding for therapists.

Mania represents the pathologically extreme of variation of dominance behaviour and competition-enhancing strategy.

At the emotional level, mania is associated with elevated mood or irritability communicating dominance to (perceived) contenders or high social rank to individuals who the manic patient recognizes as potential mates. Elevated mood in mania internally increases self-confidence, which may trigger, at the cognitive level, a false evaluation of a socially competitive situation such that the manic individual may believe he or she would succeed in virtually all activities. In a sense, in a state of mania, individuals show the opposite of what has been called 'appeasement strategy' (Price et al. 2004, 2007).

For example, a manic patient would not only fail to perceive that an important biosocial goal could be thwarted, but also believe that any goal is achievable. The escalation-motivated behaviour of manic patients is therefore a high-risk strategy (Price 1998a), which theoretically offers the chance to win in social competition, but in case of failure bears the risk of losing a lot (perhaps even expulsion from the community). The manic patient, however, is unable to recognize the risk; in terms of evaluating the relation of social investment and resource extraction, or social value and social burden, respectively, a manic individual will tend to assume that he or she deserves much more than invested, or that he or she has already invested much in the past, such that the manic individual uncritically overestimates his or her social value relative to his or her social burden. In contrast to the depressed patient who tends to derogate him- or herself, being unable to see his or her social value, the manic patient does not even consider that his or her inflated self-esteem may be inappropriate, and usually lacks completely insight into the disorder.

The escalation-motivated behaviour of manic patients is therefore a high-risk strategy, which theoretically offers the chance to win in social competition, but in case of failure bears the risk of losing a lot.

Thus, at the cognitive level, mania is associated with an impaired ability to accurately represent one's own and others' mental states, and possibly involves much more self-deception than depression. Depressed patients, unless grossly distorted by delusional ideation, have been found to be more accurate in their judgements about themselves and social circumstances compared to healthy controls, which suggests that a certain level of seeing the world more positively than it actually is could be adaptive. It is therefore conceivable that this tendency is exaggerated to a pathological extreme in mania. In a sense, manic episodes (which are on average far more infrequent than depressive episodes in bipolar affective disorder) may constitute a compensatory strategy, however inadequate and overshooting to the other extreme, to see the world as less threatening and repugnant than it actually is, at least for a brief period of time. In support of this hypothesis, mild forms of mania, hypomania, or even more dilute forms such as cyclothymia may even be reproductively advantageous (Akiskal and Akiskal 2005), which could make a case for the selection of self-deceptive abilities (see Chapter 22).

It is clinically a well-known fact that mixed states between depression and mania exist. For example, an individual can present with depressed mood but increased psychomotor activity or flight of ideas. Mixed states are particularly enlightening with regard to the representation of behaviour, mood, and cognition at three different levels of the triune brain (see Chapter 1). Mixed states are, in a sense, proof for the assumption that, at least under pathological conditions, these three levels can operate to some extent independently of one another. Thus, there is the possibility that a syndrome may occur with mania at the 'neomammalian' (cognitive) level, characterized by flight of ideas, accompanied by mania at the 'palaeomammalian' level, that is, elevated mood, yet at the 'reptilian' level by appeasement behaviours, suggestive of depression (Gardner 2001). This state is called 'retarded mania'. Correspondingly, a syndrome comprising competition-escalating behaviour, elevated mood, and inhibited thinking has been referred to as 'thought-impoverished mania'.

Mixed states are paradigmatic for the independent operation of the three levels of the triune brain.

In comparison to unipolar depression, BD and mixed states are far less well understood in terms of their neurobiological underpinnings and individual differences in reactivity of the neural circuits involved influenced by early experiences and attachment. Perhaps individuals with BD or mixed states have an even more labile emotional system, which is more strongly under genetic control and to a lesser degree dependent on environmental peculiarities than persons with unipolar disorder.

In any event, even though full-blown mania is probably not adaptive, one can imagine how traits conferring cheerfulness, inventiveness, creativity, competitiveness, stimulus-seeking, or promiscuousness could have been reproductively advantageous in the ancestral past (Gardner 1982: Wilson 1998; Akiskal and Akiskal 2005). Such dilute versions of the manic syndrome clearly reflect a 'fast' life-history pattern (Del Giudice 2014), and they seem to relate to sex differences in personality traits such as

Dilute versions of the manic syndrome reflect a 'fast' life-history pattern, and they seem to relate to sex differences in personality traits, such as dominance and vigilance, which are expressed more frequently in males compared to females.

dominance and vigilance, which are expressed more frequently in males compared to females (Del Giudice et al. 2012).

However, evolutionary explanations largely fail to explain why mood swings occur in BD—sometimes very rapidly—indicating a shift from a 'fast' to a 'slow' life-history strategy and vice versa.

9.7 **Differential diagnosis and comorbidity**

BD shares features with ADHD and BPD (Brody 2001). However, mood swings, affective instability, and impulsivity in BD are more pervasive in the latter and not restricted to distinct episodes. The differential diagnosis may be difficult in adolescents. In cases with late onset, frontotemporal dementia with behavioural disinhibition can be confused with mania or mixed states.

BD shares features with ADHD and BPD. Comorbid disorders of BD comprise ADHD, anxiety disorders, externalizing disorders such as intermittent explosive disorder, conduct disorder, and substance abuse.

Comorbid disorders of BD comprise ADHD, anxiety disorders, externalizing disorders such as intermittent explosive disorder, conduct disorder, and substance abuse.

9.8 **Course and outcome**

BD is associated with the tendency of phase acceleration and incomplete remission with increasing duration of the illness. Both bipolar I and bipolar II disorder can be disabling. High relapse rates, shortened intervals between individual episodes, and incomplete remission with residual symptoms may emerge over the course of the illness (Simhandl et al. 2014). Suicide risk is high in bipolar I and bipolar II disorder. About one-third of patients undertake suicide attempts, and lethal attempts may be more frequent in bipolar II compared to bipolar I patients.

BD is associated with the tendency of phase acceleration and incomplete remission with increasing duration of the illness.

9.9 **Treatment**

Acute mania responds to antipsychotic treatment, as do mixed states. Mood stabilizers for bipolar affective disorder include lithium, carbamazepine, valproic acid, and other anticonvulsive agents. The choice of drug depends on the symptomatology and course of the illness.

Acute mania responds to antipsychotic treatment, as do mixed states. Mood stabilizers for bipolar affective disorder include lithium, carbamazepine, valproic acid, and other anticonvulsive agents. Treatment may also involve psychoeducational means that aim at reducing the risk for relapse.

Treatment may also involve psychoeducational means that aim at reducing the risk for relapse. Much more could be done in terms of primary prevention, including educating parents about the need to give children the opportunity to develop a secure attachment, and how to reduce intrafamilial stress levels to avoid physical and emotional abuse (see Afterthought to Chapter 4).

Treatment recommendations and useful information for professionals and laypersons have been published by the APA, RCP, and RANZCP.

Chapter 10

Depressive disorders

Abstract

Depression is characterized by low mood, reduced affective responsiveness, lack of drive and initiative, and negative cognitive evaluation of circumstances and self. Delusional thinking may occur in severe cases. Behaviourally, depression reflects helplessness or appeasement that arise from feelings of inferiority, entrapment, or defeat. Non-verbal behaviour in depression resembles ancient strategies of vertebrates to signal submission. At the cognitive level, people with depression often engage in ruminating thoughts, often involving self-derogation or worthlessness. Depression may occur in situations when one's social status is threatened or an actual fall in rank has taken place. This is often accompanied by a reduction of serotonin availability. Genes conferring risk for depression when coupled with adverse early experiences may even protect against depression when associated with supportive parenting, suggesting genetic plasticity. Aside from ethological considerations, depression may also be linked to a dysfunction of the immune system.

Keywords

depression, appeasement, submission, entrapment strategy, social status, serotonin, genetic plasticity, immune system

10.1 Symptomatology and diagnostic criteria

According to DSM-5, depressive disorders comprise disruptive mood regulation disorder, major depression, persistent depression or dysthymia, depressive syndromes that occur due to other biological conditions, such as premenstrual dysphoria, and depression in the context of other medical diseases or substances.

Depressive disorders comprise disruptive mood regulation disorder, major depression, persistent depression or dysthymia, depressive syndromes that occur due to other biological conditions, such as premenstrual dysphoria, and depression in the context of other medical diseases or substances.

Disruptive mood regulation disorder has been included in DSM-5 as a new entry. It concerns a syndrome that is characterized by irritability and behavioural disinhibition with onset prior to age 10. This syndrome seems to develop into anxiety disorders or unipolar depression, but less often into BD (American Psychiatric Association 2013).

The typical signs and symptoms of major depression are low mood, reduced affective responsiveness, lack of drive and initiative, and negative cognitive evaluation of circumstances and self, including feelings of worthlessness and helplessness, that have been present for at least 2 weeks. Major depression can be accompanied by somatic symptoms such as weight loss, disturbances of the circadian rhythm, constipation, irritable bowel syndrome or other autonomic dysfunctions, as well as feelings of extreme guilt, agitation, or 'empty' mood (summarized under the term 'melancholic features').

The typical signs and symptoms of major depression are low mood, reduced affective responsiveness, lack of drive and initiative, and negative cognitive evaluation of circumstances and self, including feelings of worthlessness and helplessness. Major depression can be accompanied by somatic symptoms such as weight loss, disturbances of the circadian rhythm, constipation, irritable bowel syndrome or other autonomic dysfunctions, as well as feelings of extreme guilt, agitation, or 'empty' mood (summarized under the term 'melancholic features').

Severe depression may be accompanied by psychotic symptoms such as delusions and hallucinations. Mood-congruent delusional themes in depression comprise (inappropriate) guilt, impoverishment, physical illness (hypochondriasis), or Cotard's syndrome (*délire de negation*). Mood-incongruent delusions may be present in the form of persecutory delusions. Catatonic symptoms may also be coded among the specifiers. Seasonal affective disorder is coded as a major depressive episode with a specifier indicating a seasonal pattern.

Milder forms of depression which take a chronic course over at least 2 years are conceptualized as 'dysthymic disorder', of which the boundaries with chronic major depression, on the one side, and with depressive personality disorder, on the other, are vague. In addition, dysthymia and recurrent major depressive episodes may co-occur ('double-depression') and be more prevalent in patients who are hospitalized for depression. Recurrent episodes of depression are classified as unipolar depression.

Mood-congruent or -incongruent delusions as well as catatonic features may occur in severe psychotic depression. Dysthymic disorder concerns minor forms of mood swings.

10.2 **Epidemiology**

Major depression is very common across populations and cultures. The current life-time prevalence for major depression is between 4 and 20 percent, with women being twice as often affected as men (American Psychiatric Association 2013). Five to ten percent of the population will develop major depression within a 1-year period. Age at onset peaks around the fourth decade, with a second peak in the sixth decade. Dysthymic disorder has a 1-year prevalence rate of about 2–5 percent.

The current life-time prevalence for major depression is between 4 and 20 percent, with women being twice as often affected as men. Dysthymic disorder has a 1-year prevalence rate of about 2–5 percent.

10.3 Genetic risk factors

Studies of the genetics of unipolar depression suggest a continuum between mild (reactive) depression and severe (melancholic or endogenous) depression. First-degree relatives of patients with unipolar depression have a relative risk for the disorder that is between 1.5 and 3-fold higher than the population risk (Jones et al. 2005). The concordance rate in MZ twins is near 40 percent and in DZ twins roughly 20 percent. Prepubertal onset of depression is probably less genetically mediated compared with onset later in life. Instead, adverse environmental events are apparently more important in early-onset depression. However, the risk for depression in individuals at genetic risk who in addition have experienced a severe life event is twice as large as in those at low genetic risk (plus severe life event), suggesting additive genetic and environmental contributions to the vulnerability for depression. The risk for bipolar depression is apparently not increased for first-degree relatives of patients with unipolar depression.

First-degree relatives of patients with unipolar depression have a relative risk for the disorder that is between 1.5 and 3-fold higher than the population risk. The concordance rate in MZ twins is near 40 percent and in DZ twins roughly 20 percent. Prepubertal onset of depression is probably less genetically mediated compared with onset later in life.

Major depression is a highly heterogeneous disorder and is genetically more closely related to anxiety disorders than to BD. No gene of major effect size has been determined so far, but inconsistent findings point to a role for serotonin receptor polymorphisms (5-HT2A) in the aetiology of unipolar depression, particularly if associated with suicidal behaviour. In addition, a polymorphism of the serotonin transporter gene has been linked with increased risk for depression, but only in conjunction with traumatic life events (Caspi et al. 2003; Lesch 2004). Furthermore, the FKBP5 gene regulating expression of glucocorticoid receptors is apparently associated with recurrence of depression, but also with good response to antidepressants and frequent relapse. Conversely, a certain allele coding for the corticotropin-releasing hormone receptor 1 (CRHR1) seems to protect against depression even in individuals who as children have been exposed to maltreatment (Polanczyk et al. 2009).

Studies suggest that unipolar depression is mediated by polymorphisms of genes involved in serotonin metabolism. A polymorphism of the serotonin transporter gene has been linked with increased risk for depression, but only in conjunction with traumatic life events. Unipolar depression is genetically related to anxiety disorders.

10.4 Environmental risk factors

Losses of important relationships by death or separation represent life events that may cause depression in vulnerable individuals. Specifically, loss of the primary caregiver (usually the mother) prior to onset of puberty dramatically increases the risk for depressive disorders later in life (perhaps more important for the development of dysthymic disorder than recurrent depression). Loss of work and poverty are also important risk factors for depression, as are lack of social

Loss of the primary caregiver prior to onset of puberty dramatically increases the risk for depressive disorders later in life. Poverty, lack of social support, physical illness, and age are also important risk factors for depression.

support, physical illness, and age (Gilman et al. 2002). During gestation and the post-partum period, depression is particularly linked with teenage pregnancy, undesired pregnancy, unmarried status, separation, divorce, and marital conflict. In recurrent unipolar depression, however, the importance of life-events decreases after the third episode.

10.5 Pathophysiological mechanisms

Affective disorders are thought to arise from complex dysregulations of neurotransmitter systems, among which the catecholamines and serotonin are considered to be most important. First evidence came from observations that catecholamine-depleting drugs such as reserpine may cause depression. It is now quite well established from brain imaging and neurochemical studies that depression is associated with reduced serotonin availability in several key areas of the brain, including the hippocampal formation and the amygdala. Norepinephrine is reduced, with compensatorily enhanced expression of norepinephrine alpha-2 receptors in mesial temporal areas, the hypothalamus, frontal cortex, and locus coeruleus. Moreover, dopamine availability appears to be diminished in depression.

Affective disorders arise from complex dysregulations of neurotransmitter systems, among which the catecholamines and serotonin are most important. Early traumatization and other causes of chronic stress may lead to lability of the HPA axis via overactivation of limbic structures, which in turn induces excessive glucocorticoid activity.

Early traumatization and other causes of chronic stress may in addition lead to lability of the (HPA axis via overactivation of limbic structures, which in turn induces excessive glucocorticoid activity (Strickland et al. 2002). Exposure of the developing brain to chronic stress has neurotoxic effects, especially on the vulnerable hippocampal region (Lee et al. 2002a), which then is diminished in its ability to control the HPA system via negative feedback mechanisms. In line with this model, in some (but not all) patients with depression, cortisol and corticotropin-releasing hormone are reduced. Reduced levels of BDNF have also been linked to depression (and anxiety), but the exact role of BDNF is unclear, since it may exert opposite effects in different brain regions (Martinowich et al. 2007).

Consistent with the effects of chronic stress and defective repair mechanisms on brain tissue, there is an overall volume reduction by 10–20 percent of the hippocampal formation and the caudate region in depression, which correlates with the severity, duration, and number of depressive episodes. Grey matter and neuropil are also diminished in the OFC, PFC, and ACC in depression.

Consistent with the effects of chronic stress and defective repair mechanisms on brain tissue, there is an overall volume reduction by 10–20 percent of the hippocampal formation and the caudate region in depression, which correlates with the severity, duration, and number of depressive episodes. Grey matter and neuropil are also diminished in the OFC, PFC, and ACC in depression.

10.6 **Evolutionary synthesis**

Ethological analysis of behaviour in depression suggests that depressed individuals display non-verbal signals typical of submissive behaviour (Pedersen et al. 1988; Schelde 1998). Depressed patients often avoid eye-to-eye contact, show reduced facial expressivity and speech production, and withdraw from their social environment (Geerts et al. 2006). Submission also frequently makes use of species-specific child behaviours (traditionally labelled 'regression') or somatic complaints as involuntary signals of helplessness. Thus, although pathologically exaggerated in depression, these non-verbal behaviours aim at reducing the aggression of others that could be oriented towards the self, and avoiding harm by displaying de-escalating appeasement strategies in situations of (perceived) defeat or inferiority (Price et al. 2004).

Ethological analysis of behaviour in depression suggests that depressed individuals display non-verbal signals typical of submissive behaviour. Submission frequently makes use of species-specific child behaviours (traditionally labelled 'regression') or somatic complaints as involuntary signals of helplessness. Severe forms of melancholic depression can co-occur with catatonic features, which may represent the extreme of phylogenetically ancient defence mechanisms.

Severe forms of melancholic depression can co-occur with catatonic features, which may represent the extreme of phylogenetically ancient defence mechanisms such as tonic immobility (Abrams et al. 2009; see Chapter 8). It should be noted, however, that depressed individuals do not display the same behaviour in every social interaction. For example, they may well show signs of aggression oriented towards family members, especially spouses or children, from whom they demand instant support. Thus, while depressed individuals frequently display involuntary (non-verbal) signs of submission, they often lack signalling voluntary (verbal) submission. The study of non-verbal behaviour in depression is therapeutically highly relevant, because reduced expressivity on admission has predictive value for outcome and recurrence of depression (Geerts et al. 1996, 2006; Geerts and Bouhuys 1998; Bos et al. 2007).

Submission and dominance are inherent to socially living species with complex hierarchies like humans (although ancestral human societies are believed to have been fairly egalitarian with regard to social stratification). Thus, asymmetries in social status and competition for resources and mates, and relationships need to be negotiated (Watson and Andrews 2002). Human social groups, which also critically depend on cooperation between individuals, can only survive if a communicative system for social hierarchies exists that at least partially replaces physical contest, and allows both the winner and the loser to remain within the social group. In ancestral environments, social exclusion from the community was probably one of the most important real threats to an individual, and potentially equivalent to a death sentence.

Accordingly, submission in conflict-laden situations may in the first place be considered a life-saving strategy that evolved under ancestral condition, despite its obvious, though perhaps transient, disadvantage in terms of reproductive success. In other words, a decision over fight or flight critically depends on the evaluation of one's own power and potential alliances, and in situations where success is unlikely or escape impossible, submission and acceptance of subordination may be the best option, at least for the moment being (Rohde 2001). Depression, in this line of reasoning, represents the extreme of submission or appeasement strategy (Price et al. 2007), however inappropriate in terms of context, duration, and/or intensity, compared to adaptive submissive behaviour, and occurs foremost in situations associated with acute or chronic social stress (Nesse 2000; Gardner 2001).

In support of the assumption that depression represents the pathological extreme of a harm-avoiding strategy in socially competitive interactions, it is worth emphasizing that depression primarily occurs in social or interpersonal context, but less frequently following losses in non-social domains. In fact, separation from or loss of a close one and loss of social status are among the most common causes for depression (Price et al. 2007). Postpartum depression may be another example, showing that perceived or real loss of social support can also elicit depressive symptoms (Hagen 1999). Interestingly, it seems that depressive symptom patterns may differ according to the cause: while guilt, rumination, fatigue, and pessimism are more prevalent following the failure of important life goals, crying, sadness, and desire for social support occur more prominently following social losses (Keller and Nesse 2006).

Separation from or loss of a close one and loss of social status are among the most common causes for depression. Postpartum depression is related to the perceived or real loss of social support.

Many non-verbal signals, especially body postures of dominance and subordination, are reminiscent of ancient vertebrate behaviours, and probably mediated by phylogenetically old 'reptilian brain' structures (see Chapter 1). This behavioural repertoire is paralleled by emotional systems (represented in the palaeomammalian or limbic part of the brain) that serve, in the case of subordination, the dual purpose of signalling submission and helplessness to both dominant individuals and potential helpers (allies), and internally communicating defeat via low mood, hence rendering the individual at a lower risk of resuming social competitiveness too quickly (Price et al. 2004). Low mood is also likely one aspect of the social emotions that evolved in response to the increasing need for attachment of immature offspring; it typically occurs in offspring upon (prolonged) separation from the main caregiver or attachment figure. In the phase of despair, for example, the human infant disengages from the social environment and remains silent, which can be seen as an adaptation to not attract predators.

Low mood serves the dual purpose of signalling submission and helplessness to both dominant individuals and potential helpers (allies) and of communicating defeat. Ruminating thoughts about social issues may even be adaptive, if not excessive beyond a certain level.

Such negative emotions also profoundly influence an individual's conscious and unconscious cognitive evaluation of a given situation. Ruminating thoughts about social issues may even be adaptive, if not excessive beyond a certain level, and may foster problem solution by prioritizing the issue at stake (Andrews and Thomson 2009, 2010; Rottenberg 2014). In fact, depressed individuals sometimes even outperform non-depressed individuals in tasks involving complex decision-making (von Helversen et al. 2011). However, extremes of variation of low mood, including inappropriate contextual occurrence and abnormal intensity of duration, are characteristic for clinically relevant depression and are not adaptive, because they compromise reproductive success.

Much of the cognitive evaluation of one's own social standing is outside conscious awareness, and probably already part of the cognitive repertoire of our closest relatives in the animal kingdom (maintained by neocortical structures). For example, an individual constantly needs to examine his or her chance to succeed in social competition, and this does not necessarily pertain only to dramatic contests over a particular position on the social ladder, but also applies in situations involving subtle social exchange. Humans are highly socially investing beings, in both kin and non-kin, but of course also eager to receive returns on their investment. Thus an individual may (unconsciously) calculate how much he or she has been able to extract relative to his or her investment, and this calculation may critically depend on one's perceived social value and/or potential burden imposed on others. To be on the safe side and to minimize the risk for severe contest and potential exclusion, subordinate individuals are likely to invest more than they extract (Allen and Badcock 2003).

Subordinate individuals are likely to invest more than they extract. This bias towards increased investment relative to what one may feel one is allowed to extract is quite characteristic of at least mildly depressed or dysthymic persons.

This bias towards increased investment relative to what one may feel one is allowed to extract is quite characteristic of at least mildly depressed or dysthymic persons. Moreover, self-deception may play a role in some depressed persons who, in order to convincingly reassure a dominant individual about their subordination, need to make themselves believe that they really are inferior, commonly reflected in self-derogation and negative self-appraisal (Gilbert et al. 2002).

Individual differences in cognitive appraisal of social investment not only depend on current circumstances; for example, a person who experiences that an important biosocial goal has been thwarted may try even harder to achieve this goal by investing more, perhaps associated with self-deprecation that he or she is not worthy of receiving the return if he/she does not invest more (Beck 1999; Brown 2002).

Equally important, individual differences in vulnerability for depression can arise from differences in genetics and early environmental conditions (Caspi et al. 2003). For example, if early loss of the primary caregiver, insecure attachment, or physical and emotional abuse occurred in early childhood, individuals who faced such chronic stress situations would develop less stable coping strategies for novel stressors, such that even minor or moderate adverse events may not be dealt with appropriately (Gardner 2001). Individuals with certain allelic variants of the serotonin transporter gene (or carriers of other genetic susceptibility genes) may be particularly vulnerable to chronic alterations at the neurobiological level, but only when experiencing early adversity, whereas the same alleles confer a lower than average risk for depression when interacting with favourable (e.g. emotionally supportive) early environments. Interestingly, the s-allele of the serotonin transporter gene is more prevalent in

Early loss of the primary caregiver, insecure attachment, or physical and emotional abuse present in early childhood predispose individuals to develop less stable coping strategies for novel stressors.

cultures that value collectivism over individualism, whereby s-allele carriers have a lower risk for depression (Chiao and Blizinsky 2010; see Chapter 1, section 1.4.2 on 'differential susceptibility').

Moreover, someone who as a child could not build up a secure attachment relationship with the primary caregiver—or has even been exposed to prenatal stress (e.g. in the context of maternal depression), which can negatively impact on stress-coping capacities (Andersson et al. 2004; Brennan et al. 2008; see also Afterthought to Chapter 3)—may develop an inner working model suggesting that the (social) world is untrustworthy, such that returns on any social investment cannot be expected (Carter et al. 2001). These individuals will also perceive themselves as unlovable and not worth being cared for (Sadeh et al. 1993). At the same time they may be particularly sensitive to situations in which they are exposed to unjustified criticism or perceive themselves treated in an unfair manner. Altogether, this situation can produce a vicious circle of perceived entrapment, anger (which cannot be expressed appropriately), negative self-evaluation, feelings of guilt or shame, and, ultimately, actual rejection from the social environment (Gilbert et al. 2002, 2004; O'Connor et al. 2002; Nettle 2004). In fact, in severe states of depression, individuals apparently stop investing in social relationships, such that the quotient of social value and social burden may suddenly drop below a value of 1, which could actually lead to withdrawal of social support and increase the risk for suicidal behaviour.

Defeat in social competition or fall in social rank produces a steep decline in serotonin levels in the brain.

In addition, abundant primate research has shown that defeat in social competition or fall in social rank produces a steep decline in serotonin levels in the brain. Subordinate individuals have on average much lower serotonin levels than dominant individuals, and the former are more aggressive and emotionally labile, but explore their environment less compared to the latter. In addition, research in non-human primates has shown that early abuse or neglect may stimulate proinflammatory immune responses, which in turn increase the activation of the serotonin transporter, thus leading to reduced serotonin availability (Sanchez et al. 2007). In other words, both early life stress and chronic states of depression may foster low serotonin availability and perhaps hypersensitivity to serotonin exposure, which could, in part, explain why serotonin reuptake inhibitory drugs may enhance the risk for suicidal behaviour, perhaps especially in patients who are not 'classically' depressed but show increased hostility and irritability.

Both early life stress and chronic states of depression may foster low serotonin availability and perhaps hypersensitivity to serotonin exposure, which could explain why serotonin reuptake inhibitory drugs may enhance the risk for suicidal behaviour, perhaps especially in patients who do not behave 'classically' depressed, but show increased hostility and irritability.

Furthermore, chronic stress has long-lasting effects on brain morphology, including measurable volume reductions of the hippocampal formation and regions of the PFC. Thus, with every new stressor, an individual may be less well able to develop adequate coping strategies, which clinically manifests as phase acceleration and chronicity of the affective disorder.

Evolutionary approaches also offer an explanation for sex differences in prevalence rates of depression. Differences in vulnerability for depression between men and women probably relate to evolved sex differences in behaviour, emotion, and cognition (Troisi 2001). For example, women invest much more in potential offspring compared with men. They depend more on social support from kin and mates, and may face more adverse reactions from their social environment if they choose an escalating strategy, which, besides the chance to succeed, carries the risk of losing everything. Thus, in socially conflicting situations, especially marital discord, a woman, at least in ancestral societies but also in many present-day conditions, may not have the option to leave the undesirable situation. Feelings of being entrapped may be the result, with depression following as a pathological expression of appeasement or defeat (Price et al. 2004, 2007).

However, if failure in social competition is at the core of depression, sexual selection theory predicts that depression should be common in men. Male depression, however, is probably more likely to come 'in disguise', because appeasement and submission do not pay-off in sexual competition. For men, loss of social status is expected to be more important than for women, because social status serves as a proxy of reproductive success (Price and Wilson 2011). Therefore, job loss or other financial calamities may elicit depression more often in men than in women. However, as defeat is less acceptable for males, the clinical picture of depression in men may more often be coined by irritability and hostility oriented towards subordinates or dependent individuals.

It is commonly assumed that depression occurs twice as often in women compared with men. However, sex differences in adaptation to social competition scenarios suggest that depression in men may come in the disguise of irritability and hostility, because appeasement and submission do not pay-off in the sexually more competitive sex.

Depression is apparently on the rise worldwide and will pose a significant problem to healthcare systems in the future (Rottenberg 2014). The increasing prevalence has manifold causes, but several causes probably emerge from rising pressures to compete with strangers in many different arenas (the workplace, mating, etc.), and with the need to constantly present oneself as attractive and desirable (Hagen 2011). Moreover, at least in western societies, individualism prevails over mutual cooperation, which reduces the chance of getting social support. Depression is also an increasing problem in old age, probably partly due to the lack of social support from kin. Thus, the socio-economic dimension of depression is clearly part of the mismatch scenario between human-evolved psychology and 'modern' environments in which most individuals of our species live (see Chapter 5).

The increasing prevalence of depression worldwide has manifold causes, but several causes probably emerge from rising pressures to compete with strangers in many different arenas (the workplace, mating, etc.), and with the need to constantly present oneself as attractive and desirable.

From a life-history perspective, depression seems to be largely consistent with a strategy favouring a 'slow' life-history pattern (Del Giudice 2014). However, in light of the vast number of causal factors that can thwart the pursuit of important life goals and thus may lead to depression, it is clear that depression can occur in people at the entire continuum, from 'fast' to 'slow' life-history strategies, although those at the 'slow' end may be more susceptible to it. So, instead of rendering depression a 'slow' strategy, it might be better conceptualized as a *slowing* strategy, temporary or permanent. Thus, once depression has lifted, individuals may resume pursuing their 'slow' or 'fast' strategies.

Depression seems to be largely consistent with a strategy favouring a 'slow' life-history pattern. However, in light of the vast number of causal factors that can thwart the pursuit of important life goals and thus may lead to depression, it is clear that depression can occur in people at the entire continuum, from 'fast' to 'slow' life-history strategies.

In any event, while social factors indisputably contribute to the aetiology of depression and are related to life-history patterns in one way or the other way, there is increasing evidence suggesting that depression can also arise from dysfunction of the immune system. This hypothesis is based on observations showing that proinflammatory cytokines are elevated in the serum of many patients with depression, that medical treatment with immune modulators such as interleukin-2 or interferon alpha can cause depression, and that other immunologically relevant anti-inflammatory cytokines may reverse these effects (Rook and Lowry 2009).

Along these lines, it has been argued that the increase in prevalence of depression in developed countries may be related to alterations in immune function, whereby the latter could be caused by a reduction in exposure to pathogens early in life. According to the 'hygiene' hypothesis, the diminished exposure to pathogenic agents early in life may lead to an exaggerated immunological response, thus producing autoimmunity. Chronic elevation of proinflammatory cytokines may act on neurotransmitters in ways that lead to excessive glutamatergic activity and alterations of the serotonin turnover (Rook and Lowry 2009).

The increase in prevalence of depression in developed countries may be related to alterations in immune function, whereby the latter could be caused by a reduction in exposure to pathogens early in life.

Another hypothesis concerning the relationship of immune function and mood disorders posits that genes that predispose to depression have been retained in the gene pool of human populations in spite of the negative impact depression has on reproductive fitness, because they have important roles in immune function. In fact, it seems that several alleles that may predispose to major depression have proinflammatory properties and are involved in the defence against pathogens that might have been much more prevalent in our evolutionary past (Raison and Miller 2013).

In support of this assumption, depression shares some important features with sickness behaviour, which can be observed in animals and humans when fighting infectious diseases. Sickness behaviour is characterized by apathy, low mood, inappetence, anhedonia, and psychomotor retardation, which together contribute to saving energy and resources (Anders et al. 2013). In fact, these behavioural correlates that are also typical for depression may help reduce exposure to other pathogenic agents or stress in general, and may reduce the risk of spreading the disease to kin and important non-kin allies within the social group (Anders et al. 2013).

Finally, the link of depression to immune function may explain the seasonal peak pattern of depression in winter and spring, when exposure to environmental pathogens is particularly high (Anders et al. 2013), which is also reflected in seasonal variation of serotonin turnover (Luykx et al. 2013).

In summary, an evolutionary view on depressive disorders suggests that these syndromes are highly heterogeneous in nature. A key 'message' sent non-verbally by patients with depression often concerns the need to conserve resources and energy in the broadest sense, akin to sickness behaviour in animals, and to avoid harm by choosing a de-escalating submissive social strategy. However, as the example of depression may illustrate, similar phenotypic manifestations may have very different underlying causes, ranging from interactions of genes involved in serotonin and monoamine turnover with environmental adversity, such as child neglect, to complex interactions of immunologically relevant processes with exposure to pathogens or other stressors. All this is open to empirical testing, which may eventually help to improve individually tailored therapy.

10.7 **Differential diagnosis and comorbidity**

Major depression may be mimicked by frontal lobe disorders or other 'organic' brain disorders. Thus, 'organic' causes of depression must be ruled out (Swartz et al. 1997). Depressive episodes with psychotic symptoms are sometimes difficult to distinguish from acute schizophrenia, particularly in first-episode patients. A thorough longitudinal observation is warranted, because treatment differs in terms of relapse prevention. Depression is thought to be a risk factor for Alzheimer's disease, but may also precede the onset of dementia. Depressive disorders occur comorbidly with anxiety disorders and substance dependence. There is also considerable comorbidity of depression with eating disorders and personality disorders (American Psychiatric Association 2013).

A variety of 'organic' brain disorders can imitate depression or BD. Depression occurs comorbidly with anxiety disorders, substance dependence, and personality disorders.

10.8 **Course and outcome**

Major depression has a substantial tendency for recurrence, with relapse rates being high following pharmacological and psychological treatment (Steinert et al. 2014). Relapse rates for major depression are 25 percent within the first 6 months following recovery, with up to 75 percent recurrence after 5 years. Recurrent unipolar depression is associated with the tendency of phase acceleration and incomplete remission with increasing duration of the

Recurrent depression is associated with high relapse rates. Over the course of the illness, depression is associated with the tendency of phase acceleration and incomplete remission.

illness. Fifteen percent of patients suffering from major depression will eventually die from suicide.

10.9 Treatment

Several forms of treatment for depression have become available, including a broad spectrum of antidepressant substances with differences in receptor profiles. The most recommended substances are reuptake inhibitors of serotonin, norepinephrine, and dopamine. In addition, psychotherapy is effective in many forms of depression and may be combined with antidepressant pharmacotherapy. The evolutionary perspective may suggest that special attention is paid to dealing with the causes of depression using psychotherapy, rather than choosing a symptom-based approach, including encouragement of the patient to negotiate conflict, seek compromises, and perhaps give up unrealizable goals.

Several forms of treatment for depression have become available, including a broad spectrum of antidepressant substances with differences in receptor profiles. The most recommended substances are reuptake inhibitors of serotonin, norepinephrine, and dopamine. In addition, psychotherapy is effective in many forms of depression and may be combined with antidepressant pharmacotherapy.

In light of the high relapse rate, recurrence of depression can be prevented by administration of lithium or several anti-epileptic substances.

Treatment of depression may also involve psychoeducational means that aim at reducing the risk for relapse. Much more could be done in terms of primary prevention of depression, including educating parents about the need to give children the opportunity to develop a secure attachment, and how to reduce intrafamilial stress levels to avoid physical and emotional abuse (see Afterthought to Chapter 4).

Treatment recommendations and useful information for professionals and laypersons have been published by the APA, RCP, and RANZCP.

Chapter 11

Anxiety disorders

Abstract

Anxiety disorders comprise a group of syndromes that revolve around fear or worry elicited by specific situations and objects (i.e. phobias), or occurring independently of specific triggers (general anxiety disorder). They are accompanied by autonomic nervous system activation, including sweating, tachycardia, tremor, and nausea. Avoidance of the precipitating stimulus is typical. Anxiety disorders occur in response to perceived danger or threat. Accordingly, flight or freezing may follow. At the cognitive level, anxiety disorders are associated with increased uncertainty about future threats, and at the emotional level with feelings of uncontrollability and unpredictability. Like depression, anxiety disorders are concerned with harm avoidance and defence. Fear and anxiety are among the most common evolutionarily conserved emotions. Following the analogy of the smoke detector, thresholds for fear responses are low, which may explain why so many false alarms occur. Threshold-lowering factors include impending abandonment or the perception of social threat.

Keywords

anxiety, fear, phobia, generalized anxiety, flight, freezing, harm avoidance, defence, smoke detector

11.1 Symptomatology and diagnostic criteria

Anxiety disorders have in common feelings of intense distress, anticipation of impending danger, and entrapment. At the physiological level, these symptoms are accompanied by the activation of the autonomic sympathetic system, which includes tachycardia, hyperventilation, dizziness and nausea, and sweating. Cognitive symptoms include excessive worry, fear of being humiliated, rejected, or abandoned, and fear of losing control or dying. Duration and intensity of these symptoms vary greatly between different forms of anxiety disorders, from relatively short periods of time with the greatest intensity in panic disorder

Anxiety disorders have in common psychological symptoms of subjectively highly distressing and excessive worry, and anticipation of impending danger and entrapment. At the physiological level, these symptoms are accompanied by tachycardia, hyperventilation, dizziness and nausea, and sweating.

(PD), to enduring worrying of minor intensity in generalized anxiety disorder (GAD). Moreover, there are differences with regard to the situational circumstances that may elicit symptoms of anxiety. In phobic disorders, the precipitating situational context is part of the definition, whereas in PD and GAD these situations are less well determined or absent.

Accordingly, the definitional criteria of the anxiety disorders emphasize different aspects of the symptomatology. DSM-5 now features among the anxiety disorders separation anxiety disorder, selective mutism, specific phobia, social anxiety disorder (SAD), PD, agoraphobia, GAD, substance-induced anxiety disorders, and anxiety due to another medical condition (American Psychiatric Association 2013).

DSM-5 features among the anxiety disorders separation anxiety disorder, selective mutism, specific phobia, SAD, PD, agoraphobia, GAD, substance-induced anxiety disorders, and anxiety due to another medical condition.

Separation anxiety disorder typically manifests in childhood. It is characterized by the fear of being separated from attachment figures and persistent fears about being harmed, being kidnapped, or about something dreadful happening to the attachment figure.

Selective mutism also manifests in childhood. It often co-occurs with SAD. Individuals with selective mutism fail to speak in specific social situations, whereas speech is normal in more familiar situations.

Phobias are object- or situation-related fears, whereby the object (snakes, spiders, etc.) or situation (receiving an injection, etc.) triggers immediate fear or anxiety. Avoidance behaviour with regard to the fear-eliciting object or situation is typical. Agoraphobia is separated from the other 'specific phobias', although the mechanism involved is similar, in that open space or enclosed places provoke anxiety.

PD concerns physical symptoms that occur abruptly and include sweating, tachycardia, trembling, nausea, paraesthesias, shortness of breath, intense fear (of dying), and derealization.

GAD occurs independent of specific triggers. It is characterized by persistent worry about different 'everyday' circumstances or events. It is associated with physical symptoms such as elevated muscle tension, restlessness, and sleep disturbances.

11.2 **Epidemiology**

As a group, anxiety disorders have a life-time prevalence of up to 30 percent and a 12-month prevalence of about 15 percent, but with considerable cultural variation. SAD, formerly known as 'social phobia', is the most common anxiety disorder, with a life-time prevalence rate of around 15 percent (den Boer 2000; Wittchen and Fehm 2001). Other specific phobias are also quite common in the general population (around 7–9 percent), but appear less often in clinical settings. Agoraphobia, which is frequently associated with PD, is also common, whereas GAD is the least common of the classic anxiety disorders, with a life-time prevalence of about 5 percent (Kessler et al. 2001). Prevalence of the newly introduced syndromes 'separation anxiety disorder' and 'selective mutism' has been reported to figure around

Anxiety disorders are among the most common psychiatric disorder, with a life-time prevalence of up to 30 percent and a 12-month prevalence of about 15 percent. SAD is the most common anxiety disorder. Anxiety disorders are twice as likely to affect women as men.

1–2 percent in adults for the former and 0.03–1 percent for the latter. Separation anxiety disorder is believed to be the most common anxiety disorder in prepubertal children, with rates declining from childhood to adulthood (American Psychiatric Association 2013). Selective mutism occurs in young children, with little knowledge about its development over the life-time.

Anxiety disorders are twice as likely to affect women as men. Onset of anxiety disorders is difficult to determine, because many individuals who later seek treatment for anxiety disorder had 'precursor' symptoms as children, including 'inhibited' temperament and avoidance behaviour. The average age at clinical manifestation is around adolescence or early adulthood and anxiety disorders peak towards the end of the third decade. Exceptions to this are separation anxiety disorder and selective mutism, which typically manifest in childhood.

11.3 **Genetic risk factors**

Family and twin studies into anxiety disorders have revealed mixed results. First-degree relatives of index subjects have a three to five times higher risk of developing a disorder compared to controls. In all anxiety disorders, both shared and individual-specific environmental conditions play a major role (Marks 1986). The least genetic influence is probably found in GAD, which, however, shares some genetic risk factors with major depression, as GAD is increased in relatives of patients with major depression compared with controls. PD and GAD apparently do not share genetic diathesis, nor does genetic susceptibility between PD and major depression greatly overlap. Concordance rates for PD in MZ twins have been reported between 40 and 70 percent, as compared to 0 and 20 percent in DZ twins. Agoraphobia shares genetic vulnerability with PD. SAD is two to six times more prevalent in first-degree relative of patients compared with relatives of controls. SAD may overlap, genetically, with selective mutism. All phobias seem to share some genetic vulnerability with one another, as well as with PD, but not with GAD or major depression.

Studies into the genetics of anxiety disorders suggest a heritable component, which differs considerably between subtypes of anxiety disorders. Phobias seem to share some genetic vulnerability with one another, as well as with PD, but not with GAD or major depression.

Candidate genetic polymorphisms for anxiety disorders have been the promoter region of the serotonin transporter (Sen et al. 2004), of which a short-form allele leads to decreased serotonin availability and of the gene controlling the degradation of monoamines (Deckert et al. 1999). Studies into polymorphisms of GABA-synthesizing genes and genes involved in stress regulation via the HPA axis, two potential candidate mechanisms of anxiety disorders, have received mixed results. Animal studies suggest that allelic variation of genes coding for the social-bonding hormones oxytocin and vasopressin may be candidates for further research in humans.

Candidate genetic polymorphisms for anxiety disorders have been the promoter region of the serotonin transporter, of which a short-form allele leads to decreased serotonin transporter expression, and of the gene controlling the degradation of monoamines. The contributions of genes involved in GABA regulation, stress hormone regulation, and pro-inflammatory substances such as cholecystokinin are less well buttressed by empirical studies.

The promoter region of the cholecystokinin-coding gene has been associated with PD, which is interesting because cholecystokinin can produce panic attacks in healthy individuals.

11.4 **Environmental risk factors**

Early traumatization, including emotional and sexual abuse, parental neglect, heightened parental anxiety, and social inhibition in parents, comprises the most significant environmental risk factor for anxiety disorders (Otto et al. 2001; Bandelow et al. 2002). Likewise, loss or early separation from a caregiver is overrepresented in individuals with anxiety disorders (Preter and Klein 2008). In addition, accidents, experience of violence, and chronic exposure to life-threatening events constitute important risk factors. Insufficiently developed coping strategies for stressful events, including low self-efficacy and feelings of poor control, enhance the risk for anxiety disorders, but may be the consequence of poor social support and discouraging parenting behaviour.

Early traumatization, including emotional and sexual abuse, parental neglect, and heightened anxiety in parents, comprises the most significant environmental risk factor for anxiety disorders.

11.5 **Pathophysiological mechanisms**

Current knowledge of the pathophysiology of anxiety disorders is fuelled by studies into the mode of action of psychotropic drugs, animal studies, and brain lesions studies. Even though there are differences between the subtypes of anxiety disorders, research has focused on three neurotransmitter systems involved in the pathophysiology of anxiety disorders, namely serotonin, norepinephrine, and GABA.

The main neurotransmitter systems involved in the pathophysiology of anxiety disorders regulate the turnover of serotonin, norepinephrine, and GABA.

Serotonin is widely distributed in the brain. It has, by and large, dampening effects on neurotransmission, but this depends on the specific receptor type and binding site. It is well established that serotonin reuptake inhibitory substances have anti-anxiety potential. Conversely, drugs that cause the release of serotonin, such as lysergic acid diethylamide (LSD) and fenfluramine, have pro-anxiety effects. Early adversity interacts with genetic variation of the serotonin transporter gene and can lead to increased anxiety sensitivity (Stein et al. 2008).

Norepinephrine is synthesized in the locus coeruleus, from which pathways project to the neocortex and other brain areas. Norepinephrine regulates arousal and attention. Direct stimulation of the locus coeruleus produces fear responses in animals, whereas destruction of this area blocks adaptive responses to fear-inducing stimuli. Drugs that stimulate beta-adrenergic neurons produce anxiety, similar to antagonists at the alpha-adrenergic receptor. On the other hand, beta-receptor antagonists ('beta-blockers') and alpha-receptor agonists such as clonidine can reduce pathological anxiety.

GABA is the most abundant inhibitory transmitter in the brain. It is known that GABAergic substances such as the benzodiazepines are potent anti-anxiety drugs, but the exact contribution of the GABA system to anxiety disorders is not entirely clear.

A central role in fear and anxiety is ascribed to the amygdala and its reciprocal connections, particularly with the OFC and hippocampal formation (Davidson 2002; Charney 2003; Blair et al. 2005; Deussing and Wurst 2007; Milad and Rauch 2007). The famous animal lesion studies by Klüver and Bucy, in which they bilaterally ablated the temporal lobes (including the amygdala) in rhesus monkeys, revealed that operated animals lost their natural fear response, accompanied by several other behavioural abnormalities. In humans, damage to the amygdala due to Urbach–Wiethe disease, in which calcium deposition destroys the amygdala, results in the inability to accurately decipher fear from facial expressions (Adolphs et al. 1994). The amygdalae also contribute to the detection of gaze direction and, hence, behaviour monitoring of other individuals (Allman and Brothers 1994). The OFC contributes to the emotional evaluation of potentially threatening stimuli and is involved in fear-conditioning, whereas the medial PFC is involved in extinction of conditioned fear responses.

A central role in fear and anxiety is ascribed to the amygdala and its reciprocal connections with the OFC and hippocampal formation.

Brain imaging studies in patients with anxiety disorders show inconsistent results. Anatomical abnormalities of the temporal lobes and parahippocampal gyrus have been shown in PD (Brambilla et al. 2002). In functional brain imaging studies the amgydalae are overactive when individuals evaluate threat-related stimuli (Etkin and Wager 2007).

PD is associated with anatomical abnormalities of the temporal lobes and parahippocampal gyrus. The amgydalae are overactive when individuals evaluate threat-related stimuli.

11.6 **Evolutionary synthesis**

Behavioural observation of patients with anxiety disorders suggests that these disorders—as a group—reflect exaggerated responses to internal or external signals of perceived danger or threat. The autonomic part of the anxious response pattern prepares the organism for one of several behavioural options how to terminate the anxiety-eliciting situation, namely flight, immobility, submission, or aggression (Marks and Nesse 1994). More specifically, ethological analyses of the non-verbal behaviour of people with anxiety disorders (foremost SAD) reveal that individuals often present with a 'fear grin', an expression that can also be observed in other primates. In contrast to a genuine smile, it is characterized by the exposure of the teeth, whereby the mouth corners are retracted (Harrigan and Taing 1997; Troisi 1999). This expression conveys the meaning of subordination or appeasement (Price et al. 2004). Excessive fear may also induce 'freezing' and tonic immobility, a 'primitive' response to life-threatening situations, which serve the purpose to reduce detection by predators (see Chapter 8 on catatonia).

Anxiety disorders reflect exaggerated responses to internal or external signals of perceived danger or threat.

Fear and anxiety are so intrinsic to human nature that the distinction between 'normal' and 'pathological' can be difficult to draw. With regard to terminological issues, it is consensus that 'fear' reflects an adaptive response to threat, whereas 'anxiety' concerns pathological exaggerations of fear responses in terms of duration, intensity, or situational appropriateness. In any event, mechanisms involved in anxiety disorders are clearly related to evolved defence mechanisms.

Anxiety disorders also share important features with depression (Stein and Bouwer 1997). Depression is often a response following perceived or actual danger, whereas anxiety concerns threat or impending danger, that is, the anticipatory phase, although both depression and anxiety may operate in synergistic ways to manage social conflict (Price 2013). In contrast to depression, anxiety attacks usually cease automatically, and often aim more directly at eliciting care from others (like in PD or agoraphobia). Moreover, situations causing anxiety can better be avoided than those leading to depression.

Anxiety disorders share important features with depression. Depression is often a response following perceived or actual danger, whereas anxiety concerns threat or impending danger, that is, the anticipatory phase.

Indeed, most anxiety disorders occur in social contexts (like in SAD) or concern social matters (e.g. fear of abandonment, as in cases with separation anxiety and PD, or worry about future threats, as in GAD). Some forms of fear-related behaviours may even be altruistically motivated. For example, alarm calls are found in many primate species and can be truly seen as altruistic behaviour, because the call is clearly at the cost of the alarming individual, which runs the risk of attracting the attention of predators, and because the alarming individual has no immediate pay-off from warning its conspecifics. In a similar vein, social anxiety can perhaps contribute to reducing hostile competition for rank within social groups (Kahn 2013), and worry about future threat may be motivated by protection of close kin (as in GAD).

Phobic fears of specific situations are the most prevalent forms of anxiety disorders, and much of the associated behaviours are inherited from our mammalian ancestors (LeDoux 1996). For example, during normal human ontogeny, separation from the primary caregiver, heights, and strangers are among the strongest fear-evoking situations, to which the human infant is biologically prepared to respond (Bowlby 1973). These fear responses are particularly prevalent during certain developmental periods: separation distress occurs soon after birth, fear of heights emerges when the infant starts to crawl, and fear of strangers occurs when the toddler begins to give up physical closeness to the mother for brief periods of time.

These fear reactions operate on actual sources of fear that were persistent enough in the EEA to select for adequate (adaptive) anticipatory anxiety. Their ways of functioning have been likened to the principle of a 'smoke detector' mechanism, which works optimally if the threshold is low enough to reliably produce a response to potentially life-threatening stimuli at the cost of some false alarms, but high enough to limit the costliness of too many energetically expensive false alarms. Here, it needs to be emphasized that not responding to a genuine threat (e.g. in a predation situation) is most expensive, because it may cause death of the individual; thus, behaviour too dauntless would readily be eliminated by natural selection, and a lack of fearfulness would not translate into greater reproductive fitness (Nesse 2001).

In primates, including humans, phobic fear reactions are acquired not only through direct conditioning experiences, but also through vicarious experiences, in which an individual witnesses the response of another individual to fear-relevant stimuli (Mineka

1987). This is probably the most important mechanism by which biologically predisposed fears become actually manifest (Olsson and Phelps 2007). For example, fear of snakes is most likely not 'innate' in primates, but requires observation of fear responses of conspecifics to the sight of a snake. However, although conditioning seems to be necessary, biological preparedness is also likely involved, because no such reactions can be experimentally conditioned when using flowers instead of snakes as conditioned stimuli (Mineka 1987).

Fear reactions operate on actual sources of fear that were persistent enough in the EEA to be selected. Phobic fear reactions are acquired not only through direct conditioning experiences, but also through vicarious experiences, in which an individual witnesses the response of another individual to fear-relevant stimuli.

Even though these conditioning models may be more valid for between-species fears than same-species (social) phobic fears, it is most obvious that normal fear-conditioning and pathological phobia and other anxiety disorders occur along a continuum. Normal fear conditioning takes place early in life. For example, a young primate may easily acquire fear of snakes through attending to its mother's reaction (Mineka 1987). The extraordinary importance of physical closeness for young primates and humans supports the assumption that individual differences in attachment exert long-lasting effects on how young infants and children learn to cope with fear-inducing situations. If, for instance, the primary caregiver is unresponsive to the infant's needs or even unavailable, insecure attachment is likely to develop. Consequently, ambivalently or avoidantly attached infants are more vulnerable to develop anxiety disorders later in life. In line with this, patients with various forms of anxiety disorders have experienced early losses more often than controls, report rejection by parents more frequently, or have experienced extremely inadequate caregiving more often compared to controls.

This makes sense in light of the hypothesis that insecurely attached individuals are prepared through adverse early experiences to develop mistrustful inner working models and to see the world as a hazardous place (see Chapter 3). Gene–environment interactions leading to anxiety disorders seem to predispose these individuals to assume behavioural strategies aiming at harm avoidance and acquiring defence strategies associated with internalizing symptoms (which explains the frequent comorbidity of anxiety disorders with depression). In line with this assumption, carriers of the short polymorphic version of the serotonin transporter gene have been found to develop depression or anxiety disorder after negative life events more often than individuals who lack this allele variant (Canli and Lesch 2007).

Insecurely attached individuals are more vulnerable to develop anxiety disorders later in life. Carriers of the short polymorphic version of the serotonin transporter gene have been found to develop depression or anxiety disorder after negative life events more often than individuals who lack this allele variant, suggesting important gene–environment interactions.

Early experiences may, therefore, 'shape' the responsivity of neurobiological circuits involved in fear responses. For example, evidence from brain imaging studies suggests exaggerated sensitivity of the amygdalae to fearful stimuli in patients with SAD (Amaral 2002). In addition, the reduced control over fear responses may be augmented by a diminished emotional evaluation of threat signals (projected from the amygdala to PFC areas) and insufficient integration of representation of past experiences (via the hippocampal formation). In other words, in sensitized individuals, irrespective of whether sensitization is genetically predisposed, acquired through aversive experience, or both, the amygdala may lose its inhibitory control through which it normally controls the approach of novel objects or other organisms (including individuals of the same species). Instead the amygdala responds in a dysregulated or hyperactive fashion such that benign environmental stimuli may be perceived as dangerous. Put another way, in anxiety disorders there is exaggerated uncertainty about future threat, which leads to an inflated estimate of potential threat costs, as well as a heightened feeling of unpredictability and uncontrollability (Grupe and Nitschke 2013). All this may result in exaggerated avoidance behaviour and subjectively overwhelming feelings of intense fear in vulnerable individuals (Amaral 2002).

In sensitized individuals the amygdala loses its inhibitory control through which it normally controls the approach of novel objects or other organisms.

Conceivably, humans may be particularly susceptible to dysregulation of fear circuits for several reasons, which may account for the high prevalence rates of anxiety disorders. First, since humans are exceptionally social, but physically vulnerable, they may be inclined to constantly check their environment for potential sources of threat (both from outside and from within the social group). This may include not only predatory or physical threat, but also threat of social status and loss of resources (Lerner and Keltner 2001). If feelings of social safeness are threatened (real or imagined), social anxiety or panic may emerge (Grupe and Nitschke 2013; Kahn 2013). In support of this assumption, the neuroanatomical structures involved in the evaluation of potentially dangerous situations have increased in size over evolutionary time, which underscores their importance in terms of survival and reproductive success.

Second, newborn humans critically depend on intense nurturance and care, such that a stable affectional bond with a primary caregiver is outstandingly vital for survival. If, however, stability of an affectional bond is unattainable or disrupted (e.g. by loss of the primary caregiver), a hypersensitive and constantly overaroused fear system may result. Such a situation may dramatically worsen if physical or emotional abuse is involved, with which an immature human infant can hardly cope.

Third, humans have evolved the capacity to anticipate future scenarios, which, on the one hand, has certainly been highly adaptive with regard to foreseeing food shortages or other potentially perilous situations, including changing alliances between contenders; on the other hand, exaggerated anticipation of threat and danger seems to be immanent to various forms of anxiety disorders, which may, in part, explain why patients often report fear of recurrence of anxiety (anticipatory anxiety; Chua et al. 1999; Grupe and Nitschke 2013).

Humans may be particularly susceptible to dysregulation of fear circuits, because they are physically vulnerable, and may therefore constantly check their environment for potential sources of threat; because as immature infants they extremely rely on secure attachment ties and may be hypersensitive to potential threats if insecurely attached; and because humans have evolved the capacity of anticipating future events, including possible scenarios associated with danger.

Finally, it could be that in modern societies the diminished necessity to cope with fear-inducing situations—simply due to a reduced number of dangerous encounters with poisonous animals or predators—renders the neurobiological system involved in the evaluation of potential hazards more labile and 'unprepared' to accurately respond to real-life confrontation with spiders, snakes, or heights. However, a notable exception could be potential or actual harm caused by conspecifics. In modern societies, individuals frequently meet other people whom they have never seen before, and whose intentions are much harder to determine than in familiar people. This may cause problems particularly for those individuals who have developed mistrustful inner working models and are cognitively biased towards assuming malicious intents in others. In fact, patients with anxiety disorders frequently complain that others can virtually see what is wrong with them, and of being observed or stared at (in contrast to delusional beliefs, patients with anxiety disorders do not report incorrigible conviction that this is true; continua between extreme anxiety and paranoid ideation may, however, exist; Kahn 2013).

Although the preceding paragraphs have dealt with anxiety disorders as if they were different manifestations of a singular diathesis, they differ, to some extent, in neurobiology and precipitating events.

PD may reflect a false suffocation alarm.

PD is perhaps the most 'primitive' of the anxiety disorders. For example, PD has been interpreted as false suffocation alarm, because carbon dioxide inhalation or lactate infusion may produce panic attacks in vulnerable (healthy) individuals. Moreover, PD occurs more frequently in individuals with heightened partial pressure of carbon dioxide (pCO_2) levels, for example, during sleep, during the premenstrual period, and in patients with respiratory disorders. On the other hand, PD is less common in physiological states associated with lowered PCO_2, including pregnancy and delivery.

Although there is some evidence that genetic vulnerability is most prominent in PD compared to other anxiety disorders, additional environmental factors, such as loss of an attachment figure, may be equally important in that such events may lower the suffocation alarm threshold (Bandelow et al. 2002). Panic attacks may therefore be seen as the extreme version of a preparatory set of physiological changes typical of immediate flight or escape behaviours. Anticipatory anxiety is often the result of recurrent panic attacks. Thus, at the cognitive level, PD involves the mental representation of future negative events. From a neurobiological perspective, PD probably involves hyperexcitability of norepinephrine pathways and reduced serotonergic and GABAergic dampening of limbic structures. In light of the putative association of PD with separation distress, a link with abnormal oxytocin turnover is conceivable (Preter and Klein 2007).

Agoraphobia, which often accompanies PD, reflects an exaggerated response to avoid open space, or fear of being in an enclosed space (claustrophobia). Agoraphobia, like PD, is probably the pathological extreme of an evolutionarily conserved behavioural pattern that is common to many animal species, and helps to protect the organism from entering unknown terrain that could yield a predatory threat or hostile attacks from conspecifics. Whether or not agoraphobia differs from PD in neurobiology or simply represents a more severe and complex form of PD is debatable.

Agoraphobia is the extreme of variation of fear associated with entering unknown terrain.

Shared genetic vulnerability between agoraphobia and PD and associations with similar precipitating life events may support the latter assumption.

SAD is characterized by intense fear of social situations in the presence of an authoritative person (den Boer 2000). Social phobia can be interpreted as an exaggerated submissive gesture triggered by situations that may potentially lead to humiliation and loss of social status (Stein et al. 2004). There are some phenomenological parallels or overlap with normal blushing, which, in extreme forms, may develop into erythrophobia, the fear of reddening of the skin as a visible signal of the subjective state of embarrassment (Darwin 1872). SAD causes a dilemma, especially in its generalized form, because fear and anxiety usually elicit care and comforting behaviour in others, which the affected individual cannot tolerate. In fact, heightened attention from others may even aggravate the phobic reaction.

SAD can be interpreted as an exaggerated submissive gesture triggered by situations that may potentially lead to humiliation and loss of social status.

The difference to other anxiety disorders is that SAD patients tend to exaggerate the evaluation of mental states of others. Unlike patients with autism or schizophrenia who have difficulties in representing the mental states of others (reduced mentalizing in the former, inaccurate hypermentalizing in the latter), patients with social phobia are well able to appropriately reason about other persons' mental life; in specific situations, which are perceived as posing a threat to social status and reputation, however, they negatively interpret the social signals of others, and may overanticipate a personally appalling outcome of social encounters (Kahn 2013).

More specifically, people with SAD resemble those with depression in that they engage in a variety of submissive behaviours that are accompanied by cognitive distortions related to the fear of being evaluated by others (both negatively and positively), possibly to minimize the risk of social exclusion (Weeks et al. 2009). Interestingly, fear of positive, rather than negative evaluation, seems to be associated with concerns of social reprisal by dominant others, suggesting that concerns of being 'too good' may foster cognitive tendencies of self-derogation in people with severe SAD (Weeks and Howell 2012). In addition, in experimental settings they evaluate hypothetical threat scenarios as more dangerous and choose more often escape as a potential response to such scenarios compared to controls (Mesquita et al. 2011).

Taken together, these findings suggest that people with SAD are concerned with potential social threat, because they experience themselves as having a lower social rank and being inferior to others, which may affect how they perceive intimacy and closeness to others (Aderka et al. 2009; Weisman et al. 2011).

Consistent with these studies, research in animals and humans strongly suggests a central role of amygdala dysfunction in SAD (Amaral 2002). This dysfunction may be mediated by reduced availability of GABA and serotonin, as well as by impaired regulation of affiliative behaviour and social attachment via oxytocin (Insel 2002). Moreover, reduced inhibition of amygdalar function through glutamatergic prefrontal efferents (via GABAergic interneurons) has been identified as potential proximate causation of SAD.

In contrast to phobic anxiety, GAD is not explicitly associated with particular precipitating events. GAD rather reflects an overall tendency towards excessive worry and hypervigilance, probably forming a continuum with avoidant personality disorder. It is the least heritable anxiety disorder, and therefore depends even more than the other anxiety disorders on early aversive subjective experiences and learned behaviour. Chronic hyperexcitability, restlessness, and increased muscle tension are likely to involve the HPA axis, which may induce secondary somatic problems, including chronic arterial hypertension and other stress-related disorders.

GAD rather reflects an overall tendency towards hypervigilance.

In summary, anxiety disorders represent pathologically exaggerated defence mechanisms, which primarily manifest at the emotional but also at the corresponding and interconnected behavioural and cognitive level. Anxiety is perhaps one of the most profound emotions that deeply root in our evolved repertoire to deal with threat or anticipated threat. Anxiety disorders differ to some extent in their genetic underpinnings and environmental causation. However, all anxiety disorders have in common that they can be triggered by social experiences and are influenced by different modalities of associative (social) learning. Unlearning the conditioned response is sometimes hard to manage, such that preventive measures, including prevention of early traumatization and strengthening of resilience, are crucial aspects of any therapeutic effort.

11.7 **Differential diagnosis and comorbidity**

Differential diagnoses of anxiety disorders comprise many somatic disorders, including endocrinological disorders such as hypoglycaemia, hypocalcaemia, cardiac problems, and epileptic aura. Moreover, anxiety can accompany almost every other psychiatric disorder, including substance withdrawal syndromes and psychosis. In particular, panic attacks may serve as an index of severity of psychiatric conditions in general, not just among the anxiety disorders.

Differential diagnoses of anxiety disorders comprise endocrinological disorders, cardiac problems, epileptic aura, and substance withdrawal. Comorbidity of anxiety disorders with depression or substance abuse is very common. In patients with anxiety disorders the risk for suicidal behaviour is substantial. Anxiety disorders co-occur comorbidly with one another.

Comorbidity of anxiety disorders with depression is very common (Wittchen et al. 1994). The life-time prevalence of depression in PD, for example, figures around 50–70 percent. Conversely, PD is prevalent in patients with unipolar and bipolar depression in 10–60 percent. Comorbid cases are usually more severe, and age at onset is earlier than in both disorders alone. Suicidality is often underestimated in patients with anxiety disorders, because it is erroneously believed that anxious people also have an exaggerated fear of dying. However, the actual suicide rate in anxiety disorders is about tenfold higher compared to the general population risk, and further increases in cases with comorbid depression or substance abuse. Substance abuse, particularly alcohol abuse or dependence, is common in patients with anxiety disorders. Alcohol dependence has been reported in up to 30 percent of in-patients who were treated for anxiety disorder. On the other hand, anxiety disorders may be comorbidly present in over 40 percent of patients with alcohol abuse.

Comorbidity within the anxiety spectrum disorders is frequently observed. For example, SAD and agoraphobia co-occur in almost 50 percent of cases. Similarly, PD occurs comorbidly with agoraphobia in 20 percent, and with SAD in roughly 10 percent. Also, PTSD is accompanied by specific phobias or agoraphobia in up to 20 percent of cases.

PTSD, somatic symptom disorder, and illness anxiety disorder are also important differential diagnoses to several of the anxiety disorders featured in this chapter.

11.8 **Course and outcome**

Course and outcome vary greatly between different types of anxiety disorders. Separation anxiety disorder usually decreases with age, and most adults, who as children had separation anxiety disorder, are functionally unimpaired. Specific phobias may change focus with age, whereby older adults may attribute their concerns to somatic problems. Social anxiety disorder may remit spontaneously, though it may take years in some individuals (American Psychiatric Association 2013). The severity of PD and agoraphobia tends to decline after the fourth decade. However, in a considerable number of patients the disorder takes a chronic course, with incomplete remission and impaired social and occupational functioning, which may be complicated by comorbid disorders such as substance abuse or depression.

Anxiety disorders frequently take a chronic course with incomplete remission, or change focus with age.

11.9 **Treatment**

For severe anxiety disorders a combined psychotherapeutic and pharmacological treatment is recommended, depending on the patient's preferences and potential side-effects. Acute treatment may often include the administration of benzodiazepines, whereas this substance group is not helpful in maintenance treatment (Goddard et al. 2004). Among the antidepressants, selective serotonin reuptake inhibitors (SSRI) are usually tolerated best. Some patients respond to tricyclic antidepressants (TCI) or monoamine oxidase inhibitors (MAOI).

For severe anxiety disorders, a combined psychotherapeutic and pharmacological treatment is recommended, depending on symptom severity, patient's preferences, and potential side-effects.

Among the various forms of psychotherapy, cognitive behavioural therapy (CBT) focusing on exposure to fear-inducing cues and cognitive restructuring is most widely recommended in anxiety disorders (Clark 1999). Education for patients with anxiety disorders is most advanced compared to other psychiatric disorders in providing comprehensible models of the disorder, which (often implicitly) include the evolutionary background of natural defence mechanisms, or may at least benefit thereof (Bateson et al. 2011). This greatly helps to reduce stigmatization, and patients are usually grateful for explanations of the biological and sociopsychological dimension of anxiety.

Detailed treatment guidelines for anxiety disorders are available on the internet published by the APA, RCP, and RANZCP.

Chapter 12

Obsessive-compulsive and related disorders

Abstract

Obsessive-compulsive and related disorders comprise several syndromes, to which repetitive thoughts or behaviours are central. Compulsive behaviour is concerned most with hygiene, orderliness, checking, grooming, and hoarding, whereas obsessive thoughts (rumination) focus on harm avoidance and cultural taboos. Compulsive behaviours resemble stereotypic movements seen in animals or cultural rituals. Cognitively, anticipating potential future risk scenarios may help in minimising threat, suggesting that obsessive-compulsive disorder may be a by-product of foresight. Obsessive-compulsive disorder is often linked to life events that require heightened vigilance for threat, including sexual maturation (puberty), pregnancy, and childbirth. While most individuals with obsessive-compulsive disorder follow a 'slow' life-history strategy, cases with increased impulsivity and reduced inhibitory control seem to pursue a 'fast' life-history strategy.

Keywords

obsessive-compulsive disorder, repetitive behaviour, rituals, harm avoidance, foresight, rumination

12.1 Symptomatology and diagnostic criteria

Obsessive-compulsive and related disorders comprise OCD, body dysmorphic disorder, trichotillomania, and excoriation disorder, as well as medication-induced obsessive-compulsive symptoms, and symptoms that occur due to another medical condition, such as Sydenham's chorea and autoimmunological diseases.

Obsessive-compulsive and related disorders comprise OCD, body dysmorphic disorder, trichotillomania, and excoriation disorder, as well as medication-induced obsessive-compulsive symptoms, and symptoms that occur due to another medical condition, such as Sydenham's chorea and autoimmunological diseases.

OCD is characterized by repetitive thoughts, feelings, and patterns of behaviour that are usually perceived as unwanted and unpleasant, whereby the cognitive component is referred to as 'obsessions' and 'compulsions' concern the behavioural dimension. Obsessions often involve the cognitive anticipation of situations that are perceived as dangerous and need to be controlled, whereas compulsive behaviour is enacted to reduce fear and anxiety, often in an extremely time-consuming fashion.

OCD is characterized by repetitive thoughts, feelings, and patterns of behaviour that are usually perceived as unwanted and unpleasant. OCD usually involves hygiene, orderliness, symmetry, taboos, or harm.

Content-wise, OCD usually involves certain 'themes', including hygiene, orderliness, symmetry, taboos, and harm. In contrast to people with delusional disorder, individuals with OCD usually perceive such thoughts and behaviours as ego-dystonic, although some overlap between the two syndromes may exist (Fear and Healy 1997; O'Dwyer and Marks 2000). DSM-5 has therefore introduced specifiers for insight/delusional beliefs. Even absent insight or presence of delusional beliefs in OCD do not qualify for the diagnosis of a psychotic disorder (American Psychiatric Disorder 2013). In any event, individuals with OCD have a strong tendency to keep their rituals secret. This often leads to a substantial delay of diagnosis and treatment (Rapoport and Fiske 1998).

Body dysmorphic disorder (dysmorphophobia) concerns a condition in which individuals are excessively preoccupied with their physical appearance and perceive flaws or defects that are not observable by others. People with the condition can have preserved or poor insight or delusional conviction that they look ugly or deformed (American Psychiatric Association 2013).

Body dysmorphic disorder (dysmorphophobia) concerns a condition in which individuals are excessively preoccupied with their physical appearance. Hoarding disorder describes a syndrome that is characterized by exaggerated accumulation of possessions. Trichotillomania (hair-pulling) and excoriation disorder (skin-picking) refer to manipulation of hair or skin, resulting in hair loss or skin lesions.

Hoarding disorder describes a syndrome that is characterized by exaggerated accumulation of possessions, whereby individuals have profound difficulties in abandoning their possessions, irrespective of their actual value. By definition, the collection of items in hoarding disorder is not the result of obsessions. Discarding items causes marked distress. Collections may concern newspapers, clothes, books, and even animals.

Trichotillomania (hair-pulling) and excoriation disorder (skin-picking) refer to manipulation of hair or skin, resulting in hair loss or skin lesions. They are usually experienced as an irresistible urge to pull out one's hair or pick one's skin, with attempts to conceal or camouflage the lesions (American Psychiatric Association 2013).

12.2 **Epidemiology**

OCD has a life-time prevalence rate of about 2–3 percent (Bebbington 1998; Horwath and Weissman 2000). In addition to idiopathic forms of OCD, OCD-related symptoms may accompany disorders involving dysfunction of the basal ganglia, including infectious disorders such as encephalitis lethargica (von Economo), chorea minor (Sydenham), and toxoplasmosis; degenerative disorders, such as Huntington's disease and Parkinson's disease; and other

OCD has a life-time prevalence rate of about 2–3 percent. Age at onset of OCD is around 20 years, but cases with childhood onset are not uncommon.

idiopathic disorders, such as GTS (Frankel et al. 1986; Swedo et al. 1989a, 1989b; Cummings and Cunningham 1992; Alegret et al. 2001).

Age at onset of OCD is around 20 years, but cases with childhood onset are not uncommon.

Prevalence rates for body dysmorphic disorder, trichotillomania, and excoriation disorder hover around 1 and 2 percent, whereby body dysmorphic disorder seems to be slightly more common. Reliable figures for hoarding disorder do not exist. Women are slightly more often affected from all obsessive-compulsive and related disorders than men (American Psychiatric Association 2013).

12.3 **Genetic risk factors**

OCD is associated with a polygenic heritable component, which is particularly obvious if subsyndromal cases are included (Pauls and Alsobrook 1999; Pato et al. 2001). It might be that genetic factors are more relevant for OCD with childhood onset (Pauls et al. 2014). GTS and chronic tic disorders are also several times more common in patients with OCD compared with controls.

OCD is associated with a polygenic heritable component, which is particularly obvious if subsyndromal cases are included.

Linkage studies have identified several loci on different chromosomes, with the strongest finding pointing to a locus on chromosome 1p (Pauls et al. 2012). OCD has been linked with polymorphisms of the serotonin transporter gene and the serotonin 2A receptor. In addition, the dopamine D4 receptor could be involved, with the counterintuitive finding that OCD seems to be associated with the 7-repeat variant, which is typical of ADHD (see Chapter 7). Other dopamine turnover-relevant genes comprise the dopamine transporter and the DRD3 receptor. In males with OCD, an association was also found with the methionin variant of the COMT coding gene and the MAO-A coding gene (Pooley et al. 2007). GWAS have revealed inconclusive results (Pauls et al. 2012).

12.4 **Environmental risk factors**

Early traumatization, including emotional and sexual abuse, is associated with an increased risk for OCD. In particular, body dysmorphic disorder seems to be highly associated with childhood neglect or abuse.

Early traumatization, including emotional and sexual abuse, is associated with an increased risk for OCD.

12.5 **Pathophysiological mechanisms**

Two different frontostriatal pathways seem to be involved in OCD, whereby a 'direct' positive feedback loop is normally under control of an 'indirect,' mainly negative, feedback loop. In OCD, a hyperactivity of unknown cause in these cortical–subcortical pathways is thought to induce a response bias toward stimuli relating to 'socioterritorial' concerns, such that individuals with OCD are 'captured' and unable to switch tasks or change behavioural routines (Saxena and Rauch 2000).

OCD involves a dysfunction of frontostriatal pathways. OCD may be associated with reduced grey matter volumes in the medial frontal gyrus, the medial orbitofrontal gyrus, and the left insular–opercular region.

A recent study of structural brain abnormalities in patients with OCD revealed reduced grey matter volumes in the medial frontal gyrus, the medial orbitofrontal gyrus, and the left insular–opercular region. In contrast, grey matter volumes in the ventral striatum and anterior cerebellum were larger in OCD patients compared to controls (Pujol et al. 2004).

A substantial number of functional brain imaging studies have shown an elevated metabolism (as indicated by an increased regional blood flow) in the OFC, the ACC, the basal ganglia, and the thalamus in patients with OCD (Saxena and Rauch 2000). A functional brain imaging study using a symptom provocation paradigm in patients with OCD revealed a significant bilateral activation of the anterior and posterior orbital gyri, the superior, middle, and inferior frontal gyri, the ACC, the temporal cortices, the right caudate and left lenticulate nuclei, and the left insula and bilateral amygdala (Breiter et al. 1996). In contrast, another study found a reduced cerebral blood flow in the right lateral OFC of OCD patients, which correlated with the severity of the OCD symptomatology (Busatto et al. 2000). In addition, a treatment study of patients with OCD using the SSRI paroxetine revealed a significant decrease of glucose metabolism in the anterolateral OFC after treatment in responders, but not in non-responders (Saxena et al. 1999). The authors suggested that SSRI may reduce excitatory activity in orbitofrontal–subcortical pathways.

12.6 Evolutionary synthesis

Compulsive behaviours associated with OCD and related disorders typically concern hygiene, orderliness, checking, grooming, and hoarding, whereas obsessions involve ruminating thoughts about harm avoidance and taboos. From an evolutionary point of view, it therefore appears straightforward to render these signs and symptoms as exaggerations of adaptive processes that are concerned with risk aversion (Abed and de Pauw 1998; Woody and Szechtman 2011; Glass 2012).

Signs and symptoms associated with OCD represent the pathological extremes of adaptive processes that are concerned with risk aversion. Compulsions are similar in appearance to stereotypies seen in animals under physical restraint.

At the cognitive level, individuals with OCD seem to be preoccupied with the generation of risk scenarios that aim at minimizing future harm.

Ethological interpretations emphasize the similarities of compulsive behaviour with stereotypic movements in animals, as well as with human rituals and ritualized behaviour at large (Insel 1988). For example, animal stereotypies, which often occur in conditions associated with physical restraint (such as restricted locomotion in small cages), share with compulsions the features of excessive performance, inappropriateness to context, or both (Nurnberg et al. 1997). Similarly, animal stereotypies resembling ritualized patterns of behaviour can experimentally be induced by the administration of dopamine agonists, which partly respond to treatment with SSRI (Szechtman et al. 1998). There is also superficial similarity of compulsive behaviour with so-called displacement activities. Displacement activities occur when two opposing motivational drives are simultaneously activated (such as fight or flight), whereby the drive typically 'sparks over' to species-characteristic behaviour involving locomotion or self-grooming (Tinbergen 1952).

Compulsions phenotypically overlap with human rituals, which serve social purposes and help contain fear, anxiety, or perceived threats.

More specifically, compulsive behaviours in OCD resemble culture-bound human rituals, because the latter are also displayed repetitively and often performed in exaggerated and highly stereotyped ways (Eibl-Eibesfeldt 1995). Furthermore, many rituals serve social purposes and help contain fear, anxiety, or perceived threats (Fiske and Haslam 1997). In contrast to compulsions, however, rituals are accepted as culturally implemented patterns of behaviour, and often serve the purpose of enhancing group cohesion and identification with one's social group (Polimeni et al. 2005). Interestingly, rituals also play a crucial role in healing (Fabrega 1997), whereby trance induced by stereotypic repetition of movements or ritual formulas may actually strengthen the immunological response against pathogens (Hanna 1995). Another feature that distinguishes compulsions from rituals pertains to the termination of the behaviour, which is what OCD patients cannot control.

The cognitive processes involved in obsessive thinking and rumination of thoughts concern difficulties in set shifting, decision-making, and prioritizing behavioural routines (Marks and Nesse 1994; Rapoport and Fiske 1998; Saxena and Rauch 2000). Consistent with this, individuals with OCD seem to be preoccupied with the generation of risk scenarios (Abed and de Pauw 1998) that aim at minimizing future harm (Marks and Nesse 1994). In fact, the imaginative generation of future risk scenarios may help to develop harm-avoiding behavioural strategies without the person being subjected to real-life dangers. However, avoiding potential low-frequency hazards involves the detection of subtle cues without external feedback, indicating that ruminating about future threats can be terminated (Woody and Szechtman 2011; Del Giudice 2014), which may explain the emergence of obsessions. According to the hypothesis that an overactive 'risk scenario generating system' (Abed and de Pauw 1998) is at the core of OCD, such obsessive thoughts should be rare in individuals who habitually engage in risky activities, such as people with psychopathy and antisocial personality disorder. Conversely, people with OCD should tend to be socially compliant and rule-abiding in order to avoid social risks, and the severity of OCD should correlate with measures of harm avoidance.

Finally, life events should exacerbate the symptoms of OCD (Abed and de Pauw 1998), which may be more prevalent in women (Del Giudice 2014). Indeed, biologically vulnerable periods across the human lifespan, such as puberty, pregnancy, and childbirth, where increased vigilance to potential threats makes biological sense, increase the risk of developing or worsening obsessive-compulsive symptoms (Williams and Koran 1997; Leckman and Mayes 1999; Lochner and Stein 2001).

In extension to this, it seems plausible to assume that obsessive ruminating is a costly by-product of the human ability of foresight. The imagination of future events and the representation of past experiences (episodic memory) provide us with the ability to 'travel' mentally in time (Suddendorf and Corballis 1997). Mental time travel seems to be fairly unique to humans. Unlike anticipatory behaviour in hibernating animals, for example, which is purely instinct-driven and independent of experience (i.e. hibernators collect foods already in their first hibernating season), 'foreseeing' future risks or needs requires the metarepresentation of events that may or may not happen in the future, that is, the cognitive representation of the anticipatory process (Suddendorf and Corballis 1997). Earlier research suggested that apes are relatively constrained in their cognitive capacity to represent episodic memories and that they live in a rather restricted 'present' (Köhler 1921). The evolution of mental time travel in humans certainly brought about advantages in terms of survival, because it allowed for anticipating future food shortages. As Suddendorf and Corballis (1997) put it, a full-bellied lion might not be dangerous to potential prey; however, a full-bellied *Homo sapiens* might well remain dangerous and continue to hunt to prevent future famine (Suddendorf and Corballis 1997).

Following this line of reasoning, OCD may involve excessive metarepresentation of anticipated potential risks for self and others in order to increase controllability and predictability of future events (Brüne 2006). In support of this hypothesis, studies in non-clinical populations examining beliefs about worry, as well as beliefs about the meaning, consequences, controllability, and dangers of thoughts, revealed that these metacognition processes were positively correlated with the number of obsessive-compulsive symptoms (Myers and Wells 2005).

OCD may involve excessive metarepresentation of anticipated potential risks for self and others in order to increase controllability and predictability of future events.

Along similar lines, there is evidence to suggest that brain regions involved in anticipating future events have disproportionally increased in size during human evolution. In primates, the dorsolateral PFC, the OFC, the ACC, the supplementary motor cortex, pallidostriatal structures, and parts of the thalamus all contribute to the execution of flexible behaviour, where striatum and thalamus operate as filter stations and project back to different areas of the frontal cortex (Pitman 1989; Saint-Cyr et al. 1995; Bradshaw and Sheppard 2000).

Interestingly, the brain regions presumably associated with the pathogenesis of OCD closely match those that are selectively involved in future action planning and episodic memory retrieval in healthy subjects (Okuda et al. 1998; Lepage et al. 2000). In a study using PET, Lepage and colleagues (2000) demonstrated that episodic memory retrieval was associated with enhanced brain activity in the ACC, PFC, dorsolateral PFC, and dorsal PFC. Almost identical activation patterns were found in a paradigm involving 'prospective memory'—the ability to keep in mind something that needs to be carried out in the future (Okuda et al. 1998). Likewise, a PET study of anticipatory anxiety in healthy subjects found activation of the right superior temporal sulcus, bilateral insular cortices, the left fusiform gyrus, and the left ACC, which partially correlated with the score on the Spielberger State and Trait Anxiety Inventory (Chua et al. 1999).

Taken together, these findings suggest that early gene–environment interaction prepares the organism to more readily activate systems involved in the anticipation of future threats. Individuals may then be more vulnerable to decompensate in situations that require greater attention to potential threat to self and others. Accordingly, it makes sense that precipitating events for OCD include situations that are associated with the acceptance of novel social roles, that is, sexual maturation (puberty), pregnancy, childbirth, etc. (Maina et al. 2001).

Early gene–environment interaction prepares the organism to more readily activate systems involved in the anticipation of future threats.

Biologically vulnerable periods across the human lifespan, such as puberty, pregnancy, and childbirth, increase the risk of developing or worsening obsessive-compulsive symptoms.

All this is typical for a 'slow' life-history pattern, as described in Chapter 3. In line with this interpretation, adult OCD seems to be more prevalent in women (Fontenelle and Hasler 2008).

Moreover, OCD is associated with high levels of harm avoidance and conscientiousness, and this also pertains to obsessive-compulsive personality disorder (Samuel and Gore, 2012; Del Giudice 2014). In addition, people who judge past and future scenarios in fatalistic ways are often more aggressive, depressed, or anxious (Zimbardo and Boyd 1999), all of which are part of the OCD symptom spectrum. Conversely, individuals who rate past and future events in more hedonic ways usually score higher on novelty-seeking and sensation-seeking. Both novelty- and sensation-seeking are usually not part of OCD spectrum disorders.

However, Del Giudice (2014) raises the possibility that not all OCD spectrum disorders follow a 'slow' life-history pattern, which makes sense in light of the heterogeneity of the syndromal spectrum. For example, OCD is often characterized by increased impulsivity and reduced motor inhibition, and there is even comorbidity with ADHD, all of which are indicative of a 'fast' life-history strategy (Sheppard et al. 2010; Del Giudice 2014).

A possible explanation for these associations may reside in the distinction between autogenous and reactive obsessions (Lee and Kwon 2003). While autogenous obsessions have sexual, aggressive, and/or blasphemous content, reactive obsessions deal with fears of contamination and issues concerning order. Moreover, autogenous obsessions are associated with schizotypal traits, disorganized thought, reduced inhibitory control, and higher levels of hostility and substance abuse (Lee et al. 2005a), whereas reactive obsessions are associated with perfectionism and high levels of conscientiousness (Moulding et al. 2007). This could suggest that within the OCD spectrum, both 'slow' and 'fast' life-history patterns can occur which differ with regard to the association with defensive as opposed to more aggressive strategies, an interpretation that is further supported by findings with regard to socio-economic status, which is particularly high in people with obsessive-compulsive personality disorder (Del Giudice 2014).

Most cases of OCD seem to follow a 'slow' life-history pattern. However, OCD is often characterized by increased impulsivity and reduced motor inhibition, which is indicative of a 'fast' life-history strategy.

In summary, OCD and related disorders cover a heterogeneous spectrum of disorders, the majority of which concern evolutionarily relevant themes associated with harm avoidance, security, and, in contrast to other anxiety disorders, precautionary measures of preventing future threat. Cognitive symptoms such as persistent rumination of thoughts about future danger can be explained within this framework. Compulsions resemble and share important features with human rituals, and serve the purpose to fend off situations that may disturb social harmony or pose a threat to oneself or close kin.

Similar to depression and anxiety disorders, there may also be relevant immunological factors (not discussed here; see Chapter 11 for details) that contribute to the initiation or persistence of obsessive-compulsive symptoms.

Comorbidly occurring signs and symptoms may render OCD spectrum disorders to correspond to either a 'fast' or 'slow' life-history pattern, which may be empirically tested more directly.

12.7 **Differential diagnosis and comorbidity**

Anxiety disorders are, like OCD, often accompanied by avoidant behaviours and excessive worry. Worrying in anxiety disorders, however, seems to concern more 'real-life' events than in OCD. Rumination is also characteristic of depression, whereby the ruminating thoughts in depression are usually mood congruent and less distressing than in OCD.

OCD may comorbidly occur with anxiety disorders or depression. OCD is frequently observed in children with streptococcal infections (Sydenham's chorea), and also in various disorders affecting the basal ganglia, including Parkinson's disease, Huntington's disease, GTS, chronic tic disorder, and frontal lobe degeneration.

OCD is frequently observed in children with streptococcal infections (Sydenham's chorea), and also in various disorders affecting the basal ganglia, including Parkinson's disease, Huntington's disease, GTS, chronic tic disorder, and frontal lobe degeneration. Compulsory behaviours are also typically found in eating disorders, which frequently co-occur with OCD. Distinguishing OCD from psychosis can be difficult, especially in cases with poor insight or delusional beliefs. Hallucinations and formal thought disorder in the form of derailment are not typical for OCD, although some circumstantiality may occur in OCD.

Body dysmorphic disorder shares some important features with eating disorders (preoccupation with physical appearance) and psychosis (delusional conviction of one's distorted appearance). Hoarding may occur in psychosis, mainly caused by delusions or severe negative symptoms. If so, a diagnosis of hoarding disorder is inappropriate. Trichotillomania and skin-picking may also occur in psychosis, whereby the behaviours are caused by hallucinations and/or delusions (such as in delusional parasitosis). Trichotillomania and excoriation disorder frequently co-occur with OCD (American Psychiatric Association 2013).

12.8 **Course and outcome**

OCD with childhood onset may remit in a substantial number of cases by adulthood. In most cases, however, OCD is likely to take a chronic course, particularly if undetected and insufficiently treated. Around 50 percent of people with OCD have at some point suicidal thoughts. Individuals with body dysmorphic disorder are particularly at risk for suicide, particularly in cases with age at onset under 18 years (American Psychiatric Association 2013). Comorbid depression increases the risk for suicide attempts in all obsessive-compulsive and related disorders.

OCD with childhood onset may remit in a substantial number of cases by adulthood. In most cases, however, OCD is likely to take a chronic course.

12.9 **Treatment**

SSRI often work for patients with OCD, but most need higher doses of SSRI compared to patients with depression or anxiety disorders. Moreover, response to treatment occurs later (after 10–12 weeks, up to 6 months) compared with anxiety disorders. In OCD, low-dose co-medication with second-generation antipsychotic (SGA) drugs may be helpful in reducing obsessions and compulsions. Apart from drug treatment, CBT has proven successful in OCD (Hand 1998).

SSRI often work for patients with OCD, but most need higher doses of SSRI compared to patients with depression or anxiety disorders. Apart from drug treatment, CBT has proven successful in OCD.

Detailed treatment guidelines for anxiety disorders are available on the internet published by the APA, RCP, and RANZCP.

Chapter 13

Trauma- and stressor-related disorders

Abstract

Trauma- and stressor-related disorders occur following exposure to a traumatic or other stressful event. They differ according to the timing of exposure and age at manifestation. Post-traumatic stress disorder (PTSD) develops following exposure to actual or threatened death, serious injury, or sexual assault. Intrusions, distressing dreams, dissociative reactions (flashbacks), intense psychological distress, and physiological stress responses at exposure to internal of external cues that symbolize aspects of the traumatic event are typical for PTSD. Behaviourally, PTSD reflects a strategy of defence involving avoidance, attentive immobility, withdrawal, aggressive defence, appeasement, and tonic immobility, some of which are ancient vertebrate heritage. These defence mechanisms are preceded by heightened vigilance and risk assessment. Persistent stress responses often occur when important biosocial goals had been thwarted by the traumatic event. Species with long life-history patterns may be more vulnerable to developing PTSD than species with short life cycles.

Keywords

trauma, post-traumatic stress disorder, defence, vigilance, risk assessment, biosocial goals

13.1 Symptomatology and diagnostic criteria

Trauma- and stressor-related disorders comprise a group of syndromes that occur following exposure to a traumatic or other stressful event. Childhood trauma- and stressor-related disorders comprise two syndromes directly related to social neglect or deprivation, namely reactive attachment disorder and disinhibited social engagement disorder (DSM-5; American Psychiatric Association 2013). Reactive attachment disorder concerns a condition that is characterized by emotionally withdrawn behaviour. The affected child does usually not seek comfort when distressed and is emotionally unresponsive to contact with caregivers. Quite the opposite pattern occurs in disinhibited social engagement disorder,

Trauma- and stressor-related disorders comprise a group of syndromes that occur following exposure to a traumatic or other stressful event.

where children lack normal shyness when interacting with unfamiliar adults (American Psychiatric Association 2013).

The other syndromes pertaining to the category of trauma-related disorders occur at any time during one's life-time and comprise acute stress disorder, PTSD, and adjustment disorder. Acute stress disorder and PTSD differ mainly by time of onset and duration, whereas adjustment disorder does not meet the full criteria of the former two.

Acute stress disorder and PTSD are characterized by exposure to actual or threatened death, serious injury, or sexual assault, which can take the form of directly experiencing the traumatic event, witnessing such events, or learning that something dreadful has happened to a close family member or friend. In addition, experiencing exposure to aversive details of horrible events (e.g. collecting human remains after a natural or man-made disaster) can cause acute stress disorder or PTSD. Involuntary distressing memories (intrusions), distressing dreams, dissociative reactions (flashbacks), intense psychological distress, and physiological stress responses at exposure to internal or external cues that symbolize aspects of the traumatic event may occur, whereby affected individuals undertake efforts to avoid thoughts, memories, and feelings associated with the traumatic event. Distorted cognitions about the cause or consequences are frequently associated with acute stress disorder and PTSD, often involving self-blame and negative expectations about oneself or others.

Acute stress disorder and PTSD are characterized by exposure to actual or threatened death, serious injury, or sexual assault, which can take the form of directly experiencing the traumatic event, witnessing such events, or learning that something dreadful has happened to a close family member or friend. Involuntary distressing memories (intrusions), distressing dreams, dissociative reactions (flashbacks), intense psychological distress, and physiological stress responses at exposure to internal or external cues that symbolize aspects of the traumatic event may occur.

People with PTSD also show signs of emotional detachment (numbing) from others and an inability to experience positive emotions. Both acute stress disorder and PTSD are typically characterized by dysregulated arousal, expressed by hypervigilance, exaggerated startle response, sleep disturbance, and poor concentration (Cantor 2009). In PTSD, irritability, reckless behaviour, or self-destructive behaviour may occur (American Psychiatric Association 2013). Emotional responses following the traumatic event are quite heterogeneous. They may be either more fearful, such as the experience of helplessness or horror, or aversive, including anhedonia (inability to experience pleasure) and dysphoric mood states. Moreover, externalizing aggressive behaviours may occur. Children with PTSD may re-enact traumatic events during play or in dissociative states. Moreover, regression to developmentally younger stages can be observed. In adults, PTSD can be associated with pseudo-hallucinations, paranoid ideation, and difficulties in emotion regulation and in maintaining trustful interpersonal relationships (American Psychiatric Association 2013).

13.2 **Epidemiology**

Reactive attachment disorder and disinhibited social engagement disorder seem to be quite rare in the general population, but occur in higher frequency among children in foster care. PTSD is, by definition, highly dependent on environmental factors. In western countries, about 60 percent of men and 50 percent of women experience a severe traumatic event at some point during their life-time, and it is estimated that the life-time prevalence of PTSD is 5 percent for men and 10 percent for women (Vermetten and Lanius 2012). Rates of acute stress disorder and PTSD are higher among people who are more frequently exposed to potentially traumatizing events, including military personnel, fire fighters, and emergency medical personnel. The highest rates of adult PTSD are found among survivors of sexual assault, war, and captivity, exposure to politically or religiously motivated persecution, and humanitarian catastrophes such as genocide (Yehuda et al. 1998).

In western countries, about 60 percent of men and 50 percent of women experience a severe traumatic event at some point during their life-time, and it is estimated that the life-time prevalence of PTSD is 5 percent for men and 10 percent for women.

In addition to adult onset of PTSD, children exposed to neglect or abuse are at elevated risk of developing PTSD or other disorders that share important features with PTSD, including personality disorders and enduring personality change.

13.3 Genetic risk factors

Although at first sight counterintuitive, PTSD is linked with genetic risk factors. PTSD is more likely to occur in MZ than DZ twins, and also is more common in twins of patients with GAD. Candidate genes involved in PTSD comprise the 'short' variant of the serotonin transporter coding gene and genes involved in controlling dopamine turnover, however, studies have produced inconsistent results (Almli et al. 2014; Navarro-Mateu et al. 2013). One of the most promising candidate genes is concerned with the regulation of glucocorticoid sensitivity. For example, the FKBP5 gene (involved in glucocorticoid signal transduction) may alter sensitization of the stress-response pathway during early development, such that individuals who have experienced child abuse may face an increased risk for PTSD when exposed to other traumatic experiences later in life (Binder et al. 2008). There is also limited evidence to suggest contributions of genes involved in neuropeptide turnover, BDNF, and other loci, including the cannabinoid receptor gene and apolipoprotein E (APOE) (Pitman et al. 2012; Almli et al. 2013).

PTSD is more likely to occur in MZ than DZ twins, and also is more common in twins of patients with GAD. Candidate genes involved in PTSD comprise the 'short' variant of the serotonin transporter coding gene, genes involved in controlling dopamine turnover, and genes concerned with the regulation of glucocorticoid sensitivity.

Epigenetic factors such as DNA methylation through exposure to traumatic events may further increase the risk for PTSD, and explain transgenerational transmission of epigenetic changes to gene expression (Perroud et al. 2014a, 2014b). Epigenetic gene methylation may, for instance, contribute to the upregulation of immunological responses and downregulation of neurogenesis. It may also explain altered

Epigenetic factors such as DNA methylation through the exposure to traumatic events may increase the risk for PTSD.

fear-conditioning, by modulating the activity of a gene involved in oestrogen turnover in the brain (Pitman et al. 2012). Moreover, there is evidence to suggest that early adversity can lead to increased gene methylation (Murgatroyd et al. 2009).

13.4 Environmental risk factors

Early traumatization, including emotional and sexual abuse, parental neglect, and heightened anxiety in parents, comprises the most significant environmental risk factor for trauma- and stressor-related disorders. In addition, accidents, violence, and chronic exposure to life-threatening events constitute important risk factors for PTSD. Insufficiently developed coping strategies for stressful events, including low self-efficacy and feelings of poor control, enhance the risk for anxiety disorders, but may be the consequence of poor social support and discouraging parenting behaviour (Meaney 2001).

Early traumatization, including emotional and sexual abuse, parental neglect, and heightened anxiety in parents, comprises the most significant environmental risk factor for trauma- and stressor-related disorders.

13.5 Pathophysiological mechanisms

Internal and external stressors activate a cascade of neuronal and hormonal responses that involve the autonomic nervous system and the HPA axis. As a rule of thumb, physiological stressors (e.g. hypoglycaemia, decreased blood volume, low blood pressure, and altered thermoregulation) activate more the sympathetic system, whereas responses to external stressors (threat) are more strongly mediated by steroids. The sympathetic response to stress occurs within seconds, and involves the secretion of epinephrine and norepinephrine, followed by a slower response involving the hypothalamic release of corticotrophin-releasing hormone (CRH), and the secretion of pituitary adrenocorticotropic hormone (ACTH). Over the course of minutes, glucocorticoid (GC) secretion is stimulated and gonadal steroid secretion generally declines (Sapolsky et al. 2000). GCs suppress the stress response and protect the system from pathological overactivation. They also have important functions in the regulation of metabolic and immunological processes. For example, cortisol contributes to the regulation of arousal, vigilance, focused attention, and memory formation; at the same time, it inhibits growth reproduction (Sapolsky et al. 2000).

The sympathetic response to stress occurs within seconds, and involves the secretion of epinephrine and norepinephrine, followed by a slower response involving the hypothalamic release of CRH, and the secretion of pituitary ACTH.

Anatomically, the rapid catecholaminergic response is regulated via the activation of the locus coeruleus projecting to the PFC, the amygdalae, and the hippocampus. The hippocampus is particularly stress-sensitive. Chronic stress especially in the context of PTSD is associated with a reduction of the hippocampal volume by up to 12 percent after sexual trauma (Bremner 1999), relating to neurotoxic effects of GCs that may induce hippocampal atrophy, which in turn may account for memory deficits in PTSD (Vermetten and Lanius 2012).

There is also evidence to suggest that gene–environment interaction is importantly linked to PTSD in both directions, that is, increased vulnerability (Mehta and Binder 2012) as well as resilience (Ressler et al. 2011) via epigenetic mechanisms (Yang et al. 2013).

Chronic stress in the context of PTSD is associated with a reduction of the hippocampal volume, relating to the neurotoxic effects of GCs that may induce hippocampal atrophy.

Functional brain imaging has shown that individuals with PTSD have reduced activity in the PFC and increased activity in the insular cortex when processing emotional stimuli (Pitman et al. 2012), which may contribute to difficulties in differentiating salient from less salient stimuli with regard to threat evaluation (Jankord and Herman 2008). Chronic stress can also permanently alter the activity of the autonomic nervous system by compromising the function of the myelinated vagus (see Chapter 2). Conversely, neuropeptide Y and testosterone may act in protective ways and enhance resilience against stressor-related disorders (Russo et al. 2012).

13.6 **Evolutionary synthesis**

Acute stress disorder and PTSD occur upon the experience of a single or recurrent severe traumatizing, life-threatening event(s). As regards the content of the trauma, events that threaten the pursuit of important biosocial goals are more likely to produce acute stress disorder and PTSD than events that do not interfere with biosocial goals.

Events that threaten the pursuit of important biosocial goals are more likely to produce acute stress disorder and PTSD than events that do not interfere with biosocial goals. PTSD involves several defences, including avoidance, attentive immobility, withdrawal, aggressive defence, appeasement, and tonic immobility, which are associated with heightened vigilance and risk assessment.

Behaviourally, PTSD can be viewed as a strategy of defence (Cantor 2005, 2009). PTSD involves several defences, which appear hierarchically organized. These include avoidance, attentive immobility, withdrawal, aggressive defence, appeasement, and tonic immobility, which are associated with or preceded by heightened vigilance and risk assessment (Cantor 1999). All can be conceptualized as ancient survival mechanisms, some of which evolved in our vertebrate ancestors millions of years ago. Others reflect more closely our primate heritage and human-specific aspects of memory formation (Cantor 1999). In fact, there are several reports suggesting that PTSD may occur in captive non-human primates following traumatization through early separation of infants from their mothers, single housing in small cages, and recurrent anaesthetizing for biomedical research (Brüne et al. 2006; Bradshaw et al. 2008; Ferdowsian and Merskin 2012).

Several defence mechanisms found in PTSD are not specific for PTSD, but occur also in depression (appeasement), anxiety disorders (heightened vigilance, withdrawal, tonic immobility), and OCD (exaggerated risk assessment) (Marks 1987; see Chapters 10–12).

In any event, elevated levels of vigilance help detect potential dangers; thus vigilance may in the first place serve the purpose of preparing the organism for impending danger

(Cantor 2005). From an ethological point of view, vigilant observation of the environment may have evolved to avoid predatory threat. In species living under constant predatory threat, alertness of this kind is adaptive, and chronic predatory threat does not cause dysfunction of the stress response system (Boonstra 2013). It seems that chronic stress responses are more likely to occur in species with long life histories, whereas short-lived species (such as voles) do not develop signs of chronic stress (Boonstra 2012).

Chronic stress responses are more likely to occur in species with long life histories, whereas short-lived species do not develop signs of chronic stress.

Avoidance is a relatively 'primitive' response of the 'reptilian brain' (see Chapter 2) that helps save energy by avoiding fight or flight. Avoidance is pre-emptive in that it occurs prior to exposure (real or imagined) to a predatory attack (whereby in humans 'predatory' may symbolize the encounter with an abusive or otherwise violent conspecific, including caregivers in children).

If avoidance fails and the encountering threat is impending or inevitable, attentive immobility may occur. Attentive immobility (which is different from tonic immobility) involves vigilant (selective) attention, cardiac deceleration, analgesia, and startle (Cantor 1999). Attentive immobility or freezing prepares the organism to choose among different routes of action, including withdrawal, flight, aggressive defence, or appeasement. Withdrawal and flight are similar to avoidance, but occur post-hoc, that is, after exposure to a perceived threat. Aggressive defence involves signalling of anger or, in case of escalation, fight. Irritability and outbursts of anger of PTSD patients fall into this category.

Appeasement is a somewhat counterintuitive response to persisting threat. It concerns submissive behaviour oriented towards the source of threat, that is, flight from the abusive or otherwise harmful perpetrator (Cantor 1999, 2005). Appeasement occurs in situations in which escape from a dominant oppressor is impossible. It is therefore typical for children who have experienced abuse or adults entrapped in an inescapable situation. The diagnosis of disinhibited social engagement disorder may be mainly expressed by appeasement behaviour. Similarly, cases diagnosed with 'Stockholm syndrome', so named after the behaviour of freed hostages after a bank robbery in Sweden, reflect fear-driven appeasement (Cantor 2005). Along similar lines, it is conceivable that individuals may pursue a mating strategy, akin to 'assortative mating', based on their traumatizing experiences, whereby abused women choose as partners abusive antisocial men (Marmorstein et al. 2004).

Finally, tonic immobility concerns a 'last resort' (Cantor 2005), which occurs in situations of imminent predatory threat. In human PTSD subjects, tonic immobility has frequently been found in victims of sexual assault (Cantor 1999).

As regards the psychological dimension of PTSD, emotional numbing, a state of emotional detachment from close others, seems to be linked to withdrawal or aggressive defence. In contrast, intrusive recollections of the traumatic event represent episodic memories that may be linked to hypervigilance or, in the form of flashbacks and other dissociative symptoms, accompany tonic immobility (Cantor 1999).

Taken together, the signs and symptoms associated with PTSD suggest that they represent exaggerated (pathological) defences following the experience of life-threatening events, whereby perceived helplessness and horror are so intense that individuals seek out ways to avoid retraumatization in the future. So, with regard to the development of PTSD signs and symptoms over time (with the possibility of delayed onset of symptoms), a possible mechanism explaining the persistence of PTSD symptoms could reside in the effort to preserve autonomy and attain controllability over potential threat, even though many individuals with PTSD fail in this endeavour (Cantor 1999).

A possible mechanism explaining the persistence of PTSD symptoms could reside in the effort to preserve autonomy and attain controllability over potential threat.

This situation seems to be similar to OCD, however, with the difference that the manifestation of PTSD is, by definition, preceded by a severe traumatic event—in OCD, real danger may have never been encountered. Remembering past situations associated with threat or actual harm is certainly adaptive in that it helps to avoid similar future negative experiences (i.e. the adaptive function of mental time travel; Suddendorf 2013). In PTSD, however, this mechanism is pathologically hyperactive to the extent that it may actually preclude adaptive responses, but instead gives way to phylogenetically primitive fear reactions such as 'freezing' and dissociative states (regarding catatonic/dissociative behaviours see Chapter 8).

Similar to OCD, many individuals suffering from PTSD perceive intrusive thoughts and memories as uncontrollable, and usually generate strong autonomic arousal, chronically heightened vigilance, and persistent feelings of impending danger. It would seem that individuals with PTSD are unable to disentangle past, present, and future threat scenarios in that they re-experience in the present what frightened them in the past. Hence, at the physiological level PTSD represents a hyperactivity of the alarm system associated with chronic upregulation of the HPA axis, which, in turn, impairs integration of traumatic experiences and appropriate memory consolidation. Moreover, even though the amygdala is hyperactive during recollection of traumatic events, normal threat evaluation is impaired such that the affected individual is less well able to distinguish between relevant and irrelevant stimuli as potential sources of danger. In addition, the communication between the right ('emotional') and left ('rational') hemisphere seems to be functionally disrupted in PTSD, such that traumatic memories may be experienced as ego-alien, because the emotional aspects of the traumatic experience cannot be appropriately verbalized.

With regard to the developmental age at which traumatization occurs, it is plausible to assume that changes at the physiological and neuroanatomical level in PTSD differ between early and late traumatic experiences. Early childhood trauma, for instance, may induce pervasive alterations of neural circuits underlying emotion processing and emotion regulation. Individual genetic make-up may then interact with negative environmental contingencies in ways that predispose the individual to be more responsive to stress. In the wording of life-history theory, early adversity may lead to an acceleration of life-history strategies, which lead to more opportunistic interpersonal orientation, increased stress responsivity, and pro-inflammatory disposition.

Evidence from brain imaging studies suggests exaggerated sensitivity of the amygdalae to fearful stimuli in patients with PTSD. In addition, poor control of fear responses may be exacerbated by a diminished emotional evaluation of threat signals (projected from the amygdala to PFC areas) and insufficient integration of representation of past experiences (via the hippocampal formation). In other words, in sensitized individuals, the amygdala may lose its inhibitory control, which normally regulates approach or avoidance of novel objects or organisms (including individuals of the same species). Instead, the amygdala responds in a dysregulated or hyperactive fashion, such that benign environmental stimuli may be perceived as dangerous (Vermetten and Lanius 2012).

Evidence from brain imaging studies suggests an exaggerated sensitivity of the amygdalae to fearful stimuli in patients with PTSD.

Immunologically, elevated corticosterone levels over a prolonged period of time can have deleterious effects on immunity and cognitive abilities, and cause important metabolic changes (Altemus et al. 2006). For example, skin and gastric mucosa are known to be involved in immunological defences against pathogens, and there seems to be an important cross-talk between the endocrinological and immune systems (Ottaviani 2011). Conversely, skin and gastric problems are common in individuals with PTSD (Burges Watson et al. 1992), and patients with PTSD have reportedly poorer physical health than traumatized persons without PTSD (Vermetten and Lanius 2012). All this renders PTSD a psychosomatic condition, which may be decisively linked to the action of ancient molecules involved in defences against pathogens (Burges Watson et al. submitted).

Immunologically, elevated corticosterone levels over a prolonged period of time can have deleterious effects on immunity and cognitive abilities, and cause important metabolic changes.

A different pathway leading to PTSD could emerge after the experience of traumatic events later in life which strike unexpectedly. That is, in contrast to early adversity interacting with plasticity genes, which may 'prepare' an organism to deal with future threat and unpredictable conditions (i.e. to pursue a 'fast' life-history strategy), an individual that grew up in a secure environment may be particularly ill-equipped to cope with sudden perilous situations that thwart or endanger the pursuit of important biosocial goals, because the traumatizing event may profoundly interfere with the individual's 'slow' pattern. However, although PTSD is regarded as a heterogeneous disorder (Cantor 1999; Vermetten and Lanius 2012), possible differences at the neurobiological level between early and late traumatization are insufficiently clear. In any event, individuals who grew up in relatively safe conditions (with regard to attachment, i.e. emotional availability of caregivers) may be all but immune against PTSD, even if used to frequent encounters of danger and threat.

An individual that grew up in a secure environment may be particularly ill-equipped to cope with sudden perilous situations that thwart or endanger the pursuit of important biosocial goals, because the traumatizing event may profoundly interfere with the individual's 'slow' life-history pattern.

Interestingly, when looking at traditional cultures (hunter-gatherers or horticulturalists) as model societies for ancestral 'environments of evolutionary adaptedness', it seems that PTSD is not uncommon, but occurs in less severe forms. That is, even though a substantial number of individuals in traditional cultures died by homicide (with large cross-cultural differences ranging from about 30 percent of children of the Ache people to 4 percent in the !Kung San) or warfare (around 25 percent of Melanesian men in New Guinea died in combat; Diamond 2012), as assault and violence were much more prevalent in these cultures, PTSD has been reported in the !Kung San but is associated with less avoidance behaviour (McCall and Resick 2003). The ritualization of mourning may prevent many from developing more severe post-traumatic symptoms (Schiefenhövel 1995). These insights from traditional cultures may shed light on practices in our cultures in order to deal with trauma. Lack of social support in the aftermath of a traumatizing event may contribute to the persistence of stress responses and the development of PTSD. For example, victims of rape often experience rejection from partners and families, which intensifies feelings of guilt and anxiety.

In summary, PTSD is a heterogeneous condition that is characterized by ancient, as well as more recently evolved defence mechanisms against life-threatening events. While some signs and symptoms associated with PTSD may be adaptive below a subsyndromal threshold, the full-blown picture causes severe suffering and functional impairment. Gene–environment interaction may account for differences in vulnerability to PTSD. Traumatization during early developmental stages may be associated with different neurobiological consequences compared to late traumatization, and differentially interfere with life-history strategies.

13.7 **Differential diagnosis and comorbidity**

PTSD is frequently associated with other psychiatric disorders, including depression, substance abuse, and personality disorder. It may also co-occur with other anxiety disorders, somatic symptom disorder, and psychosis. Even though the risk of completed suicide in PTSD does not seem to be generally elevated, PTSD has been found to be associated with an increased rate of suicide attempts (Krysinska and Lester 2010). Conversely, comorbid PTSD greatly impacts on adherence to therapy, quality of life, frequency of relapse and hospitalization, symptom severity, morbidity, and mortality (Cavalcanti-Ribeiro et al. 2012).

PTSD is frequently associated with other psychiatric disorders, including depression, substance abuse, and personality disorder. It may also co-occur with other anxiety disorders, somatic symptom disorder, and psychosis.

13.8 **Course and outcome**

Acute stress disorder improves spontaneously in most cases. Development or transition to PTSD may occur, but this depends on peritraumatic factors, trauma characteristics, and post-traumatic social support (Keane et al. 2006). Response to psychotherapy is generally good, and many patients with PTSD recover or experience symptom reduction. However, a substantial number of patients have residual symptoms, although longitudinal follow-up studies over at least

Acute stress disorder improves spontaneously in most cases. Development or transition to PTSD may occur, but this depends on peritraumatic factors, trauma characteristics, and post-traumatic social support.

2 years are scarce (Bradley et al. 2005). Untreated PTSD bears the risk of symptom persistence and reduced quality of life even 10 years after the traumatizing event (Priebe et al. 2009).

13.9 Treatment

The most effective treatment for PTSD is psychotherapy. Psychotherapeutic techniques comprise CBT (including exposure elements), eye movement desensitization and reprocessing (EMDR), and biofeedback (Vermetten and Lanius 2012). Pharmacological treatment has only modest effects and focuses mainly on individual symptoms or comorbid disorders. For example, mood stabilizers and SGA drugs may help reduce intrusions and flashbacks. SSRI may be helpful in reducing depressive symptoms and hyperarousal. There is some evidence to suggest that anti-adrenergic drugs (e.g. propranolol) can help prevent the manifestation of PTSD when given shortly after the traumatizing event (Pitman et al. 2002). Experimental evidence also suggests that neuropeptides and steroids can increase resilience and potentially help cope with stressor-related disorders (Russo et al. 2012).

The most effective treatment for PTSD is psychotherapy. Anti-adrenergic drugs (e.g. propranolol) can help prevent the manifestation of PTSD when given shortly after the traumatizing event.

Chapter 14

Somatic symptom and related disorders

Abstract

Somatic symptom disorders are characterized by the presentation of somatic complaints (somatization), often, but not necessarily, in the absence of a medical explanation of these sensations. The level of concern is generally disproportionate in relation to the severity of the somatic illness. Behaviourally, somatic symptom disorder entails signals that call for help and attention from others. Evolutionary considerations of why people present with somatic symptoms in the absence of a medical cause suggest that this behaviour could reflect a strategy to manipulate others in order to evoke care. Signals that aim at eliciting care from others are more persuasive if the 'real' intention is hidden from conscious awareness. Thus, self-deception may be involved in the presentation of somatic symptoms. Within the spectrum of somatic symptom and related disorders, the degree of self-deception may vary from high, as in illness anxiety disorder, to relatively low, as in factitious disorder.

Keywords

somatic symptom disorder, illness anxiety, care-eliciting behaviour, self-deception, factitious disorder

14.1 Symptomatology and diagnostic criteria

Somatic symptom disorder and related syndromes share the common feature of prominent somatization, often, but not necessarily, in the absence of a medical explanation of these sensations. Accordingly, central to somatic symptom and related disorders is not the lack of a somatic correlate of the patient's subjective complaints, but the way in which or how symptoms are presented and interpreted. Somatic symptom disorder can therefore co-occur with somatic problems, whereby the level of concern and worry is disproportionate in relation to the severity of the somatic illness. Normal bodily

Somatic symptom disorder and related syndromes share the common feature of prominent somatization, often, but not necessarily, in the absence of a medical explanation of these sensations.

sensations are frequently attributed to physical illness, and many patients with somatic symptom disorder fear that physical activity can aggravate bodily harm. Accordingly, they often seek medical help, yet reassurance of somatic integrity does not last. In somatic symptom disorder, pain is among the most frequently reported symptoms; others may include gastrointestinal sensations, vertigo, fatigue, and multiple chemical sensitivity. Disease conviction may sometimes be extreme and resistant to counter-factual evidence, such that the diagnosis of delusional disorder, somatic type, may be considered.

The category of somatic symptom and related disorders also includes illness anxiety disorder (overlapping, to some degree, with hypochondriasis), conversion disorder (functional neurological symptoms), factitious disorder (formerly known as Münchausen's syndrome; deceptive falsification of medical or psychological symptoms in oneself or others, which can include exaggeration, fabrication, simulation, and induction of such symptoms), and psychological factors affecting other medical conditions, which complicate the course of the medical condition (American Psychiatric Association 2013).

The category of somatic symptom and related disorders also includes illness anxiety disorder (overlapping, to some degree, with hypochondriasis), conversion disorder (functional neurological symptoms), factitious disorder (formerly known as Münchausen's syndrome), and psychological factors affecting other medical conditions, which complicate the course of the medical condition.

Patients with illness anxiety disorder present mainly with worry and concern about health, but somatic symptoms are absent or only mild. Accordingly, most patients formerly diagnosed with hypochondriasis now fall into the category of somatic symptom disorder, rather than illness anxiety disorder. Conversion disorder concerns neurological symptoms, such as muscular weakness and paralysis, anaesthesia, speech problems, and seizures, which are unexplained by neurological examination. Non-epileptic seizures may be difficult to diagnose in patients who suffer from epilepsy. Factitious disorder is characterized by the surreptitious production of medical or psychological signs and symptoms imposed on self or (dependent) others such as children (formerly called factitious disorder by proxy), which occurs in the absence of external rewards. Such action may include the ingestion or injection of substances to induce abnormal laboratory tests or sepsis, and repetitive venous puncture to induce anaemia.

14.2 **Epidemiology**

The exact prevalence of somatic symptom disorder is unknown. It is estimated that around 5–7 percent of the adult population fulfils the criteria of somatic symptom disorder, with women being more frequently affected than men. The prevalence of illness anxiety disorder is even less well known, with estimates between 1 and 10 percent of the adult population. Conversion disorder is supposed to be relatively rare (in contrast to observations over a century ago, where the French neurologist Charcot became famous for his case presentations of conversion disorder). Similarly, the frequency of factitious

It is estimated that around 5–7 percent of the adult population fulfils the criteria of somatic symptom disorder, with women being more frequently affected than men.

disorder is unknown, because most patients are treated in somatic hospitals and rarely referred to a psychiatrist (and if so, many patients refuse psychiatric assessment and treatment (American Psychiatric Association 2013)).

14.3 Genetic risk factors

Research into genetic factors contributing to somatic symptom disorder is scarce, although early reports have suggested that somatic symptom disorder runs in families (Guze 1993; Limer et al. 2008). Putative candidates comprise genes involved in the regulation of the opioid receptor expression, due to the role of the opioid system in pain sensitivity (Landa et al. 2012). Indirect evidence for other candidates comes from studies into alexithymia and attachment, because poor parenting and insecure attachment have been identified as factors predicting somatic symptom disorder (Landa et al. 2012).

Putative candidates comprise genes involved in the regulation of the opioid receptor expression due to the role of the opioid system in pain sensitivity.

Early distress, if pervasive, may lead to alterations in pain sensitivity later in life, though the evidence for heightened immune responses in somatic symptom disorder is mixed.

14.4 Environmental risk factors

There is a paucity of knowledge of environmental risk factors that predispose to the development of somatic symptom or related disorders. It seems that the personality trait 'neuroticism' is associated with the presentation of somatic symptoms; in addition, anxiety disorders and depression are often expressed by or associated with somatic symptoms. Poor education and low socio-economic status appear to be related to somatic symptom disorder, as well as recent life events. Illness anxiety disorder, conversion disorder, and factitious disorder are more frequently associated with a history of childhood abuse and neglect. Generally, somatic symptom disorder (with pain) seems to be associated with insecure attachment (Landa et al. 2012).

It seems that the personality trait 'neuroticism' is associated with the presentation of somatic symptoms; in addition, anxiety disorders and depression are often expressed by or associated with somatic symptoms.

14.5 Pathophysiological mechanisms

Somatic symptom disorders share important features with anxiety disorders in depression with regard to their pathophysiological underpinnings (Stein and Muller 2008). For example, evidence suggests that catecholamines and the opioid system are involved in somatic symptom disorders, especially when associated with the experience of pain. Conversely, research has shown that depression and somatic symptom disorder differ in their biological profile with regard to inflammatory responses, activity of the HPA axis, availability of catecholamines, and genetics involved in serotonin turnover (Rief et al. 2010).

Catecholamines and the opioid system are involved in somatic symptom disorders, especially when associated with the experience of pain. Depression and somatic symptom disorder differ in their biological profile with regard to inflammatory responses, activity of the HPA axis, availability of catecholamines, and genetics involved in serotonin turnover.

Neuroimaging has shown that when people evaluate painful stimuli in terms of type, location, and intensity of the pain, they activate a 'pain matrix' involving the ventral posteromedial and posterolateral nuclei of the thalamus, which relay the information to the primary and secondary somatosensory cortices (S1 and S2) (Craig 2003; Singer et al. 2004). In addition, the unpleasantness of the aversive stimuli is processed by the mediodorsal and parafascicular nuclei of the thalamus, the ACC, and the amygdala, which in primates also involves the AI cortex (Craig 2003; Singer et al. 2004). Patients with somatic symptom disorder seem to be more vulnerable (perhaps triggered by early adverse experiences such as abuse or neglect) to somatization and catastrophizing pain. This may also pertain to people with anxiety disorders or depression, who, under stress, often experience heightened pain sensitivity and somatic symptoms (Stein and Muller 2008). In general, given the heterogeneous nature of somatic symptom disorder and related syndromes, the findings from neuroimaging studies are quite diverse and perhaps not specific to any one of the syndromes subsumed in this category (Wood 2005; García-Campayo et al. 2009).

Unpleasantness of the aversive stimuli is processed by the mediodorsal and parafascicular nuclei of the thalamus, the ACC, the amygdala, and the anterior insula.

14.6 Evolutionary synthesis

Somatic symptom disorder and related disorders have in common that they clearly entail verbal and non-verbal signals that call for help and attention from others, sometimes expressed by appeasement displays (Price et al. 2004). This is obviously similar to anxiety disorders and depression (Stein and Muller 2008), yet in somatic symptom disorder and related syndromes, activities that elicit care and support from others are more subtle and indirect, often even unconscious to the affected individual. Many subjects with somatic symptom disorder have experienced adversity during childhood. Insecure attachment, fear of abandonment, or other (interpersonal) stressors may trigger alterations in pain sensitivity (Landa et al. 2012). Pain is actually among the features that somatic symptom disorder shares with anxiety disorders and depression and also may explain why these syndromes often occur comorbidly. A possible distinction from the latter two can, however, best be understood in a frame of reference focusing on the evolutionary development of reciprocal altruism (see Chapter 1).

Somatic symptom disorder and related disorders have in common that they entail verbal and non-verbal signals that call for help and attention from others, sometimes expressed by appeasement displays. Insecure attachment, fear of abandonment, and other (interpersonal) stressors may trigger alterations in pain sensitivity.

Reciprocal altruism occurs in group-living species where individuals are highly dependent on mutual aid and cooperation (Trivers 1971). The tendency to act altruistically towards non-kin bears, however, the risk of being exploited, such that cognitive mechanisms evolved to identify and counteract deception. Leaving aside moral issues, an evolutionary perspective suggests that disease simulation can be seen as a specific kind of deception. As we will explore, somatic symptom and related disorders differ from one another in conscious awareness of the veridicality of the somatic cause of the body sensation. Pretending to be sick is a form of social manipulation that evokes care, which is costly to the helper (Troisi and McGuire 1990). Both care for invalid conspecifics and disease simulation have been described in many social animals, foremost non-human primates, suggesting that neither is a human-specific evolutionary novelty (de Waal 1996). Evolutionary scenarios predict that deception increases in frequency if it pays off reproductively, that cheating detection mechanisms evolve to thwart and punish deception, and that self-deception can further escalate this 'arms race', in that self-deception helps conceal the deceptive motivation from the perpetrator (Trivers 2000; von Hippel and Trivers 2011). Put another way, deceptive signals become more persuasive if the deceptive nature of the behaviour is hidden from the conscious awareness of the deceiver.

Self-deception may play a role in somatic symptom and related disorders.

As somatic symptom disorder and related disorders differ in voluntary control over symptoms, one could argue that differences in control covary with the degree of self-deception. In somatic symptom disorder, illness anxiety disorder, and conversion disorder, self-deception seems to be quite pronounced. An extreme case of self-deception may be reflected in patients with somatic (hypochondriac) delusions. In contrast, in factitious disorder (or even more obvious in malingering) patients seem to be more 'inventive' in the production of symptoms, possibly because the effect of self-deception is weaker. That is, if the deceptive intention to elicit care from others is not so strongly repressed into the unconscious, any effort needs to be taken to show signs of illness that potential helpers take seriously (Troisi and McGuire 1990).

Whether or not this sociobiological explanation holds for all kinds of somatic symptom disorders remains a contentious issue. In traditional societies, for example, the boundaries between somatic and psychiatric illness are much more obscure than in western societies (Fabrega 1990). In fact, as Fabrega (1990) pointed out, in traditional societies, which may be more similar to ancestral hunter-gatherer communities, the concept of 'self' is recognized in less individualistic terms, but as part of 'social and cosmic realities', thereby rendering illness as a social affair (Fabrega 1990). It is therefore less likely that in traditional societies, individuals presenting with what we render somatic symptom disorder are perceived as being 'not ill' and, hence, deserving less or no care or treatment. In particular, in traditional societies the containment of pain, including psychological pain, is achieved through highly ritualized ceremonies, which may help shorten periods of grief and mourning (Schiefenhövel 1995).

In traditional societies, individuals presenting with what we render somatic symptom disorder are perceived as being 'ill' and, hence, deserve care or treatment.

Moreover, similar to depression and anxiety disorders, immunological factors may play a role in somatic symptom disorder. For example, early stressors, including danger signals related to attachment, may contribute to an overactivation of the immune system. Animal research suggests that isolation alters cytokine expression and may therefore increase the vulnerability to sickness behaviour (Landa et al. 2012; see Chapter 10). Early distress, if pervasive, may thus lead to alterations in pain sensitivity later in life, though the evidence for heightened immune responses in somatic symptom disorder is mixed (Rief et al. 2010; Landa et al. 2012).

These considerations can have profound implications for dealing with 'medically unexplained' somatic symptoms (Oyama et al. 2007; Landa et al. 2012).

In summary, the new category of somatic symptom and related disorders is heterogeneous both clinically and neurobiologically. From a life-history perspective, somatic symptom disorder and illness anxiety disorder seem to be best explained as a 'slow' strategy. This might be different in individuals with factitious disorder, where the production of psychological or physical signs of illness seems to be more closely linked to the pursuit of short-term goals.

Anxiety disorders and depressive disorders are the most relevant differential diagnoses of somatic symptom disorder. Conversion disorder can co-occur with neurological disease such as epilepsy, which makes it sometimes difficult to diagnose conversion disorder.

14.7 **Differential diagnosis and comorbidity**

Anxiety disorders and depressive disorders are the most relevant differential diagnoses of somatic symptom disorder. Somatic symptom disorder may also be difficult to distinguish from illness anxiety disorder, as the distinction largely depends on the severity of somatic symptoms. Somatic symptoms may be part of delusional disorder, which differs from somatic symptom disorder by the firmness and incorrigibility of the beliefs concerning the somatic symptoms. Body dysmorphic disorder shares with somatic symptom disorder the preoccupation with the 'wrongness' of the body, but in dysmorphic disorder it is the physical appearance, rather than bodily function, that is the focus of concern. Somatic symptom disorder is often comorbidly associated with anxiety disorders and depression, as well as with somatic disorders, the symptoms of which are overinterpreted, and the preoccupation with somatic symptoms can negatively affect functional impairment (American Psychiatric Association 2013).

Illness anxiety disorder has in common with OCD the presence of intrusive thoughts about physical or mental illness, whereby individuals with illness anxiety disorder are concerned with fears that they have a disease, whereas people with OCD project such fears into the future. Illness anxiety disorder can comorbidly occur with other anxiety disorders and depression.

Conversion disorder can co-occur with neurological disease such as epilepsy, which makes it sometimes difficult to diagnose conversion disorder. The boundaries of conversion disorder with dissociative disorders are imprecise, and in some individuals both diagnoses need to be coded. Similar to other disorders of the group of somatic symptom and related disorders, conversion disorder can comorbidly be associated with depression and anxiety disorders, as well as with personality disorders.

Factitious disorder may be difficult to distinguish from malingering, where the presentation of symptoms is more clearly related to immediate personal gains. Intentional self-harm is also a frequent symptom found in BPD; however, the deceptive intent is usually lacking in borderline disorder. Both factitious disorder and BPD can comorbidly occur (American Psychiatric Association 2013).

14.8 **Course and outcome**

Generally speaking, little is known about the course and outcome of somatic symptom and related disorders. There is some evidence to suggest that somatic symptom disorder is underdiagnosed in older individuals, because the prevalence of somatic disorders increases with age, and symptoms associated with somatic symptom disorder may be concealed by physical illness. Illness anxiety disorder is considered to frequently take a chronic course. The condition may become more frequent with age, and in older individuals the preoccupation may focus on memory loss. Conversion disorder seems to peak in the third and fourth decades. It may be transient or persistent, often depending on the acuity of repressed conflict. Factitious disorder manifests often after hospitalization for a medical condition, or may be imposed on another (by proxy) after the treatment of a medical condition. The condition may persist throughout life (American Psychiatric Association 2013).

There is some evidence to suggest that somatic symptom disorder is underdiagnosed in older individuals, because the prevalence of somatic disorders increases with age, and symptoms associated with somatic symptom disorder may be concealed by physical illness.

14.9 **Treatment**

Treatment recommendations for somatic symptom disorder comprise pharmacological approaches and psychotherapy. Among pharmacological agents, antidepressants such as duloxetine and mirtazapine may be of some help (Kroenke 2007), though the effect size seems to be fairly small (Kleinstäuber et al. 2014). However, serotonin and noradrenaline reuptake inhibitors (SNRI) may be more effective that SSRI in cases with predominant pain symptoms, whereas SSRI are perhaps more useful in illness anxiety disorder and body dysmorphic disorder (Somashekar et al. 2013). Similarly, psychotherapeutic approaches, including CBT, seem to show some effect, but, again, effect sizes of available studies have been small (Sharma and Manjula 2013; van Dessel et al. 2014).

Treatment recommendations for somatic symptom disorder comprise pharmacological approaches and psychotherapy.

Chapter 15

Feeding and eating disorders

Abstract

Feeding and eating disorders comprise syndromes occurring in childhood or in people with intellectual disability, as well as the classic eating disorders, namely anorexia nervosa, bulimia, and binge-eating disorder. Individuals with anorexia nervosa are preoccupied with body weight and shape. They engage in diverse activities aimed to reduce body weight. People with bulimia have normal body weight, and have episodes of uncontrolled intake of food (binge eating). Both anorexia and bulimia are associated with the desire to gain control over pressures to fulfil sociobiological role models. Paradoxically, these disorders occur more often in societies where food is abundant. Eating disorders are much more prevalent in females than males. It is unclear whether amenorrhoea is key to the control of one's reproductive potential, and whether this behaviour is maternally induced to promote 'help at the nest'. Alternatively, thinness, as in anorexia, may be a by-product of intrasexual competition for mates.

Keywords

anorexia, bulimia, binge eating, amenorrhoea, food abundance, intrasexual competition

15.1 Symptomatology and diagnostic criteria

The diagnostic group concerning feeding and eating disorders comprises eating disturbances that primarily occur in childhood or in individuals with intellectual disability, and the classic syndromes referred to as 'anorexia nervosa', 'bulimia', and 'binge-eating disorder'. Pica (the Latin word for 'magpie') is characterized by persistent eating of inedible substances. These may include paper, soap, hair, and faeces. Rumination disorder concerns repeated regurgitation (and reingestion) of food, which is unrelated to a gastrointestinal disease. Avoidant/restrictive food intake disorder describes a feeding or eating disturbance in which individuals lack interest in eating or refuse to eat due to the smell, appearance, temperature, etc. of food. It leads to

Feeding and eating disorders comprise disturbances that primarily occur in childhood or in individuals with intellectual disability, and the classic syndromes referred to as AN, BN, and binge-eating disorder.

a significant weight loss or failure to thrive, a significant nutritional deficiency, and dependence on enteral feeding or supplementation of nutrition.

Anorexia nervosa (AN) is characterized by a preoccupation with body weight and shape. Patients restrict their calorie intake to achieve a much lower than average body weight. Body image is usually distorted in a way that, even though the actual body weight may be dangerously low, patients perceive themselves as overweight or have fears of gaining weight or becoming fat. The individual engages in behaviours that prevent weight gain, such as excessive exercising, misuse of laxatives, diuretics, or enemas, and self-induced vomiting. A restricted type in which individuals control their body weight by fasting, dieting, or exercising can be distinguished from a binge-eating/purging type, which involves the misuse of substances that lead to weight loss or the occurrence of episodes of binge eating.

AN is characterized by a preoccupation with body weight and shape, calorie restriction, and distorted body image. BN has many similarities with AN. BN is associated with normal body weight and episodes of binge eating. AN and BN can be subdivided according to the presence or absence of purging behaviours.

Bulimia nervosa (BN) shares several symptoms with AN. In contrast to AN, however, patients with BN usually have normal body weight and more frequent episodes of binge-eating, during which they consume large amounts of food. In addition, individuals with BN experience a lack of control over eating during these episodes (American Psychiatric Association 2013). Compensatory behaviours (purging) are common in BN. Also, self-evaluation in terms of body weight or shape is exaggerated.

Binge-eating disorder is characterized by the occurrence of binge-eating episodes; however, the disorder lacks the compensatory behaviour found in AN and BN.

In addition to the cognitive and behavioural symptoms, patients with eating disorders often have difficulties in recognizing their own emotional states, which has been referred to as 'alexithymia'. Thus, they may appear inhibited in expressing emotions or display problems in emotion regulation.

15.2 **Epidemiology**

Pica and rumination disorder occur most frequently in individuals with intellectual disability, whereby exact prevalence rates are unknown. Likewise, epidemiological data are missing for avoidant/restrictive food intake disorder. In developed countries, AN has a life-time prevalence of about 1–2 percent, with BN being twice as common in the general population. Accordingly, AN is the third most common chronic disorder in adolescent girls in western countries. Both AN and BN are much less common in developing countries, although increasingly observed in countries in economic transition.

Pica and rumination disorder occur most frequently in individuals with intellectual disability. In developed countries, AN has a life-time prevalence of about 1 percent, with BN being twice as common in the general population. A much larger percentage of the population shows subthreshold manifestation of the disorders. Ninety to 98 percent of affected individuals are female.

A much larger percentage of the population shows subthreshold manifestation of the disorders. For example, in the USA as many as 5–15 percent of adolescent girls control their body weight by making use of purging behaviours. Both AN and BN in males are exceptionally rare; 90–98 percent of affected individuals are female. The typical age at onset is around puberty for AN and late adolescence for BN (American Psychiatric Association 2013).

15.3 **Genetic risk factors**

Since AN and BN share several clinical features, and longitudinal studies suggest a continuum between the two, there is some evidence that both disorders have, in part, a common genetic basis (Eley et al. 2005). AN is more common in families with BN probands, and vice versa. In addition, twin studies, although scarce, point to heritable factors in AN and BN (Ben Dor et al. 2002). The relative risk for AN in first-degree relatives is approximately ten times higher than in the general population. For BN, the relative risk is about two- to threefold increased compared to control probands. Moreover, childhood obesity seems to predispose to BN.

AN and BN run in the same families. The risk for developing AN is approximately ten times higher in first-degree relatives of AN patients compared with the general population. For BN, the relative risk is about two- to threefold increased. Polymorphisms of serotonin receptor-coding genes, the COMT gene, and BDNF have been associated with AN.

In AN, a polymorphism of the promoter of the 5-HT2A serotonin receptor gene has inconsistently been associated with the disorder. Similarly, one study has found an association of AN with allelic variation of the COMT gene. Moreover, there is some evidence of an association between a polymorphism of the BDNF coding gene and eating disorders, which is assumed to be particularly prevalent in AN with purging behaviours (Gorwood et al. 1998; Gorwood et al. 2003; Ribasés et al. 2004; Hashimoto et al. 2005). However, a recent GWAS in patients with AN produced inconclusive results, possibly because the study was statistically underpowered (Boraska et al. 2014).

15.4 **Environmental risk factors**

Several obstetric complications have been linked to a heightened risk for AN and BN. Specifically, maternal anaemia, diabetes mellitus, pre-eclampsia, placental infarction, neonatal cardiac problems, and hyporeactivity may increase the risk for AN; placental infarction, neonatal hyporeactivity, early eating difficulties, and low birth weight seem to be predictive for later BN (Favaro et al. 2006). Research into attachment has shown that patients with eating disorders frequently report poor parental care and invalidating parental behaviour (Waller et al. 2007). Specifically, fathers of patients with eating disorders are often described as emotionally unavailable, whereas mothers are described as overprotective and dominant, with a tendency towards perfectionism (Ward et al. 2001). Striving for independence and autonomy is often suppressed by both parents. These early

Obstetric complications have been linked to a heightened risk for AN and BN. Patients with eating disorders frequently report poor parental care, emotional unavailability of fathers, and perfectionist mothers. Traumatization may play a role, but this is not associated with greater symptom severity in eating disorders. Social attitudes towards thinness contribute to the high prevalence of eating disorders.

family conditions may lead to the development of dismissive or unresolved attachment styles (Delvecchio et al. 2014), which promote dissatisfaction with one's body (Troisi et al. 2006).

Moreover, childhood sexual abuse has been identified as a non-specific risk factor for eating disorders (Wentz et al. 2005). Traumatization is, however, not necessarily associated with greater symptom severity of the eating disorder. On the other hand, traumatic experiences increase the risk for comorbid disorders, and subclinical PTSD may be a risk factor for BN (Brewerton 2007; Sansone and Sansone 2007). Impulsivity has also been identified as a predictor of eating disorders in general (Favaro et al. 2005), but perhaps more so for BN.

There is also a clear influence of social attitudes towards thinness (Abed and de Pauw 1998). Interestingly, in developing countries, adolescent girls and young women are particularly vulnerable to developing AN or BN if they come from a high-income and high-education background, and have difficulties in accepting traditional role models.

15.5 Pathophysiological mechanisms

The pathophysiological mechanisms involved in eating disorders are only partially understood. It is largely agreed that most abnormalities at the physiological level are secondary to the extreme restriction of food intake, which, however, perpetuates the effects on neuroendocrinological systems.

Abnormalities at the physiological level are secondary to the extreme restriction of food intake, which, however, perpetuates the effects on neuroendocrinological systems. Evaluation of the organism's energy balance and signalling of satiety, to which several hormones contribute, is dysregulated in AN and BN. Hypothalamic dysregulation is also involved in hypertrichosis, amenorrhoea, and reduced sexual interest during periods of starvation.

Animal models have shown that the lateral hypothalamus (LH) is involved in regulating appetitive behaviours and that damage to the LH produces anorexia. The ventromedial hypothalamus (VMH), by contrast, is critical in evaluating the organism's energy balance. The VMH contains insulin-sensitive cells and is able to integrate information about the status of peripheral energy stores. This function is mediated, in part, by secretion of leptin and other neuropeptides. The hypothalamus is anatomically close to the pituitary gland, which secretes hormonally active neuropeptides involved in energy regulation of the body, such as thyroxine, growth hormone (GH), cortisol, and leptin. In AN, there is usually an excess of GH activity, whereas the insulin-like growth factor I is often found to be reduced (Gianotti et al. 2002). GH interacts in complex ways with somatostatin, and may also be influenced by leptin and ghrelin secretion (the latter being a gastric somatotropin-stimulating hormone).

Other neuropeptides such as orexin and neuropeptide Y are involved in regulation of food intake. Neuropeptide Y has been found to be elevated in the cerebrospinal fluid (CSF) of patients with BN. Stress increases the level of neuropeptide Y, which may cause abdominal fat deposition (Jimerson and Wolfe 2004). Moreover, cholecystokinin, which is secreted by the gut to signal satiety, is decreased in BN. This reduction in satiety signalling may, therefore, be part of the pathology of binge eating.

Interestingly in terms of the AN phenotype, the VMH is not only involved in the regulation of food intake. It also controls female sexual receptivity, which may explain why patients with AN experience reduced sexual interest when starving. Also, hypertrichosis, amenorrhoea, and a more male-type physiognomic phenotype are the result of complex dysregulations of the neuroendocrine circuits, which, however, remit upon restoration of a sufficient amount of body fat. This suggests that most pathophysiological mechanisms involved in AN and BN are the result rather than the cause of the disorder.

Similarly, at the anatomical level, chronic reduction of food intake to the point of starvation may lead to cortical atrophy and ventricular enlargement (Herholz 1996). This is believed to be a consequence, rather than cause, of eating disorders, and partly remits following weight gain.

15.6 **Evolutionary synthesis**

Eating disorders comprise phenotypically diverse manifestations of problems with the regulation of food intake and body weight. Interestingly, Pica and rumination disorder have repeatedly been described in captive non-human primates, including great apes, probably as a consequence of sensory understimulation and boredom (summarized in Brüne et al. 2004, 2006).

AN and BN are associated with a strong desire to gain control over pressures to fulfil sociobiological role models. From an evolutionary point of view, the prevalence of eating disorders poses a paradox in two respects. First, there is an inverse relationship of food availability and the prevalence of eating disorders across societies. Historically, AN has anecdotally been reported in the Hellenistic era, but was 'rediscovered' only in the 17th century (Pearce 2004). It would seem, ironically, that food abundance in western societies is associated with high prevalence rates of eating disorders, especially when subsyndromal manifestations are being considered, whereas eating disorders are almost absent in less developed countries (Katzman et al. 2004). Second, irregularities of the menstrual cycle or amenorrhoea, which frequently occur in eating disorders, counteract any reproductive effort.

The prevalence of eating disorders poses an apparent paradox to evolutionary theory, because prevalence rates correlate inversely with the availability of food, and because amenorrhoea counteracts reproductive success.

How can this be consistent with an evolutionary explanation of behaviour? A couple of hypotheses exist that take into account female preponderance in eating disorders. For example, eating disorders manifest around the time at which female fertility peaks. Moreover, some findings point to the fact that some peculiarities of the family environment may increase the risk for young females to engage in food restriction and control of body weight. These hypotheses, based on evolutionary theory, share the assumption that the suppression of reproduction (i.e. amenorrhoea) is the main 'function' of eating disorders, rather than being a by-product of the symptomatology (Mealey 2002). It needs to be emphasized, however, that eating disorders do not convey any adaptive value in the strict sense. Instead, it is plausible to assume that runaway processes associated with voluntary starvation lead to a 'point of no return' at which one's individual fitness is severely compromised by pervasive metabolic and endocrinological alterations (Ploog and Pirke 1987).

At the proximate level, the avoidance of food and efforts to reduce body weight are strong signals sent by the affected individual, indicating, at the very least, conflict over resource allocation, where the addressee of these behaviours is most likely the nuclear family or the social group at large (Gatward 2007). Studies suggest that mothers of adolescent girls with AN tend to be overprotective, dominating, and monopolizing. Patients with AN, on the other hand, are often overcompliant and worry excessively about the well-being of the family. Consistent with this is the observation that anorexic females often dismissively negate family problems (Ward et al. 2001; Vidovic et al. 2005). AN is also associated with low self-esteem, introversion, pronounced harm avoidance, and reduced novelty-seeking, and the co-occurrence with anxiety disorders and depression suggests that patients with eating disorders unconsciously assume the behavioural strategy of a subordinate individual, to which genes may contribute heritable susceptibility. Seen through the lens of life-history theory, this suggests that AN is compatible with a 'slow' life-history strategy (Del Giudice 2014). Conversely, the association of BN with high impulsivity, sensation-seeking, novelty-seeking, and BPD is more suggestive of a 'fast' life-history strategy (Cassin and von Ranson 2005; Del Giudice 2014).

AN could reflect behaviour of subordinate individuals whose reproductive potential is inhibited by the presence of dominant females, which is compatible with a 'slow' life-history strategy. Conversely, the association of BN with high impulsivity, sensation-seeking, novelty-seeking, and BPD is more suggestive of a 'fast' life-history strategy.

Reproductive inhibition in subordinates is common in non-human primates, and this is often the result of active manipulation by higher-ranking females. Elevated stress levels in subordinates, for example, are known to contribute to the suppression of ovulation, and such a scenario is similarly conceivable in humans. Moreover, women may also suppress the reproductive potential of other women by cultural means, for instance, by unconsciously promoting that the 'ideal' female figure is one of below-average weight. This is confounded by the tendency to perceive thinness as an indicator of youth. As youth signals attractiveness, there is intrasexual competition in women for looking thin, which may, to some extent, enhance the preference for thinness not only by men but also by women (Abed et al. 1998). In fact, a competing evolutionary hypothesis posits that intrasexual competition for mates is at the core of eating disorders, which may be more relevant for BN than AN (Faer et al. 2005; Abed et al. 2012). Consistent with this assumption, female patients with AN do not perceive female faces as rewarding and avoid looking at faces and eyes (Watson et al. 2010).

Suppression of reproduction in adolescent girls could be in the interest of mothers, who need them as 'helpers at the nest', particularly in the presence of male siblings.

Coming back to the idea of suppressed reproduction in eating disorders, it might in some cases even be possible that suppressed reproduction is not due to the interference of an unrelated higher-ranking female, but that the mother of the affected adolescent girl is the source of manipulation. From a genetic point of view, the logic behind this hypothesis could be that the mother suppresses reproduction in her own daughter such that the daughter may serve as a 'helper at the nest' (Voland and Voland 1989). In other words, altruistic behaviour of adolescent girls may be imposed upon the daughter by the mother, particularly in the presence of younger (male) siblings. Theoretically, the reproductive success of a male descendant exceeds that of a female, at least under favourable environmental conditions (see Chapter 1), which could explain why AN is especially prevalent in upper-middle and upper class girls in socially stratified societies. Since the affected individual would indirectly benefit from supporting her mother at the expense of her own reproduction, this sort of altruism in female individuals with AN would be typical of kin-selected behaviour.

There may be, however, another reason for mothers (and fathers) to suppress fertility in adolescent daughters. In western societies, the abundance of nutrient-rich food has accelerated sexual maturation over the last decades. Suppression of premature sexual activity in adolescent girls may well be in the interest of parents in order to increase their daughters' reproductive success in the long run. This possibility may be accentuated in families in which the father is absent. Unlike other primates, father absence in humans is associated with earlier maturation and sexual activity. In other words, the presence of fathers (and high paternal investment) postpones sexual maturation in girls, perhaps as a reflection of a K-selected reproductive strategy (see Chapter 3). Accordingly, in families with fathers being absent, manipulation of girls to restrict food intake may indirectly serve the function to turn an early maturer into a late maturer, that is, to decelerate life-history strategies.

Suppression of premature sexual activity in adolescent girls (which in western societies is fostered by earlier sexual maturation due to supply of energy-rich nutrients) may be in the interest of parents to increase their daughters' reproductive success in the long run.

Similar interest in delaying reproduction could also be on the side of the adolescent girl. The onset of eating disorders is often preceded by (unwanted) first sexual experiences. Thus AN may be seen as a counter-strategy to avoid premature pregnancy. Moreover, the increase of eating disorders in western societies and threshold countries may reflect changes in social structure associated with increased sexual competition between females. Therefore, under adverse environmental conditions, which, above all, may include the absence of emotional availability of significant others and lack of social support, long-lived iteroparous species like humans may be better off by postponing reproduction until the conditions are more favourable.

Delay of reproduction could be in the interest of young girls if current environmental conditions are poor, but predictably improves in the future. Such behaviour does not pay off for older women, which may explain why the onset of eating disorders peaks in adolescence or early adulthood.

At the proximate level, this is maintained by reducing the amount of body fat. In contrast to male fertility, ovulation ceases if the amount of body fat undercuts 15 percent of body weight. This makes sense from an evolutionary perspective, because in times of food scarcity the likelihood of successfully raising offspring declines sharply, such that the hypothalamus stops producing gonadotropin-releasing hormone. Moreover, the fall of oestrogen and extreme loss of body weight leads to a reduction of secondary sexual characteristics in women, such that in extreme cases women become sexually less attractive for males. Consistent with this, sexual interest often declines in young women with AN, which further reduces the risk of unwanted pregnancy.

However, such a strategy pays off reproductively only if the probability of improved conditions in the future is predictably high. This is the case in western societies in which, on average, adult mortality is low (accordingly, within western societies the prevalence of eating disorders is predicted to be low in neighbourhoods with high criminality and homicide rates). Again, this notion is supported by the evidence that eating disorders occur more frequently in socially well-situated families. By contrast, if the likelihood that future environmental conditions will improve is low, it does not make sense to postpone reproduction, which may explain the low prevalence of AN and BN in developing countries and in socially disadvantaged people. Furthermore, the hypothesis of reproductive delay is plausible to explain why eating disorders manifest in adolescence or early adulthood; for older women, postponing reproduction would be too risky a strategy, because it could preclude reproduction at all.

This hypothesis also explains why for males such a strategy would not pay off. According to parental investment theory, male reproduction is theoretically constrained by the number of sex partners, whereas females invest more in individual offspring; hence their reproductive success is limited by a much lower theoretical maximum number of offspring that corresponds with the number of fertile cycles, social support, and inter-birth intervals (see Chapter 1). Accordingly, for young women, optimal environmental conditions, including the presence of a male partner who is willing to invest in offspring, are much more important than for young men. Conversely, in light of the lower paternal investment and the more intense male–male competition, it does not make sense for males to postpone reproduction.

From an evolutionary perspective, male anorexia does not make sense due to evolved differences in parental investment and sexual strategies.

As already pointed out, these hypothetical models of the evolutionary background of eating disorders hinge upon the proposition that amenorrhoea is the (unconscious) goal or function of eating disorders, which is achieved by restricted food intake, weight control, excessive exercising, and/or other compulsive behaviours. However, a substantial number of patients with eating disorders, particularly BN, do not stop ovulating and show promiscuous behaviour.

Moreover, women with a history of eating disorder have a greatly elevated risk of hyperemesis during pregnancy, they more often deliver children with lower birth weight and smaller head circumference, and have significantly more miscarriages and caesarean deliveries compared to women without a history of eating disorder (Kouba et al. 2005). The elevated number of birth complications is not compensated for by a greater number of children or number of pregnancies. There is, therefore, little evidence that postponing reproduction pays off for women with a history of eating disorder (Bulik et al. 1999).

Furthermore, research into perinatal risk factors for the development of AN or BN has revealed that maternal anaemia, diabetes mellitus, pre-eclampsia, placental infarction, neonatal cardiac problems, and hyporeactivity independently predicted the development of AN later in life, with similar, though less pronounced risks for BN (Favaro et al. 2006). Also, intergenerational studies of attachment in patients with AN and their mothers have shown that insecure attachment, dismissive attachment styles, and poor reflexive functioning ('mentalizing') may be 'transferred' from mother to daughter (Ward et al. 2001). In addition, the risk of childhood trauma is increased in eating disorder. Drawing on attachment theory and life-history theory (see Chapter 3), these findings suggest poor parental investment that is conserved over successive generations.

The consequences of AN (and less so of BN), namely a visible waste of resources and profoundly health-threatening behaviour, can therefore be interpreted as a correlate of parent–offspring conflict. In parent–offspring conflict, the child has only a limited set of behavioural strategies at hand to increase parental investment. One such strategy is the expression of temper tantrums, which typically occur during the weaning period. The 'logic' behind such behaviour is that it threatens not only the health of the offspring, for example, by attracting predators, but also that of the parents, because the latter would lose all resources they have already invested. Confronting a parent or both parents with the risk of losing a child through deliberate starvation is therefore one of the strongest conceivable signals of the child to mobilize parental investment. The timing or onset of the behaviour peaks around or precedes the time of maximum fecundity of adolescent girls and young women, and thus constitutes the maximum threat to the inclusive fitness of both parents. If the parent, however, is unable or unwilling to provide additional investment, the situation is self-perpetuating, and a vicious circle may result that can only be resolved through therapeutic interventions fostering greater independence of parental investment in the child.

The visible consequences of AN (and less so of BN), namely a waste of resources and profoundly health-threatening behaviour, can be interpreted as a correlate of parent–offspring conflict. Deliberate starving in offspring poses a threat to the inclusive fitness of parents, such that parents are forced to increase parental investment.

Eating disorders are so heterogeneous in aetiology that none of the hypothetical models can embrace all clinical and neurobiological facets. In some patients with eating disorders, it is plausible to assume that the affected individual carries the burden of maladaptive consequence of suppressed fertility, which benefits others, perhaps including the patient's own mother. Other patients with AN may be forced to postpone reproduction if environmental conditions are unfavourable, with the expectation that conditions will predictably improve in the future. Finally, in some patients with eating disorders, the symptomatology may be an exaggeration of behavioural consequences related to parent–offspring conflict to increase parental investment. None of these behavioural 'strategies' involves conscious awareness of the underlying conflict. Nor do they convey a reproductive advantage; on the contrary, eating disorders can be seen as emergency strategies that emerge in young women who struggle with the achievement of biosocial goals, among which the search for social security is imperative.

Aside from the classical eating disorders featured in DSM-5, it is surprising that virtually nothing is said in the latest edition about one of the most pressing health issues world-wide: obesity. Secular trends in obesity represent a growing health issue in developed countries, with profound impact on adult health. Since the 1880s or so, the body mass index (BMI) has constantly increased in developed countries, with figures of obesity having constantly risen since the 1980s. Adult obesity often originates in childhood. The prevalence of childhood obesity is currently below 5 percent in African countries, with figures of around 20 percent in Europe, and over 30 percent in the USA. It is non-existent in traditional societies of hunter-gatherers, which have served as models of Palaeolithic human societies.

Obesity occurs mainly due to an increase in energy consumption and decrease in physical activity. The oversupply of energy and the lack of physical activity and exercise is an example of an evolutionary mismatch.

Among the most 'obesogenic' factors are increasing energy consumption, mainly foods rich in fat and sugar, and decreasing physical activity. The oversupply of energy and the lack of physical activity and exercise is an example of an evolutionary mismatch. For most of their evolutionary history, humans have lived in conditions where the availability of food could change dramatically. Food scarcity and famine probably occurred much more often than times of food abundance. According to the 'thrifty gene' hypothesis (Neel 1962), humans have therefore evolved mechanisms of maximizing the extraction of energy from food, and store energy in fat depots, which now turns into a disadvantage with regard to health. Transition to farming was associated with frequent famines that hindered the adjustment of the genome to the newly established, mostly carbohydrate diet. So, arguably, a mismatch between a Palaeolithic genome and a Holocene diet is key to the obesity epidemic we observe today (Cordain et al. 2005; Eaton et al. 2010; Brüne and Hochberg 2013).

Overweight and obesity may, however, also be linked to the intrauterine environment, which, through 'foetal programming' (see Chapter 3), prepares the organism's expectations of future resource availability. This makes sense from an evolutionary perspective, because an organism that is adaptively prepared before birth for optimally dealing with conditions after birth has a greater chance for survival (and reproduction). Excessive maternal intake of calories during pregnancy, for instance, may influence the development of the foetus's first fat lobules in utero. Intrauterine and postnatal stress may also act on fat deposition by increasing an organism's allostatic load (McEwen 2002; see Chapter 3). Moreover, there is evidence suggesting that childhood maltreatment is an important risk factor for obesity (Danese and Tan 2014).

Foetal programming may be involved in the development of postnatal obesity by preparing the baby's organism for excess calorie intake.

Consistent with such a scenario, life-history theory would predict that personality traits indicative of a 'fast' life-history strategy would be highly prevalent in people with obesity. Indeed, it has been demonstrated that neuroticism, impulsivity, and reward dependence (all indicative of a 'fast' life-history strategy; Del Giudice 2014) are risk factors for weight gain, whereas conscientiousness and self-control (akin to a 'slow' strategy) protect against excessive weight gain (Gerlach et al. 2015). Moreover, dysregulated dopaminergic neurotransmission in the striatum seems to be involved in opportunistic eating behaviour in obesity (Guo et al. 2014).

Therefore it seems that obesity shares several important features with the classical eating disorders, foremost BN and binge-eating disorder. This extends to the neurophysiological level, as indicated by similarities in dysfunction of executive control across eating and weight conditions (Fagundo et al. 2012). Thus obesity treatment warrants an interdisciplinary approach, which should essentially include evolutionary considerations such as insights from life-history theory (Ellis and Del Giudice 2014).

15.7 **Differential diagnosis and comorbidity**

Differential diagnoses for Pica and rumination disorder include factitious disorder and self-injurious behaviour in personality disorders. In rumination disorder, gastrointestinal medical conditions need to be ruled out. Pica and rumination disorder are often associated with intellectual disability and ASD. Avoidant/restrictive food intake disorder may occur in conditions affecting attachment, as well as in psychosis depression, OCD, and factitious disorder imposed on another (American Psychiatric Association 2013). The main differential diagnoses to AN comprise disorders associated with pronounced weight loss, including tumours and other causes of endocrinological abnormalities.

The main differential diagnoses to AN comprise disorders associated with pronounced weight loss, including tumours and other causes of endocrinological abnormalities. Eating disorders occur comorbidly with anxiety disorders, OCD, substance abuse, and depression. BPD can occur comorbidly particularly in individuals with a history of traumatization.

The prevalence of anxiety disorders in patients with eating disorders is exceptionally high (Kaye et al. 2004). OCD occurs comorbidly in up to 40 percent of patients with AN. Social phobia is present in up to 20 percent of patients, and other types of anxiety disorders figure around 10–15 percent. Patients with AN and BN differ significantly with respect to comorbid PTSD, which is more frequent in BN (Brewerton 2007). Comorbid substance abuse and depression are also common in patients with eating disorders. In patients with a history of early traumatization, comorbidity of eating disorders with personality disorders, above all BPD, is common. High trait-levels of harm avoidance and low novelty-seeking are often found in AN, whereas high impulsivity and high novelty-seeking are more characteristic of BN (Tomotake and Ohmori 2002; Cassin and von Ranson 2005).

There has been some discussion about the association of eating disorders with ASD, but this comorbidity is probably rare, as is the association of eating disorders with psychosis.

15.8 **Course and outcome**

Little is known about the course and outcome of Pica and rumination disorder, Both may take a chronic course, occur episodically, or remit spontaneously. In AN, the recovery rate after 5 years is around two-thirds of cases (Keski-Rahkonen et al. 2007). Twenty-five to 33 percent of patients with AN and BN develop a chronic disorder (Patel et al. 1998). Mortality estimates range from 6 to 20 percent, including death from suicide or starvation, particularly in patients with AN. Suicide attempts occur in 10–20 percent of patients with AN and 25–35 percent in BN. These figures are associated with comorbid depression, substance abuse, and a history of childhood abuse (Franko and Keel 2006).

Twenty-five to 33 percent of patients with AN or BN develop a chronic disorder. Mortality estimates range from 6 to 20 percent, including death from suicide and starvation.

15.9 **Treatment**

Treatment of eating disorders requires interdisciplinary consultation, particularly in the presence of weight loss below 85 percent of the estimated healthy body weight. Severe restriction of food intake and starvation can affect virtually every organ system. Low blood levels of potassium can produce dangerous and potentially fatal cardiac arrhythmia. Gastrointestinal signs may include reflux, Mallory–Weiss syndrome, and constipation; anaemia, muscle weakness, dental caries due to vomiting, and reduced pulmonary capacity may also be observed. Hospitalization may be necessary to prevent medical instability. In AN, treatment goals may entail restoring weight and normalizing eating patterns, and initiation of formal psychotherapy. Antidepressants may be useful if comorbid depression or anxiety disorder is present. SSRI are usually tolerated best. In BN, SSRI can also be prescribed to reduce the frequency of binge-eating attacks and vomiting, with dosages being usually higher than those administered to treat depression.

Treatment of eating disorders requires interdisciplinary consultation, particularly in the presence of weight loss below 85 percent of the estimated healthy body weight. Antidepressants may be useful if comorbid depression or anxiety disorder is present, or to reduce the frequency of binge eating. Psychotherapy is essential.

Psychotherapy is essential.

Treatment guidelines and recommendations have been published by the APA and RANZCP. For lay persons and carers, useful information can also be found online via links provided by the RANZCP.

Chapter 16

Sexual dysfunctions

Abstract

Sexual dysfunctions comprise heterogeneous disorders that are characterized by disturbed sexual responsiveness, reduced sexual desire, or problems in experiencing sexual pleasure. Women more frequently have problems in experiencing sexual arousal and pleasure, whereas men more often suffer from erectile dysfunction or dysfunctional ejaculation. From an evolutionary point of view, many sexual dysfunctions are caused by conflict relating to intra- and intersexual competition or cultural practices of controlling sexual activity of the opposite sex. Suppression of sexual interest in women may, for example, occur in patrilocal societies, where curbing one's daughter's sexual activity before her arranged marriage may eventually increase the parents' reproductive success. Evolutionary hypotheses of female orgasm suggest that the function of orgasm in women could signal satisfaction and fidelity to their male partners. Premature ejaculation in men may relate to performance anxiety. Finally, hormonal contraceptives impact on the experience of sexual pleasure and mate choice in relevant ways.

Keywords

sexual desire, arousal, intrasexual competition, intersexual competition, orgasm, premature ejaculation, hormonal contraceptives

16.1 Symptomatology and diagnostic criteria

Sexual dysfunctions comprise a heterogeneous set of disorders in males and females that are characterized by disturbed sexual responsiveness, reduced sexual desire, or problems in experiencing sexual pleasure. In women, the most common sexual dysfunctions include problems in experiencing sexual interest and arousal, orgasmic disorder, and experiencing sexual intercourse as painful (penetration disorder). In men, erectile dysfunction, delayed or premature ejaculation, and hypoactive sexual desire disorder are the most frequent sexual dysfunctions.

Sexual dysfunctions comprise a heterogeneous set of disorders in males and females that are characterized by disturbed sexual responsiveness, reduced sexual desire, and problems in experiencing sexual pleasure.

DSM-5 distinguishes between acquired and lifelong sexual dysfunctions, as well as between generalized and situational, depending on the type of stimulation, contextual factors, or partners. In addition, there are several factors that may impact on the expression of sexual dysfunction, including partner factors (e.g. whether or not the partner has sexual problems), quality of the relationship in terms of communication patterns, individual factors such as a history of abuse, cultural and religious factors, and medical factors (American Psychiatric Association 2013).

All sexual dysfunctions have in common that a diagnosis can only be made if the condition occurs in all or nearly all (i.e. in 75–100 percent) occasions of sexual activity.

16.2 **Epidemiology**

Sexual dysfunctions seem to be relatively common in the USA and European societies. Given the huge variation in attitude toward sexual activity among different cultures, religions, and ethnicities, it is very difficult to give exact prevalence rates for any one of the sexual dysfunctions. For example, female sexual interest/arousal disorder seems to increase with age (as do other sexual dysfunctions). Genito-pelvic pain/penetration disorder may occur in up to 26 percent of women. Female orgasmic disorder reportedly occurs in up to 35 percent of adult women, with about two-thirds of women complaining about desire problems (Pereira et al. 2013).

Sexual dysfunctions seem to be relatively common in US and European societies. Given the huge variation in attitude towards sexual activity among different cultures, religions, and ethnicities, it is very difficult to give exact prevalence rates for any one of the sexual dysfunctions.

Female orgasmic disorder reportedly occurs in up to 35 percent of adult women, with about two-thirds of women complaining about desire problems. In men, the prevalence of erectile disorder increases with age, with some 2 percent of men younger than 40 years reporting frequent problems with erection, and between 40 and 50 percent of men over 60–70 years complaining of erectile dysfunction.

In men, the prevalence of erectile disorder increases with age, with some 2 percent of men younger than 40 years reporting frequent problems with erection, and between 40 and 50 percent of men over 60–70 years complaining of erectile dysfunction. Delayed ejaculation is apparently quite rare, whereas 1–3 percent of men are affected by premature ejaculation (within the first minute of vaginal penetration). Hypoactive sexual desire disorder is quite uncommon in men; it is also clearly related to age, with some 6 percent of younger men (in their 20s) and 40 percent of older men (over 60–70) reporting problems with sexual desire (American Psychiatric Association 2013).

16.3 **Genetic risk factors**

Genetic risk factors for sexual dysfunction are unknown (except those factors involved in comorbid disorders such as depression, anxiety disorders, etc.).

16.4 Environmental risk factors

Sexual dysfunctions seem to occur more frequently in individuals with mood or anxiety disorders. There is some controversy about whether genito-pelvic pain disorder is associated with a history of abuse in childhood (Buster 2013).

Orgasmic disorder in women can be linked to concerns about pregnancy, gender role expectations, and relationship problems. Premature ejaculation seems to be more specifically related to social anxiety disorder. Organic factors such as hysterectomy, vaginal infections, and other medical conditions such as diabetes mellitus may contribute to or cause sexual dysfunction.

Genetic risk factors for sexual dysfunction are unknown. Sexual dysfunctions seem to occur more frequently in individuals with mood or anxiety disorders. There is some controversy about whether genito-pelvic pain disorder is associated with a history of abuse in childhood.

16.5 Pathophysiological mechanisms

Sexual functioning is under the control of sex hormones such as testosterone, oestrogen, and progesterone, and is influenced by neuropeptides, foremost vasopressin and oxytocin (Bancroft 2005). Panksepp (1998) highlights the distinction between organizational and activating aspects of human sexuality. The former concern early influences of hormones on brain development, whereas the latter refer to the initiation of sexual activity.

Sexual functioning is under the control of sex hormones such as testosterone, oestrogen, and progesterone, and is influenced by neuropeptides, foremost vasopressin and oxytocin.

Importantly, the 'default mode' of the brain is female. Accordingly, it is the action of hormones that guide brain development toward a male phenotype. In the absence of such hormonal influence, the brain retains its female organization. The Y chromosome contains a gene coding for a testis-determining factor, which induces the male gonads to produce testosterone. Testosterone is converted to oestrogen in the brain and to dihydrotestosterone in the periphery. Oestrogen is the molecule that induces the masculinization of the brain.

Several brain areas are sexually dimorphic (see Chapter 2). The ones involved in sexual behaviour include the ventromedial hypothalamus, the periaquaeductal grey (PAG), and the spinal cord. These areas contain a high number of oestrogen receptors. Damage to the ventromedial hypothalamus seems to be more detrimental to female than male sexuality.

Sex steroid receptors are also abundant in the medial areas of the amygdala, which play a role in aggression. The male brain contains higher levels of vasopressin. Areas rich in vasopressin comprise the amygdala, the anterior hypothalamus, and the septal area. Vasopressin is released from the pituitary gland during sexual arousal in males, and drops after ejaculation. The female brain contains more oxytocinergic neurons than the male brain and the production of oxytocin is controlled, in part, by oestrogen. Oxytocin seems to promote erectile function in males. It is released in large quantities during orgasm and its action lasts for some time after sexual climax (Panksepp 1998). In essence, vasopressin seems to be more involved in sexual aggression in both sexes, whereas oxytocin promotes nurturance and sexual pleasure. In fact, vasopressin is involved in intrasexual, including territorial, aggression in males, but also maternal protection of offspring.

A broad spectrum of psychological and physical factors can intervene with sexual functioning. Diseases affecting sex steroid production, as well as diseases impacting on vascularization, such as diabetes mellitus and atherosclerosis, can compromise sexual functions in both men and women.

A broad spectrum of psychological and physical factors can intervene with sexual functioning. Diseases affecting sex steroid production, as well as diseases impacting on vascularization, such as diabetes mellitus and atherosclerosis, can compromise sexual functions in both men and women. Among the most relevant psychological factors, mood disorders, anxiety, and marital discord influence sexual function.

16.6 **Evolutionary synthesis**

Few topics are more relevant for life in an evolutionary perspective than sexuality. Given the large differences between males and females with regard to strategies that maximize reproductive success, it is not surprising that culture impacts greatly on human sexuality. Such cultural factors may actually range from cruel rituals, including mutilation of the genital organs (e.g. infibulation, clitoridectomy), to advertisement of one's mate value by means of enhancing one's physical and psychological attractiveness. The former is mainly imposed on females by males to control women's sexuality in terms of sexual desire, chastity, and faithfulness, whereas the latter concerns both sexes in all cultures (Buss and Schmitt 1993).

Culture impacts greatly on human sexuality. Such cultural factors may actually range from cruel rituals, including mutilation of the genital organs (e.g. infibulation, clitoridectomy), to advertisement of one's mate value by means of enhancing one's physical and psychological attractiveness.

Intra- and intersexual competition profoundly influences how individuals can act out their sexual desires or suppress them. Inhibition of sexuality occurs in cultures in which female kin (e.g. virgin daughters) are traded for property or status. This kind of sexual inhibition of own female offspring may be relevant in cultures that are patrilocal and practice female exogamy. Exogamy is biologically meaningful, because it reduces genetic risks associated with inbreeding. In fact, recent evidence from genetics suggests that arranged marriages and reciprocal exogamy was the evolved societal structure in hunter-gatherer societies, where polygyny was relatively rare (Walker et al. 2011). In societies that practice female exogamy, it can therefore be in the interest of parents to temporarily suppress sexual activity of their daughters (before marriage) to maximize their own reproductive success (Wenegrat 1990).

In societies that practise female exogamy, it can be in the interest of parents to temporarily suppress sexual activity of their daughters (before marriage) to maximize their own reproductive success. Sexuality-hostile environments promote difficulties in experiencing sexual interest and arousal.

Along similar lines, unfaithfulness decreases a partner's reproductive fitness, such that vigilance towards fidelity has been selected in both males and females (Buss 1999). Accordingly, rigid control of female sexuality is more prevalent in patriarchal societies in which men control the resources that are necessary to raise children; in matriarchal societies, the need to curb female sexuality is less important for parents and male partners, such that women experience greater freedom from sexual restrictions (Wenegrat 1991).

Following this line of reasoning, discouraging own offspring from engagement in (premature) sexual activity or preventing it can be adaptive if it ultimately increases the offspring's mate value. So, it is conceivable that sexuality-hostile environments promote difficulties in experiencing sexual interest and arousal, as well as sexual activity as something rewarding. For example, anorgasmia is a prevalent condition, mostly in women. Psychiatric conditions such as depression, substance dependence, and traumatic experiences, including rape, increase the risk for orgasmic disorder.

From a phylogenetic perspective, it is important to note, however, that orgasm in females is reportedly absent in most non-human animals, including primates, perhaps with the exception of bonobos (de Waal and Lanting 1997). Another difference between humans and non-human primates is that human women are sexually receptive for most of their menstrual cycle (though intercourse is avoided during menstruation in most cultures), whereas some non-human primates are sexually receptive only for a few hours around mid-cycle (Hrdy 2000). Except humans, bonobos are exceptional in regard to sexual activity, because they use sexual contact for conflict resolution, whereby genito-genital 'rubbing' occurs among females and anal penetration among males (de Waal and Lanting 1997). Concealed ovulation is another adaptation that evolved during human evolution (see Chapter 1). So, human females may experience vaginal penetration far more frequently than any other primate, except bonobos.

In any event, the experience of orgasm is highly variable and depends on sexual practices concerning foreplay with extensive clitoral stimulation. Accordingly, the frequency of orgasmic experiences following sexual stimulation should vary greatly depending on cultural conventions. Several theories exist why female orgasm evolved in humans. One is that female orgasm has no reproductive function but occurs as a by-product due to the anatomic homology with the male sexual organ. Another hypothesis revolves around ideas that female orgasm encourages women to engage in sexual activity via activation of the reward system.

Several theories exist why female orgasm evolved in humans. One is that female orgasm has no reproductive function but occurs as a by-product due to the anatomic homology with the male sexual organ. Another hypothesis revolves around ideas that female orgasm encourages women to engage in sexual activity via activation of the reward system. Female orgasm may also serve as a test of the male's affection to engage in extensive foreplay and therefore investment in partnership.

Female orgasm may also serve as a test of the male's affection to engage in extensive foreplay and therefore investment in partnership. Related to this, female orgasm may signal to the male sexual satisfaction and fidelity (Symons 1979), and may therefore serve to reduce tension between partners (Hrdy 2000). In line with this assumption, it seems that women frequently pretend orgasm, perhaps to reassure their male partners about their satisfaction. Finally, it has been suggested that female orgasm may increase the likelihood of conception by producing an 'upsuck' response of the male's sperm, and that orgasm occurs more frequently during sexual intercourse with men who carry 'good genes' (Baker and Bellis 1995). In any event, it seems that anorgasmia and experiencing sexual intercourse as painful has a communicative meaning in those cases in which organic causes can be excluded. As Wenegrat (1984) suggests, for many men the experience of a sexual climax by their female partners seems to be an index of their male sexual competence. Conversely, male sexual problems such as erectile dysfunction and premature or delayed ejaculation may, in part, arise from performance anxiety. These problems may be accentuated in human males, also, because the duration of sexual intercourse is much longer than in other primates. In addition, humans lack a penile epidermal spine (see Chapter 1), which renders penile function more vulnerable to psychological stress. In cases of premature ejaculation (often associated with social anxiety disorder), the duration of genital stimulation is shortened, which increases the likelihood that the female does not experience sexual climax, which, in turn, may reduce the male's mate value (Wenegrat 1984).

Erectile dysfunction and premature or delayed ejaculation may, in part, arise from performance anxiety. These problems may be accentuated in human males, also, because the duration of sexual intercourse is much longer than in other primates. In addition, humans lack a penile epidermal spine, which renders penile function more vulnerable to psychological stress.

Another issue that needs to be mentioned in the context of evolutionary approaches to human sexuality concerns the revolutionary developments of birth control. Humans have practised birth control ever since. In the not so distant past, the decision over accepting or rejecting offspring was sometimes postponed after birth, which led to neonaticide, mainly in the first 24 hours after parturition. Abortion has also been practised widely (Hrdy 2000). With the discovery of pharmacological contraception and widespread availability of birth-control pills in the 1960s, the risk for women of unwanted pregnancy has dramatically decreased. Greater sexual freedom has certainly influenced sexual activity and practice of women in modern societies. It may also have impacted on males' vigilance over the females' sexual faithfulness and on the males' mate-guarding strategies.

Pharmacological birth control through hormonal contraceptives has lead to greater sexual freedom of women in modern societies. It may also have impacted on males' vigilance over females' sexual faithfulness. However, women's risk of experiencing sexual dysfunction, including orgasmic disorder, and loss of sexual desire and arousal may increase under hormonal contraceptives.

Ironically, even though hormonal contraception frees women of fears of an unwanted pregnancy, it seems that women's risk of experiencing sexual dysfunction, including orgasmic disorder and loss of sexual desire and arousal, is greater relative to women who do not use hormonal contraceptives or other methods of birth control such as condoms (Wallwiener et al. 2010). This is understandable, because hormonal contraception mimics pregnancy, during which most women experience a decrease in sexual desire (Yeniel and Petri 2014), though it need not necessarily be an adaptation. In fact, evidence suggests that the woman's immune system is activated by seminal fluid, and that the female immune system facilitates optimal female reproductive investment and helps to maximize the offspring's fitness by evaluating the male partner's reproductive fitness and tissue compatibility (Robertson 2010). The use of hormonal contraceptives seems to interact with the evaluation of tissue compatibility of sexual partners, however. Women who take hormonal contraceptives seem to prefer the odour of men who are similar to their own, suggesting that, in a state of imitated pregnancy, women seek proximity of close kin (Hrdy 2000). Freely ovulating women, in contrast, prefer the scent of men different from their own, suggesting that they favour men with immunological attributes that differ from their own (Wedekind and Füri 1997). Men, on the other hand, perceive their female partners to be more attractive around mid-cycle (i.e. shortly before ovulation), compared to other time points of the menstrual cycle or when their partners take oral contraceptives (Roberts et al. 2014). Taken together, the use of hormonal contraceptives may have profound implications for mate choice and fitness of offspring, as well as on the expression of sexual dysfunction in both sexes.

Women who take hormonal contraceptives seem to prefer the odour of men who are genetically similar to themselves. Freely ovulating women, in contrast, prefer the scent of men with immunological attributes that differ from their own.

16.7 **Differential diagnosis and comorbidity**

Sexual dysfunction seems to be quite prevalent in western societies. The most important differential diagnoses of primary dysfunction (lacking an organic causation) refer to somatic disorders affecting the genitals directly (e.g. endometriosis), the endocrinological system (sex hormones), and disease that indirectly impacts on sexual function (diabetes mellitus, atherosclerosis). SSRI profoundly impact on sexual function (see Chapter 23) and may be the cause of delayed ejaculation. Other psychotropic drugs, including antipsychotics and tricyclic antidepressants, also negatively influence sexual arousal and the experience of sexual pleasure.

The most important differential diagnoses of primary dysfunction (lacking an organic causation) refer to somatic disorders affecting the genitals directly (e.g. endometriosis), the endocrinological system (sex hormones), and diseases that indirectly impact on sexual function (diabetes mellitus, atherosclerosis).

16.8 **Course and outcome**

Little is known about the course and outcome of sexual dysfunctions. It is likely that most forms do not remit spontaneously and take a chronic course.

16.9 **Treatment**

The most widely prescribed drug for erectile dysfunction is sildenafil. Sildenafil is a phosphodiesterase (PDE5) inhibitor, which produces vasodilation and, thus, increased blood flow into the corpus cavernosum of the penis. The substance does not work in the absence of sexual arousal.

A broad array of psychotherapeutic interventions has been tried for female sexual dysfunction with mixed success, ranging from masturbatory training to couples therapy and CBT, whereby the main focus of therapies is anxiety reduction and improvement of sexual desire and arousal. The bottom line of the classic sex therapies (Masters and Johnson) has been the experience of orgasm, with less improvement in sexual desire (reviewed in Pereira et al. 2013). Efficacy rates of psychotherapeutic interventions range from around 30 percent for penetration disorder, with larger success rates for sexual desire disorder of around 75 percent (Pereira et al. 2013). In light of the substantial heterogeneity of sexual dysfunctions and difficulties in recruitment of sufficiently large samples, there is still a need for more controlled studies.

The most widely prescribed drug for erectile dysfunction is sildenafil. A broad array of psychotherapeutic interventions has been tried for female sexual dysfunction, with mixed success.

Chapter 17

Substance-related and addictive disorders

Abstract

Substance-related and addictive disorders concern the misuse or dependence of psychotropic substances. Substance misuse or dependency is often accompanied by hazardous behaviour and legal problems. Substance dependence is characterized by the development of tolerance following recurrent exposure to the substance and increment of the consumed quantities. Behaviourally, individuals with substance-related disorders show significant craving and an inability to resist efforts to reduce the dose or terminate the intake of the substance. While psychotropic substances that can cause misuse or dependence are widespread in nature, the availability of large quantities has emerged only recently, suggesting an evolutionary 'mismatch'. Most psychotropic substances causing misuse or dependence usurp the brain's reward system (mainly dopaminergic substances) or the attachment system (mainly opioidergic substances). Research of gene–environment interaction has shown that social status and separation from caregivers or abusive behaviour of caregivers promotes the development of misuse or dependence.

Keywords

substance misuse, dependence, reward system, dopamine, attachment system, opioids, social status, separation

17.1 Symptomatology and diagnostic criteria

The misuse of psychotropic substances represents a maladaptive pattern of behaviour that is associated with recurrent failure at work, school, or home. Recurrent and continuing substance misuse is usually accompanied by physically hazardous behaviour and often leads to legal problems. Surprisingly, people with substance use disorders continue consumption in spite of mounting social, interpersonal, or financial problems.

The misuse of psychotropic substances represents a maladaptive pattern of behaviour that is associated with recurrent failure at work, school, or home.

Substance misuse often evolves into substance dependence. Substance dependence is characterized by the development of tolerance due to repetitive exposure to psychotropic substances in shortening intervals, such that increasing quantities are needed to produce the desired effects, including euphoria, calmness, and relief from anxiety.

Substance dependence is characterized by the development of tolerance due to repetitive exposure to psychotropic substances in shortening intervals, such that increasing quantities are needed to produce the desired effects, including euphoria, calmness, and relief from anxiety.

Withdrawal syndromes occur if consumption of the substance is promptly terminated, and typically comprise instability of vegetative functions and psychological disturbances such as confusion, hallucinations, irritability, and intense anxiety or rage.

In contrast to substance misuse, in substance-dependent individuals a withdrawal syndrome occurs if consumption of the substance is abruptly terminated. Withdrawal syndromes typically comprise instability of vegetative functions, including blood pressure, heartbeat rate, and sweat production, as well as psychological disturbances, such as confusion, hallucinations, irritability, and intense anxiety or rage. Thus, a substance-dependent individual is forced to take the same or pharmacologically similar substances to relieve or avoid withdrawal symptoms—resulting in a vicious circle.

Individuals with substance dependence spend a lot of time acquiring and using the substance, often in a compulsory manner, or recovering from intoxication; social and occupational functioning further deteriorates. Substance-dependent people continue intake of psychotropic substances in spite of potentially severe physical harm and psychological problems caused by substance use, sometimes to the point of self-destruction. Moreover, even after successful detoxification and treatment of withdrawal symptoms, the rates of relapse are incredibly high across all psychotropic substances.

Accordingly, DSM-5 features impaired control (of the substance use), social impairment, risky use, and pharmacological criteria as central to all substance use disorders (American Psychiatric Association 2013). Alcohol, caffeine, cannabis, hallucinogens, inhalants, opioids, sedatives, stimulant, tobacco, and other substance classes are the most common causes of substance use disorders.

Alcohol, caffeine, cannabis, hallucinogens, inhalants, opioids, sedatives, stimulant, tobacco, and other substance classes are the most common causes of substance use disorders. In addition to substance use disorders, DSM-5 lists Gambling Disorder as the only behavioural addiction, mainly because there is insufficient research on other behavioural manifestations of addiction.

In addition to substance use disorders, DSM-5 lists Gambling Disorder as the only behavioural addiction, mainly because there is insufficient research on other behavioural manifestations of addiction (American Psychiatric Association 2013). Gambling disorder, like substance use disorders, is characterized by irritability when the individual attempts to stop the behaviour. Preoccupation with the behaviour and numerous attempts to control the behaviour, concealment of the behaviour before others, and social isolation are also typical for behavioural addiction.

17.2 **Epidemiology**

In the developed countries millions of people fulfil the criteria for substance dependence, and an even greater number of unreported cases misuse one or more psychotropic substances.

Alcohol and nicotine are probably the most widespread legal drugs, but the consumption of illegal substances such as cocaine, heroin, and modern designer drugs is on the rise and poses a huge problem for both medical and legal systems. In Europe and the USA it is estimated that 5–10 percent of adult men and 3–5 percent of adult women have alcohol dependence, with the number of people at risk being perhaps ten times higher. Substance misuse and dependence usually develops over months or years. Its typical onset is insidious, and manifestation of first withdrawal symptoms occurs in the third or fourth decades of life. The prevalence of gambling disorder is estimated to reach 0.4 percent, with males being more often affected than females (American Psychiatric Association 2013).

In Europe and the USA it is estimated that 5–10 percent of adult men and 3–5 percent of adult women have alcohol dependence, with the number of people at risk being perhaps ten times higher.

17.3 Genetic risk factors

High concordance rates of alcoholism in MZ male twins of 20–80 percent and 10–60 percent in DZ male twins suggest heritable risk factors, with lower figures of 10–50 percent in MZ female twins and 5–40 percent in DZ female twins. In males, those who start to drink alcohol at an early age (before 25 years) have been found to differ from those who start drinking later with regard to the personality traits 'novelty-seeking' (pronounced in the former), 'harm avoidance', and 'reward dependence' (both more expressed in the latter group). Adoption studies have shown that these differences in personality and consummatory behaviour are associated with differential genetic risks (Cloninger 1987). Individuals who start drinking early in life with high scores of novelty-seeking are at greater genetic risk, yet, in turn, are less influenced by adverse childhood experiences such as increased alcohol consumption in parents. This elevated genetic risk may be associated with allelic variation of the MAO-A coding gene, specifically in alcohol-dependent men with antisocial behaviour. Moreover, polymorphic variation of the COMT coding gene has been associated with elevated risk for developing alcoholism in some, but not all, populations studied (Enoch 2006; Sery et al. 2006).

Concordance rates in MZ and DZ twins suggest heritable factors involved in alcohol dependence. People who commence drinking before age 25 probably have a higher genetic load compared to late drinkers.

Furthermore, linkage studies have revealed susceptibility loci on chromosome 4, close to the beta-1-GABA receptor gene locus, the GABA-A receptor gene on chromosome 5, and a region on chromosome 11 adjacent to DRD4 (particularly in American Indians). Polymorphisms of the alcohol dehydrogenases (ADH) and acetaldehyde dehydrogenase (ALDH) have been suggested to be involved in alcohol dependence in some populations (particularly Asian), with a possible protective locus on chromosome 4 near the ADH cluster.

Genes regulating the dopamine turnover and the enzymatic degradation of alcohol have been associated with an increased risk for alcohol dependence. It is assumed that the heritability of drug abuse is lower compared to alcoholism.

The genetic contributions to misuse and dependence on illicit drug are less well researched compared to alcoholism. In general, the heritability of drug misuse is probably lower; thus the development of drug dependence is even more strongly associated with adverse environmental conditions, particularly during early childhood. For heroin, polymorphisms of the mu opioid receptor and the cytochrome CYP2D6 enzyme coding genes have been researched, with inconsistent results across populations. Cannabis misuse may be associated with allelic variation of the endogenous cannabinoid receptor system. Misuse of stimulants and cocaine is most likely to involve the dopamine transporter (DAT) system, as well as the norepinephrine and serotonin transporter systems (Heinz et al. 2004).

17.4 Environmental risk factors

Impoverishment, parental alcohol or drug abuse, and other adverse environmental conditions, including lack of a stable attachment figure, are important risk factors for alcohol and drug misuse later in life. One particular environmental problem lies in the widespread availability of alcohol and easy access to lifestyle drugs. Early consumption of alcoholic beverages or illicit 'soft' drugs such as cannabis in adolescence increases the risk for the development of tolerance and dependence (American Psychiatric Association 2013).

Impoverishment, parental alcohol or drug abuse, and other adverse environmental conditions, including lack of a stable attachment figure, are important risk factors for alcohol or drug abuse later in life.

17.5 Pathophysiological mechanisms

The pathophysiology of alcohol and drug abuse and dependence involves multiple neurochemical pathways in the brain that interact in many ways. Alcohol and many other psychotropic drugs activate the brain's dopaminergic pathways that connect the midbrain with the PFC (Bainton et al. 2000). Repetitive stimulation leads to alterations of receptor sensitivity, such that tolerance and dose increase are necessary to produce the desired effect. Excessive stimulation of the dopamine system also affects associative learning, so that previously unconditioned stimuli may be attributed salience. When re-exposed to these stimuli, individuals may feel compelled to re-ingest the psychotropic substance to which the stimulus has been linked.

Alcohol and many other psychotropic drugs activate the brain's dopaminergic pathways that connect the midbrain with the PFC. Repetitive stimulation leads to alterations of receptor sensitivity, such that tolerance and dose increase are necessary to produce the desired effect.

Moreover, alcohol stimulates GABAergic receptors, which explains its dampening effects on many brain functions. Ethanol is catalysed by the enzyme ADH to produce acetaldehyde, which is further metabolized by ALDH to yield acetate. Some slow-acting polymorphisms of the alcohol-degrading enzymes cause accumulation of acetaldehyde, which itself is toxic and produces nausea and vomiting. Individuals who are slow metabolizers are therefore to some extent protected from excessive alcohol intake and may be less vulnerable to developing alcohol dependence.

Alcohol withdrawal produces symptoms that can be explained in terms of excessive activity of hypersensitized dopaminergic and GABAergic systems. Visual hallucinations, disorientation, poor concentration, and intense anxiety are characteristic of delirium tremens. In predisposed individuals, chronic exposure to ethanol produces upregulation of dopaminergic receptors, causing alcohol hallucinosis, which at times is indistinguishable from paranoid schizophrenia, or delusional jealousy.

Alcohol withdrawal produces symptoms that can be explained in terms of excessive activity of hypersensitized dopaminergic and GABAergic systems. Visual hallucinations, disorientation, poor concentration, and intense anxiety are characteristic of delirium tremens.

At the macro-anatomical level, continuous alcohol consumption may cause brain atrophy, associated with cognitive decline and personality change. More specifically, alcohol and stimulant misuse may cause damage to the PFC. Korsakoff syndrome is characterized by irreversible loss of short-term and autobiographical memory caused by chronic vitamin B1 deficiency-induced lesions of the corpora mamillaria.

Heroin addiction affects the brain's endogenous opioid receptors, which are part of the 'social affiliation' system.

17.6 **Evolutionary synthesis**

A synthetic approach to the understanding of the high prevalence of alcohol and drug abuse and dependence in western populations needs to take into account the widespread availability of psychoactive substances, as well as individual differences that contribute to the vulnerability (or resilience) for misuse and dependence (Hall 2002; Hill and Newlin 2002).

Psychotropic substances are widespread in nature. Toxic alkaloids, for example, evolved in plants to prevent consumption of plant material by animals; others substances such as sugar derivates attract frugivorous animals to disperse seeds. ADH and ALDH are phylogenetically ancient enzymes already found in fruit flies and other invertebrates. In anatomically modern humans, the activity of ADH and ALDH varies between ethnic groups, which suggests adaptive variation to geographically different diets in the past 100,000 years or so.

Psychotropic substances are widespread in nature. Toxic alkaloids, for example, evolved in plants to prevent consumption of plant material by animals; others substances such as sugar derivates attract frugivorous animals to disperse seeds. Ripe fruit can produce considerable quantities of ethanol (up to 5 percent) by fermentation of sugar. Sugars and ethanol are energy-rich nutrients. Accordingly, millions of years ago, enzymes evolved in animals to digest these substances. ADH and ALDH are phylogenetically ancient enzymes already found in fruit flies and other invertebrates (Wolf and Heberlein 2003). The diet of human ancestors, like the one of extant apes, was probably rich in fruit, depending on seasonal availability. Even modern hunter-gatherers subsist to a considerable extent on fruit consumption. Thus it is parsimonious to conclude that small quantities of ethanol were part of the natural diet of early humans (Dudley 2000, 2002).

In anatomically modern humans, the activity of ADH and ALDH varies between ethnic groups, which suggests adaptive variation to geographically different diets in the past 100,000 years or so. Some East Asian peoples, for example, possess an ALDH isozyme that metabolizes acetaldehyde slower than the isozyme found in Caucasians.

Slow metabolizing of alcohol leads to an accumulation of acetaldehyde, which in turn produces an aversive reaction accompanied by nausea and sickness. This could in part explain lower prevalence rates of alcoholism in some East Asian peoples, because people readily get sick after drinking small quantities of ethanol. However, the activity of ethanol-degrading enzymes cannot account for the susceptibility to alcoholism alone. In indigenous North Americans, for instance, the activity of ALDH is similar to that in Caucasians. The odds of becoming addicted to 'firewater' are, however, proverbial in many Native North American peoples.

In any event, despite evolved genetic differences between human populations in enzymatic alcohol degradation, and the presence of ethanol-containing food throughout human history, it is the availability of large quantities of ethanol and other psychotropic substances that has created the problem of alcohol misuse and dependence in modern environmental conditions. In other words, substance misuse and dependence are clearly examples of the mismatch of evolved human traits with modern environmental conditions (St John Smith et al. 2013; see Chapter 4).

Despite evolved genetic differences between human populations in enzymatic alcohol degradation, and the presence of ethanol-containing food throughout human history, it is the availability of large quantities of ethanol and other psychotropic substances that has created the problem of alcohol misuse and dependence in modern environmental conditions.

Until quite recently (in evolutionary standards), industrial mass production of ethanol-containing beverages was virtually absent. Obtaining highly concentrated ethanol requires the technical knowledge of artificial fermentation and distillation. This is not to say that early humans in ancestral environmental conditions did not intentionally ingest psychotropic substances for various purposes. Betel nut (*Areca catechu*) chewing, for example, increases brain acetylcholine levels; cocaine, the active alkaloid in *Erythroxylum coca*, is a powerful reuptake inhibitor of norepinephrine and dopamine. So, consuming relatively small quantities of substances that alter the activity of neurotransmitters may have even been adaptive to some extent (Sullivan and Hagen 2002). It is conceivable, for example, that the psychotropic effects of these substances could have enhanced group cohesion and cooperation when used in rituals and ceremonies. Psychotropic drugs may have also been ingested for controlling pain (Saah 2005).

In ancestral environmental conditions, early humans almost certainly ingested psychotropic substances for various purposes. Betel nut (Areca catechu) chewing, for example, increases brain acetylcholine levels; cocaine, the active alkaloid in Erythroxylum coca, is a powerful reuptake inhibitor of norepinephrine and dopamine. It is conceivable that the psychotropic effects of these substances could have enhanced group cohesion and cooperation when used in rituals and ceremonies.

By contrast, flooding the brain with substances that exert various effects on brain metabolism is certainly not adaptive, because it exceeds the organism's detoxification potential by orders of magnitude. Indeed, psychotropic substances unfold their effect on brain metabolism by 'usurping' evolved brain systems involved in adaptive signalling of reward and social attachment (Panksepp et al. 2002). These systems interact in many ways. For didactical reasons, however, they will be examined separately.

Perhaps best understood is the motivational system that has imprecisely been termed the 'reward system', for which the expression 'incentive salience system' is a better term. It refers to the observation that it is not necessarily the subjectively pleasurable or rewarding effect of substance consumption itself, but the relevance attributed to potentially fitness-increasing stimuli associated with the activation of this system that lies before the consummatory act (Lende and Smith 2002).

Psychotropic substances unfold their effect on brain metabolism by 'usurping' evolved brain systems involved in adaptive signalling of reward and social attachment.

The motivational system operates largely via dopaminergic pathways. Dopaminergic neurons originate in the ventral tegmental area (VTA), a phylogenetically old brain region (Wolf 1999). They project to the ventral corpus striatum, precisely the nucleus accumbens (NAc), and further to the PFC, with which important feedback loops exist (Robbins and Everitt 1999). This ascending mesolimbic/mesocortical dopamine system stimulates appetitive behaviour such as foraging and sexual appetence. It is also involved in guiding attention, decision-making, and internal signalling of emotional content (Bechara et al. 2001). The PFC exerts top-down control and projects back to the limbic proportion of the motivational system. The PFC provides contextual information through associative learning. For instance, the experience that alcohol consumption provides positive feelings in certain circumstances may trigger craving in conditions reminiscent of the original situation (Wrase et al. 2007). In other words, intake of psychotropic substances such as alcohol produces an unconditioned stimulus in the ascending dopaminergic system. The PFC then adds contextual information from particular reward-signalling situations, hence sensitizing the dopamine system by signifying incentive salience. This by no means needs to pass the threshold of conscious experience. Even the smell of alcohol may activate the VTA and NAc in people with alcohol dependence, and it is reasonable to assume that sometimes simply the scent of alcoholic beverages or passing the pub where one used to drink may lead to relapse.

The ascending mesolimbic–mesocortical dopaminergic system is involved in reward prediction. Repetitive consumption of psychotropic substances downregulates the dopaminergic pathways, such that simultaneous desensitization and reward-seeking require dose increment to produce the same effect.

One problem of the ascending dopamine system is that it has no built-in stopping device. It was simply unnecessary in evolutionary times to select for such a mechanism, because in natural conditions the exhaustion of resources terminated the activation of the ascending dopamine system, and the appetitive or seeking behaviour ceased automatically. With psychotropic substances available in abundance, the activation of the mesolimbic/mesocortical dopamine system is abnormal in terms of both degree and duration (Nesse and Berridge 1997). The continuing activation of the VTA and NAc anticipates a salience signal (attribution of relevance) from the PFC. With repetitive consumption of psychotropic substances the dopaminergic neurons become downregulated, such that simultaneous desensitization and salience or reward-seeking require dose increment to produce the same effect, hence promoting tolerance. This may be particularly relevant for individuals who rapidly metabolize dopamine or carry genetic variations of catecholamine-depleting enzyme activity.

Aside from the dopamine system involved in appetitive behaviour, alcohol in particular enhances the inhibitory effect of GABA and decreases excitatory glutamate activity at the NMDA receptor subtype. Glutamate is produced from the amino acid glutamine; decarboxylation of glutamate by the enzyme glutamic acid decarboxylase leads to GABA. Thus, under physiological conditions, excitatory and inhibitory neurotransmission can easily be balanced by the organism.

GABA is abundant in the human cerebral cortex, especially in the primary sensory cortex, Heschl's gyrus, and the ACC. Extended cortical inhibition represents an evolutionary novelty that is crucial for controlling upcoming impulses from lower brain centres. Conditions of overly enhanced inhibition and decreased excitation of neuronal activity by alcohol can produce sedation, poor concentration, and even coma.

In the 1980s, researchers found receptor binding sites that are specific to benzodiazepine (BDZ)-like substances. BDZ receptors are abundant in brain regions that are functionally associated with the regulation of fear (these receptors are also present in the neocortex). The lateral and central areas of the amygdala connect downwards to the anterior and medial hypothalamus and further down to the PAG; these pathways are rich in BDZ receptors. Alcohol, barbiturates, and benzodiazepines bind to these receptors. By dampening neural transmission, these substances exert powerful anxiolytic effects. Conversely, rapid withdrawal of these substances, if recurrently used, produces rebound or withdrawal symptoms, with dramatic increase in arousal and anxiety, and lowered threshold of startle reactions. One important function of the amygdala is to control the associative learning of fear-inducing situations. Fear conditioning takes place in the central part of the amygdala mediated by the action of glutamate. Inhibition of glutamatergic action may therefore reduce fear conditioning in people with alcohol dependence. Reduced fear and increased risk-taking behaviour are often found in patients with chronic alcoholism, and the aggressive behaviour of intoxicated individuals is a major cause of admissions to psychiatric services.

Alcohol, barbiturates, and benzodiazepines bind to GABAergic receptors. By dampening neural transmission, these substances exert powerful anxiolytic effects. Conversely, rapid withdrawal of these substances, if recurrently used, produces rebound or withdrawal symptoms, with dramatic increase in arousal and anxiety, and lowered threshold of startle reactions.

From an evolutionary point of view, it makes sense that fear and anger are intimately linked at the neuroanatomical level. In dangerous situations, an animal has to swiftly decide whether flight or fight is the appropriate response. Short distances between brain centres involved in such decision-making are therefore advantageous. In fact, the neuronal pathways concerned with the expression of aggressive behaviour originate in the medial area of the amygdala and connect to lower centres in the brain of the PAG via the hypothalamus. Many psychotropic substances, including alcohol and opioids, exert

Many psychotropic substances, including alcohol and opioids, exert strong anti-aggressive effects. Withdrawal of these substances may lead to aggression due to the absence of neural inhibition, which may further be incited if missing reward or salience signals from the PFC lead to frustration.

strong anti-aggressive effects. Withdrawal of these substances may lead to aggression due to the absence of neural inhibition, which may further be incited if missing reward or salience signals from the PFC cause feelings of frustration. In other words, disorders of the subtle balance between inhibition and excitation in amygdaloid circuits and the close functional and anatomic relationship of the fear and anger systems can explain aggression in both acute alcohol intoxication and rebound and withdrawal syndromes.

Another brain system involved in substance misuse and dependence is naturally controlled by endogenous opiates and neuropeptides (Insel 2003). This brain system evolved, partly, to signal social affiliation, attachment, and absence of potentially fitness-decreasing situations. In experimental conditions, opioids at non-sedating doses, as well as oxytocin, reduce separation distress in social animals. Thus, the consumption of substances stimulating the opioid system may falsely indicate social security. Individuals, for instance, who as children had formed insecure social bonds with their primary attachment figures may be particularly at risk of developing misuse and dependence of opioidergic substances, and this assumption has been confirmed in many studies in opiate addicts. When tolerance to repetitive administration of opiates emerges, the pleasant feeling of social security insidiously wears off, leading to dysphoria and consequently the urge to consume higher doses.

The endogenous opioid system is involved in social affiliation and attachment. Opioid addicts may seek to stimulate this system, because they often lack secure attachment. Insecurely attached children, for example, due to poor parental care, especially those who experienced physical or emotional abuse, tend to perceive the world as perilous and unpredictable, and therefore may adopt opportunistic behavioural strategies.

The neuropeptide oxytocin is critically involved in the formation of social bonds, sexual arousal, and mother–infant interaction. Oxytocin increases the sensitivity of opioid neurones, and can inhibit the development of tolerance in people with opiate dependence. Clinically, opioid withdrawal syndromes are characterized by highly aroused negative emotional states such as irritability, despair, and pain—strikingly similar to symptoms associated with separation anxiety (Panksepp 1998). Avoidance of such aversive emotional states is most desirable, and individuals who as infants and children were insecurely attached may be particularly at risk of adopting maladaptive strategies to shun negative emotional states.

Opioid withdrawal syndromes are characterized by highly aroused negative emotional states such as irritability, despair, and pain—strikingly similar to symptoms associated with separation anxiety.

Insecurely attached children, for example, due to poor parental care, especially those who experienced physical or emotional abuse, tend to perceive the world as perilous and unpredictable. As adolescents they may adopt behavioural strategies of immediate resource extraction, which could have been a successful strategy in the environment of evolutionary adaptedness in environmentally harsh conditions. In contrast to well-predictable conditions, where benefits may be obtained in the long term at the cost of delaying immediate reward, insecure environmental conditions predispose to greater risk-taking and opportunistic behaviour in order to increase short-term fitness gains. Individuals who are insecurely attached are therefore perhaps more inclined to sensation-seeking behaviour, easier frustrated, intolerant to social pressure and norms, and more likely to exhibit impulsive behaviour and emotional instability in situations where immediate gains are thwarted (see Chapter 3).

Consequently, people who strive for immediate fitness benefits also tend to manipulate others, as can be observed in opiate addicts. At the same time, however, they tend to restrict their behavioural repertoire to patterns that are easy to control. This could, for example, explain some situations in which relapse occurs; despite enhanced novelty-seeking, individuals who anticipate situations to be dangerous have difficulties in tolerating the prospect of a potentially negative outcome, and try to gain control by something familiar—which could be calming down and inducing feelings of security and pleasure by the consumption of psychotropic substances.

If opiates, in part, have the potential of substituting emotional states normally associated with reliable social bonds and attachment, people addicted to such substances may not experience the need to integrate into conventional social groups. Rather, they occupy an ecological niche where social competition is reduced and their peers adopt the same fragile strategy: that is, immediate resource extraction for short-term benefits at the cost of poor behavioural inhibition, and neglect of potentially negative outcome in the long run, including severe physical damage (Lubman et al. 2004; Lende 2008). Pathological risk-taking, including precarious (and precocious) sexual behaviour, manipulation, and poor impulse control may account for the high rate of deviant behaviour and high prevalence of sexually transmitted diseases in drug addicts (Martins et al. 2004). Put another way, this pattern of behaviour reflects a 'fast' life-history strategy (Del Giudice 2014).

If opiates have the potential of substituting emotional states normally associated with reliable social bonds and attachment, people addicted to such substances may not experience the need to integrate into conventional social groups.

In a more general vein, socially disadvantaged individuals may be particularly vulnerable to drug-intake (Lende and Smith 2002). Research into non-human primates has revealed that environmental conditions influence the dopaminergic system in dominant and subordinate individuals differently (Morgan et al. 2002). Individually housed monkeys have been shown to possess a hyper-reactive dopamine system. Interestingly, in experimental conditions this hyperactivity returned to normal when formerly isolated monkeys were introduced in social groups, but only in those individuals who became dominant; the dopamine system remained hyperactive in subordinate individuals, who, in addition, self-administered higher amounts of cocaine in social housing conditions (Kuhar 2002). Social separation has also been shown to increase alcohol consumption in non-human primates (Kraemer and McKinney 1985). These models could therefore provide a powerful explanation as to why underprivileged and socially isolated humans maintain substance consumption and become engaged in a vicious circle.

In addition to environmental factors such as adverse early rearing conditions, the development of substance dependence is clearly genetically influenced. Individual vulnerability to substance dependence is polygenetically inherited. Among other candidate genes, a polymorphism of the dopamine D2 receptor has been linked to the risk for alcoholism. Carriers of the A1 allele of the dopamine D2 receptor are apparently at higher risk of their motivational system being occupied by unnatural reward-signalling substances. Findings that the genetic susceptibility to alcoholism interacts with exposure to stress in pre-adolescence emphasizes the existence of strong gene–environment interactions in the emergence of substance dependence. Likewise, it has been demonstrated in a non-human primate model that serotonin transporter gene variation is linked to the amount of alcohol consumption, depending on rearing conditions (Barr et al. 2004). Individuals who are separated from their mothers and reared in peer-groups drink more alcohol when carrying a certain serotonin transporter allele compared to non-carriers, which is explained by differences in anxiety regulation and responsiveness of the HPA axis.

At present, we do not know why these genetic differences evolved. Several dopamine receptor polymorphisms associated with increased risk for substance dependence also seem to be involved in the regulation of novelty-seeking and impulsivity, particularly in men. In the ancestral environment of early humans, such behavioural tendencies may well have conferred fitness advantages in terms of access to food or sexual partners in uncertain conditions (see Chapter 7 on ADHD).

Dopamine receptor polymorphisms associated with increased risk for substance dependence also seem to be involved in the regulation of novelty-seeking and impulsivity, particularly in men. In the ancestral environment of early humans, such behavioural tendencies may well have conferred fitness advantages in terms of access to food or sexual partners in uncertain conditions.

Furthermore, sex differences in the propensity of developing substance dependence in favour of males may be linked to divergent evolved behavioural strategies in men and women, which may in turn explain sex differences in drug sensitivity (Lynch et al. 2002). For example, men have evolved behavioural dispositions to compete with each other for access to fertile women. Thus men are selected to engage in risky behaviour to display their genetic quality. Also, due to divergent parental investment in potential offspring, men are predicted to receive higher gains from pursuing short-term goals. Thus, impulsivity and opportunistic behaviour should be more prevalent in men (including the respective genetic predisposition).

In contrast, substance dependence relating to replacement of secure emotional bonds may be found in both sexes at similar rates. Evidence is accumulating that women progress to dependence more rapidly than men, which may be associated with the action of oestrogen or X-chromosome-linked genes involved in habit formation. These effects may, on the other hand, be mitigated by women's superior inhibitory control and harm avoidance as a consequence of greater parental investment in potential offspring.

In sum, the proximate and ultimate mechanisms causing substance misuse or dependence (which lie on a continuum) can be seen as the extreme of variation of traits associated with novelty-seeking and poor social attachment. As such, they require an integrative approach, taking into account both the genetic and behavioural dimension, which contribute to the maladaptive phenotypic expression.

17.7 **Differential diagnosis and comorbidity**

Alcohol and drug abuse or dependence can develop secondary to anxiety disorders, depression, ADHD, and disorders associated with poor inhibitory control such as schizophrenia, frontotemporal dementia, and Huntington's chorea. Many individuals misuse or are addicted to more than one substance, a situation that complicates treatment (American Psychiatric Association 2013).

Alcohol and drug abuse or dependence can develop secondary to anxiety disorders, depression, ADHD, and disorders associated with poor inhibitory control such as schizophrenia, frontotemporal dementia, and Huntington's chorea.

17.8 **Course and outcome**

Alcohol and drug dependence are chronic disorders with high relapse rates. Alcoholism is one of the leading causes of disability in the developed countries, and, as yet, there is no cure for either alcoholism or drug dependence. However, relapse rates decline with increasing duration of abstinence.

Alcohol and drug dependence are chronic disorders with high relapse rates.

17.9 **Treatment**

Acute intoxication with alcohol or illicit drugs may require monitoring in an intensive care unit. Withdrawal symptoms need differential treatment depending on the nature of the dependence. Alcohol withdrawal syndrome can be treated with benzodiazepines or clomethiazol (not approved in the USA and several other countries). Hallucinatory behaviour may be contained by administration of antipsychotic drugs. Drugs that help reduce the negative emotional experiences of drug withdrawal syndromes may include oxytocin agonists, dopamine agonists, and noradrenergic agonists such as clonidine, but such treatment options are to date largely experimental (e.g. Pedersen et al. 2013). In addition, drugs such as disulfiram that cause aversive reactions by increasing the toxic effects of alcohol derivatives (acetaldehyde), glutamate antagonists such as acamprosate, and the opioid antagonist naltrexone may be useful in the reduction of craving, if combined with a socially rewarding therapeutic setting.

Treatment of acute intoxication or withdrawal syndromes is symptom-oriented. Drugs that help reduce the negative emotional experiences of drug withdrawal syndromes may include oxytocin agonists, dopamine agonists, and noradrenergic agonists such as clonidine, but such treatment options are to date largely experimental. Drugs such as disulfiram that cause aversive reactions by increasing the toxic effects of alcohol derivatives (acetaldehyde), glutamate antagonists such as acamprosate, and the opioid antagonist naltrexone may be useful in the reduction of craving, if combined with a socially rewarding therapeutic setting.

Prevention is certainly the best option, by fostering the development of secure attachment and social bonds in early childhood to reduce the likelihood of adopting high-risk behavioural strategies. For example, family intervention studies have shown that parental attitudes impact substantially on the treatment outcome of children who displayed problem behaviour including drinking (Nye et al. 1999). Moreover, careful screening for comorbid disorders and treatment of comorbid conditions are essential.

Self-help maintained by various organizations and counselling by experienced social workers are helpful for relapse prevention.

Detailed treatment guidelines are available online from the APA website. Recommendations for carers and lay persons are accessible via the website of the RCP.

Chapter 18

Neurocognitive disorders

Abstract

Neurocognitive disorders affect a broad array of cognitive domains, but produce also emotional and behavioural signs. Dementia is most prevalent among the neurocognitive disorders, with Alzheimer's disease being the most common form. Neurocognitive dysfunction is related to aging and senescence. Evolutionary considerations suggest that senescence has escaped selection, because most individual of a population would die before the onset of senescence. However, there is some evidence that longevity has been positively selected during human evolution. It is possible that the human isoforms of the ApoE gene, ApoE2 and E3, were positively selected during periods of rapid increase in brain size some 1.5 million years ago, and that they may have evolved as an adaptation to the increasing intake of a protein-rich diet (i.e. meat). A-beta and neurofibrillary tangles may, on the other hand, have antimicrobial properties, which could tell a different story with regard to the evolutionary history of dementia.

Keywords

neurocognitive disorder, dementia, Alzheimer's disease, senescence, aging, ApoE isoforms, longevity, protein-rich diet, antimicrobial properties

18.1 Symptomatology and diagnostic criteria

Neurocognitive disorders comprise delirium, major neurocognitive disorders, and mild neurocognitive disorders (DSM-5: American Psychiatric Association 2013). These disorders have in common that their primary manifestation is in one or several cognitive domains, including sustained attention, executive function, learning and memory, language, perception, and social cognition (American Psychiatric Association 2013). Major neurocognitive disorder, commonly referred to as dementia, is characterized by an insidious and progressive loss of memory, disorientation, cognitive decline in other domains, and affective flattening. It is often accompanied by neuropsychological deficits such as aphasia, apraxia, and agnosia, and disturbances in

Dementia is characterized by an insidious and progressive loss of memory, disorientation, cognitive decline, and affective flattening. It is often accompanied by neuropsychological deficits such as aphasia, apraxia, agnosia, and disturbances in executive functioning. Behavioural symptoms such as withdrawal, depression, delusions, motor restlessness, wandering, and aggression may complicate dementia in advanced stages of the disorder.

executive functioning, including planning, organizing, and sequencing of events in a logical fashion. Neurocognitive disorder affecting the frontal lobes is primarily characterized by impairment in social cognition and understanding social rules and norms, whereas memory loss is less dominant (Gregory et al. 2002; Snowden et al. 2002; Lough et al. 2006).

Behavioural symptoms such as withdrawal, depression, delusions, motor restlessness, wandering, and aggression may complicate dementia, particularly in advanced stages of the disorder. These behavioural symptoms may occur, in part, secondary to loss of orientation and memory, with loss of autobiographic memory perhaps being most devastating. A patient, for example, who is impaired in retrieving past social interactions from autobiographical memory or recalling other relevant personal information may be more likely to respond with increasing irritability or anxiety in situations that are actually or perceived unfamiliar. Such a patient may perhaps choose a 'safety first' strategy or remain captured in indecisiveness, which could manifest in ruminated thinking and stereotyped behaviour, or displacement activities expressing motivational conflict and ambivalence. In any event, the combination of memory loss with other cognitive disturbances certainly leads to a profound deterioration of social competence.

It is also noteworthy that, in addition to the problems the patients have themselves, which they generally deny except in the earliest stages of the disorder (anosognosia), dementia creates a substantial burden on patients' spouses, children, and other carers. The most common causes of major neurocognitive disorder are Alzheimer's disease (AD), frontotemporal dementia (FTD), Lewy body disease (LBD), vascular dementia (VD), traumatic brain injury, substance dependence, infectious diseases such as HIV, prion disease, and other neuropsychiatric conditions including Parkinson's and Huntington's disease (American Psychiatric Association 2013).

The most common causes of major neurocognitive disorder are AD, FTD, LBD, VD, traumatic brain injury, substance dependence, infectious diseases such as HIV, prion disease, and other neuropsychiatric conditions, including Parkinson's and Huntington's disease.

18.2 **Epidemiology**

AD accounts for approximately two-thirds of all major neurocognitive disorders. A definitive diagnosis can only be made post mortem, although standardized clinical diagnostic criteria and biological markers in the cerebrospinal fluid (CSF) may produce reliable results during a patient's lifetime (Bibl et al. 2007). Men and women are affected in nearly equal numbers, although brain pathology seems to be more severe in women with AD (Barnes et al. 2005).

AD accounts for approximately two-thirds of all major neurocognitive disorders. The prevalence rate of AD increases steadily, from about 1 percent in people 65 years of age to over 20 percent in the ninth decade. The male to female ratio of AD is nearly 1:1.

The prevalence rate of AD increases steadily, from about 1 percent in people 65 years of age to over 20 percent in the ninth decade (Hendrie 1998). The male to female ratio of AD is nearly 1:1, if differential survival rates and longevity differences between males and females are taken into account. AD is infrequent in the presenium, but progresses in sporadic or familial cases probably more rapidly. It is currently under debate whether or not the incidence of AD declines in the tenth decade, but studies have revealed inconsistent results.

In some populations worldwide the rates for AD have been reported to be lower than in western countries, but such differences may have been masked by different survival rates and diagnostic conventions (Ineichen 2000). Recent research shows, however, that people of African ancestry in Brazil have lower prevalence rates of AD (Schlesinger et al. 2013). Conversely, other studies suggest increased prevalence rates for AD in some populations, independent of apolipoprotein E (APOE) genetics (Farrer et al. 2003). Overall, determining precise prevalence rates has proven difficult (Kukull and Bowen 2002). If only we would grow old enough, perhaps everyone might develop AD at age 120 or so. This could suggest that dementia could be the extreme of variation of normal aging and senescence. Consistent with this assumption, the conversion rate of mild cognitive impairment (MCI) to dementia is between 25 and 50 percent at 2- to 3-year follow-up.

LBD is often associated with parkinsonism, visual hallucinations, fluctuating vigilance, and intolerance of antipsychotic drugs (Graeber and Müller 2003).

VD is the second-most common form of major neurocognitive disorder in countries with high prevalence of atherosclerosis, figuring around 20 percent of cases, with overlap between AD and VD at both the behavioural and neuroanatomical level. Fluctuations in cognitive performance are more common in VD than AD.

FTD comprises a spectrum of non-AD affecting the frontal lobe, with predominating behavioural symptoms and personality change (fvFTD), the temporal lobe associated with aphasia (semantic dementia), and progressive aphasia. Characteristically, these symptoms usually precede the onset of cognitive decline. Onset of FTD is between the fourth and seventh decade. FTD is generally rare, but accounts for up to 20 percent of dementia cases in the presenium (Hodges and Miller 2001).

LBD is often associated with parkinsonism, visual hallucinations, fluctuating vigilance, and intolerance of antipsychotic drugs. VD is the second-most common form of neurocognitive disorder in countries with high prevalence of atherosclerosis. FTD comprises a spectrum of non-AD affecting the frontal lobe, with predominating behavioural symptoms and personality change.

18.3 **Genetic risk factors**

The risk for developing AD is increased in first-degree relatives of patients with AD, suggesting a heritable component. By age 90, relatives of AD patients have a cumulative risk of 15–20 percent for developing AD, compared to 5 percent in controls. If both parents are affected, the risk for offspring may rise to over 50 percent at age 80. Twin studies suggest double concordance rates in MZ twins of 30–80 percent compared to 10–40 percent in DZ twins. In a minority of AD cases, particularly those with early onset, an autosomal dominant inheritance pattern has been described. However, familial AD accounts for only 13 percent of early-onset cases and less than 0.01 percent of all AD (Liddell et al. 2005).

Most cases of AD are sporadic, although family studies suggest a heritable component. In familial cases, mutations of the APP coding gene on chromosome 21, and the presenilin 1 and 2 genes on chromosome 14 and 1, respectively, have been identified. Late-onset AD is associated with polymorphisms of the ApoE family.

In familial AD, mutations of the amyloid precursor protein (APP) coding gene on chromosome 21, and the presenilin 1 and 2 genes on chromosomes 14 and 1, respectively, have been identified (Rademakers et al. 2003; Bertram and Tanzi 2008). Late-onset AD is associated with polymorphisms of the apolipoprotein-E (ApoE) family on chromosome 19, with ApoE4 conveying the greatest risk for developing AD (up to 50 percent of homozygous individuals develop AD until age 80, but not in all populations studied; Evans et al. 2003; Ewbank 2004), whereas ApoE2 is supposed to have protective effects. However, the possession of an ApoE4 allele is neither necessary nor sufficient to develop the disorder. Overall, ApoE4 contributes about 17 percent to the population variance in susceptibility for AD. Several other genetic susceptibility loci have been discussed, of which the functional significance is poorly understood (Lendon et al. 1997; Bertram and Tanzi 2008). For example, genes involved in cholesterol turnover do not seem to play a major role in AD (Riemenschneider et al. 2004).

FTD has been linked with polymorphisms of the tau-protein coding gene on chromosome 17 (Hodges and Miller 2001), though cases with uncertain genetic contribution may be more common (Goldman et al. 2004).

18.4 **Environmental risk factors**

Age is the most significant risk factor for AD. People with Down syndrome who carry an extra chromosome 21 (on which the APP gene is located) often develop AD in their 40s. Moreover, poor education and oestrogen depletion at menopause have been discussed as putative risk factors for AD. Interaction of ApoE and oestrogen may also be relevant for males, because in the brain, testosterone is converted into oestrogen. Whether or not the risk of AD is linked to exposure to aluminium or heavy metals is not entirely clear.

Age is the most significant risk factor for AD. Poor education and oestrogen depletion at menopause have also been suggested as putative risk factors for AD, whereas the role of exposure to aluminium or heavy metals is unclear.

Age and risk factors for atherosclerosis, such as hypertension, diabetes, and smoking, increase the risk for AD, but also VD (Ballard et al. 2011). No environmental risk factors are known for LBD and FTD.

18.5 **Pathophysiological mechanisms**

The pathophysiological mechanisms involved in AD are only partially understood. Several pathways have been identified that lead to the accumulation of neurotoxic substances and neuronal cell death. ApoE, presenilin, and APP interact in complex ways (Anliker and Müller 2006). ApoE is synthesized in brain and liver tissue. It is sensitive to hormonal activity, and serves as a transporter of cholesterol into steroid-producing cells (Herz and Chen 2006). Neurons, like all other cells, can produce their own cholesterol.

Humans possess three isoforms of ApoE, namely ApoE2, ApoE3, and ApoE4. The ApoE isoforms differ with respect to their binding potential to cholesterol fractions. The most common isoform in humans is ApoE3. In Caucasians about three-quarters of the population have the ApoE3 isoform; ApoE4 has been found in 15 percent and ApoeE2 in about 8 percent of the population. In Europe, a north-to-south gradient of the ApoE4 has been described, but there is considerable variation of allele frequencies between different populations (in Pygmies, for instance, about 54 percent have the ApoE3 allele and about 41 percent carry the ApoE4 isoform, whereas in Mayans, 91 percent have the ApoE3 isoform).

The pathophysiology of AD is intimately linked to the accumulation of neurotoxic substances and neuronal cell death, which depends on complex interactions between ApoE, presenilin, and APP.

ApoE4 preferentially binds to low density lipoprotein (LDL) and very low density lipoprotein (VLDL), and the ApoE4 load is associated with a significantly higher risk of developing AD and coronary heart disease. ApoE3 and ApoE2 have a higher affinity to high-density lipoprotein (HDL) cholesterol, which relatively protects from atherosclerosis. The risk of developing AD is significantly lower in ApoE2 and ApoE3 carriers compared to ApoE4 carriers (Conejero-Goldberg et al. 2014). ApoE3 is also known to slow down aging-related neuronal demyelination. High levels of intracellular cholesterol enhance the production of A-beta, because cholesterol accelerates proteolysis of APP into A-beta (Nelson and Alkon 2005). ApoE also interacts with oestrogen. Oestradiol itself has neuroprotective effects in several ways. It increases cholinergic neurotransmission and sprouting of neurons. In ApoE knock-out mice, oestradiol-induced sprouting of hippocampal neurones is reduced, but returns to normal when a human ApoE3 transgene is introduced. In vitro, oestradiol inhibits the secretion of amyloid A-beta-peptide in neurones.

A-beta is usually produced in a minor pathway of APP metabolism through the action of beta- and gamma-secretase. The presenilins are presumably involved in the cleavage of APP by gamma-secretase (Marx 1996). At physiological concentrations, A-beta impairs synaptic transmission via glutamatergic NMDA receptors. If, however, the A-beta region of the APP is altered due to a mutation in the coding gene, the secretases involved in APP processing excessively produce abnormal A-beta, which aggregates to form neuritic plaques in the extracellular space. This aggregation of A-beta leads to an inflammatory reaction and the production of neurofibrillary tangles (NFTs). NFTs consist of hyperphosphorylated tau-protein and ultimately cause neuronal death. Since APP has manifold functions, possibly including membrane stabilization, a vicious circle may induce more production of APP, thus leading to a further increase of its pathogenic cleavage product A-beta, a process known as the 'amyloid cascade hypothesis'.

A-beta is usually produced in a minor pathway of APP metabolism through the action of beta- and gamma-secretase, mediated by the availability of intracellular cholesterol. Excessive production of abnormal A-beta leads to the formation of neuritic plaques. Aggregation of A-beta leads to production of NFTs, which consist of hyperphosphorylated tau-protein, and ultimately causes neuronal death.

Neuritic plaques and NFT can be found—to some degree—in normal aging, yet the neurobiological substrates of normal aging and dementia seem to differ in important ways (Morrison and Hof 1997). The number of NFTs correlates better with the severity of AD than the number of plaques, but neuritic plaques are more specific to AD pathology. Accumulation of NFT and neuritic plaques is most prominent in ApoE4 homozygous carriers, whereas there is no clear evidence for an association of the ApoE genotype with cholinergic transmission in AD (Tiraboschi et al. 2004).

The neuropathological changes in AD first affect the entorhinal cortex and hippocampus. In addition, the nucleus basalis of Meynert, which contains a large number of cholinergic neurons, degenerates early in the course of AD. In later stages, cortical atrophy, particularly of the parietal cortex, is characteristic for AD.

The neuropathological changes in AD first affect the entorhinal cortex and hippocampus.

Pathologies of the tau-protein have also been found in FTD, but, in general, the pathophysiology of FTD is less well understood. Brain atrophy is more pronounced in frontal and/or temporal regions (Snowden et al. 2002). Recent animal and human studies suggest that altered expression of micro-RNA may change the levels of alpha-amino-3-hydroxy-5-methyl-4-isoxazolepropionic acid (NMDA) receptors in the PFC, and may explain changes in social behaviour (Gascon et al. 2014).

18.6 **Evolutionary synthesis**

Brain disorders that cause cognitive decline are highly heterogeneous in nature. They involve multiple genetic effects, which interact with environmental factors, including nutrition and perhaps exposure to toxic substances. Above all, however, most major neurocognitive disorders are ultimately linked to aging and senescence, processes that sexually reproducing organisms inevitably undergo. By definition, senescence, as opposed to aging, is characterized by increasing deterioration of the body functions. The immunological competence of the body and the ability to repair damaged tissue, for example, decreases with age; thus prevalence of autoimmune diseases and cancer increase with age. The same steady functional decline may occur with regard to cognition, emotion, and behavioural flexibility, though emotional regulation seems to improve with age, suggesting that selection has, to some point, operated against senescence (Carstensen and Löckenhoff 2003). Strictly speaking, however, for most body functions, human senescence sets in shortly after puberty, and the pattern of senescence in humans does not seem to deviate from that of other primates (Bronikowski et al. 2011).

Most neurocognitive disorders are ultimately linked to aging and senescence, processes that sexually reproducing organisms inevitably undergo.

One reason why senescence occurs is that natural selection does not operate on genes that cause senescence, because in the wild all individuals would die from natural hazards, such as starvation or predation, before senescence could decrease an individual's inclusive fitness. In other words, most individuals of a population would not live to the day when senescence sets in. This account of senescence, however, is only to a certain extent plausible. It predicts that in wild populations, senescence would almost be absent (Nesse 1988). Research in wild populations suggests that the mortality rate in many animal species, rather than being constant as would be expected in a hypothetical state of absence of senescence, increases with age. Thus, escape from selection alone is not sufficient to explain senescence. It is much more likely that, in addition, genes have been selected which exert pleiotropic effects: such genes convey fitness advantages early in life, while having deleterious effects at advanced ages (Williams 1957; Kirkwood and Rose 1991). In particular, one would expect that the beneficial effects of pleiotropic genes causing senescence are highest at the peak reproductive period of a species (Nesse 1988). For instance, a hypothetical gene that acts on calcium metabolism by facilitating bone calcification, thus making young individuals more resistant against bone fractures, may trigger atherosclerosis in older adults. Likewise, genes favouring a strong immune system early in life may induce autoimmune diseases in older individuals and hence accelerate senescence (Nesse and Williams 1994).

Selection has operated on genes that convey fitness advantages early in life while having deleterious effects later in life. Conversely, selection for longevity should be balanced against selection for genes that cause senescence.

Moreover, senescence could result from selection *against* anti-aging genes, because anti-aging effects are relatively irrelevant for young individuals (Kirkwood and Rose 1991). Conversely, selection for longevity should be balanced against selection for genes that cause senescence. In fact, breeding experiments have demonstrated that in fruit flies artificial selection for longevity decreases early fecundity and increases late fecundity. In flour beetles, artificial selection for early reproduction decreases longevity, probably due to the action of pleiotropic genes.

With respect to senescence and longevity in humans, the evolution of ApoE polymorphisms in primates reveals interesting insights. Recent research in non-human primates and other vertebrates suggests that an ApoE4-like allele is the ancestral form from which ApoE3 and subsequently ApoE2 are derived (Mahley and Rall 1999). The human isoforms E2 and E3 differ from ApoE4 by only two amino acids at position 112 and 158 in the polypeptide chain. In ApoE4 both positions code arginine (CGC), whereas in ApoE3 a transition at codon 112 to TGC replaces arginine by cysteine. ApoeE2 comprises an additional C to T transition at codon 158, thus coding for another cysteine. All non-human primate species examined so far exhibit CGC codons at a position homologous to 112 and 158 in humans. Moreover, biochemically the transition from C to T is easier than the reverse, which would be necessary to derive ApoE4 from ApoE3. Thus, it is more parsimonious to conclude that ApoE3 derived from ApoE4, and ApoE2 from ApoE3, rather than the opposite way (Fullerton et al. 2000).

ApoE2 and ApoE3 possibly emerged in the human lineage when brain size and longevity increased dramatically, perhaps in order to postpone senescence and compensate for changes in the human diet towards larger amounts of protein and fat.

Although the fossil record of early humans does not contain sufficient genetic material to exactly date back the evolutionary origin of the ApoE3 and ApoE2 variants, it is plausible to assume that these polymorphisms emerged at some point in human evolution that was accompanied by a rapid increase in brain size (Kosik 2000). Since brain size correlates with longevity (see Chapter 2), it is plausible to assume that longevity was also a target of selection (Martin 2002). These evolutionary changes affecting brain size and the human life-history pattern could have emerged around 1.5 mya with the appearance of *Homo ergaster*. Brain size in *Homo ergaster* had already doubled since the split of the chimpanzee and the human lineage from a common ancestor about 5–6 mya. Such a big brain was already energetically expensive and required large amounts of high-quality diet, including large amounts of protein. In addition, it took several years longer for *Homo ergaster* to reach sexual maturity compared to chimpanzees, and the need of transgenerational transfer of knowledge (through culture) increased rapidly in successive *Homo* species.

This scenario suggests that the increasing duration of dependence of infants on their mothers (and their mother's survival) created a selection pressure of expanding the human lifespan. It is then reasonable to assume that it became advantageous for early humans to survive sufficiently long enough beyond ceasing reproduction to raise offspring born shortly before menopause (Finch and Sapolsky 1999). A life history of a female who gave birth at age 40 and died before her offspring was socially mature (some 20 years later) would certainly not have been favoured by natural selection. In fact, modern *Homo sapiens* women have by far the longest post-reproductive lifespan of all primates (Sapolsky and Finch 2000). Experiencing and living beyond menopause is rare in non-human primates, but in humans there is perhaps 20–30 years to come after ovulation has terminated (see Chapter 3).

In anatomically modern humans, at birth infants are essentially immature. This reflects an evolutionary compromise between the size of the infant's brain (and head) and the diameter of its mother's birth canal (see Chapter 3). In contrast to non-human primates the human brain continues to grow after birth at the same pace for more than a year. Brain maturation (synaptic pruning and myelination) and developing adult social competence are extended well into the third decade of life, requiring extended periods of parental care. Thus, in addition to experiencing longer lifespans themselves, mothers (and their offspring) could have benefited from additional help from their own mothers—hence grandmothering evolved (Hrdy 2000). Among primates, grandmothering is quite unique to humans. In hunter-gatherer societies grandmothers contribute a substantial proportion of calories to the diet of their grandchildren. In addition, human grandmothers help pass on social skills to subsequent generations—certainly another fitness advantage of postponing senescence (Hrdy 2000). Thus, by analogy, the emergence of ApoE3 and ApoE2 polymorphisms in humans may have occurred by sporadic mutation at some point of human evolutionary history, which were favoured by selection in order to delay senescence, thereby selecting against an early onset of AD-like pathology (Finch and Sapolsky 1999; Sapolsky and Finch 2000).

Moreover, in light of their regulatory effects on cholesterol metabolism, the new ApoE variants may have been selected in response to an increasing amount of meat and fat of the human diet (Finch and Stanford 2004). Captive chimpanzees, for example, are extremely susceptible to developing hypercholesterolaemia and atherosclerotic plaques when fed a diet rich in protein and fat. However, they develop less often neoplasia compared to humans (Finch 2010). In their natural habitat, however, chimpanzees consume a diet that usually contains low amounts of animal tissue. An increasing meat intake of human ancestors that was probably advantageous in terms of protein supply for growing big brains would predict, in reverse, a shorter lifespan—given the atherogenic effect and high load of infectious particles of (raw) meat. The differential binding potential of ApoE variants to cholesterol fractions may therefore be an adaptive response to both changing diet in early humans and the need of postponing senescence (Finch and Stanford 2004).

Interestingly with respect to human life history, some studies suggest that men with a homozygous ApoE3 genotype have more children compared with men carrying other ApoE allele combinations (Gerdes et al. 1996). In addition, there is some evidence for the functional significance of APP for sperm mobility (Fardilha et al. 2007); however, how this exactly relates to mutations at the APP locus is, at present, unclear (Shoji et al. 1990; Harrison 1995). A speculative explanation could be that different APP polymorphisms affect sperm function in different ways, which may support the assumption of a trade-off (balanced polymorphism) between reproductive success early in life and dementia after cessation of the reproductive period. In line with this speculation, women who have at least one ApoE4 allele (E4/E4 or E4/E3) reach menopause earlier than women with other ApoE genotypes (Koochmeshgi et al. 2004).

There is some evidence suggesting that the possession of an ApoE2 or ApoE3 allele pays off reproductively.

Finally, the ApoE genotype seems to play a role in the variation of life expectancy in European populations (Ewbank 2004), but such an effect seems to disappear in the oldest old (over 100 years of age), perhaps by escaping the forces of selection. These findings therefore support the assumption of a putative fitness advantage of non-ApoE4 genotypes over ApoE4 homo- or heterozygosity, although it has been speculated that ApoE4 could protect against some viral infectious diseases in the sense of a balanced morphism (reviewed in Finch 2010).

Consistent with this scenario, the onset of AD-like neuropathology corresponds with the beginning of senescence in humans and some other primate species. Senile plaques have been found in a variety of other mammals, and extracellular and vascular A-beta deposits are common in chimpanzees at age 30 (although chimpanzees do not develop Alzheimer-like cognitive decline; Finch and Sapolsky 1999). Conversely, it could well be that A-beta has beneficial effects related to its antimicrobial properties and dampening effect on excitatory neurotransmission (reviewed in Glass and Arnold 2012). Human-type NFTs, by contrast, are absent in non-human primates, but similar neurocytoskeletal abnormalities may occur in carnivores, which could reflect common dietary characteristics (Sapolsky and Finch 2000). NFTs primarily occur in neurons containing large amounts of neurofilament protein, which is part of the cytoskeleton of certain neurons. Like A-beta, NFTs may not always be harmful but may protect the cell body from apoptotic death (Glass and Arnold 2012).

ApoE4 is believed to protect against viral infection. Moreover, A-beta could have antimicrobial properties.

Now, why do memory, orientation, and executive planning deteriorate first in AD? Generally speaking, the human brain may be particularly susceptible to senescence because of its extremely high oxidative metabolism and cellular stress induced by oxygen radical formations. This could particularly hold for brain regions that underwent recent adaptive modifications in human evolution. The basal forebrain is, however, an ancient brain structure. It contains cholinergic nuclei of which the nucleus basalis of Meynert is the

The human brain may be particularly susceptible to senescence because of its extremely high oxidative metabolism and cellular stress induced by oxygen radical formations.

most important one. Ninety per cent of neurons of the nucleus basalis of Meynert use cholinergic synaptic signal transmission. These neurons are the major source of cholinergic projections to the neocortex, and project also to the amygdala, the hippocampus, and the brainstem. Input from the neocortex to the nucleus basalis is by comparison sparse.

In functional terms, the cholinergic system is important for sustaining attention, motivation, and learning. Projections to the pontine reticular fields are involved in sleep regulation. In primates the size and complexity of the cytoarchitecture of the nucleus basalis of Meynert correlates with the neocortex size, indicating an allometric expansion.

Similarly, the entorhinal cortex which degenerates early in the course of AD has allometrically greatly enlarged in humans in relation to body weight, and its architecture is much more complex compared to insectivores and non-human primates. The most important efferent projections of the entorhinal cortex terminate in the hippocampus. The retrocommissural part of the hippocampus is allometrically also vastly expanded in humans. In functional terms, the entorhinal cortex and the hippocampus are critically involved in memorizing (see Chapter 2).

Moreover, VENs located in the medial wall of the cingulate gyrus are particularly vulnerable to degeneration in AD and FTD (with a loss of approximately 60 percent of neurons), perhaps due to their richness in neurofilament protein (Allman et al. 2011). The density and size of VENs increased over evolutionary time and are greatest in humans. Experiments in non-human primates have shown that the ACC is active during voluntary vocalization and electric stimulation in monkeys. Lesions to the ACC in humans produce mutism. The ACC is also crucial for emotional self-control and problem-solving capacity, but the exact role of VENs is as yet unknown.

In sum, the distribution of brain lesions in AD at the cellular level explains the clinical manifestation of this type of dementia. For other causes of dementia such as VD, FTD, and rare causes of dementia, the evolutionary scenario is less well understood.

Fortunately for our species, evolution has probably selected genes postponing senescence and, hence, the onset of AD. However, these evolutionary changes have also created a burden in both economic and interpersonal terms. In light of the demographic development in western countries, expenses for care for the elderly will rise considerably in the next 50–100 years. However, if there is anything unique to humans, it is the propensity to invert the evolutionary problem of parent–offspring conflict. *Homo sapiens* is probably the only species where parental investment can be 'reversed', that is, producing commitment of the young to care for the old. In light of the higher parental investment of females, it becomes clear why the burden of care is largely on the daughters or daughters-in-law of dementia patients. However, the willingness to invest in old people is probably limited. Thus, the pressure to find a cure for AD will certainly become more intense.

The ability to invert the problem of parental investment, that is, that the young care for the old, is probably unique to humans, even though the willingness to invest in the parental generation is constrained. In light of the demographic development, the pressure to find a cure for AD will become more intense.

Aggression directed towards demented persons is a fact that must not be neglected. Rather, it is crucial to bring to consciousness the possibility that biological constraints may have an impact on caregivers' behaviour, including close relatives and professional personnel in nursing homes. Accordingly, it could be useful to integrate this perspective into psychoeducation of caregivers to improve coping with such devastating disorders.

18.7 Differential diagnosis and comorbidity

In elderly people, the most significant differential diagnosis to AD (and some cases of FTD) is depression. Severe depression can mimic dementia, particularly if associated with cognitive impairment, for which the somewhat unfortunate term 'pseudo-dementia' has been introduced. However, depression may also co-occur in patients with dementia (both AD and FTD) or precede the onset of dementia, such that longitudinal follow-up is essential to arrive at a conclusive diagnosis. If depression is present in patients with dementia, treatment should be provided for both conditions (Downing et al. 2013).

In elderly people, the most significant differential diagnosis to AD (and some cases of FTD) is depression.

18.8 Course and outcome

All forms of dementia are chronically progressive disorders, with increasing cognitive decline associated with loss of neurons. The average duration of illness in AD is 8–10 years. Causes of death are usually secondary complications to increasing frailty and bedriddenness, including pneumonia and cardiovascular decompensation (Brunnström and Englund 2009).

All forms of dementia are chronically progressive disorders, with increasing cognitive decline associated with loss of neurons.

18.9 Treatment

To date, no cure for dementia exists. Current therapeutic efforts in AD focus on the improvement of cholinergic transmission. Several acetylcholine esterase inhibitors (AchEI) have been approved for AD treatment. AchEI are also effective in LBD (Lahiri et al. 2004). Memantine, an NMDA receptor antagonist, has also been approved for treatment of AD, but is probably less effective compared to AchEIs.

Normalizing intracerebral (and cellular) cholesterol levels and oestrogen replacement therapy are currently under investigation. Oestrogen replacement therapy can improve cognitive functioning after ovarectomy in young women (without neurogenerative disorders), and may enhance cognition in women with AD who receive cholinesterase inhibitors. Acetylsalicylic acid and non-steroidal anti-inflammatory drugs (NSAIDs) have shown some beneficial effect in AD, but apparently depending on the ApoE genotype. Statins, which help normalize the level of blood cholesterol, also have anti-inflammatory effects, and have been discussed in AD and VD, with no proven effect for AD so far.

Current therapeutic efforts in AD focus on the improvement of cholinergic transmission. In light of the lifelong need of human beings for attachment and closeness with others, it might be advisable to stimulate demented persons via different sensory channels, including haptic and acoustic means. Moreover, it must not be forgotten that dementia is devastating to all kinds of relationships, such that counselling of relatives and carers should be an integral part of a 'systemic' treatment approach.

Whether dietary means, cognitive training, physical exercise, or other lifestyle characteristics may help prevent or delay the onset of AD requires further empirical investigations (Pope et al. 2003; Ballard et al. 2011).

Moreover, many demented individuals suffer from sensory deprivation, which increases with the severity of the illness. In many respects, the ontogenetic development is reversed ('retrogenesis'), such that in the most severely affected persons only basic communication by touching and caressing is possible. In light of the lifelong need of human beings for attachment and closeness with others, it might be advisable to stimulate demented persons via different sensory channels, including haptic and acoustic means. Moreover, it must not be forgotten that dementia is devastating to all kinds of relationships, such that counselling of relatives and carers should be an integral part of a 'systemic' treatment approach.

AchEI are ineffective in FTD, for which no specific drugs are available.

Treatment guidelines and other helpful information for professionals, carers, and lay persons have been published by the APA, RCP, and RANZCP.

Chapter 19

Personality disorders

Abstract

Personality disorders (PD) concern inflexible and maladaptive cognitive, emotional, and behavioural patterns, which cause significant functional impairment or subjective distress. One group of PD is characterized by 'eccentricity', another by 'dramatic' behaviour, and a third cluster by predominant anxiety. Personality traits reflect individual patterns of behaviour that serve the purpose to achieve important biosocial goals. These behaviours can be grouped according to their interpersonal meaning: dominance versus submission; competition versus cooperation; dependence versus nurturance; assertion versus avoidance; aggression versus defence; and risk-taking versus harm avoidance. From a life-history perspective, personality traits, as well as personality disorders representing the extremes of variation of normal trait distribution, can be differentiated into 'fast' and 'slow' life-history strategies. Predictions about future resource availability arise from early childhood experiences with caregivers and the interaction of these experiences with genes involved in the regulation of aggression, attachment, etc.

Keywords

personality disorder, maladaptive patterns, dominance, submission, competition, cooperation, risk-taking, harm avoidance, life-history strategy

19.1 Symptomatology and diagnostic criteria

Personality can be referred to as a construct to describe cognitive, emotional, and behavioural traits that are peculiar to a particular person. These traits are assumed to be relatively stable and enduring rather than changing over time. Current conceptualizations of personality traits favour the distinction of five major dimensions according to which a personality can be described. These are termed 'extraversion', 'neuroticism', 'agreeableness', 'conscientiousness', and 'openness' (McCrae and Costa 1987). 'Temperament' and 'character' are also widely used to describe aspects of personality. The term 'temperament' largely refers to the biological dimension of personality,

Personality can be referred to as a construct to describe cognitive, emotional, and behavioural traits that are peculiar to a particular person. These traits are assumed to be relatively stable and enduring rather than changing over time. The most widely accepted descriptive theories propose five personality dimensions, or seven temperament and character dimensions.

whereas 'character' is more related to environmental influences, above all, the socialization process during the formative years (infancy, childhood, and adolescence). Commonly used labels are 'novelty-seeking', 'harm avoidance', 'reward dependence', and 'persistence' to describe temperament, and 'self-directedness', 'cooperation', and 'self-transcendence' as the main character dimensions (Cloninger et al. 1993; Cloninger 2000).

Recent research suggests, contrary to widely held views, that there are significant sex differences in personality traits. For example, sensitivity, warmth, and apprehension are more expressed in women, whereas emotional stability, dominance, rule-consciousness, and vigilance are more typical for men (Del Giudice et al. 2012), which expectedly has profound implications for the phenotypic variation of personality disorders.

A personality *disorder* is characterized by inflexible and maladaptive cognitive, emotional, and behavioural patterns, which cause significant functional impairment or subjective distress. Patients with personality disorders have profound difficulties in self-perception and in relating to their (social) environment. Personality traits are perceived as 'ego-syntonic', which makes it sometimes difficult for patients with personality disorders to seek psychiatric help. Deviations can occur in the domain of cognition, affectivity, interpersonal functioning, and/or impulse control.

A personality disorder *is characterized by inflexible and maladaptive cognitive, emotional, and behavioural patterns, which cause significant functional impairment or subjective distress.*

Current nosological systems cluster personality disorders into three groups. Cluster A comprises personality disorders that appear 'eccentric'. Paranoid personality disorder (PPD) is characterized by distrust and suspiciousness; schizoid personality disorder (SPD) concerns a pattern of behaviour whereby the individual lacks the desire for close relationships and is detached from his or her social environment; schizotypal personality disorder (STPD) pertains to pervasive social and interpersonal deficits, magical thinking, odd thinking and speech, and eccentricity.

DSM-5 personality clusters embrace the 'eccentric', the 'dramatic', and the 'anxious' personality disorders.

Cluster B embraces the 'dramatic' disorders, that is, antisocial (APD), borderline (BPD), histrionic (HPD), and narcissistic (NPD) disorder. APD involves pervasive failure to follow social norms and moral rules, reckless behaviour, irresponsibility, and lack of remorse. BPD concerns a pattern of unstable interpersonal relationships, emotional instability, intense fear of abandonment, risk-taking behaviour, and impulsivity. Transient paranoid ideation or dissociative symptoms may occur. HPD is characterized by excessive attention-seeking and inappropriate sexually seductive or provocative behaviour. NPD involves the need for admiration and a sense of grandiosity, as well as lack of empathy.

Cluster C includes the 'anxious' disorders, which are termed avoidant (AVPD), dependent (DPD), and obsessive-compulsive (OCPD). People with AVPD are preoccupied with being criticized or rejected, are socially inhibited, and see themselves as socially inferior to others. DPD is characterized by a persistent need for being cared for, submissive behaviour, and avoidance of taking responsibility for oneself. OCPD concerns behaviours of preoccupation with orderliness, perfectionism, and control (American Psychiatric Association 2013).

In addition to the traditional clustering, DSM-5 proposes an alternative model for the classification of personality disorders. This model emphasizes that personality traits are continuous variables that differ from non-disordered states by degree, not qualitatively. Disturbances in self and interpersonal functioning are mandatory and refer to the dimensions 'identity' (experience of self as unique, with clear boundaries between self and others), 'self-direction' (ability to pursue short-term and life goals), 'empathy' (ability to take another's perspective, feelings of concern for others), and 'intimacy' (connectedness with others, need for closeness).

An alternative model to describe personality disorders concerns disturbances in self and interpersonal functioning in the dimensions 'identity' (experience of self as unique, with clear boundaries between self and others), 'self-direction' (ability to pursue short-term and life goals), 'empathy' (ability to take another's perspective, feelings of concern for others), and 'intimacy' (connectedness with others, need for closeness).

In addition, DSM-5 comprises five different personality disorder trait domains, analogous to the five personality dimensions, that is, 'negative affectivity' (vs. emotional stability or neuroticism), 'detachment' (vs. extraversion), 'antagonism' (vs. agreeableness), 'disinhibition' (vs. conscientiousness), and 'psychoticism' (vs. lucidity). These five trait domains comprise 25 trait facets. 'Negative affectivity' comprises the facets emotional lability, anxiousness, separation insecurity, submissiveness, and hostility. 'Detachment' concerns the facets withdrawal, intimacy avoidance, anhedonia, depressivity, suspiciousness, and restricted affectivity (the latter three facets can also be attributed to negative affectivity). 'Antagonism' refers to the facets manipulativeness, deceitfulness, grandiosity, attention-seeking, callousness, and hostility. 'Disinhibition' concerns irresponsibility, impulsivity, distractibility, risk-taking, and lack of perfectionism. 'Psychoticism' comprises the facets unusual beliefs and experiences, eccentricity, and cognitive and perceptual dysregulation (American Psychiatric Association 2013). This model does justice to observations that many individuals show personality traits of more than one personality disorder. Thus, if a person fulfils the criteria of more than one personality disorder, each should be diagnosed. However, the new model also allows diagnosing subthreshold personality disorders.

The new DSM-5 dimensional model of personality traits can be used to describe 'slow' and 'fast' life-history features. BPD comprises features of both 'fast' and 'slow' strategies.

19.2 **Epidemiology**

Personality disorders as a whole occur in 10–20 percent of the general population. A recent survey found prevalence rates of 5.7 percent for cluster A, 1.5 percent for cluster B, and 6.0 percent for cluster C personality disorders, with 9.1 percent for any personality disorder. However, due to classification problems and divergent approaches (e.g. categorical versus dimensional), all prevalence rates of personality disorders should be cautiously considered as relatively rough estimates (Grant et al. 2004). Usually, personality disorders manifest around adolescence or early adulthood.

Personality disorders as a whole occur in 10–20 percent of the general population. In psychiatric populations, the prevalence of comorbid personality disorders is much higher and may range around 50–60 percent.

In psychiatric populations, the prevalence of comorbid personality disorders is much higher and may range around 50–60 percent. Individual traits associated with personality disorders are even more prevalent in both the community and psychiatric populations.

Within cluster A, the prevalence of PPD is estimated at 0.5–2.5 percent in the general population, with figures for SPD and STPD being around 7.5 percent and 3 percent, respectively. PPD is perhaps slightly more common in women, whereas the opposite may be true for SPD and STPD.

Among cluster B personality disorders, the prevalence of APD is about 3 percent for males and 1 percent for females. By comparison, BPD affects about 1–2 percent of the general population. Women are two to three times as often diagnosed with BPD as men. In clinical populations, up to 15 percent of psychiatric patients are diagnosed with BPD, and in clinical samples with personality disorders, the majority (roughly 50 percent) may have BPD. The prevalence of HPD is estimated to be 2–3 percent, with figures around 10–15 percent in psychiatric in-patient samples. HPD is more often diagnosed in women. NPD has been found in less than 1 percent of the general population. Again, the prevalence rate of NPD is higher in clinical samples.

Cluster C personality disorders are considered to be most common. AVPD has been found in 2.5 percent of the general population. DPD is assumed to occur in 0.5–2.5 percent of the general population. OCPD is perhaps the most common cluster C personality disorder, with prevalence estimates of about 8 percent. AVPD and DPD are more often diagnosed in women.

19.3 **Genetic risk factors**

Research into the genetic contributions to different personality dimensions has shown that individuals from the same families resemble each other in the expression of extraversion, neuroticism, conscientiousness, agreeableness, and openness. This is attributed to similarities in genetic make-up (42–46 percent), rather than shared environment, the impact of which contributes a much smaller proportion (about 7 percent) to resemblance in personality (Bouchard 1994; Bouchard and Loehlin 2001).

Individuals from the same families resemble each other in the expression of extraversion, neuroticism, conscientiousness, agreeableness, and openness, which is attributed to similarities in genetic make-up (42–46 percent), rather than shared environment.

The largest contribution to the population variance of personality traits is, however, made by non-shared environmental variation (Plomin et al. 2005). With respect to temperamental factors, a polymorphism of the dopamine D4 receptor coding gene has been associated with 'novelty-seeking'. Fast metabolism of the catecholamines by the val/val allele of the COMT genotype has been found to be associated with 'sensation-seeking' in women but not men, whereas the slow metabolizing variant has been linked to 'harm avoidance' and 'neuroticism' in females (Lang et al. 2007). Similarly, a functional polymorphism of the serotonin

Different allelic variants of genes involved in regulating the dopamine turnover have been associated with the expression of 'novelty-seeking', 'sensation-seeking', and 'harm avoidance'.

transporter coding gene has been linked to the trait 'neuroticism' in some but not all studies.

Cluster A personality disorders have been found in relatives of patients with schizophrenia at elevated rates. It has therefore been suggested to incorporate PPD, SPD, and STPD in a broader concept of schizophrenia spectrum disorders. For example, STPD and schizophrenia share susceptibility loci on chromosomes 5q, 6p, 6q, 9q, 8p, and 10p. Moreover, the val/val allele of the COMT coding gene has been associated with schizotypy scores in males, and neuregulin-1, a gene locus suggested to be involved in the pathogenesis of schizophrenia, has been associated with a perceptual aberrance component in schizotypal adolescents.

Cluster A personality disorders probably share genetic susceptibility with schizophrenia.

APD is considerably heritable. First-degree relatives of males with APD are five times more likely to develop APD, and in relatives of females with APD the risk is even ten times higher compared to the general population. Moreover, if antisocial behaviour is indexed by criminality, adopted-away offspring of biological criminal fathers raised by non-criminal fathers has been found to be 20 percent, compared to roughly half of this figure in adoptees with no family history of criminal behaviour. The incidence of BPD among relatives of index cases is about 10 percent. There is now considerable evidence for an association of a low-activity variant of the MAO-A coding gene in cluster B personality disorders (Jacob et al. 2005). Conversely, there is no association between serotonin transporter polymorphisms and serotonin receptor 1B alleles with BPD (Amad et al. 2014). Data on heritability of HPD and NPD are sparse, except that there is evidence for a genetic influence on the personality trait 'extraversion', which may be overexpressed in HPD and NPD.

Cluster B personality disorders are highly heritable and have been associated with polymorphisms of the MAO coding gene.

Research into heritable or genetic aspects of cluster C personality disorders have been complicated by the fact that these disorders are often difficult to distinguish from anxiety or depression. For example, AVPD may be genetically related to anxiety disorders, and OCPD may overlap with OCD, but evidence for particular genetic associations is, at present, mixed. Polymorphisms of the promoter sequence of the serotonin transporter coding gene have been inconsistently linked with neuroticism and harm avoidance, both of which represent anxiety-related personality traits and are thus overrepresented in cluster C personality disorders (Sen et al. 2004), but not in all population studies (Umekage et al. 2003).

Cluster C personality disorders may be genetically related to axis-I anxiety disorders, but evidence in favour of this assumption is mixed.

19.4 **Environmental risk factors**

Young adulthood, low socio-economic status, and marital status other than being married have been identified as non-specific risk factors for personality disorders. More specifically, traumatic life experiences, including neglect and abuse during childhood, predispose to the development of personality disorders (Zanarini et al. 2000). Evidence for an association of personality disorder with childhood trauma and insecure attachment is empirically supported best for cluster A and cluster B disorders. In cluster C disorders, evidence for the assumption of a link between trauma, neglect, and abuse with the development of personality disorder is mixed, which is most likely due to the fact that cluster C personality disorders are often difficult to distinguish from anxiety disorders and depression (Lenzenweger et al. 2007).

Traumatic life experiences, including neglect and abuse during childhood, predispose to the development of personality disorders.

Within cluster A disorders, PPD is most strongly associated with sexual, physical, and emotional abuse in childhood.

Within cluster B, a large number of individuals with APD (estimated about 90 percent) have experienced prolonged periods of absence of the primary attachment figure, often in association with physical abuse or harsh discipline during childhood. In APD, separation from the caregiver is more often the result of divorce rather than death, antisocial behaviour in fathers, or neglect by emotionally unavailable mothers. Adults with APD often display unresolved or dismissive state of minds with respect to attachment, and a subset of individuals with APD tends to devalue attachment figures or experiences with primary caregivers. An estimated 70–80 percent of patients who later develop BPD (similar to individuals with dissociative disorders) have a history of early physical or sexual abuse, half of which have experienced trauma before age 7. Moreover, a significant proportion of patients with BPD report prolonged separation from their primary caregivers, and also more often than other clinical patients a history of emotional neglect (Goldberg et al. 1985; Bezirganian et al. 1993; Bierer et al. 2003).

A large number of individuals with APD (estimated about 90 percent) have experienced prolonged periods of absence of the primary attachment figure, often in association with physical abuse or harsh discipline during childhood. An estimated 70–80 percent of patients who later develop BPD (similar to individuals with dissociative disorders) have a history of early physical or sexual abuse, half of which have experienced trauma before age 7.

Environmental risk factors for cluster C disorders are probably similar to those associated with depression (see Chapter 10) and anxiety disorders coded on DSM-IV axis-I (see Chapter 11).

19.5 **Pathophysiological mechanisms**

Personality disorders are mainly conceptualized as consequences arising from adverse early experiences, including maltreatment, abuse, and neglect, as well as overprotection or otherwise poor parenting. Adverse childhood experiences are, however, not sufficient to produce any kind of personality disorder (Bouchard 1994). Nor is any one factor specific for personality disorders in general, or a particular type of personality disorder. For example, although childhood maltreatment is an important risk factor for cluster B personality disorders such as APD, most maltreated children do not become antisocial or delinquent. Rather, there is now increasing evidence for important

There is now increasing evidence for important gene–environment interactions involved in the development of personality disorders, including complex interplays between mothers' personality and children's temperament.

gene–environment interactions involved in the development of personality disorders, including complex interplays between mothers' personality and children's temperament (Clark et al. 2000). Overall, there is good evidence to suggest that early adversity leaves a neurobiological mark on the stress axis. For example, cortico-releasing factor has been found to be elevated in the CSF of individuals with a history of childhood trauma (Lee et al. 2005b).

Genes that are assumed to play a role in personality disorders are those that control the production, enzymatic degradation, and reuptake of the biogenic amines (dopamine, norepinephrine, and serotonin), the polymorphic variations of which have, however, statistically small effect sizes. In addition, genes involved in the regulation of attachment and stress regulation seem to play a role in personality disorders, but perhaps in opposite directions for males and females (Cicchetti et al. 2014).

Cluster A personality disorders are perhaps genetically similar to the schizophrenia spectrum. The role of early neglect and abuse has recently regained attention, but gene–environment interactions are poorly understood.

A low-activity variant of MAO-A has been linked to cluster B personality disorders and to several of their behavioural correlates, such as aggressiveness, antisocial behaviour, suicidal behaviour impulsivity, and hostility, as well as comorbid disorders such as drug dependence (Jacob et al. 2005). Conversely, a high-activity variant has been associated with anxiety disorders. The low-activity variant of MAO-A has only been found predictive for APD, if associated with childhood maltreatment, whereas low activity of this enzyme in the absence of maltreatment does not predict antisocial behaviour later in life (Caspi et al. 2002).

These interactions are, however, far from being completely understood. Low activity of MAO-A leads to elevated levels of dopamine, norepinephrine, and serotonin, yet increased aggression has also been associated with low levels of serotonin in the brain. Polymorphisms of the serotonin transporter gene that differ in repeat length in the transcriptional control region regulate expression and reuptake of serotonin. The 'short' allele variant results in lower transcriptional activity and thus reduced serotonergic transmission. This variant has repeatedly been linked to violent behaviour in homozygous carriers, whereas homozygosity for the 'long' variant exerts protective effects against aggressiveness. Similar to MAO-A polymorphisms, the negative effect of the short allele of the serotonin transporter gene was only present in association with adverse events during childhood, whereas the negative behavioural effect was absent when early rearing conditions were more favourable (van Ijzendoorn et al. 2012).

Cluster A personality disorders are perhaps genetically similar to the schizophrenia spectrum. The role of early neglect and abuse has recently regained attention, but gene–environment interactions are poorly understood.

A low-activity variant of MAO-A has been linked to cluster B personality disorders and to several of their behavioural correlates, such as aggressiveness, antisocial behaviour, suicidal behaviour, impulsivity, and hostility, as well as comorbid disorders such as drug dependence. Polymorphic variation of the MAO-A and serotonin transporter genes mediate emotional responsivity to stress and may therefore be associated with different behavioural outcomes, including susceptibility to depression, anxiety, and aggression.

Thus, gene expression in the brain critically depends on environmental input in differential ways. It seems that polymorphic variation of the MAO-A and serotonin transporter genes mediate emotional responsivity to stress and may therefore be associated with different behavioural outcomes, including susceptibility to depression, anxiety, and aggression (Bennett et al. 2002; Canli and Lesch 2007; Stein et al. 2008; for more details see Chapter 1). Moreover, callous–unemotional personality traits may be linked to methylation of the oxytocin receptor gene, but more so in individuals with low levels of internalizing problems, whereas in people with high levels of internalizing problems, prenatal factors, such as partner violence, are more relevant than oxytocin gene receptor methylation (Cecil et al. 2014).

A number of brain imaging studies have revealed structural abnormalities in personality disorders. Cluster A disorders, mainly schizotypy, are associated with reduced grey matter volume in frontotemporal areas and smaller volumes of striatal structures (Koo et al. 2006). Overall, these abnormalities support the assumption of a continuum of cluster A personality disorders with schizophrenia.

Cluster A disorders, mainly schizotypy, are associated with loss of grey matter in frontotemporal areas and smaller volumes of striatal structures (similar to schizophrenia). In cluster B personality disorders, imaging studies suggest amygdalar–orbitofrontal dysconnectivity. The pathophysiology of cluster C personality disorders may be similar to that observed in depression and anxiety disorders.

In cluster B personality disorders, imaging studies suggest that a small number of patients with APD have lesions to the OFC ('acquired sociopathy'). Primary APD is associated with abnormal fearlessness, as indicated by absent autonomic responses to fear conditioning (Blair 2001; Dolan and Park 2002). Patients with APD also have shown abnormal response inhibition and executive planning deficits, suggesting increased impulsivity, which may be modulated by reduced serotonin availability in the ACC.

There is, however, growing evidence that different pathways can lead to antisocial behaviour. For example, while early adversity and hyperactivity of the HPA axis may predispose to antisocial behaviour in the absence of callous–unemotional traits in children, hypoactivity of the HPA axis in conjunction with high levels of callousness may produce antisocial behaviour in the absence of early adversity (Hawes et al. 2009). With regard to BPD, there is evidence for amygdalar–orbitofrontal dysconnectivity, as well as increased grey matter volume in the amygdala bilaterally, but reduced in the hippocampal formation and ACC, perhaps as the result of chronic stress early in life (Driessen et al. 2000; Minzenberg et al. 2008; New et al. 2007), and abnormal reward processing (Völlm et al. 2004, 2007). These functional and anatomical deviations from a statistical norm could explain patients' difficulties in emotion regulation, particularly in response to aversive stimuli, and problems in appreciating own and others' mental states, whereby an evolutionary approach does not necessarily render such deviant brain structures as pathological (see section 19.6).

With regard to the influence of gene–environment correlation on the expression of BPD traits, evidence suggests that childhood sexual abuse alone is a strong predictor of BPD, whereas other adverse events interact more with the genetic load. Notably, the genetic make-up of an individual with BPD features also predicts the likelihood of experiencing adversity, suggesting a two-way interaction of genotype and phenotype (Distel et al. 2011).

The pathophysiology of cluster C personality disorders may be similar to that observed in depression and anxiety disorders (see Chapters 10 and 11), suggesting dimensional rather than categorical differences.

19.6 **Evolutionary synthesis**

Personality traits reflect pervasive, individual-specific behavioural strategies that serve the purpose to achieve major biosocial goals, which include the need to elicit care from others, to provide care for others, to secure one's social status, to form coalition and friendships, and to find a suitable mate (see Chapter 1). The set of theoretical behavioural strategies an individual has at hand to accomplish biosocial goals can be divided along the following lines, which, however, considerably overlap: dominance versus submission; competition versus cooperation; dependence versus nurturance; assertion versus avoidance; aggression versus defence; and risk-taking versus harm avoidance.

Personality traits reflect pervasive, individual-specific behavioural strategies that serve the purpose to achieve major biosocial goals, which include the need to elicit care from others, to provide care for others, to secure one's social status, to form coalition and friendships, and to find a suitable mate.

These behavioural strategies are paralleled by adaptive cognitive and emotional biases, which guide the individual's perception and information processing, for instance, with regard to the response to reward or punishment expectations (Carver and White 1994). Individuals, for example, who engage in risk-taking behaviours, tend to not perceive defensive emotions such as fear and sadness; nor do they show heightened vigilance to potential threats. Instead, they may display increased levels of anger and impulsivity, empathize less with others, and show signs of self-aggrandisement (Lerner and Keltner 2001). Contrariwise, individuals who aim at reducing the risk of being harmed will display heightened attention towards possible cues of threat and inhibit aggressive responses. They may also tend to derogate themselves and assume submissive postures. None of these strategies is necessarily pathological, but rather part of the normal within-species variation of primates and humans. In fact, the main human personality dimensions can be found in non-human primates in almost identical ways (Clarke and Boinski 1995; Lilienfeld et al. 1999; Gosling 2001; Gosling et al. 2003; Capitanio 2004), including great apes (Uher and Asendorpf 2008; Uher 2008), as well as across human cultures, whereby intracultural differences exceed intercultural differences (Poortinga and van Hemert 2001).

Personality *disorders* are conceptualized as extremes of normal variation of strategies, which are pursued in a rigid, inflexible, or excessive way. The classification of behaviour as a 'disorder' critically depends on the presence of maladaptive consequences of the behaviour (here the term 'maladaptive' is used in its common sense, not its evolutionary meaning; Beck 1999). Maladaptiveness of behaviour may be accentuated if an important biosocial goal is thwarted, forcing the individual to try harder to achieve that goal, however, using an inappropriate strategy, which may eventually cause a vicious circle.

Personality disorders *are conceptualized as extremes of normal variation of strategies, which are pursued in a rigid, inflexible, or excessive way.*

Maladaptiveness of behaviour may be accentuated if an important biosocial goal is thwarted, forcing the individual to try harder to achieve that goal, however, using an inappropriate strategy, which may eventually cause a vicious circle.

The actual strategy an individual chooses (unconsciously) as part of a more enduring type of personality (as opposed to situational behavioural responses) depends on several other intimately linked factors, which include genetic predispositions, rearing conditions, and socialization throughout childhood and adolescence. Although some personality traits are probably more closely linked to certain genetic predispositions than others, early experiences during infancy and childhood are critical in shaping an individual's expectations and predictions about future resource availability.

These predictions, in turn, lead to different behavioural strategies in terms of interpersonal orientation, such as trust versus mistrust in interpersonal relationships, and attempts to immediately extract resources versus the ability to tolerate delay of reward. For example, a person who has experienced poor parental care and neglect or abuse during childhood will be more likely to develop a mistrustful attitude towards interpersonal relationships, and therefore value short-term gains more than long-term benefits, because these specific early environmental conditions may have primed the individual to expect unstable conditions in the future, in which long-term investment in relationships does not pay off. Put another way, individuals who have formed negative expectations about future resources tend to pursue 'fast' life-history strategies (Belsky et al. 1991; Ellis et al. 2011a; Del Giudice 2014). Predictably, such behavioural dispositions have profound consequences on how an individual will interact with peers, partners, colleagues, and kin (Feeney and Collins 2001; see also Chapter 3).

Early experiences during infancy and childhood are critical in shaping an individual's expectations and predictions about future resource availability. These predictions lead to different behavioural strategies in terms of interpersonal orientation, referred to as life-history strategies. Individual genetics play a role in that allelic variation interacts with early experiences during infancy and childhood in complex ways.

Individual genetics play a role in that allelic variation interacts with early experiences during infancy and childhood in complex ways. Evidence suggests that cluster B personality disorders are associated with certain allele variations of catecholamine-depleting enzymes, but that these genetic peculiarities only phenotypically manifest as antisocial behaviour in the presence of adverse environmental conditions such as neglect and abuse during childhood (Caspi et al. 2002). In other words, neither the genetic endowment nor environmental conditions alone 'determine' the development of personality or personality disorder (Bouchard and Loehlin 2001). Such complex gene–environment correlation and interaction are probably similarly true for cluster A and cluster C personality disorders, but are less well researched to date.

In a general vein, cluster A disorders are characterized by low-risk strategies and heightened vigilance towards possible threats from the social environment, suggestive of a 'slow' life-history strategy (Del Giudice 2014). Individuals with cluster A personality disorders tend to perceive their social environment as untrustworthy and unpredictable, and a number of patients with cluster A personality disorders may have experienced abuse or neglect. In contrast to persons with cluster B disorders, however, patients with SPD, STPD, and PPD choose defensive behavioural strategies and usually avoid direct confrontation, with the exception that

Cluster A disorders are characterized by low-risk strategies and heightened vigilance towards possible threats from the social environment. Individuals with cluster A personality disorders tend to perceive their social environment as untrustworthy and unpredictable, and a number of patients with cluster A personality disorders may have experienced abuse or neglect.

aggressive outbursts may occur. Patients with cluster A personality disorders rather try to maintain autonomy by distancing themselves from others, at the expense of reduced intimacy and reciprocity.

By contrast, cluster B personality disorders can be conceived of as high-risk strategies (i.e. a 'fast' life-history pattern) to maximize the likelihood to attain important biosocial goals. Evolutionary life-history theory (for further details see Chapter 3) predicts that individuals with low future expectations engage more in risky behaviours compared to individuals with high future expectations. APD, for example, represents a strategy that aims at maximum short-term resource extraction with little investment in reciprocal relationships. Cheating and interpersonal manipulation are part of the antisocial phenotype, which is also associated with a lack of experiencing social emotions such as love, shame, guilt, and empathy (Troisi 2005). As children, individuals with APD have frequently experienced emotional neglect, violence, or other forms of abuse, as well as loss of a parent through desertion, divorce, or separation. As outlined in section 19.5, those with low MAO-A activity or reduced serotonin turnover mediated by a short serotonin transporter allele may be particularly at risk of developing APD, if combined with adverse early childhood experiences.

Cluster B personality disorders can be conceived of as high-risk strategies (i.e. a 'fast' life-history pattern) to maximize the likelihood to attain important biosocial goals by means of deception and interpersonal manipulation. In contrast to APD, BPD is more strongly linked with internalizing problems, which may explain its high comorbidity with depression and anxiety disorders.

Similarly, BPD often develops on the basis of adverse early childhood experiences and low MAO-A activity (Pally 2002). BPD is associated with a history of ambivalent or resistant attachment style and a preoccupied state of mind with regard to important relationships. In contrast to APD, BPD is more strongly linked with internalizing problems, which may explain its high comorbidity with depression and anxiety disorders. Patients with BPD aim at eliciting maximum nurturance and care from their primary caregiver or from surrogate attachment figures, and sometimes enforce help and support by using self-injurious behaviours or temper tantrums. Traumatized patients with BPD tend to disregard their own and others' mental states, especially when emotionally aroused, which may happen in situations associated with impending retraumatization or traumatic memories (flashbacks; see Chapter 17). Similar to behaviours observed in patients with eating disorders, self-injury and emotional tantrums can be seen as threats to the inclusive fitness of the patient's parents.

A possible ultimate explanation is that human life-history patterns are such that, on a timescale, care for individual offspring is extremely expanded. Hence, self-imposed threat to the physical existence by offspring is perhaps the strongest signal on the side of the offspring to increase parental care and nurturance. On the other hand, a subset of patients with BPD may prematurely engage in short-term sexual relationships, which supports the assumption that a behavioural tendency towards immediate resource extraction exists as a result of reduced future fitness expectations (i.e. akin to a 'fast' life-history strategy).

Similar to behaviours observed in patients with eating disorders, self-injury and emotional tantrums in BPD can be seen as threats to the inclusive fitness of the patient's parents.

Thus APD and BPD share several features, including certain genetic polymorphisms, a possible history of abuse, and inadequate parenting, including the use of harsh reinforcement of discipline. On the other hand, dismissive states of mind occur more often in disorders that involve turning away attention from one's feelings (such as APD), whereas preoccupied states of mind are more often associated with disorders in which the individual is absorbed by his or her own feelings (anxiety, depression, BPD). These tendencies to externalize or internalize problems may reflect evolved sex differences in behaviour and personality traits (Del Giudice et al. 2012), which account for differences in prevalence of APD and BPD in men and women. In other words, similar gene–environment correlations may phenotypically manifest as APD in men and as BPD in women (Paris 1997, 2004).

NPD and HPD are less well understood, but, similar to APD and BPD, they seem to be characterized by a lack of reciprocity. Instead, patients with NPD display exaggerated competitive behaviour associated with self-aggrandisement, whereas HPD typically involves exaggerated courtship behaviour, which at times appears manneristic.

Disorders of cluster C are in some respects similar to cluster A disorders in that both make use of defensive strategies. During childhood, threats of loss of an attachment figure and instability of attachment are frequently associated with separation anxiety. Thus, in contrast to cluster A, cluster C personality disorders tend to increase help provided by significant others (DPD), to gain control through ritualization and anticipation of future threats (OCPD), or to avoid interaction despite the wish to socialize with others (AVPD). Although manipulation of others' behaviour is commonly conceptualized as part of cluster B disorders, patients with cluster C disorders (especially those with DPD) may also unconsciously act in manipulative ways to increase help and nurturance from others.

Cluster C personality disorders tend to increase help provided by significant others (DPD), to gain control through ritualization and anticipation of future threats (OCPD), and to avoid interaction despite the wish to socialize with others (AVPD). Although manipulation of others' behaviour is commonly conceptualized as part of cluster B disorders, patients with cluster C disorders (especially those with DPD) may also unconsciously act in manipulative ways to increase help and nurturance from others.

This is particularly interesting from a population-genetic point of view, because the success of a particular strategy critically depends on its frequency in a population. There is usually more than one strategy to accomplish a certain biosocial goal, for example, getting social support or tightening the bonds between mates, and an individual may have the option to choose between alternatives. If alternative behavioural strategies are not equally successful in terms of reproductive fitness consequences, one may regard the less successful strategy as an attempt to 'make the best of a bad job'. Depression or anxiety-associated submissive strategies may fall into this category.

In general, the fitness consequences associated with a strategy normally increase as its frequency in the population declines, and this may well apply to personality traits and extremes of variation of personality traits. For example, antisocial behaviour, which can be seen as exploitative strategy at the cost of other individuals, can only be maintained in a population at low frequency (Mealey 1995). If the frequency of genes associated with antisocial behaviour increases, because antisocial behaviour conveys a reproductive advantage, it no longer will be associated with greater fitness in a human population depending on mutual aid and reciprocity. Genetics and prevalence rates of APD are consistent with the assumption of frequency-dependent selection.

Moreover, the model also explains sex differences in expression of antisocial traits. Evolutionary theory suggests that the variance in reproductive capacity is greater in males compared to females due to the differential parental investment in potential offspring (see Chapter 1). Therefore males are more vulnerable to environmental contingencies during early childhood, which to some degree canalize the individual life-history strategy (see Chapter 3). Conversely, the genetic 'load' that is necessary to phenotypically express antisocial behaviour must be greater in females, which is consistent with the observation that first-degree relatives of antisocial women have a tenfold increased risk of developing APD relative to the general population, compared to a fivefold increased risk in relatives of men with APD.

A similar case can probably be made for other behavioural strategies in which exploitation and deception play a role. These behavioural strategies are usually outside conscious awareness, and individuals use self-deceptive strategies (i.e. repression of selfish motives; see Chapters 14 and 22) to enhance deception of others. For example, patients with cluster B personality disorders may be particularly vulnerable to developing depression and depressive adjustment disorders or to committing suicide attempts if their high-risk strategies fail. Similarly, chronic depression (dysthymia) may sometimes reflect a strategy that aims at maximizing help and support from others.

Display of helplessness and 'regressive' behaviours are probably among the strongest signals to elicit supportive behaviours in others, particularly in close kin, but also in medical professionals.

Display of helplessness and 'regressive' behaviours are probably among the strongest signals to elicit supportive behaviours in others, particularly in close kin, but also in medical professionals. In the developed countries, and at an increasing rate in developing countries, depression may actually be the most successful strategy to achieve biosocial goals that otherwise seem unattainable. In light of the rising number of depressed people worldwide, unveiling the hidden goals behind the clinical phenotype of depression, and finding appropriate therapeutic options for the divergent motivational conflicts associated with depression and personality disorders in general, may be among the most pressing tasks of psychiatrists in the near future.

All this suggests that, phenotypically, personality disorders represent life-history strategies that differ vastly in terms of 'slow' and 'fast' features. Specifically, the new DSM-5 dimensional model of personality traits can be used to describe 'slow' and 'fast' life-history features. For example, among the 25 trait facets, emotional lability, intimacy avoidance, anhedonia, suspiciousness, restricted affectivity, manipulativeness, deceitfulness, grandiosity, attention-seeking, callousness, hostility, irresponsibility, impulsivity, distractibility, risk-taking, and lack of perfectionism can be attributed to a 'fast' life-history strategy, whereas anxiousness, submissiveness, and depressivity are more typical of 'slow' life-history strategies (see Chapter 3).

In fact, many personality disorders seem to follow a specific life-history pattern, with both 'fast' and 'slow' components (Brüne 2014a). For example, key features of BPD concern emotion dysregulation, impulsivity, and risk-taking behaviour, which can be conceptualized as behavioural expression of high-stress responsivity. High-stress responsivity typically promotes a fast life-history strategy in dangerous and unpredictable contexts, by increasing vigilance to threat and downregulating sensitivity to social feedback (Boyce and Ellis 2005). Consistent with this interpretation, early adversity is associated with persistent changes of stress responsivity, possibly via epigenetic mechanisms (Murgatroyd et al. 2009), and alterations of the HPA axis in BPD correlate with symptom severity and a history of childhood trauma (Carvalho Fernando et al. 2012).

Along similar lines, patients with BPD display heightened vigilance or avoidant reactions to fear and anger (Jovev et al. 2012; Brüne et al. 2013). At the same time, patients with BPD have difficulties in reflecting upon own and others' emotions, whereby alexithymia seems to correlate with stress intolerance and impulsivity (Gaher et al. 2013). In further support of the view that BPD concerns a pathological variant of a 'fast' life-history strategy, patients with BPD are poor in tolerating delay of gratification, that is, they prefer immediate (lower) gains over (higher) future monetary gratification (Völker et al. 2009).

Moreover, life-history theory predicts that a 'fast' life-history strategy is associated with extraversion, openness to experience, and neuroticism (Del Giudice 2012), which correlate with promiscuous behaviour, risk-taking, and disruptive behaviour in both humans (Del Giudice 2014) and non-human primates (Wolf et al. 2007). Indeed, patients with BPD seem to score higher on novelty-seeking and lower on cooperativeness compared to non-clinical and clinical controls (Fossati et al. 2001). Studies using neuro-economic paradigms have revealed that patients with BPD have lower trust in others and cooperate less with other players (King-Casas et al. 2008), and that oxytocin exerts trust-lowering effects (Bartz et al. 2011; Ebert et al. 2013), which may support the idea of a prevailing 'fast' life-history strategy in BPD.

Neuroimaging findings in BPD suggest that early adversity, rather than producing brain lesions, may prepare an individual's neurobiology to cope with future adversity. Seen this way, it becomes plausible why childhood maltreatment is associated with reductions in the volume of limbic areas (e.g. Dannlowski et al. 2012; Teicher et al. 2012) and the corpus callosum (Teicher et al. 2003), and why impulsivity in BPD is associated with alterations in blood flow in frontal cortical regions (Wolf et al. 2012). Put another way, early adversity may elicit 'a cascade of stress responses that organizes the brain to develop along a specific pathway selected to facilitate reproductive success and survival in a world of deprivation and strife' (Teicher et al. 2003).

Neuroimaging findings in BPD suggest that early adversity, rather than producing brain lesions, may prepare an individual's neurobiology to cope with future adversity. Accordingly, it becomes plausible why childhood maltreatment is associated with reductions in the volume of limbic areas.

While a 'fast' life-history strategy is prevailing in BPD, the condition is also associated with traits following a 'slow' pattern, which may, to some degree, reflect (dysfunctional) coping strategies (Brüne 2014a). This could relate to the fact that risky strategies yield large gains in the case of success, but may incur enormous costs in the case of failure (Del Giudice 2014). Accordingly, BPD is associated with several defence mechanisms, partly related to efforts to avoid (feelings of) abandonment (American Psychiatric Association, 2013).

With regard to personality traits, patients with BPD score highly on harm avoidance (Fossati et al. 2001) and low on extraversion (Wischniewski and Brüne 2013). Many also have the tendency to invalidate themselves, which may underlie feelings of emptiness and self-disgust. Indeed, self-disgust in BPD is linked to the severity of traumatizing experiences (Rüsch et al. 2011). Seen through the lens of life-history theory, this could make sense, because insensitivity to disgust may bear the risk of contracting sexually transmitted diseases (Del Giudice 2014), all the more as many patients engage in promiscuous behaviour. Following this line of reasoning, feelings of disgust would be a clear sign of a 'slow' life-history strategy. This view is also supported by evidence from ethological studies. For example, when analysing patients' facial expressions during therapeutic interaction, Benecke and Dammann (2004) found that BPD patients displayed high amounts of anger, contempt, and disgust. Similar findings emerged in another study in BPD during an attachment-related task, revealing traumatization by attachment figures (Buchheim et al. 2007).

Life history theory also explains the non-genetical transgenerational transmission of personality traits. As regards BPD, there is evidence to suggest that insensitive and invalidating parenting and poor emotional availability, or even frightening behaviour on the side of parents when interacting with their children, profoundly influence children's inner working models, and may hence inadvertently promote the development of insecure attachment and emotional dysregulation (Stepp et al. 2012).

Life-history theory explains the non-genetical transgenerational transmission of personality traits. As regards BPD, there is evidence to suggest that insensitive and invalidating parenting and poor emotional availability, or even frightening behaviour on the side of parents, may promote the development of insecure attachment and emotional dysregulation.

Taken together, personality disorders comprise behavioural phenotypes that can be differentiated according to their prevailing patterns, reflecting divergent life-history strategies. An important message from an evolutionary point of view is that even neurobiological findings do not necessarily reflect 'defects', but may be seen as part of a preparatory 'strategy' that is gauged according to (early) environmental contingencies, from which predictions are made in regard to future resource availability. These insights may have profound implications for psychotherapy (see Chapter 22).

19.7 **Differential diagnosis and comorbidity**

Personality disorders frequently co-occur with one another. Up to 40 percent of patients fulfil the criteria of more than one personality disorder. Within cluster A personality disorders the main axis-I differential diagnosis is psychosis. PPD may sometimes be difficult to distinguish from APD. SPD and STPD share many features, but SPD lacks the bizarre perceptual, behavioural, and communicative characteristics of STPD. SPD may overlap with AVPD; however, the latter usually wish to engage in social interaction, which is untypical for SPD. Cluster B personality disorders often occur comorbidly with substance abuse. APD may overlap with the broader concept of 'psychopathy'. Individuals with psychopathy, however, do not necessarily have APD and may function well (Hare 1996).

Personality disorders frequently co-occur with one another. Up to 40 percent of patients fulfil the criteria of more than one personality disorder. Cluster B personality disorders often occur comorbidly with substance abuse. A subset of patients with BPD may have chronic PTSD, especially those with a history of childhood sexual abuse.

BPD may be associated with psychotic-like features, but lacks 'first rank' symptoms. BPD is often associated with recurrent depression. A substantial number of patients with BPD have features of PTSD. It has been claimed that a subset of patients with BPD may in fact have chronic PTSD, especially those with a history of childhood sexual abuse. APD and BPD may also be more prevalent in adults with persistent ADHD. HPD may be difficult to differentiate from BPD. HPD is believed to be more prevalent in patients with somatization disorder.

Cluster C disorders largely overlap with anxiety disorders traditionally encoded on axis-I. DPD is relatively non-specific and may also occur at increased prevalence rates in patients with substance abuse and depression. AVPD and social anxiety disorder have been suggested to lie on a continuum, such that the validity of differential encoding on separate axes has been questioned. A similar case has been made for OCPD in relation to OCD.

19.8 **Course and outcome**

Most personality disorders are chronic, and psychosocial functioning may be impaired lifelong. Cluster A disorders mainly remain stable over time or develop into schizophrenia. About 10 percent of patients with STPD commit suicide. Personality disorders of cluster B are generally difficult to treat, though symptom severity may decline with increasing age. Suicidal behaviour is present in many patients with BPD, especially if combined with high levels of novelty-seeking, impulsivity, and hostility. About 1 in 10 patients with BPD eventually dies from suicide. It seems that those with aggressive–impulsive features are particularly at risk of committing suicide, whereas harm avoidance seems to protect from severe suicidal behaviour in this group (McGirr et al. 2007). Moreover, cluster B disorders are associated with elevated risk of fatal car accidents, probably reflecting increased risk-taking behaviour in these patients.

Most personality disorders are chronic, and psychosocial functioning may be impaired lifelong. The risk of committing suicide is increased in all clusters.

Patients with cluster C disorders may function quite well in protected environments, unless a failure of the social support system occurs. Suicidal ideation may be quite prevalent in cluster C disorders, but the actual risk of suicide is only increased in DPD, but not

AVPD or OCPD (Chioqueta and Stiles 2004; Krysinska et al. 2006). Co-occurrence of personality disorders from different clusters seems to be associated with an elevated risk for suicide (Schneider et al. 2006).

19.9 **Treatment**

Symptomatic pharmacological treatment may include the administration of SSRI in patients with affective dysregulation, irritability, or poor impulse control. Cognitive–perceptual symptoms may be treated with low-dose second-generation antipsychotics, but psychotropic medication is generally less helpful to treat specific symptoms aside from comorbidities.

Instead, patients with personality disorders usually need extended psychotherapy to achieve improvement in social functioning and interpersonal relationships. In severe cases, adjunct pharmacotherapy may be warranted to reduce affective instability, impulsivity, self-injurious behaviour, and suicidality. Several psychotherapeutic approaches are available, and the choice of psychotherapy may depend on individual preferences and availability of therapy. Psychodynamic therapy (PDT), CBT, and dialectic behavioural therapy (DBT) are currently most widely used for treatment of personality disorders. In particular, the efficacy of DBT has been established in BPD (Linehan 1993), though transference-focused therapy and other psychodynamic therapies have also proven useful (Bateman and Fonagy 2004, 2006; Stone 2006).

Patients with personality disorders usually need extended psychotherapy to achieve improvement in social functioning and interpersonal relationships. In severe cases, adjunct pharmacotherapy may be warranted to reduce affective instability, impulsivity, self-injurious behaviour, and suicidality.

Regardless of the choice of a specific psychotherapeutic 'school', psychotherapists may want to consider evaluating which biosocial goals are being thwarted in the patient's experience, and what the patient's non-verbal behaviour tells about his or her unconscious motives to seek therapeutic help. In addition, it might be helpful to encourage patients to appreciate their own and others' mental states (mentalization-based treatment), depending on the extent to which a secure base can be established in therapy (Bateman and Fonagy 2004). Moreover, transgenerational transmission of borderline personality traits can be ameliorated by indicated preventive measures for mothers with BPD (Stepp et al. 2011).

Detailed treatment guidelines are available for BPD published by the APA, and for lay persons by the RCP.

Part III

Special topics

Chapter 20

Suicidal and self-injurious behaviour

Abstract

Suicidal behaviour is defined as a conscious, intentional act that aims at terminating one's life. Parasuicidal or deliberate self-injurious behaviour usually has no terminal intent. Self-injurious behaviour may be appellative or ambivalently motivated. Suicidal behaviour expresses the desire to reduce emotional pain or anger directed towards self or others. Moreover, abnormal perception and interpretation of one's own situation may be causally related to suicidal behaviour. Thus, suicidal behaviour or suicide attempt usually have a communicative meaning. Childhood adversity and psychiatric disorders increase the risk for suicidal behaviour, possibly by destabilizing stress-coping abilities through gene methylation. Moreover, genes involved in serotonin turnover seem to have a specific role in suicidal behaviour. Non-verbal behaviour of suicidal individuals, particularly signs of motivational ambivalence, is an important source of information with regard to the estimation of suicide risk.

Keywords

suicide, parasuicidal behaviour, emotional pain, anger, communicative meaning, stress-coping mechanisms, serotonin, non-verbal behaviour

20.1 Introductory remarks to suicidal and self-injurious behaviour

Suicidal behaviour is defined as a conscious, intentional act that aims at terminating one's life. DSM-5 lists 'Suicidal Behaviour Disorder' among the conditions for further study (American Psychiatric Association 2013). This category does not include suicidal ideation, or preparatory acts. The behaviour must not be carried out in a state of delirium or confusion, and not undertaken for political or religious reason. Attempted suicide is common in patients with psychiatric disorders, and may also occur in individuals with physical health problems.

Suicidal behaviour is defined as a conscious, intentional act that aims at terminating one's life. Suicide, even when completed, is not without meaning. Suicidal ideation is often triggered by feelings of hopelessness or social isolation.

Suicide, even when completed, is not without meaning. Suicidal ideation is often triggered by feelings of hopelessness or social isolation. Individuals who commit suicide have usually indicated their wish to die, either directly or indirectly prior to the suicide attempt. Persons who undertake suicide attempts usually go through the stages of contemplating suicidal ideas as a possibility to terminate intense suffering, which is followed by a period of ambivalence and narrowing of perceived alternative options, before a final decision is made. Suicide attempts with terminal intent can be classified as desperate or impulsive. In a minority of cases, suicide is altruistically motivated, and such behaviour may not necessarily be associated with psychopathology.

In contrast to suicidal behaviour, parasuicidal or deliberate self-injurious behaviour usually has no terminal intent. Self-injurious behaviour may be appellative or ambivalently motivated. It often conveys more overtly than suicidal behaviour the unconscious wish to punish oneself or a person with whom the affected individual has had a close, though conflict-laden, relationship. Non-suicidal self-injury may also be motivated by the wish to get relief from negative feelings, whereby the desired state is achieved immediately or shortly after the self-injurious act (American Psychiatric Association 2013).

People who show parasuicidal behaviour are usually younger, more often female, choose 'soft' methods of committing suicide more frequently, and act out interpersonal conflict more overtly compared to people who commit suicide attempts with terminal intent.

People who show parasuicidal behaviour are usually younger, more often female, choose 'soft' methods of attempting suicide more frequently, and act out interpersonal conflict more overtly compared to people who commit suicide attempts with terminal intent. However, parasuicidal and suicidal behaviour form a continuum and cannot reliably be distinguished as 'potentially harmful' or 'harmless'. On the contrary, repeated self-injury increases the risk that individuals become practised and accustomed regarding suicide and may eventually lose fear and engage in increasingly dangerous self-harm.

20.2 **Epidemiology**

The WHO estimated that in 2001 about 850,000 people world-wide died from suicide. Extrapolation of this figure suggests that in the year 2020, 1.2 million people will die from suicide. Thus, in developed countries more people die from suicide than from car accidents.

Suicide rates vary with ethnicity and social background. The average suicide rate in Europe figures around 25 per 100,000 people, with pockets of higher rates in Hungary, and lower rates in southern Europe and the USA. Suicide is the third leading cause of death in young adults and among the ten leading causes in the developed countries.

Suicide rates vary with ethnicity and social background. The average suicide rate in Europe figures around 25 per 100,000 people, with pockets of higher rates in Hungary, and lower rates in southern Europe and the USA. The suicide risk is higher in persons with high social status, but a recent fall in social status also increases the risk of suicide. Suicide is the third leading cause of death in young adults, and among the ten leading causes in the developed countries. In the developed countries, the suicide rate in adolescents and young adults has increased over the past couple of decades.

Specifically, cross-cultural research indicates that in Asian populations the suicide rate has a first peak around age 20, with rates of about 50 per 100,000 people. In men, suicide rates peak after age 45, whereas in women the rate peaks after 55 years of age. In western societies, men commit suicide at least three times more often than women, and more often choose 'hard' methods such as hanging and shooting, compared to 'soft' methods such as taking an overdose of psychoactive drugs or a poison. Contrariwise, the rate of attempted suicide is about four times higher in women. However, in Asian populations suicide is at least equally common in females, and occurs in some peoples of Papua New Guinea even exclusively in women.

The incidence of parasuicidal behaviour is probably 10–20 times as high as the rate of suicide attempt with terminal intent.

The incidence of parasuicidal behaviour is probably 10–20 times as high as is the rate of suicide attempt with terminal intent. Overall, self-injurious behaviour is common in psychiatric patients with personality disorders and patients with substance dependence. Repetitive cutting occurs about 50 times more often in psychiatric patients compared to the general population.

20.3 **Genetic risk factors**

Twin and family studies suggest that genetic factors are involved in the transmission of suicide risk. The concordance rate for death by suicide is between 10 and 20 percent in MZ twins compared to less than 1 percent in DZ twins. The concordance rate for attempted suicide is somewhat higher in both MZ and DZ twins, and the estimated genetic effects lie within the range of that associated with environmental factors. The genetic risk factors for suicide are not merely associated with the genetic risk for psychiatric disorders in which suicide is common; rather, there is apparently an independent genetic component that contributes to suicide.

The genetic risk for suicide is independent of genetic factors for psychiatric disorders. Genes regulating serotonin turnover have been associated with the risk for suicidal behaviour.

Allelic variation of genes that regulate the serotonin turnover have been identified to play a role in suicidal and self-injurious behaviour, but also in impulsive aggressiveness. The short allele of the serotonin transporter gene on chromosome 17q has repeatedly been shown to convey increased risk for suicidal behaviour compared to the long variant. Moreover, a polymorphism of the tryptophan hydroxylase (TPH) coding gene on chromosome 11q has been associated with increased suicide risk. Studies linking suicide with polymorphic variation of the COMT coding gene have revealed mixed results, with some evidence for an association of low COMT activity with violent suicide in men, but not women. Moreover, an allelic variation of a gene involved in neurogenesis (called 14-3-3 epsilon) was recently found upregulated in the amygdala of suicide victims (Yanagi et al. 2005).

20.4 **Environmental risk factors**

Factors that increase the risk for suicide include aggression and violence towards others, impulsiveness, feelings of hopelessness, shame and humiliation, agitation, anhedonia, chronic insomnia, panic attacks, and specifically previous suicide attempts (Zahl and Hawton 2004; Joiner et al. 2005). Childhood trauma, sexual abuse, recent traumatic experiences, marital discord, divorce, and adoption also convey an increased risk of suicide, suicide attempts, or self-injurious behaviour (Glover et al. 1995; Dube et al. 2001; Slap et al. 2001; Roy et al. 2007). Neglectful parenting seems to increase the life-time suicide risk especially in females (Ehnvall et al. 2008).

Factors that elevate the risk for suicide include aggression towards others, negative affect, traumatic experiences, psychopathology, and previous suicide attempts.

Age is a risk factor for suicidal behaviour, but probably mediated by psychosocial features such as lack of social support, poor relationship with family, widowhood, and cognitive characteristics such as reduced executive functioning and loss of physical health. Moreover, rigid cognitive style, dichotomous thinking, impulsivity, and a change of time perspective may contribute to an elevated suicide risk in older people.

The presence of a psychiatric disorder is probably the most significant risk factor for suicidal behaviour. In particular, adolescent men (but not women) who committed suicide or severe suicide attempts had psychiatric problems at age 8 (Sourander et al. 2009). About 90 percent of completed suicides are associated with a diagnosable disorder at the time of death. The risk for successful suicide is particularly increased in patients with affective disorders, substance dependence, schizophrenia, cluster B personality disorders, and PTSD (Hills et al. 2005; Krysinska et al. 2006; Schneider et al. 2006; Krysinska and Lester 2010). Life-time suicide rates for depression, bipolar affective disorder, alcohol dependence, and schizophrenia have been estimated around 10–20 percent, and a substantially larger number of patients with these disorders attempt suicide. In BPD, 50 percent of patients make at least one severe suicide attempt, and many undertake repeated suicide attempts or deliberately injure themselves. Impulsivity, emotional dysregulation, and aggression also convey elevated suicide risk in APD (Krysinska et al. 2006).

Self-injurious behaviour is often associated with the diagnosis of BPD, dissociative symptoms, and depression (Glover et al. 1995; Osuch et al. 1999), but boundaries with suicidal behaviour are shaky.

20.5 Pathophysiological mechanisms

One of the most robust findings in suicidal behaviour and self-injurious behaviour is a reduction in 5-HIAA in the CSF of both suicide attempters and suicide completers. 5-HIAA is one of the major metabolites of serotonin. The reduction of 5-HIAA seems to be specific, as the metabolites of the other monoamines (homovanillin acid (HVA) and 4-hydroxy-3-methoxyphenyl glycol (MHPG)) are not reduced in the CSF of suicidal individuals. There is some evidence that the level of 5-HIAA correlates inversely with the lethality of the suicide attempt and with the level of impulsivity (Kamali et al. 2001; Joiner et al. 2005).

5-HIAA, one of the major metabolites of serotonin, has consistently been found to be reduced in the CFS of suicide attempters and completers. Individuals with a history of childhood trauma, which represents an important risk factor for later suicidal behaviour alone, are at a greater suicide risk if they are carriers of a 'slow' variant of the serotonin transporter.

Similarly, suicidal behaviour has been linked to two genetic polymorphisms of the TPH coding gene (called A218C and A779C), both of which are believed to be associated with slower serotonin synthesis.

Fenfluramine challenge studies in suicidal patients have shown an attenuated prolactin response compared to non-suicidal subjects. Fenfluramine stimulates serotonin release and inhibits reuptake, which can indirectly be measured by levels of prolactin. Suicide attempters who chose 'hard' methods had a more blunted prolactin response compared to 'soft' method attempters. This reduced fenfluramine-induced prolactin response has also been demonstrated in patients with elevated impulsivity and aggression.

Recent research has revealed that a polymorphism of the serotonin transporter coding gene is involved in depression, suicidal ideation, and suicide attempts if associated with adverse early childhood experiences. Subjects who experienced childhood trauma, which represents an important risk factor for later suicidal behaviour alone, were shown to be at an even greater suicide risk if they were carriers of a 'slow' variant of the serotonin transporter (Roy et al. 2007).

Interestingly, individuals with low cholesterol blood levels are also at greater risk of committing suicide and violent crimes (Golomb et al. 2000; Coryell 2006). Smith–Lemli–Opitz syndrome is associated with a mutation in a gene involved in cholesterol metabolism, leading to a reduced cholesterol synthesis. Carriers of this mutation have a much greater risk for suicide, self-injurious behaviour, and aggression compared to controls (Lalovic et al. 2004). There is a close link between peripheral cholesterol levels and CSF levels of 5-HIAA, which suggests that the actual suicide risk is mediated by a reduced serotonin turnover rather than by cholesterol itself (Buydens-Branchey et al. 2000; Hillbrand et al. 2000). Conversely, upregulation of genes involved in neurogenesis, such as 14-3-3 epsilon, may reflect a compensatory reaction to stress-induced decreased serotonergic neurotransmission.

Extremely low cholesterol levels and dysregulation of the HPA axis have also been linked with an increased risk for suicidal behaviour.

Dysregulation of the HPA stress axis may also contribute to the pathophysiology of suicidal behaviour. A hyperactive HPA axis is characterized by non-suppression of cortisol in response to the administration of dexamethasone. Although the evidence for an association of a hyperactive HPA axis and suicidal behaviour is mixed, non-response to the dexamethasone suppression test (DST) is apparently more common in suicidal patients, and an abnormal DST may even have predictive value of suicidal behaviour later in life (Coryell and Schlesser 2001).

20.6 **Evolutionary synthesis**

Suicide, parasuicide, and self-injury are complex behaviours, which involve a broad array of psychological mechanisms and occur under numerous diverse circumstances. Suicidal behaviour and self-injury are not categorically distinct, but continuous traits associated with various degrees of ambivalence towards one's death and lethality of the behaviour (Jones and Daniels 1996).

In the majority of cases, suicidal and self-injurious behaviours are causally linked to life events, which may (unconsciously) reactivate traumatic experiences that happened in the past. Infancy and childhood are certainly vulnerable periods of life, during which the ground for the ability to cope with interpersonal conflict is laid. Thus, suicide—whether completed, attempted, or just contemplated as a possible way to end feelings of hopelessness, humiliation, and suffering—is not without meaning. In many cases, suicidal behaviour expresses the desire to reduce emotional pain or anger directed towards self or others (Joiner et al. 2005). In other cases, abnormal perception and interpretation of one's own situation may be causally related to suicidal behaviour, for example, when a patient with psychotic depression falsely assumes that he has ruined his family. Only a few suicide attempts result from taking stock of one's life perspective.

In the majority of cases, suicidal and self-injurious behaviours are causally linked to life events, which may (unconsciously) reactivate traumatic experiences that happened in the past.

Assessment of a person's suicide risk, either before or after a suicide attempt has taken place, is one of the most difficult tasks for clinicians. It is widely agreed upon that suicide assessment scales have low predictive value and do not provide a reliable estimate of individual suicidality. One possible explanation for the poor reliability of suicide assessment scales could be that patients with persistent suicidal intent might try to conceal their real intentions from the interviewer and tell him/her 'what he/she wants to hear'. In other words, a patient's verbal report may or may not reflect what is going on in the patient's mind.

Suicide assessment scales have low predictive value and do not provide a reliable estimate of individual suicidality. Therefore careful behavioural observation should become an integral part of every psychiatric examination of suicidality.

In contrast to spoken information, non-verbal behaviour can much less be brought under conscious control. For example, a patient may deny further suicidal intent, but the experienced clinician may recognize a great deal of fidgety movements, frequent change of body posture, or avoidance of eye contact, which may alarm the clinician to continue assessment and to seek third-party information from family members or friends. The use of non-verbal behaviour in establishing a diagnosis has probably received much less attention than it deserves. However, the frequency of displacement activities suggestive of motivational conflict, such as between fight and flight, may substantially aid the clinician's judgement of a patient's level of suicidality (Troisi 2002). Thus, careful behavioural observation should become an integral part of every psychiatric examination of suicidality (see Chapter 5).

Establishing a therapeutic alliance between therapist and patient is, of course, of the essence in the assessment of suicidal or self-injurious behaviour. This can, however, be extremely difficult to achieve in interaction with patients with a history of recent or past traumatization. Individuals with a history of childhood abuse or neglect are not only at an increased risk for suicide and parasuicidal behaviour later in life, but also vulnerable to acquire insecure attachment styles. Thus, many early-traumatized persons have developed mistrustful inner working models and see the world as a dangerous place in which others cannot be trusted. Individuals with a history of traumatization have therefore difficulties in acknowledging that the clinician wants to offer help to escape the situation that has led to the suicidal behaviour.

Suicidal behaviour and deliberate self-harm may be the consequence of an individual's wish to terminate his or her life, or may be motivated by feelings of revenge. Instead of harming significant others, a person may turn his or her aggression against the self (which is, in ethological terms, referred to as 'redirected activity').

Individuals with a history of traumatization may have difficulties in acknowledging that the clinician wants to offer them help to escape the situation that has led to suicidal behaviour.

At the neurophysiological level, suicidal or parasuicidal behaviour is often paralleled by altered serotonin turnover (Kamali et al. 2001). Decrease in serotonin availability is associated with heightened levels of aggression, impulsivity, and risk-taking behaviour, as well as suicidal behaviour and self-harm. Modulatory activity of serotonin on behaviour is complex and critically depends on gene–environment interaction. Individuals with less-efficient genetic variants involved in enzymatic degradation or synaptic re-uptake of serotonin display elevated levels of aggression towards self and others only if associated with adverse childhood experiences, such as emotional neglect or abuse (Roy et al. 2007). By contrast, carriers of alleles, which are associated with greater serotonin efficiency, seem to be protected from developing aggressive tendencies, even if they have grown up under unfavourable circumstances. In other words, polymorphisms involved in regulating monoamine turnover are part of the normal variation within populations and—under average environmental circumstances, that is, absence of severe adverse events during early childhood—selectively neutral (hence, there is no 'gene for suicidality'), even though different alleles convey subtle individual differences in stress responsivity. That is, early adversity may actually destabilize stress-coping mechanisms through dysregulation of the HPA axis via methylation and inflammatory processes (Preti 2011; Turecki 2014).

Carriers of alleles, which are associated with greater serotonin efficiency, seem to be protected from developing aggressive tendencies, even if they have grown up under unfavourable circumstances.

Serotonin turnover is, however, not only mediated by 'fixed' interindividual genetic variation, but contingent upon an individual's social status and success. Research in various monkey species, for example, has shown that chronic social stress leads to a reduction in serotonin availability in the PFC (Barr et al. 2004). Moreover, social dominance is associated with elevated serotonin levels compared to subordinate individuals, whereas experimentally induced loss of dominant status is accompanied by a fall in serotonin. Interestingly, dominance has been found to be distinct from aggression. Dominant primates usually engage more in prosocial interaction and behave less aggressively towards subordinates, whereas individuals who experienced a recent loss in social rank are more aggressive. Aggression can also be induced experimentally by feeding a low-cholesterol diet. Monkeys fed a low-cholesterol diet not only behave more aggressively, but also have lower 5-HIAA CSF levels compared to monkeys fed a high-cholesterol diet (Kaplan et al. 1994). This makes sense in an evolutionary perspective, because low serotonin may increase an individual's food-seeking behaviour and willingness to take greater risks (Allman 1999).

In terms of suicidal or self-injurious behaviour, it is therefore conceivable that some persons who experience or perceive a loss of social status may turn their aggression towards themselves, especially in situations associated with feelings of shame and humiliation.

In a more general vein, however, an evolutionary perspective on suicidal behaviour suggests that the intent to terminate one's life runs counter to the biological imperative to maximize one's fitness. At first sight, suicide maximally reduces an individual's fitness. However, when looking at inclusive fitness as the extended fitness of the individual and its kin, there may be situations in which suicide may convey a net fitness increase, especially when one's own reproductive potential is estimated to be low (De Catanzaro 1995).

One such theoretical model identifies perceived burdensomeness towards kin as a risk factor for altruistically motivated suicidal behaviour. There is considerable evidence that suicide attempts with a high risk of lethal outcome are sometimes motivated by the desire to make others better off (Joiner et al. 2002). 'Hard' suicide attempts differ in that respect from 'soft' suicide attempts, even though the degree of hopelessness and emotional pain do not differ between suicide completers and attempters, as far as the content of suicide notes is concerned. These findings support the view that even completed suicides may have interpersonal motives. It needs to be emphasized that humans are by no means 'fitness maximizers' in that they consciously calculate potentially selective advantages over alternative strategies (see Chapter 1). Nor does the evolutionary perspective suggest that suicidal behaviour has been selected. However, humans are by nature social beings, and emotional attachment towards kin can be such a powerful bond that in some circumstances self-sacrifice is a behavioural option (Ribeiro and Joiner 2009).

Humans are by nature social beings, and emotional attachment toward kin can be such a powerful bond that in some circumstances self-sacrifice is a behavioural option.

Even less frequently observed is suicide as a means of third-party punishment. Humans have evolved social rules and norms that have been critical throughout human evolution to maintain group cohesion and cooperation between genetically unrelated individuals within a social group. Human societies are generally intolerant against violations of social rules and moral principles, such that individuals—contrary to any logic—are willing to punish cheating behaviour even if the punishing act incurs costs to the punisher. This behaviour, referred to as 'altruistic punishment', may in extreme cases include the willingness to sacrifice one's life for the better of the group. Kamikaze fighters and suicide bombers are examples of completed suicide as a function of altruistic punishment (Atran 2003; Townsend 2007).

These scenarios occur usually outside any clinical context. Parasuicide or self-harm, by contrast, are frequently encountered in clinical and emergency settings. Similar to completed suicide, there may be manifold reasons for poisoning, overdose, or cutting, but one particular message that may be conveyed by suicide attempts and self-injurious behaviour is threat to the inclusive fitness of close kin. Self-injury is often seen in patients with BPD, which is characterized by emotional dysregulation and unstable interpersonal relationships. Patients with BPD either overidealize or derogate relationships. In times of perceived or actual rejection, patients with BPD may turn to drastic reinforcement of another's commitment (often close kin) by overtly threatening their own lives, and, hence, the inclusive fitness of close ones (Hagen et al. 2008). Such 'dramatic' behaviour pays off in species with long dependence of the offspring on parental care. Thus, temper tantrums are part of the behavioural repertoire of all primate species, and self-harm and parasuicide can be seen as an extension to the extreme of behaviours oriented towards close kin to increase nurturance and care (Taylor et al. 2011; see Chapter 19). A similar motivation may, in some cases, lie behind anorexic behaviour (see Chapter 15). Such a scenario can certainly be transmitted to therapeutic relationships, and therapeutic work may be necessary to unveil the unconscious motivation behind self-injurious behaviour.

Patients with BPD either overidealize or derogate relationships. In times of perceived or actual rejection, patients with BPD may turn to drastic reinforcement of another's commitment (often close kin) by overtly threatening their own lives.

Sex differences in evolved psychological mechanisms may explain the greater propensity of men to engage in externalizing behaviours (and perhaps greater prevalence of 'hard' suicide attempts, partly depending on the availability of violent means), and the internalizing behaviour in women, which may contribute to the larger prevalence of 'soft' suicide attempts without terminal intent.

20.7 **Course and outcome**

Individuals who previously attempted suicide have an elevated life-time risk of dying from suicide of up to 30 percent. Repetitive deliberate self-harm increases the risk for suicide considerably (Zahl and Hawton 2004). After 1 year, the risk of dying from suicide is 0.5–2 percent, and over 5 percent at follow-up after 9 years. Thus, suicide risk among individuals with repetitive parasuicidal behaviour is several hundreds of times higher than in the general population.

Suicide risk among individuals with repetitive parasuicidal behaviour is several hundreds of times higher than in the general population.

Protective factors against suicide comprise positive social support, children in the household, life satisfaction, good problem-solving skills, and a positive therapeutic relationship.

20.8 **Treatment**

The most important treatment goal is, of course, secondary prevention of further suicidal behaviour in patients who have committed suicide attempts. Equally important is primary prevention of suicide in people who are at risk of committing suicide attempts. Suicide prevention includes the reduction of access to the means to commit suicide, such as detoxification of domestic gas, car exhaust, availability of pesticides, and weapons. In several countries, suicide prevention programmes have consistently shown that the number of completed suicides can effectively be reduced by implementation of specialized hotlines and primary care centres, as well as by antisuicide campaigns designed to inform the public about the significance of the problem.

Careful evaluation of individual suicide risk must include asking the patients about suicidal ideation, suicide intent, and lethality of plan. It is compulsory to ask for past suicide attempts, self-injurious behaviour, and family history of suicidal behaviour. Hospitalization may not always be required, but is usually essential if the patient is acutely suicidal, has carried out violent suicide attempts, regrets surviving, is agitated or psychotic, or lacks social support. Assessment of comorbidity is essential (Chioqueta and Stiles 2004; Coryell 2006; Schneider et al. 2006). Careful repetition of suicide assessment is necessary, and a treatment plan should be established (Zahl and Hawton 2004). The evolutionary perspective suggests that it may be advisable that the clinician judiciously asks the patient who could potentially benefit from the patient's death (evaluation of feelings of burdensomeness or otherwise altruistically motivated suicide).

Suicide prevention programmes can effectively reduce the number of completed suicides by implementation of specialized hotlines and primary care centres, as well as by antisuicide campaigns designed to inform the public about the significance of the problem.

Detailed information on how to assess suicidal patients is available via the home-pages of the APA and RANZCP.

Afterthought: the puzzle of altruistic suicide

Lethal forms of self-sacrifice, including ritualized forms of self-killing, and suicide for altruistic reasons, such as kamikaze or, more recently, suicide bombing, are poorly understood in terms of their underlying motivation and biology. What brings people—mainly young individuals with hopes, desires, emotions, and compassion to others—to the point of sacrificing their lives? From a purely biological perspective, terminating one's life at an age when an individual's reproductive potential peaks runs counter to the laws of natural and sexual selection. Or doesn't it?

Insight is provided by evolutionary game theory. Evolutionary game theory proposes that *Homo sapiens* has evolved psychological mechanisms to deal with cooperation between genetically unrelated individuals, which includes rules of reciprocal exchange (Trivers 1971). If such a mechanism regulating reciprocality is to be positively selected and evolutionarily stable, because it increases the average individual reproductive fitness within a social group, the mechanism must entail the ability to detect and censure non-cooperative strategies to keep the proportion of 'free-riding' morphs within the group at a low rate (Trivers 1971; Mealey 1995).

One particular mechanism involved in reinforcing social norms that has intensely been researched in recent years is called 'altruistic punishment'. The most extraordinary thing about altruistic punishment is that it does not follow any *prima facie* rational logic. Altruistic punishment benefits the group rather than the individual, a fact that at first sight is counterintuitive to modern evolutionary theory, which emphasizes the role of inclusive fitness. Instead, by definition, altruistic punishment incurs costs to the punisher, for whom the prospects of ever receiving anything in return are at best dubious (Fehr and Fischbacher 2004a, 2004b; Fehr and Rockenbach 2004). Kamikaze fighters and suicide bombers, from this perspective, pursue an extreme form of an altruistic punishment strategy by (apparently) deliberately taking the risk of never being given credit or reciprocated, thus bearing enormous costs (Atran 2003).

Altruistically motivated self-killing as an extreme of variation of altruistic punishment, however, is not only puzzling for its extreme costs to the punisher; it also yields several issues that have been disregarded in standard evolutionary game theory research to date. First, the rules of *who* decides over what, or who deserves altruistic punishment by whatever means, are pre-established in standard experimental evolutionary game theory protocols. For example, classic evolutionary game theory implicitly holds that there is consensus from 'moral standards' within the social group over which behaviour ought to be punished, and which should not. In the case of suicide bombing, however, no such consensus exists. On the contrary, the decision over what and who is to be punished is made by a minority; in other words, the decision to punish or not to punish is not shared by the majority of either group. Nor are the means generally accepted. Altruistic punishment by terrorist acts almost always affects innocent people, and one may argue that such atrocity is intended to increase the 'moral' pressure on the targeted party.

Second, in statistical terms, findings reported from evolutionary game theory studies have mainly been based on mean group effect size, whereas individual differences in performance on evolutionary game theory tasks have been underresearched. This, however, may be the most intriguing part of future evolutionary game theory research agendas. For example, individuals who themselves are highly cooperative or altruistic may have different attitudes or motives towards punishing free-riders, compared to persons who are less dependent on the cooperation of others. With regard to altruists who kill themselves, one may speculate that those who actually carry out the assault are prone to obey social rules and norms, whereas those behind the scene, who decide whom to punish and who the 'chosen' perpetrator of the suicide attack is, are perhaps less cooperative and altruistic than they want to be believed they are. In line with this speculation, Merai et al. (2009) reported that 'would-be' Palestinian suicide terrorists (individuals whose suicide attack had failed) had lower levels of ego-strength, a more dependent and avoidant personality style, or more impulsive and emotionally unstable personalities compared to non-suicide terrorists. On the other hand, suicide attackers may not be suicidal at all, but, as argued earlier, driven by other motives (Townsend 2007).

Third, a problem that makes altruistic self-killing an unusual case of altruistic punishment is that the aim of altruistic punishment is somewhat unclear to the punished party (or perhaps to both the punisher and the punished). In ordinary in-group altruistic punishment scenarios it is implicitly assumed that reinforcement of social norms and rules of exchange is the target of altruistic punishment. In the case of kamikaze and suicide bombing no such universally accepted between-group 'moral' basis seems to exist, such that the prevailing answers to terrorist threats are dominated by pre-emption or deterrence (Arce and Sandler 2005).

These issues notwithstanding, insights from evolutionary game theory may contribute to developing scenarios for possible solutions to terrorism. Biologically speaking, it cannot be in the interest of either conflict party—let alone individual perpetrators—to waste large amounts of human and non-human resources. Furthermore, evolutionary game theory suggests that cooperation pays off over extended periods of time rather than mutual defection. A lesson to learn from evolutionary psychology of human behaviour might be that the most optimistic answer to the problem of mutual defection is to find a common basis of moral standards and to reduce an individual's interest in self-sacrifice. However, the make-up of human psychology sets the benchmarks to succeed in such an endeavour: mutual acceptance of needs, respect, and trust; a scenario—inconceivable as it may be for many—that is supported by recent evolutionary game theory approaches (Keet 2003).

These days, we have witnessed an outbreak of suicide bombing attacks. Suicide bombing has become 'fashionable' because of its horrific impact on thousands of innocent victims, and because of its uncontrollability. There is certainly no excuse for such atrocities. From a psychiatrist's point of view, however, one may ask whether or not those who commit suicide attacks do so on the basis of free decision-making, or because they are psychologically dependent, manipulated, and promised a better 'life'. Here, the vagueness of boundaries between rational and delusional belief evaluation may be all too obvious. Moreover, PTSD is likely to occur on all sides: the victims' families and the perpetrator's families, as well as all those people who accidentally witness the killings.

Chapter 21

Forensic aspects of psychiatric disorders

Abstract

Forensic psychiatry involves the role of the psychiatrist as expert witness, or court-mandated evaluations of patients' mental states or witnesses' credibility. Forensic psychiatry also deals with questions of responsibility, treatment of psychiatrically ill offenders, and prediction of dangerousness of delinquents. Aggressive delinquency of patients with psychosis is about five times higher compared to the general population. Conversely, the risk for individuals with schizophrenia to become a victim of violence is several times higher than that of committing a violent crime. While aggression is part of human nature, mediated, in part, by the interaction of genes and childhood experiences, there is no reason for exculpation of delinquency based on the fact that criminal behaviour has also a biological dimension. Criminal offences often concern decisions based on one's life-history strategy or evolved psychological mechanisms gone awry, including partner violence (homicide, sexual assault, stalking), paraphilic disorders, and infanticide.

Keywords

forensic psychiatry, responsibility, aggression, life-history strategy, partner violence, paraphilic disorders, infanticide

21.1 Introductory remarks to forensic aspects of psychiatric disorders

Forensic psychiatry is the branch of psychiatry that deals with questions pertaining to the interface of law and psychiatry. In its broader meaning, forensic psychiatry embraces problems relating to patients' involuntary hospitalization, or confidentiality psychiatrists may sometimes be obliged to breach, especially in cases of suspected child abuse or intended homicide by clients. More narrowly defined, forensic psychiatry involves the role of the psychiatrist as a witness of fact or expert witness, or it may concern court-mandated evaluations of patients'

Forensic psychiatry is the branch of psychiatry that deals with questions pertaining to the interface of law and psychiatry. Narrowly defined, forensic psychiatry involves the role of the psychiatrist as witness of fact and expert witness, and court-mandated evaluations of patients' mental states or witnesses' credibility.

mental states or witnesses' credibility. Court-mandated evaluations include patients' competency to stand trial and patients' mental state at the time of the offence. Practitioners of forensic psychiatry usually have received special training in this area, but regulations differ from country to country.

Forensic psychiatrists are also involved in the treatment of mentally ill offenders, as well as in prevention and prediction of patients' future dangerousness. Prognostic evaluation of future delinquency is certainly one of the most difficult tasks of forensic psychiatry.

Forensic psychiatrists are also involved in the treatment of mentally ill offenders, as well as in prevention and prediction of patients' future dangerousness.

The role of the forensic psychiatrist in criminal law is to examine whether an individual can be found not guilty of committing an offence by reason of insanity (note that 'insanity' is a legal not a medical term). It is implicitly assumed that adults are morally responsible for and have control over what they are doing. This premise is based on the proposition of a 'free will' or, better, of the ability to make conscious decisions on future behaviour for which an individual has full responsibility (see Afterthought to this chapter). Both psychiatry and the law are aware of the vague definition of 'free will' and therefore use a 'pragmatic' definition of responsibility and guilt in the juridical sense. Accordingly, it is believed that severe psychiatric disorders can cause an impaired sense of justice and an inability to follow socially accepted rules of conduct. Moreover, cognitive and emotional disorders may impair an individual's decision-making, by poor impulse control, defective reasoning, or poor insight.

Both psychiatry and the law are aware of the vague definition of 'free will', and therefore use a 'pragmatic' definition of responsibility and guilt in the juridical sense.

Exculpation for reasons of insanity can be justified in severely psychotic patients or patients with mental retardation. Deculpation (diminished responsibility) is an option in some countries where the law does not prescribe to strictly dichotomize between exculpation and full responsibility. One of the most controversially debated issues, however, is the expert opinion regarding offences carried out by people with personality disorders. Reasons for exculpation can usually not be assumed, but, as stated, in some countries the law allows deculpation on the basis of severe impairment of impulse control, extreme emotional distress, or dissociative states of consciousness at the time of the criminal deed.

Aside from homicide or suicide–homicide, sexually motivated criminal acts are among the most relevant in forensic psychiatric contexts. For example, paraphilic disorders are frequently associated with forensic consequences. DSM-5 lists among the Paraphilic Disorders the following: Voyeuristic Disorder (sexual arousal when observing others in privacy), Exhibitionistic Disorder (exposing one's genitals), Frotteurism (sexual arousal when touching or rubbing against another non-consenting person), Sexual Masochism (sexual arousal associated with one's own humiliation), Sexual Sadism Disorder (sexual arousal associated with someone else's humiliation), Paedophilic Disorder (sexual focus on prepubertal children), Fetishistic

Aside from homicide or suicide–homicide, sexually motivated criminal acts are among the most relevant in forensic psychiatric contexts.

Disorder (sexual arousal from non-living objects), and Transvestism (sexual arousal from cross-dressing) (American Psychiatric Association 2013).

21.2 **Epidemiology**

Aggressive delinquency of patients with psychosis is about five times higher compared to the general population, with quite large regional differences depending on patients' social environment and provision of individual case management. Schizophrenia patients with sexual delusions (delusional jealousy or erotomania) tend to commit more often aggressive offences compared with non-delusional patients. However, in light of the average prevalence rate of schizophrenia of about 1 percent in the general population, the risk of becoming a victim of an aggressive schizophrenic patient is about 20 times lower than that of being attacked by a non-psychotic criminal. Moreover, the risk for individuals with schizophrenia to become a victim of violence has been estimated to be several times higher than that to commit a violent crime (Walsh et al. 2002).

In spite of the elevated risk for violent behaviour in schizophrenia, the risk of becoming a victim of a schizophrenic patient is about 20 times lower than that of being attacked by a non-psychotic criminal. In general, the risk of violent behaviour is increased particularly in those patients with psychotic disorders who have comorbid substance abuse or a history of antisocial behaviour since childhood.

Individuals with affective disorders are also at an increased risk of delinquent behaviour. Patients with mania, for example, although less likely than schizophrenic patients to commit capital crimes such as manslaughter, are at risk of perpetrating sexual harassment. Patients with psychotic depression may sometimes attempt homicide–suicide and may be charged with manslaughter after successful homicide, yet failed suicide. In general, the risk of violent behaviour is increased particularly in those patients with psychotic disorders who have comorbid substance abuse or a history of antisocial behaviour since childhood (Eronen et al. 1998).

Alcohol and substance abuse is highly prevalent among individuals who commit violent crimes. Differences in prevalence rates exist depending on the nature of the violent act, cultural background, and availability of psychotropic substances.

Personality disorders are extremely prevalent among inmates. Specifically, APD has been found in up to 90 percent of prisoners. PPD may occasionally lead to aggression against the perceived persecutor. On the other hand, the diagnosis of personality disorder must not lead to criminalization of these individuals.

APD has been found in up to 90 percent of prisoners. Sexually deviant behaviour in delinquents, especially paedophilia, is often associated with personality disorders, mental retardation, or substance abuse.

The prevalence of paraphilic disorders is generally considered to be low, although exact rates are missing for most paraphilic disorders. While most paraphilic disorders seem to decline in frequency with increasing age, paedophilia is deemed a lifelong disorder. Sexually deviant behaviour in delinquents, especially paedophilia, is often associated with personality disorders, mental retardation, and substance abuse. These and other sexually motivated offences, such as sexual coercion, rape, sexually motivated homicide, and child sexual abuse, are particularly prevalent among patients who are treated in high-security hospitals for mentally ill. Prognostication of the risk for re-offences is a particularly sensitive issue, and release of patients from mental hospitals is highly disparaged in public opinion.

In general, sex differences in the propensity to commit violent crimes are profound. Inmate populations are on average 80 percent or more male. Among those who commit capital crimes, the sex ratio in favour of males is even larger. Similar discrepancies in prevalence of violence can be found between males and females with psychiatric disorders, which may, in part, reflect differences in prevalence between the sexes regarding substance abuse and APD.

Sex differences in the propensity to commit violent crimes are profound, with inmate populations being on average 80 percent or more male. Similar figures are found in forensic psychiatric populations.

21.3 **Genetic risk factors**

Much of what can be said of genes predisposing to violence has already been summarized in the respective sections of the chapters on personality disorders and suicidal behaviour (see Chapters 19 and 20). In particular, polymorphic variation of the serotonin transporter gene on chromosome 17q seems to be associated with both increased risk for suicidal behaviour and violent aggression. Moreover, individuals with low cholesterol levels tend to be more aggressive than individuals with higher cholesterol levels (Golomb et al. 2000; Hillbrand et al. 2000; extremely low cholesterol levels are associated with Smith–Lemli–Opitz syndrome. Carriers of the genetic abnormality have a several times greater risk for committing suicide or violent offences (Lalovic et al. 2004)). The risk of violent behaviour associated with chromosomal abnormalities such as in XYY males is usually overestimated. However, theoretically, male individuals with an extra Y chromosome may be more likely to behave aggressively because of an excess production of testosterone. It is well known that elevated levels of testosterone are associated with increased aggression, but the effect is small and clearly depends on social factors such as social status.

Polymorphic variation of the serotonin transporter gene on chromosome 17q is associated with violent aggression. The risk of violent behaviour associated with chromosomal abnormalities such as in XYY males is usually overestimated.

21.4 **Environmental risk factors**

John Bowlby's pioneering work with delinquent juveniles in the 1940s can be regarded as one of the first studies to provide evidence that harmful early rearing conditions, above all poor parental care and neglect, can have long-lasting negative effects on behaviour later in life (Bowlby 1944). In other words, adverse early experiences can profoundly impair an individual's sensitivity to social rules and norms. Among individuals with APD, a large proportion have been separated from attachment figures at an early developmental age, and many have as children experienced physical abuse (Lang et al. 2002). Maternal depression and antisocial traits in fathers seem to be independent risk factors for conduct disorder in children, as well as for later delinquency (Kim-Cohen et al. 2005). Conduct disorder itself has been shown to be a risk factor for delinquent behaviour later in life, independent of the presence or absence of ADHD symptoms.

Adverse early experiences can profoundly impair an individual's sensitivity to social rules and norms. Among individuals with APD, a large proportion have been separated from attachment figures at an early developmental age, and many have as children experienced physical abuse.

Recent research has confirmed the hypothesis that among inmates (regardless of whether or not suffering from mental illness) the prevalence of a history of childhood maltreatment is considerably higher than in the general population, with sexual abuse figuring as high as around 60 percent in male prisoners. Moreover, a considerable number of delinquents fulfil partial or full criteria for PTSD (Ruchkin et al. 2001, 2002).

Among inmates (regardless whether or not suffering from mental illness) the prevalence of a history of childhood maltreatment is considerably higher than in the general population, with sexual abuse figuring as high as around 60 percent in male prisoners. Moreover, a considerable number of delinquents fulfil partial or full criteria for PTSD.

Other risk factors for delinquent behaviour include poor academic performance, deviant peer relationships, impoverished neighbourhoods with high levels of crime, and the availability of psychotropic drugs (Herrenkohl et al. 2000).

21.5 **Pathophysiological mechanisms**

Aggression is part of human nature, just as reconciliation and cooperation are. Testosterone, substance P, and norepinephrine increase aggression, whereas oestrogen, serotonin, and oxytocin reduce aggressive tendencies. With regard to human (pathological) behaviour, interaction between genetic variants associated with low serotonin availability and adverse experiences during early childhood have been shown to reliably predict aggression, antisocial behaviour, and substance abuse later in life (Caspi et al. 2002; Reif et al. 2007). Genes involved in serotonin turnover include the MAO-A and the serotonin transporter coding gene. Serotonin deficiency in the brain, for example, causes poor inhibitory control and emotional lability.

Testosterone, substance P, and norepinephrine increase aggression, whereas oestrogen, serotonin, and oxytocin reduce aggressive tendencies. Interaction between genetic variants associated with low serotonin availability and adverse experiences during early childhood have been shown to reliably predict aggression, antisocial behaviour, and substance abuse later in life.

Gene–early environment interaction producing serotonin-mediated cognitive and emotional dysfunction may have particularly long-lasting effects if striking the developing organism. Animal models suggest that separation of animals from their parents at an early developmental age can alter the expression of serotonin and dopamine receptors, particularly in brain regions involved in emotion regulation and motivated behaviour, and that social isolation may exert persistent effects on amygdalar–prefrontal connectivity. Although at this stage fairly speculative, anatomical *in vivo* findings of volume reductions in the right amygdala, bilateral hypothalamus, septal regions, and striae terminalis in paedophilic offenders, as well as findings that childhood emotional and/or sexual abuse and family dysfunction comprise risk factors for sexual offending later in life, clearly suggest that similar gene–environment interactions may be present in humans (Lee et al. 2002b).

In a more general vein, damage to the PFC has repeatedly been shown to be associated with violent behaviour. For example, the ventromedial part of the orbitofrontal cortex (VMOFC) appears to be essentially involved in the appreciation of moral rules and norms. Individuals with a record of criminal behaviour display reduced neuronal activity in frontotemporal regions. Strikingly, individuals with damage to the VMOFC, while being capable of reasoning about rule violations, are unable to act upon their knowledge, presumably because they are unable to attach emotional valence to social interaction (i.e. to empathize with others; Dolan 1999). Again, this seems to be, in part, an age-specific effect, because effects on behaviour are the more profound the earlier the traumatic injury of the VMOFC occurred in an individual's life-time.

Damage to the PFC has repeatedly been shown to be associated with violent behaviour.

The OFC and parts of the ACC have also been found to be underactive in psychopathic individuals, specifically males, during performance of tasks requiring cooperation, and when processing negative emotions such as fear and sadness (Blair 2001; Sommer et al. 2006). Moreover, structural abnormalities in amygdalar–orbitofrontal areas have been revealed in male schizophrenia patients with a history of antisocial behaviour from childhood onwards, but not in schizophrenic men without a history of childhood deviant behaviour (Naudts and Hodgins 2006a, 2006b).

21.6 **Evolutionary synthesis**

Forensic psychiatry deals with legal issues pertaining to abnormal behaviour that leads to the violation of a society's rules and norms. In addition to its medical and jurisdictional foundation, forensic psychiatry clearly entails input from the social sciences. What is considered normative in a society can vary widely between cultures. In a general vein, aggression between individuals not only is part of human nature, but also constitutes an inevitable aspect of life. Aggression is indispensable for survival and reproduction. For example, predatory aggression is ubiquitous throughout the food chain. Intraspecies aggression between males secures access to fertile females, and in many animal species intersexual aggression occurs with regard to sexuality and reproduction (a special case of intraspecies aggression is male infanticide, which can happen after a new alpha-male has taken over a group of females, killing offspring he had not sired). What is at stake in the context of forensic psychiatry is aggressive behaviour that is associated with mental illness and considered pathological for its abnormal intensity, inappropriateness with regard to context, or moral unacceptability, especially if violating the rights of others.

Aggression is part of human nature. Forensic psychiatry deals with aggressive behaviour that is associated with mental illness and considered pathological for its abnormal intensity, inappropriateness with regard to context, or moral unacceptability, especially if violating the rights of others.

Aggressiveness varies between individuals, partly as a function of serotonergic activity. In primates, individuals who have recently fallen in rank are more aggressive, which is associated with low serotonin. Rising in rank is accompanied by an increase in serotonin, and high-ranking individuals are usually less aggressive than subordinates (Kaplan et al. 1994). With regard to human behaviour, this suggests that there is no sharp distinction between 'normal' aggression and pathological variants. Normal aggression and delinquency are situated on a continuum. Aggression is highly context-dependent and the degree of cultural acceptance of aggression may vary considerably. Consequently, behaviour that is being sanctioned in one culture or society is not necessarily deemed 'criminal' in another.

In spite of variation, however, many basic rules and norms are principally agreed upon across cultures. These norms include the condemnation of the violation of a person's physical integrity, property, and sexual self-determination, although the latter is probably the least universally acknowledged issue with regard to women's rights. For example, in some US states, manslaughter due to cuckoldry was acquitted until the early 1970s.

In spite of cultural variation, many basic rules and norms are universally agreed upon. These norms include the condemnation of the violation of a person's physical integrity, property, and sexual self-determination.

Beyond the normative aspect of behaviour, forensic psychiatry faces the problem of defining boundaries between an entirely intentional act, for which an individual has full responsibility and behaviour that emerged under conditions associated with poor impulse control or blurred consciousness, for which an individual possibly lacks full responsibility in the juridical sense.

Leaving these difficulties aside, from a behavioural biological perspective the majority of delinquent actions can be seen as an extreme of variation of opportunistic behaviours that aim at maximizing an individual's success in accomplishing important biosocial goals, such as securing resources, mates, or status, at the expense of other individuals. In many instances, the victims of criminal behaviour are personally known to the perpetrators, with the vast majority of delinquents being males. Put differently, delinquency often arises in the context of 'fast' life-history strategies (see Chapter 3), that is, higher levels of aggression, impulsivity, and reduced harm avoidance.

The majority of delinquent actions can be seen as an extreme of variation of opportunistic behaviours that aim at maximizing an individual's success in accomplishing important biosocial goals, such as securing resources, mates, or status, at the expense of other individuals. Opportunistic interpersonal orientation is frequently the consequence of adverse rearing conditions during childhood.

Such opportunistic interpersonal orientation is frequently the consequence of adverse rearing conditions during childhood, and ultimately linked to a reproductive strategy oriented towards early procreation at the expense of the amount of parental investment. In a sense, individuals are 'prepared' to behave selfishly, callous and unresponsive to the needs and rights of others, if their early social environment, in particular their primary caregivers, shows little interest in them, and behaves in an unempathetic and rejecting way (see Chapter 3).

Moreover, such individuals are willing to take greater risks in achieving their short-term goals, are more impulsive, and are less tolerant towards frustration (note that girls with conduct disorder mature physically early, which is entirely in line with the hypothesis of a close association between childhood experience and reproductive strategy; for details see Chapter 3). If such unfavourable early rearing conditions meet certain genetic predispositions associated with low serotonergic activity and high dopaminergic activity in the brain, the likelihood for delinquent behaviour increases considerably. Gene–environment correlation is therefore critical in the development of antisociality and psychopathy. Psychopaths are generally callous, deceptive, and opportunistic, but sometimes also superficially charming and empathetic (Hare 1996). However, they are usually inept in recognizing others' emotions, but often superior in their ability to infer mental states of others (termed 'theory of mind' or 'mentalizing'; see Afterthought to Chapter 2).

If unfavourable early rearing conditions meet certain genetic predispositions associated with low serotonergic activity and high dopaminergic activity in the brain, the likelihood for delinquent behaviour increases considerably.

It would seem that males are particularly susceptible to responding to early childhood adversities with antisocial behaviour, because they are selected to be more aggressive compared to females, because opportunistic behaviour is generally more prevalent in males, and because males are more vulnerable to engaging in aggressive peer group behaviour (Wilson and Daly 1985). All these behavioural tendencies are intimately linked with the evolutionary forces of sexual selection, above all, less parental investment in males relative to females, greater male intrasexual competition, and the problem of 'uncertain paternity' (see Chapter 1).

Men are overrepresented in forensic samples, because males are selected to compete intrasexually, to engage more often in aggressive peer group behaviour, and to solve the adaptive problem of 'uncertain paternity'.

This explains at both the proximate and the ultimate level why males are overrepresented in almost all categories of criminal behaviour, however, with some notable exceptions such as infanticide. Accordingly, men are more likely to transgress rules pertaining to others' property and physical health, but are also more likely to become victims of male violence, except crimes that violate sexual self-determination.

The same holds for forensic psychiatric patients. The majority of forensic patients are male and have been exculpated or deculpated for reasons of insanity due to lack of responsibility, or grossly reduced impulse control and lack of insight during the criminal act.

It is beyond the scope of this chapter to give a complete overview of all relevant behaviours observed in forensic psychiatric patients. It is not even possible to give a comprehensive account of the subgroup of sexually motivated delinquency associated with psychiatric disorders, but some overarching behavioural tendencies can clearly be discerned using insights from evolutionary theory. For example, crimes such as rape and other forms of sexual coercion, paedophilia, stalking, pathological jealousy, erotomania (the delusion of being loved by another person), and sexually motivated homicide are easily explicable in the context of evolutionary theory.

Sexually motivated delinquency associated with psychiatric disorders, such as sexual coercion, paedophilia, stalking, pathological jealousy, erotomania (the delusion of being loved by another person), and sexually motivated homicide, is easily explicable in the context of evolutionary theory.

Two issues need to be reiterated in this regard: first, an evolutionary explanation of behaviour does not mean that biologically motivated behaviour is to be exculpated per se ('I cannot do otherwise, it's my biology'). Nor does an evolutionary explanation suggest that behaviour is impervious to modification. Second, evolved behavioural tendencies cannot morally be justified just because they exist. This error, known as 'naturalistic fallacy', should be kept in mind especially when analysing the biology of abnormal, deviant, or delinquent behaviour (see Afterthought to Chapter 1).

Pathologies pertaining to sexual orientation and behaviour can occur at any stage of mating behaviour. For example, men are selected to find female attributes attractive that signal fecundity, such as youth and a certain waist-to-hip ratio. Youth in females is associated with paedomorphic features such as large eyes, a round face, high cheekbones, and full lips (see Chapter 2). These characteristics are also typical of juveniles and exaggerated in prepubertal children. Thus it is plausible that paedophilic tendencies reflect an extreme of variation of male preferences for female attributes indicating juvenility and fecundity (Ponseti et al. 2014). In accordance with this hypothesis, the vast majority of paedophiles are male, their victims being prepubertal children who display signs of 'cuteness'.

Paedophilic tendencies may reflect an extreme of variation of male preferences for female attributes indicating juvenility and fecundity.

This explanation does not rule out, however, that paraphilia involves complex learning mechanisms, perhaps sometimes akin to 'imprinting', nor does it imply that paraphilic behaviour is simply a by-product of selection (Feierman and Feierman 2000). At the proximate level it is noteworthy that, as children, many paedophiles have been sexually abused themselves. Sexual abuse may therefore contribute to a 'priming' effect, causing a lifelong sexual preference for physically (and psychologically) immature individuals. Exculpation for reasons of insanity, however, can usually not be assumed.

Pathologies of courtship behaviour may be prevalent in both sexes. Men, for example, tend to guard their mates more intensely in terms of sexual faithfulness than do women. The evolutionary rationale behind this behavioural tendency is that males, throughout evolution, have faced the problem of uncertain paternity. Since mate choice is on the side of females, males can never be 100 percent certain that they have actually fathered potential offspring. Thus, evolution would have eliminated sexually permissive attitudes in males, simply because, from a genetic point of view, 'jealous' males would have sired more offspring than permissive ones, and hence had greater reproductive success (Buss 1988a, 1988b, 2000).

Pathological jealousy and stalking can be seen as extremes of variation of male mate-guarding behaviours, which include psychotic variants such as delusional jealousy (most frequently associated with chronic alcoholism) and male erotomania. Spousal homicide associated with pathological jealousy or stalking is many more times committed by men compared to women.

In terms of psychopathology, pathological jealousy and stalking can be seen as extremes of variation of mate-guarding behaviours, which include psychotic variants such as delusional jealousy (most frequently associated with chronic alcoholism) and male erotomania. Consistent with this assumption, pathological jealousy and stalking are much more prevalent in men, many of which have antisocial, narcissistic, or paranoid personality traits (Mullen and Pathé 1994a, 1994b; Kurt 1995; Del Ben and Fremouw 2002). The bio-logic behind such behaviour is that human males invest much more heavily in offspring compared to most non-human males (though still less than females). Consequently, human males would have much more to lose if they invested in children they had not fathered.

Accordingly, domestic violence, including spousal homicide associated with pathological jealousy or stalking, is also many more times committed by men compared to women (Buss and Shackelford 1997). In cases where the female partner initiates spousal separation, women have been found to be especially vulnerable shortly thereafter, with almost half of lethal violence occurring within 2 months after separation. Young women and women who are considerably younger than their partners seem to be at greatest risk, which, from an evolutionary perspective, can be explained as a function of young women's greater reproductive potential relative to older women. In fact, spousal homicide drops by 50 percent in women who are postmenopausal (Wilson and Daly 1993, 1994, 1996). Pathological jealousy and stalking, especially if part of a psychotic disorder, can sometimes cause diminished responsibility or irresponsibility. However, protection of victims is most important, such that many countries have introduced antistalking laws.

Rape is one of the most devastating traumas. A significantly greater proportion of women who were victims of rape suffer from PTSD, sexual disorder, major depression, eating disorder, or anxiety disorder compared with women who survived a different life-threatening trauma, such as car accidents, physical assaults, and robberies.

Sexual coercion including rape is also typical of males and not restricted to the human species (although the term 'rape' entails psychological suffering and humiliation of victims, which has not been observed in non-human animals). Due to sex differences in the amount of parental investment in potential offspring, females are 'choosier' with respect to potential sex partners. Sexual coercion on the side of males can be seen as a behavioural strategy to circumvent the 'female choice' principle (Thornhill and Palmer 2000). Men who rape are often incompetent to attract a partner, low in social status, and unable to form stable heterosexual relationships.

From a woman's perspective, rape is one of the most devastating traumas. According to one study, an alarming number of 25 percent of young women in urban environments have experienced sexual coercion or rape in the past year (Rickert et al. 2004). Moreover, a significantly greater proportion of women who were victims of rape suffer from PTSD, sexual disorder, major depression, eating disorder, or anxiety disorder compared with women who survived a different life-threatening trauma, such as car accidents, physical assaults, and robberies (Faravelli et al. 2004). This clearly underscores that the nature of the trauma affecting women's sexual self-determination plays a causal role in producing persistent psychological distress.

The evolutionary interpretation not only suggests that the majority of rape victims are females, but also predicts that young women during their reproductive age are more likely to be victims of rape or sexual assault compared with postreproductive women, that women in their reproductive age are more severely traumatized compared with postmenopausal women, that married women suffer more severely than unmarried women, because the former face the additional risk of being abandoned by their partners, and that women with no clear physical signs of rape are psychologically more severely affected than women with physical evidence of resistance (Thornhill and Palmer 2000; Faravelli et al. 2004). These risk factors for persistent traumatization have to be kept in mind in situations in which the psychiatrist is asked to examine a rape victim. For example, questioning the fact of rape by a male physician can aggravate the traumatic experience; thus this and other insensitivities have to be strictly avoided. Male sexual coercion and rape are barely a reason for exculpating a perpetrator from punishment for reasons of insanity.

In contrast to sexual jealousy and associated behaviours such as stalking, which are much more prevalent in men, erotomania, the delusion that one is loved by another person, is typical of women. Erotomania is most frequently associated with schizophrenia, mania, and schizoaffective disorder, although several cases have been described in 'organic' psychoses. Similar to delusions in general, erotomania has long been considered as the result of repressed homosexuality and a general inability to form intimate relationships. Beyond speculation about the proximate causes of erotomania, it has long been disregarded that the patterns of behaviour and preference for certain partner characteristics in erotomania strikingly reflect a mating strategy, albeit extremely exaggerated, that is typical of women.

Erotomania, the delusion that one is loved by another person, is much more prevalent in women. Mate preferences and behaviour associated with erotomania can be seen as an extreme of variation of female courtship behaviour.

Characteristically, the 'love object' is a man of high social status who is slightly older than the erotomanic woman. Most erotomanic women are unmarried and socially isolated. Erotomanic subjects tend to harass their 'love objects' by sending countless letters expressing their affection, by phone calls, or even by 'besieging' the 'love object's' home. In contrast to male stalking, erotomanic women are hardly physically aggressive, nor do they usually show any sign of jealousy if the 'love object' is married. Rejection by the 'love object' is frequently rationalized as 'inability to show his "real" affection'. Erotomania has sometimes been referred to as 'old maid's insanity'; however, the majority of erotomanic women are biologically at the end of their reproductive period, rather than postmenopausal.

Clearly, mate preferences and behaviour associated with erotomania can be seen as an extreme of variation of female courtship behaviour (Brüne 2001a). Human females who on average invest heavily in potential offspring are selected to choose long-term mates who are willing and able to invest resources in joint offspring.

From a forensic perspective, male erotomania, though generally much less infrequent compared to female erotomania, is much more relevant, because it is often accompanied by jealousy and stalking behaviour, including possible violent attacks on the 'love object' or perceived 'rival' (Harmon et al. 1995; Dunne and Schipperhejn 2000). Again, the male pattern of erotomania reflects the evolutionary condition of uncertain paternity, which selected males to evolve strategies to minimize the risk of investing in other men's offspring. In erotomania, male sex, low social status, and associated jealousy have been found to predict forensically relevant behaviours. Consistent with this finding, the fixation on multiple objects, which is expected to be rarely associated with erotomania, and antisocial behaviour prior to onset of the erotomanic delusion also predict violent outbursts. According to the evolutionary model, the pressure on ensuring paternity should increase with the number of 'love objects', therefore leading to excessive sexual jealousy (Brüne 2003a).

In terms of the question of exculpation by reason of insanity, forensic psychiatric evaluation should focus on the firmness with which the belief of being loved by another person is held. Forensic cases with fixed delusional beliefs may qualify for being testified as reduced responsibility, whereas so-called borderline erotomania (Meloy 1989), which is associated with narcissistic or APD, may not fulfil the criteria of reduced insight or diminished impulse control justifying deculpation.

Another issue that frequently involves forensic psychiatric services is infanticide. In the USA, almost two-thirds of children who die from assault are killed by one of their parents. Homicide ranks number four among causes of death in preschool-age children, and number three in 5- to 14-year-olds. Infants younger than 12 months are at particular risk of dying through homicide (Brookman and Nolan 2006). Infanticidal behaviour can be distinguished according to the child's age.

The association of neonaticide with psychopathology is generally weak. Neonaticide occurs if the mother is extremely young or single, if the baby is defective, if the pregnancy was the result of incest or rape, or if socio-economic resources are scarce. Filicidal mothers are usually older, more frequently married, socially isolated, and were victims of domestic violence, and are often depressed, psychotic, or engage in substance abuse.

Neonaticide occurs within the first 24 hours after birth, a sensible period for the formation of attachment and bonding. Across cultures, neonaticide has been a function of differential parental investment throughout human history, and cultural preferences of one sex over the other may even impact on genes that alter sex ratios (Kumm et al. 1994; Kumm and Feldman 1997). Unlike other mammals, humans are unable to abort undesired offspring if environmental conditions are unfavourable (such as during times of food shortage). In traditional societies, female newborns have been at greater risk of being killed by their mothers, based on the evolutionary logic that males statistically produce more offspring than females. In line with this evolutionary scenario, in modern societies neonaticide occurs more often if the mother is extremely young or single, if the baby is defective, if the pregnancy was the result of incest or rape, or if socio-economic resources are scarce (Hrdy et al. 1994; Overpeck et al. 1998). The association of neonaticide with psychopathology is generally weak.

In contrast, filicide, the killing of older infants and children, deviates from the evolutionary model, as filicidal mothers are usually older, more frequently married, socially isolated, or have been victims of domestic violence (Stone et al. 2005). Moreover, filicidal mothers are more frequently depressed, psychotic, or diagnosed with substance abuse. Suicidal thoughts may occur in up to 50 percent of filicidal women. In women with postpartum depression, infanticidal ideation may occur in over 40 percent, and in one study actual infanticidal behaviour happened in one-third of patients, sometimes originally planned as homicide–suicide. These figures clearly indicate that the risk of infanticide should be closely monitored in women with postpartum depression (Spinelli 2004).

Young children are also at increased risk of being killed if brought up by parents who are not biologically related to them (Temrin et al. 2000). Some studies suggest that particularly stepfathers commit more often infanticide than biological fathers, with infants and pre-schoolers being at greatest risk. Moreover, stepfathers use more 'brutal' methods to kill their children compared to biological fathers, possibly reflecting differences in degree of resentment and antisocial personality traits (Weekes-Shackelford and Shackelford 2004). As already pointed out, this kind of aggressive behaviour may reflect a biological predisposition in males to induce sexual receptivity in females by killing offspring they had not fathered (Daly and Wilson 1988). In western societies, child abuse can perhaps be regarded as an extension to infanticide in ancestral communities (Archer 2013). Psychosis or psychotic depression at the time of committed infanticide may justify exculpation for reasons of insanity. The majority of infanticides, however, do not fall into this category.

It needs to be emphasized, again, that evolutionary biological explanations of delinquent behaviour by no means morally justify or automatically exculpate an aggressive perpetrator from responsibility. Acknowledging that humans have a biological history of many millions of years that wrought our cognitive apparatus, emotional repertoire, and behaviour in a way that increased the likelihood of leaving surviving offspring, long before moral implications came into being, may help to predict the risk for recidivism and perhaps to prevent criminal behaviour and victimization.

Evolutionary biological explanations of delinquent behaviour by no means morally justify or automatically exculpate an aggressive perpetrator from responsibility.

21.7 **Course and outcome**

Studies into the risk for criminal recidivism of psychiatrically ill offenders suggest on average rates between 20 and 40 percent for re-offences in both men and women (Putkonen et al. 2003). However, these figures vary widely depending on the diagnosis, symptomatology, comorbidity, availability of treatment, and potential for social reintegration. For example, in patients with psychosis, prognostic factors for an elevated risk of recidivism include lack of insight, presence of delusional symptoms, chronicity of the disorder, and persistent feelings of revenge. By comparison, factors such as preserved insight, treatment compliance, and stable remission of symptoms are associated with improved prognosis.

Studies into the risk for criminal recidivism of psychiatrically ill offenders suggest on average rates between 30 and 40 percent for re-offences. However, these figures vary widely depending on the diagnosis, symptomatology, comorbidity, availability of treatment, and potential for social reintegration.

In patients with personality disorders, high scores of psychopathic traits such as callousness, shallow affect, lack of empathy, remorse or guilt, impulsivity, and irresponsibility are considered to be prognostically unfavourable. Moreover, comorbid substance abuse further increases the risk for criminal recidivism in individuals with personality disorders.

In recent years, recidivism in sexual offenders has received considerable public attention. For example, in rapists the risk for re-offences has been estimated between 30 and

70 percent. High scores of psychopathic traits associated with sexual deviance are the strongest predictors for recidivism. By contrast, age seems to be inversely correlated with the risk for sexual re-offences.

21.8 **Treatment**

In ancient times, the Roman courts exculpated from punishment the 'furiosi' (maniacs), the 'mente capti' (insane), and the 'dementes' (idiots). However, most mentally ill offenders were incarcerated under inhumane conditions.

In the nineteenth century, the Italian criminologist Cesare Lombroso (1836–1909), drawing on concepts of psychiatry and eugenics, popularized the view that criminal behaviour was a heritable evolutionary throwback to more primitive stages of human evolution caused by degeneration. Accordingly, he proposed that physiognomic attributes such as atavistic stigmata were indicative of the 'born criminal's' character and personality. For these reasons Lombroso pleaded for medical treatment of criminals and strongly opposed capital punishment.

Similarly, Emil Kraepelin (1856–1926) conceptualized delinquency in general as 'social illness', even though he rejected Lombroso's ideas of observable stigmata (Hoff 1998). Kraepelin embarked on a discussion that is unresolved to the present day. That is, the difficulty, perhaps impossibility, to draw a line between full responsibility, diminished responsibility, and exculpation from punishment of criminal offenders for reasons of insanity. Kraepelin suggested that punishment ought not to serve as a society's means of revenge, but to improve a delinquent's social adjustment (Kraepelin 1880). Still, there is certainly a grey area in this regard, all the more as social therapy and rehabilitation has been shown to improve outcome in criminal offenders, regardless whether exculpated for reasons of insanity or deemed fully responsible.

In cases with schizophrenia, irresponsibility or diminished responsibility is generally assumed in acute psychotic states associated with delusions and hallucinations. Similarly, acute mania and psychotic depression usually imply reduced inhibitory control of impulses. Acute intoxication and severe withdrawal symptoms may also justify the assumption of diminished or sometimes even lack of responsibility.

In cases with schizophrenia, irresponsibility or diminished responsibility is generally assumed in acute psychotic states associated with delusions and hallucinations. Cases with stable residual symptoms are more difficult to evaluate. Similarly, acute mania and psychotic depression usually imply a reduced inhibitory control of impulses. Acute intoxication and severe withdrawal symptoms may also justify the assumption of diminished or sometimes even lack of responsibility, whereas other drug-related crimes that aim at maintaining provision with substances are more problematic to judge. Severely impaired behavioural control can sometimes be testified in individuals with severe personality disorders, particularly if associated with pathological impulsivity, comorbid substance dependence, or deprivation, and may lead to deculpation. However, there is considerable disparity across different legal systems (Simon and Gold 2010).

The psychiatric assessment has to pay special attention to the mental state at the time of the offence or the mental state at the time of trial, which both may lead to the application of mental health legislation to detain people in hospital. In case of exculpation for reasons of insanity, most countries have special hospitals for psychiatrically ill offenders or special wards within correctional facilities.

Psychiatric assessment has to pay special attention to the mental state at the time of the offence or the mental state at the time of trial, which both may lead to the application of mental health legislation to detain people in hospital.

Treatment of mentally ill offenders depends on the nature of the psychiatric disorder. Patients who are released from hospital—usually only after extensive psychiatric evaluation of prognostic factors for recidivism—are subsequently supervised in the community by a multiprofessional forensic team comprising psychiatrists, psychologists, nurses, and social workers. Teamwork aims at prevention of recurrence of violent behaviour by means of individual risk management. At the same time, the team has the responsibility to promote appropriate health care to patients.

Patients who are released from hospital are supervised in the community by a multiprofessional forensic team. Teamwork aims at prevention of recurrence of violent behaviour by means of individual risk management.

Common factors contributing to risk management include the evaluation of the patient's mental state in terms of impulsivity, psychotic symptoms, and substance abuse, as well as social support, rehabilitation, and supervision of treatment (Simon and Gold 2010).

Afterthought: remarks on the debate on 'free will' and moral responsibility in forensic psychiatry

Folk psychology suggests that humans are unconstrained in their decision-making, that is, that they possess a 'free will'. If this were actually the case, humans, under all circumstances except during states of clouded consciousness, would be fully responsible for all kinds of behaviour, including forensically relevant ones. This position, however, has been challenged from several perspectives. For centuries, philosophers have debated the issue of 'free will' without having arrived at a generally accepted position (Roth 2006). Immanuel Kant, for example, proposed that 'free will' entailed the mental causation of action, and the freedom to behave differently in otherwise identical constellations ('alternativism'), hence implying full responsibility in the moral sense. In contrast, David Hume defined 'free will' somewhat weaker as the power of acting or of not acting (Timpe 2006).

From a neuroscientific point of view, the existence of a 'free will' has been criticized for various reasons: first, human behaviour is guided by sometimes competing motivations and drives, but is certainly not free of biological constraints such as emotions. Second, research into brain function suggests that mental processes are deterministic in nature, that is, they are initiated by some neuronal activity, which measurably predates conscious awareness (Haggard 2005). For example, experimental studies suggest that the decision to move a hand is first being made subconsciously (as indicated by a 'readiness potential'), to which people later ascribe an intention. In other words, the subjective impression of having initiated a movement according to one's 'free will' is being made in retrospect (Libet et al. 1983). Moreover, the decision which hand to move can be influenced using transcanial magnetic stimulation. Depending on whether the right or the left PFC is stimulated, individuals prefer the hand contralateral to the stimulated hemisphere, while subjectively reporting that they have acted based on free choice. Third, alternativism is implausible from a neurobiological perspective, because alternative behaviour without causal motives would undermine the proposition of subjective agency based on an individual's 'free will'. Therefore the assumption of an entirely 'free will' is no longer tenable, which does not mean that 'freedom of action' is, to some extent, possible and inherent to the evolved human nature.

Within philosophy and among neuroscientists, there are different positions on the degree of determinism of behaviour (Dennett 1984, 2003). 'Hard' determinists argue that the course of the future, including future behaviour, is exclusively determined by the laws of nature. Thus, according to 'hard' determinism, 'free will' does not exist (contrariwise, indeterminism proposes that 'free will' exists *because* events are not deterministic). Another position held by compatibilists suggests that even though all action is ultimately predetermined by neural activity, unconscious motivation, and drives, freedom to make decisions exists to some degree. Moreover, the compatibilist stance assumes that determinism is a prerequisite for having the freedom of decision-making, because indeterminism (all behaviour occurs at random) would preclude any form of freedom of action. In a similar vein, people can be held responsible (also in the moral sense) for their actions because of determinism. If indeterminism were true, no one could be punished for an action or behaviour that originated from random activity of the nervous system (Timpe 2006).

Compatibilism is also consistent with evolutionary constraints of human behaviour. Humans have evolved a variety of cognitive mechanisms involved in conscious decision-making. These include the ability to experience the self as agent, to consciously reflect upon opposing motives, to plan future behaviour, and perhaps even to have the illusion of possessing a 'free will' (Haggard 2008). In terms of morality, humans have evolved universal rules of social conduct that help keep the delicate balance between selfishness and altruism (Alexander 1987). These mechanisms require a great amount of computational resources, many of which are located in the large prefrontal lobes. On the other hand, freedom of action can be constrained by a number of factors. In the early twentieth century, it was Sigmund Freud who already argued that human behaviour is largely dependent on non-conscious information processing, and that only a tiny fraction of what is going on in our minds breaches conscious awareness. Accordingly, decision-making is more or less under the control of unconscious motives, feelings, and desires. Mental states associated with intense fear or rage may even abandon the influence of conscious decision-making on behaviour, to an extent that they may preclude responsibility for forensically relevant behaviour.

Some psychopathological conditions, above all psychotic states, are associated with a diminished sense of agency. Empirical evidence from experimental studies suggests that delusions of influence are related to an individual's abnormal perception of his or her own actions, perhaps due to malfunctioning of a mechanism, referred to as the 'reafference principle' (Frith et al. 2000). A reafference copy is seen as part of goal-directed behaviour according to which an efference copy of an action is made to predict the sensory consequences of the resulting action. The reafference copy serves the purpose to signal deviations from the expected outcome of the action, such that adjustments of the movement can be made. In patients with delusions of control or influence, the representation of the desired state, the motor command, and the actual movement are intact, but the individual is apparently unaware of or unable to represent the predicted state, and hence has no feeling of being in charge of the action. This lack of self-monitoring capacity may similarly underlie other passivity symptoms observed in schizophrenia, such as auditory hallucinations in the form of hearing voices, which, in fact, represent subliminal self-generated inner speech (Frith et al. 2000). Thus, an individual with a diminished sense of being the agent of his or her action, who instead has the impression that his or her behaviour is guided by alien forces, may not be responsible for criminal behaviour if that behaviour occurred during such a delusional state.

With regard to morality, humans have evolved preferences for altruistic behaviour that is even shown towards genetically unrelated non-kin (Trivers 1971). It could be that this kind of strong altruism evolved by means of group selection, which, however, competes with selfish motives. Behaviour that benefits the group may in the long term also help the individual, but only if altruistic behaviour is being reciprocated. This is usually the case, and most people tend to punish non-cooperative behaviour, even if they only observe that others have been cheated. Game theoretical experiments have revealed that people's behavioural performance in scenarios requiring cooperation or defection does not depend on logic. Rather, the behaviour of others determines an individual's decision whether or not to cooperate.

One of the simplest rules is tit-for-tat, that is, cooperation will be reciprocated, whereas defection will be answered by defection. In more complex scenarios, however, an offer from a proposer is likely to be rejected if perceived as unfair, even if a possible net gain is foregone. For example, if player A offers player B two out of ten money units while keeping the difference, player B will decline the offer if both players receive nothing upon player B's rejection. A logic decision would have been to accept the two money units (which is better than nothing), but it would seem that feelings of injustice guide one's behaviour towards punishing unfair behaviour at one's own expense. These experiments suggest that human behaviour is strongly influenced by the reinforcement of cooperation and punishment of defection (Fehr and Gächter 2002).

At the population level, however, non-cooperative behaviour or 'free-riding' can be maintained at low prevalence. If selfish behaviour would spread in a population and become more prevalent, the population would clash. Thus, an individual's opportunistic behaviour at the expense of altruists can succeed only if a small fraction, figuring perhaps around 1 percent, of people behaves selfishly. This estimate comes close to the prevalence of psychopathy (Mealey 1995; Troisi 2005).

With regard to forensically relevant behaviour, this means that societies need to keep the number of 'free-riders' low, and thus have developed systems of punishing non-cooperative behaviour. Accordingly, the need to reinforce obedience to social rules and norms by punishment of deviant behaviour is deterministic in the sense that compatibilists use the term.

These deterministic aspects of rule-enforcement are, however, in diametrical opposition to the 'alternativism' position of jurisprudence. Jurisprudence implicitly assumes that individuals who have committed a crime could have done otherwise, because they are, at all times, aware of right and wrong. Based on the aforementioned, such a position is arguably contestable. So, in the end, was Kraepelin right in claiming to abolish the degree of punishment and replace it by medical treatment? Can we hold people responsible and punish them for their behaviours in light of the manifold constraints to freedom of action?

There is probably no definitive answer to these questions. However, a pragmatic solution could be to punish offenders based on the assumption that they share the knowledge of right and wrong in a particular culture, even if they may not be able to act upon their knowledge in every given situation. This requires a potential offender's cognitive ability to comprehend what is right or wrong, and to be (theoretically) capable of refraining from behaviours that may be sanctioned. In the past, this was not always easy. At the time of the Holy Inquisition thousands of innocent people were accused of obscure deeds, tortured, and killed. Similar trials (though not on large scales) have been performed in 'primitive' societies, which only seem to work if supernatural forces such as witchcraft are invoked. Thanks to enlightenment and the growth of the natural sciences, such atrocities are no longer imaginable in western societies. Human societies always have had means to sanction behaviours that did not comply with rules and norms. Since it is impossible to draw a line between mental health and mental illness, jurisprudence and forensic psychiatry will continue to face problems with regard to guilt versus exculpation, punishment versus treatment. Naturalizing these problems may, however, help find more conclusive answers.

Chapter 22

Psychotherapy

Abstract

Psychotherapy can be defined as the attempt to reframe consequences of maladaptive behaviour that have caused suffering in self or others by scientifically evaluated psychological interventions. The response to psychotherapy does not solely rely on the specific technique. Instead, it is the quality of the patient–client relationship that determines the outcome of psychotherapeutic interventions. In spite of the relevance of early experiences with caregivers and significant others for well-being later in life, few psychotherapeutic 'schools' explicitly refer to evolutionary theory. However, evolutionary thinking in psychotherapy has a lot to offer, beyond issues pertaining to attachment theory. The concept of self-deception can explain phenomena related to repression and how some therapeutic interventions work. The ability to mentalize is deeply rooted in our biology and is actively used in psychotherapy. In summary, integrative approaches to psychotherapy are much more in line with human evolutionary biology and neuroscience than puristic psychoanalysis or behaviourism.

Keywords

psychotherapy, maladaptive behaviour, patient–client relationship, attachment, self-deception, repression, mentalization, integrative psychotherapy

22.1 Introductory remarks to psychotherapy

Psychotherapy can be defined as the attempt to change cognitions, emotions, and behaviours in humans who suffer from maladaptive consequences of their behaviour or have caused suffering in others, by means of scientifically evaluated psychological techniques and interventions (Lambert 2004). Central to all kinds of psychotherapy is the assumption that patients or clients can develop more functional strategies to cope with interpersonal distress or other adverse conditions through learning and experience, albeit with different likelihoods of success depending on the age at onset of first symptoms, as well as on the duration and severity of the underlying disorder.

Psychotherapy is the attempt to change maladaptive cognitions, emotions, and behaviours by means of scientifically evaluated psychological techniques and interventions.

It is widely acknowledged among psychotherapists that logic in therapeutic discourse alone does not suffice to enable a patient to give up maladaptive strategies; rather, it is essential that the patient can *feel* a difference; perhaps first imaginatively, and later on, as therapy progresses, as part of his or her 'real life' experience. Even though it becomes increasingly clear that psychotherapy has the potential to induce long-lasting changes in brain activation (Etkin et al. 2005), particularly in the most recently evolved cortical midline structures involved in the representation of self and others (Northoff et al. 2007), and in phylogenetically older brain centres involved in emotion regulation, the fact that any kind of psychotherapy is deeply rooted in the evolved psychology of our species is more implicitly, rather than explicitly, approved by therapists (McGuire and Troisi 2006a, 2006b).

For example, mental representation of self and others is at the core of interpersonal and intrapersonal conflict, as well as of conflict resolution. The ability to empathize with others, to infer others' mental states, to imagine future social interactions, and to reflect upon one's own mental life may have been not only a major driving force in human brain evolution, but also a major source of cognitive distortion, excessive worry, and concern, thereby causing psychological distress and suffering (for further details see Chapters 2 and 5).

Psychotherapy has the potential to induce long-lasting changes in brain activation. Mental representation of self and others is central to interpersonal and intrapersonal conflict, as well as conflict resolution.

22.2 **Historical developments in psychotherapy**

The origins of psychotherapeutic treatment date back to the late nineteenth century when Sigmund Freud and Josef Breuer developed what later became known as psychoanalysis and psychodynamic psychotherapy. The value of many of Freud's discoveries cannot be overestimated, although some of his ideas appear scientifically flawed today. Above all, the fact that most of our mental life is unconscious and only small parts of it surface as conscious reflection or are accessible to the reflexive self have greatly changed our view of human mentality in pervasive ways. It was also Freud who emphasized the important role of phylogenetically ancient drives and motives for human psychology and behaviour. He further argued that unconscious drives and motives can be at odds with an individual's conscious desires, expectations, and self-appraisal, which may cause psychological malfunctioning and subjective distress.

One of the most important discoveries of psychoanalysis was that most of our mental life is unconscious and only small parts of it surface as conscious reflection or are accessible to the reflexive self. Even though Sigmund Freud recognized evolution as an important scientific concept to explain human psychology, his conceptualization was strongly influenced by the assumption of Lamarckian inheritance (inheritance of acquired characters).

Even though Freud recognized evolution as an important scientific concept to explain human psychology, his conceptualization was strongly influenced by the assumption of Lamarckian inheritance (inheritance of acquired characters), recapitulation theory (the repetition of phylogeny in ontogeny), and group selection (as opposed to individual and kin selection). For reasons that may have lain in his personal history (he was brought up by a nanny, while his mother remained unattainable for him), Freud came to overemphasize infantile sexuality and the Oedipal model as central to intrapsychic conflict (although it has been argued that the Oedipal situation may have evolved as an unconscious 'seductive' strategy of the infant to increase parental investment). Moreover, he did not recognize that incest avoidance was deeply rooted in biology and represents an evolved mechanism to avoid accumulation of deleterious mutations, rather than being part of a universal neurosis that manifests through repression of incestuous impulses (Erickson 2000). Today, Freud's drive theory appears at times overly mechanistic, and his overemphasis of aggressive instincts as driving forces behind human behaviour is no longer shared by most therapists (although still prevalent in many textbooks).

Freud's colleagues Carl Gustav Jung and Alfred Adler developed their ideas independent of Freud and took many of the basic psychoanalytic hypotheses further. Jung elaborated upon the phylogenetic aspects of human mental life shared by all individuals (called 'collective unconscious') represented in 'archetypes', which Jung conceived of as being much richer and more diverse compared to Freud's drive theory. By contrast, Adler focused on compensation of inherited 'inferiority feelings' as a basic psychological mechanism shaping an individual's lifestyle. In contrast to Freud, Adler recognized the importance of sociality ('community feeling') for human development, and the impact of early rearing conditions and birth order on individual psychological development.

Freud's colleagues Carl Gustav Jung and Alfred Adler developed their ideas independent of Freud and took many of the basic psychoanalytic hypotheses further. Both acknowledged the importance of unconscious information processing and the role of defence mechanisms in coping with intrapersonal conflict. Similar to Freud, they were convinced that much of an individual's unconscious mental life was brought to surface in dreams and by 'free association'. Jung elaborated upon the phylogenetic aspects of human mental life shared by all individuals (called 'collective unconscious') represented in 'archetypes', which Jung conceived of as being much richer and more diverse compared to Freud's drive theory (Stevens 2000). By contrast, Adler focused on compensation of inherited 'inferiority feelings' as a basic psychological mechanism shaping an individual's lifestyle. In contrast to Freud, Adler recognized the importance of sociality ('community feeling') for human development and the impact of early rearing conditions and birth order on individual psychological development. Both Jung and Adler believed that therapeutic success was linked to the quality of the therapeutic relationship and that a warm, accepting, and empathetic alliance with the patient was vital to psychotherapy, which to some extent differed fundamentally to Freud's more distant-analytic perspective (Stevens and Price 1996).

In the 1950s, John Bowlby and his pupils began to develop attachment theory by integrating insights from psychoanalysis with ethology, and developmental and cognitive psychology (Holmes 1993). Bowlby was struck by his observation of children in foster care who often engaged in delinquent behaviour, in spite of being provided with food and shelter (Bowlby 1944). He came to realize that the quality of an infant's emotional relationship with his or her primary caregiver, including the development of feelings of security and protection, had the potential to bias cognitive processes in terms of expectations and predictions of future interpersonal relationships throughout the lifespan (Pearce

In the 1950s, John Bowlby and his pupils began to develop attachment theory by combining insights from psychoanalysis with ethology, and developmental and cognitive psychology. Bowlby came to realize that the quality of an infant's emotional relationship with his or her primary caregiver had the potential to bias cognitive processes in terms of expectations and predictions of future interpersonal relationships in one's adult life.

and Pezzot-Pearce 2001). In other words, personality development entails the emergence of mental templates (so-called inner working models) concerning representations of self and others, which, in part, determine the way an individual unconsciously creates his or her interpersonal environment.

This focus on early actual relationships was at odds with classic analytic views that a child's primary motivation to bond with his or her mother was motivated by the infant's polymorphic sexual drives. Instead, Bowlby and co-workers saw human behaviour as guided by innate tendencies to secure survival through establishing close proximity to an attachment figure, usually, but not necessarily, the mother (Cassidy and Shaver 1999). According to attachment theory, the attachment system is automatically activated when an infant perceives threat or danger (see Chapter 3). If the caregiver is unavailable, unresponsive to the infant's needs, or even abusive, hyperactivation or deactivation of the attachment system emerge as secondary strategies to either retain proximity or distance oneself from others by denying threat to the individual's sense of security (Shaver and Mikulincer 2005). Unlike classic psychoanalysis, attachment theory sees actual interpersonal conflict and internalized models of interpersonal relationships at the core of psychological problems, rather than conflict between divergent drives, motives, and fantasies (Bowlby 1991). Attachment theory, along with related and integrative psychotherapeutic concepts such as schema-focused therapy, mentalization-based treatment, and compassion-focused therapy, is inextricably linked to the evolutionary biology of our species.

Unlike classic psychoanalysis, attachment theory sees actual interpersonal conflict and internalized models of interpersonal relationships at the core of psychological problems, rather than conflict between divergent drives, motives, and fantasies. Attachment theory, along with related and integrative psychotherapeutic concepts, such as schema-focused therapy, mentalization-based treatment, and compassion-focused therapy, is inextricably linked to the evolutionary biology of our species.

Behaviourism and cognitive social learning theories were originally formulated in diametrical opposition to psychoanalytic theory. In particular, these theories utterly denied the existence of innate behavioural predispositions. On the contrary, early behaviourists assumed that humans were born as 'blank sheets', and that behaviour was simply the result of learned or conditioned responses, which, in the case of maladaptive behaviour, could simply be unlearned (through extinction). This perspective greatly neglected the role of biological motives, individual development, and defence mechanisms in favour of situational influences on cognition and behaviour. Conditioning surely contributes to the acquisition of fear and anxiety or pathological habits, such as substance dependence and compulsive behaviour. It needs to be emphasized, however, that learning has a biological basis itself that cannot be separated from an individual's genetic endowment and early environmental contingencies, perhaps even

Early behaviourists assumed that humans were born as 'blank sheets', and that behaviour was simply the result of learned or conditioned responses, which, in the case of maladaptive behaviour, could simply be unlearned (through extinction). The role of early experience is now widely recognized among behaviour therapists, and with regard to the anxiety disorders, evolutionary ideas have been incorporated into the psychoeducational part of behaviour therapy.

those in one's foetal life. On the contrary, imprinting-like learning during an individual's foetal and early postnatal period may perhaps be most impervious to therapeutic modification later in life. The role of early experience is now widely recognized among behaviour therapists, and with regard to the anxiety disorders, evolutionary ideas have been incorporated into the psychoeducational part of behaviour therapy. Moreover, the proposition of 'cognitive schemas' by CBT is in many respects akin to the assumption of evolved information processing biases that are modified through individual experience (Beck 1999).

As the sharp distinction between analytic and behavioural concepts of personality development and psychological problems has increasingly proven impracticable and scientifically untenable, it is now time to integrate the complex interactions between early and present experience, genetics, and the evolutionary history of our species. This complex interplay sets the stage for human interaction, including patient– or client–therapist relationships. Hence, any form of psychotherapy, whatever 'school' it may belong to, ought to consider an integrative perspective, including the basic needs for security, protection, respect, and empathetic containment, which all humans share as members of the same species (Linehan 1993).

22.3 The patient– or client–therapist relationship

There has been considerable debate over the question of what actually helps a patient in psychotherapy. Although still not entirely clear, there is consensus that the quality of the patient– or client–therapist relationship (some professionals favour the term 'client' over 'patient', because the former does not exclusively invoke pathology as a source of help-seeking; here the terms are more or less interchangeably used) cannot be overestimated, whereas the particular therapeutic method is perhaps less important compared to patient and therapist variables (Troisi and McGuire 2000). The differential contributions of relationship and method to therapeutic success vary, however, according to the nature and complexity of the disorder. In the treatment of complex personality disorders, relationship-associated variables may be more important, whereas in the treatment of 'simple' phobias, the use of a manual-driven approach may prevail over therapist variables.

The role of the patient– or client–therapist relationship cannot be overestimated, whereas the particular therapeutic method is perhaps less important compared to patient and therapist variables.

Among the most important determinants of a successful basis for psychotherapy on the side of the therapist is the ability to be genuinely empathetic and accepting, and to create a therapeutic atmosphere that is as egalitarian and reciprocal as possible to foster trust, feelings of safeness, and protection from further traumatization in the patient (Bateman and Fonagy 2006; Gilbert 2006; Kellogg and Young 2006). In some respects, the therapeutic alliance should emulate the safety and stability of a kinship bond, diminish the dominance hierarchy between patient and therapist, and thus help to avoid distant professionalism (Bailey K.G. 2000). Such a therapeutic stance acknowledges the role of evolved psychological mechanisms involved in the formation of trustful interpersonal alliances, which may include 'limited reparenting', that is, creating a therapeutic situation that is characterized by the provision of safety and emotional availability (Young et al. 2003). At the same time, however, the therapist should be able to set clear boundaries and be straightforward about essential prerequisites for a trustful therapeutic alliance.

The therapeutic alliance should emulate the safety and stability of a kinship bond, diminish the dominance hierarchy between patient and therapist, and thus help to avoid distant professionalism. The therapist should simultaneously be able to set clear boundaries and be straightforward about essential prerequisites for a trustful therapeutic alliance.

For example, it should be made clear to the patient that successful therapy requires abstinence from drug and alcohol consumption, because intoxication leads to distorted reality perception and may cause inappropriate behaviour (Bateman and Fonagy 2004). Moreover, some clients may strive for a deeper relationship than is professionally acceptable or warranted, and limitations of the therapist's availability ought to be pointed out. To avoid disappointment or confusion on either side, it may be useful—depending on the nature of the disorder—to explicitly reach consensus over rules of conduct before formally commencing therapy, perhaps using a leaflet or information sheet, or even a written contract about rules of conduct. It can be assumed that all patients benefit from an unambiguous therapeutic attitude.

Beyond attitude and role models, a therapist's authenticity critically depends on his or her non-verbal behaviour. Many patients are hypervigilant to deception and may therefore quickly sense if the therapist is not sincerely interested in the patient's needs and emotional distress, or unconsciously signals ambivalent feelings toward the patient. In addition, subtle signs of hierarchizing, perhaps unconsciously expressed by an elevated sitting position or a desk put between the client's and the therapist's chairs, as well as non-verbal signs of rejection like folding one's arms or turning away from the patient, ought to be avoided. Therapists should be able to carefully self-monitor their non-verbal behaviour. On the other hand, therapists should forestall clients' perception of the therapist as being subordinate, emotionally weak, or inconsistent, because such inequality may be equally deleterious to therapeutic progress.

A therapist's authenticity critically depends on his or her non-verbal behaviour. On the patient or client's side, it is important that a patient has the genuine wish for a change, though some patients initially expect that others change attitudes and behaviour, rather than they themselves.

On the patient or client's side, it is important that a patient has the genuine wish for a change, though some patients initially expect that others change attitudes and behaviour, rather than they themselves. A useful categorization of a client's willingness to actively engage in therapy has been put forth by the school of Brief Therapy, according to which a 'visitor' does not see the therapist on a voluntary basis, has no complaints, and has no expectations regarding a change of the current situation. In such a case, therapy is impossible. A 'complainant' is subjectively distressed but expects others to change. Complainants should be encouraged to consider alternatives to their current (maladaptive) behaviour. A 'customer' is genuinely motivated to change the situation and may respond best to therapeutic interventions that aim at enabling the patient to give up dysfunctional behaviour and to pursue biosocial goals more effectively (de Shazer 1985). Active support and encouraging the patient to take a chance for a change may be warranted in patients with pronounced tendencies of regression.

In addition to determining a client's (unconscious) motivation for therapy, it may be helpful to explore the client's representation or state of mind of attachment. In adults, the way past relationships with important attachment figures are represented and verbalized corresponds with the individual's acquired attachment style in infancy. Incoherent verbalization suggests insecure attachment during infancy and childhood. Insecurely attached individuals may, for example, either have difficulties in remembering their childhood or over-idealize parents. They may have a dismissing state of mind; as children, they may have developed an avoidant attachment style. Others are quickly overwhelmed by adverse memories when asked about their relationship to parents and have preoccupied states of mind. They may switch from idealization to anger and rage when recalling aspects of the primary attachment figure. As children, they usually displayed an ambivalent attachment style. Individuals who as children experienced abuse or neglect or were otherwise traumatized due to the unavailability of a primary attachment figure and lack of protection and security often report childhood memories in a pronounced disorganized way (Cassidy and Shaver 1999; Liotti 2000; see Chapter 3).

In addition to determining a client's(unconscious) motivation for therapy, it may be helpful to explore the client's representation or state of mind of attachment, because past experiences with primary caregivers shape an individual's ability to represent self and others' mental states.

The importance of a careful evaluation of attachment representations in adult clients resides in the fact that past experiences with primary caregivers shape an individual's ability to represent self and others' mental states (Fonagy 1991). Moreover, it has a profound impact on how current relationships are formed, including the therapeutic relationship. Hence, the exploration of the client's current problems along with his or her way to arrange close relationships may help the therapist get an impression of how the therapeutic alliance may develop and how the individual therapeutic process should ideally be tailored according to the patient's needs.

The apparent paradox here is—contrary to widely held views that parents' emotional responsiveness and availability bear the risk of 'spoiling' the infant—that securely attached individuals, whose primary caregivers respond to infants' needs, are emotionally available, and provided a safe haven for infants from which they can explore the environment, are better able to move to a mature autonomous state (Bowlby 1991). Securely attached individuals are also better at reflecting upon their own and others' mental states, compared to individuals whose primary attachment figures are emotionally unavailable or even abusive. It is the latter who have more difficulties in maintaining trusting interpersonal relationships and who chronically overactivate or deactivate their attachment systems (Bateman and Fonagy 2004).

22.4 The social brain and psychotherapy

Sociality and proximity to significant others are central to human nature throughout the human lifespan (and not ones that have to be outgrown). These basic needs are ultimately linked to human immaturity at birth, long dependence on parental care, and other aspects of human life history, such as the formation of long-term pair-bonds and investment in offspring of both sexes (see Chapter 3). Human psychology is designed by nature to guide the individual in accomplishing biosocial goals, which include care-giving, care-eliciting, forming social bonds and alliances, attaining social status, and mating (Gilbert 1998). Successful accomplishment of these goals may increase the likelihood of translation into reproductive success, but humans are by no means fitness maximizers in that they were able to (consciously) calculate how to increase one's inclusive fitness (see Chapter 1). However, there is striking evidence to suggest that the quality of social relationships is the most significant predictor for decreased mortality across the lifespan (Holt-Lunstad et al. 2010).

Sociality and proximity to significant others are central to human nature throughout the human lifespan (and not ones that have to be outgrown).

Due to the complexity of ancestral human communities with the need to delicately balance selfish and altruistic motivation of behaviour, humans have evolved a set of psychological mechanisms to evaluate reciprocality and cooperation by means of detecting cheaters, collectively punishing cheaters, but also to subtly deceive others (Trivers 1971). These social manoeuvres have induced a cognitive 'armsrace', which led to sophisticated ways to predict the behaviour of others by inferring their mental states. Competition between selfish motives and altruism may be an important source of intrapersonal conflict. The emotions of shame and guilt may have specifically evolved through group-selection and to maintain reciprocal relationships. The induction of guilt and shame serve manipulative purposes to reinforce the cooperative behaviour of individuals who, under specific circumstances, are tempted to behave selfishly. However, the possibility to act in selfish ways is enhanced by the cognitive ability to conceal one's real motives before the self, referred to as 'self-deception' (Trivers 2000). Self-deception may in the first place have evolved to enhance the ability to deceive others, because if an individual is unaware of his or her selfish motives, it is easier to send more convincing signals to others so as not to recognize the individual's real intention. This assumption is intriguing because it suggests that natural selection has not favoured cognitive capacities to produce accurate images of the world, but to systematically distort conscious awareness and to block inadvertent access to non-conscious information processing (Nesse and Lloyd 1992). These mechanisms are active in distinct ways in healthy as well as disordered mental life, and therefore play an important role in psychological problems and disorders requiring psychotherapy (Allen and Gilbert 2000).

Competition between selfish motives and altruism may be an important source of intrapersonal conflict. The emotions of shame and guilt may have specifically evolved through group-selection and to maintain reciprocal relationships.

Natural selection has not favoured cognitive capacities to produce accurate images of the world, but to systematically distort conscious awareness and to block inadvertent access to non-conscious information processing. The cognitive ability to conceal one's real motives before the self is referred to as 'self-deception'.

The primary target of any therapeutic intervention, including psychotherapy, is the reduction of mental pain and subjective distress. Mental pain can be seen as an adaptive signal to alert the individual of impending or actual threats or losses. Psychopathology often arises if individuals are precluded from achieving biosocial goals and forced to use inappropriate defences as secondary strategies to achieve such goals. Excessive mental pain and suffering may result from continuing obstruction of reaching biosocial goals, and chronic activation of the physiological stress axis may lead to a vicious circle by producing anger, despair, and more distress (Gilbert 2006). The difference between adaptive mental pain and pathological mental pain causing suffering and enduring subjective distress is, however, a matter of degree, rather than category.

Mental pain can be seen as an adaptive signal to alert the individual of impending or actual threats or losses. Psychopathology often arises when individuals are precluded from achieving biosocial goals and forced to use inappropriate defences as secondary strategies to achieve biosocial goals.

Thwarting of biosocial goals may be caused by actual recent adverse or traumatic experiences, such as loss of job, divorce, or loss of important attachment figures (Gilbert 2006). However, current problems always need to be considered in light of an individual's personal history and endowment to cope with stressful life-events. Here, genetic variation, early experiences, and relationships with significant others, as well as gene–environment interaction affect an individual's actual vulnerability but also resilience against pathological stress responses.

Both healthy and disordered individuals possess several built-in means to reduce mental pain, to suppress painful memories, and to conceal unacceptable feelings or desires before the self by keeping them unconscious. The overarching mechanism through which this is achieved is commonly referred to as 'repression', a process akin to self-deception. Generally speaking, repression serves the function of actively distorting cognitive processes to decrease anxiety and keep dysfunctional pain out of conscious awareness (Northoff et al. 2007). It may also serve the purpose to inflate one's self-esteem so as to see one's role in social competition as more optimistic. Some therapeutic interventions actively promote self-deceptive processes, including those that utilize Buddhist meditative practice, such as assuming a 'non-judgemental' stance or 'radical acceptance' (Linehan 1993). This is, by no means, a bad thing, because it can help contain intense emotions and stabilize a fragile self. Repression is also ubiquitously involved in regulating important biosocial goals, including sexuality and interpersonal communication, which underscores that it increases an individual's biological fitness, unless it becomes inflexible and pervasive. This can happen, however, in situations in which an unresolved conflict remains active, and resurfaces unintentionally and repetitively in experience and behaviour.

Healthy and disordered individuals possess several built-in means to reduce mental pain, to suppress painful memories, and to conceal unacceptable or unmanageable feelings or desires before the self by keeping them unconscious. The overarching mechanism through which this is achieved is commonly referred to as 'repression'.

In its broader meaning, the term 'repression' embraces a set of self-deceptive defence mechanisms that combine denial of unmanageable feelings with different modes of representations of self and others, where the maturity of denial and representation are inversely correlated. Mature defences involve more sophisticated forms of denial, but less difficulties in self–other distinction, whereas immature defences are characterized by the inability to differentiate between own and others' mental states and, hence, loosening of ego-boundaries.

In its broader meaning, the term 'repression' embraces a set of self-deceptive defence mechanisms that combine denial of intolerable or unmanageable feelings with different modes of representations of self and others, where the maturity of denial and representation are inversely correlated. Mature defences involve more sophisticated forms of denial, but less difficulties in self–other distinction, whereas immature defences are characterized by the inability to differentiate between own and others' mental states and, hence, loosening of ego-boundaries. Accordingly, mature defence mechanisms comprise intellectualization (excessive use of abstract thinking to conceal unacceptable motives), rationalization (rational justification of emotionally motivated action), and sublimation (partial satisfaction of unconscious motives by means of culturally accepted activities), whereas introjection (internalizing values or characteristics of another person), projection (attribution of one's own desires to another person, where paranoid ideation is the psychotic extreme of projection), and projective identification (projection of one's own negative attributes to a significant other with the tendency to introject the originally projected attributes) are considered to be more ontogenetically 'primitive' and immature defence mechanisms. Other, relatively mature defence mechanisms are displacement, isolation, and reaction formation, with identification with the aggressor, dissociation, and fragmentation lying at the immature end of possible defences (Nesse and Lloyd 1992).

Since early social relationships with primary caregivers have lasting effects on an individual's attitudes towards present and future patterns of social interaction, and the way mentalities of others are appreciated, it is intuitively plausible that patients with early traumatic experiences have greater difficulties in mental state attribution, and hence use 'primitive' defence mechanisms more often than individuals who as children developed secure attachment and an autonomous state of mind.

Patients with early traumatic experiences have greater difficulties in mental state attribution, and use 'primitive' defence mechanisms more often than individuals who as children developed secure attachment and an autonomous state of mind.

However, the activation of mature versus immature defence mechanisms critically depends on the level of psychological distress. In situations associated with extreme real threats or dangers (such as warfare, being taken as hostage, and victimization through sexual coercion), perhaps everyone would tend to activate his or her attachment system, use more primitive defence mechanisms, and shut down one's mentalizing system. In other words, the activation of the attachment system inhibits mentalization in both normal and abnormal personality development (Fonagy 1991). For example, healthy individuals who fall in love tend to ignore less desirable features of the loved one. In a similar vein, people who have experienced recurrent traumata during early childhood chronically activate their attachment systems, and hence shut down their mentalizing systems. Consequently, traumatized individuals are particularly vulnerable to make use of immature defence mechanisms. Due to their impaired ability to accurately represent own and other's mental states, they may have more difficulties in distinguishing inner and outer reality, be more intolerant of alternative perspectives, or tend to constructing mental images of the world that no longer resemble reality. For example, a person with a history of childhood abuse may as an adult tend to identify with an abuser, disavow the abuser's malicious intents, or even direct negative affect towards the self in the way that he or she 'deserves' maltreatment. This may be particularly relevant if the abusive person is among the victim's own kin (Erickson 2006).

These examples may illustrate that mentalizing is at the core of evolved human psychology and individual development. As the costly side of the coin, the mentalizing system may be particularly vulnerable to dysfunction (see Chapters 3 and 4). However, this does by no means imply therapeutic nihilism. Rather, because the development of mentalizing abilities critically depends on environmental input, this cognitive capacity is one of the most 'open programmes', and therefore flexible enough to be reframed and modulated later in life. Mentalizing is essentially involved in regulation of social interaction between individuals, and should accordingly be actively encouraged and maintained in psychotherapeutic discourse. The therapist has the difficult task, however, to find the appropriate balance between inspiration of mentalizing in the patient and activation of the patient's attachment system.

The development of the mentalizing system critically depends on environmental input and one of the most 'open programmes'. Accordingly, it can be assumed that the mentalizing system is flexible enough to be reframed by therapeutic means. The therapist has the difficult task, however, to find the appropriate balance between inspiration of mentalizing in the patient and activation of the patient's attachment system.

Treating patients with severe personality disorders may therefore require a careful examination of the patient's ability to mentalize (Fonagy 1999). Poor mentalizers tend to focus on external social factors and the physical environment, and are often preoccupied with social rules and norms. At the same time, they may have difficulties in expressing anger when norms are violated by others. Poor mentalizers also tend to generalize and express rigidity or inappropriate certainty about thoughts and feelings of others. A possible explanation could be that emotionally unresponsive or unavailable primary caregivers, who themselves have difficulties in appreciating their child's mental states, may tend to overly induce shame and guilt in the child to sanction the child's selfish behaviour. Individuals who were reared in emotionally unresponsive conditions may then tend to obey those rules that are acceptable for the parent, but unconsciously act upon repressed selfish motives, and appreciate own and others' mental states only in an inflexible one-sided way. As adult patients or clients, these individuals may perhaps express overconfidence in their mental state attributions to others and deny objective realities that are not consistent with their self-interests and preferences.

Mentalizing in psychotherapy entails a process of joint attention focusing on the patient's mental states. This often requires an active role of the therapist by questioning and constructing images of the patient's mental states. The main goal is to help the patient access and explore his or her mental life and to encourage him or her to think about alternative perspectives on interpersonal processes (Bateman and Fonagy 2006). However, as mentalizing and attachment are inversely related, mentalizing may be discouraged when the patient is overwhelmed with emotions in favour of empathy and

As mentalizing and attachment are inversely related, mentalizing may be discouraged when the patient is overwhelmed with emotions in favour of empathy and support. A patient's ability to accept mentalizing interventions depends on his or her experience of the therapeutic relationship as a 'secure base'.

support. A patient's ability to accept mentalizing interventions depends on his or her experience of the therapeutic relationship as a 'secure base'. From such a base, patients may be able to adopt alternative, more trustful models of interpersonal relationships, to give up dysfunctional modes of repression, and to improve emotion regulation (Bateman and Fonagy 2004; Kellogg and Young 2006).

Focusing on the therapeutic relationship and mentalizing processes emphasizes the view that psychotherapy in general may benefit from insights of human cognitive and emotional evolution, and that one of the most recently evolved human capacities may be actively used to reduce subjective distress and suffering. Most 'schools' of psychotherapy, not only psychodynamic approaches, acknowledge that the quality of the therapeutic relationship influences outcome and prognosis of the therapeutic process (Linehan 1993; Beck 1999; Young et al. 2003). Likewise, working with patients' and therapists' mental states is part of many forms of psychotherapeutic interventions. Encouraging patients to apprehend their own mental states and those of significant others is certainly a useful tool across psychotherapeutic modalities, but should be carefully monitored, regardless of whether psychodynamic or cognitive–behavioural intervention techniques are preferred. Integrative therapies such as schema-focused therapy or mentalization-based therapy seek to focus on attachment issues and modes of how patients create inner models of their social environment. For example, schema therapy posits that individuals can operate in different modes, depending on their early experiences with caregivers. Accordingly, individuals who experienced their caregivers as emotionally unavailable or even abusive may enter the mode of an 'abandoned child', 'an aggressive and impulsive child', or a 'detached protector'. Others may be more prone to express a 'punitive parent mode', based on pathological identification and internalization of a rejecting and invalidating parenting style (Kellogg and Young 2006).

Integrative therapies such as schema-focused therapy or mentalization-based therapy seek to focus on attachment issues and modes of how patients create inner models of their social environment. Dysfunctional mentalization may emerge from adverse early experiences, such that patients 'regress' to more immature modes of mentalization.

Dysfunctional mentalization may emerge from adverse early experiences, such that patients 'regress' to more immature modes of mentalization. For example, individuals may be overwhelmed by re-experiencing traumatic memories, and enter a 'psychic equivalence mode' in which inner and outer reality become indistinguishable. Others may engage in 'pseudo-mentalization' ('pretend mode') and derogate themselves without any anchoring in 'real life'. Finally, 'teleological thinking' may occur as another dysfunctional mode of coping with distress, whereby inner states, such as feelings of psychological pain, are acted out through self-injurious behaviour (Bateman and Fonagy 2004).

Another issue that deserves clinical attention relates to patients' difficulties in being self-compassionate, which, again, is highly relevant for traumatized individuals. In fact, many patients seeking psychotherapy experience shame and guilt and are highly self-critical. In addition, many are sensitive to cues of rejection or criticism. Both may lead to the experience of a hostile internal and external environment (Gilbert 2009). Compassion-focused therapy is a therapeutic approach that focuses on the development of feelings associated with secure attachment, such as contentment, soothing, and self-compassion, which facilitate the development of more positive emotional experiences (Gilbert 2009, 2010, 2014; Kelly et al. 2012). Compassion-focused therapy explicitly refers to attachment theory and evolutionary concepts of threat perception, attachment, and motivation. It may be useful for reducing dissociative symptoms (Gilbert 2013), and in rehabilitation after psychotic episodes (Brähler et al. 2013).

Compassion-focused therapy is a therapeutic approach that focuses on the development of feelings associated with secure attachment, such as contentment, soothing and self-compassion, which facilitate the development of more positive emotional experiences.

In summary, integrative approaches to psychotherapy are much more in line with human evolutionary biology and neuroscience than puristic psychoanalysis or behaviourism. It seems that they can do justice better to many patients' needs and have better outcomes, at least in patients with BPD (e.g. Giesen-Bloo et al. 2006), even though more face-to-face comparison studies are warranted (Stoffers et al. 2012). Moreover, there is also a need for more 'objective' outcome measures of treatment, which may include changes in heart rate variability (as a sign of stress reduction) and other autonomic parameters (Bär et al. 2004; Garakani et al. 2009).

Collectively, integrative psychotherapy may help clients understand and change their (dysfunctional) individual life-history strategies. To reiterate, the term 'strategy' does not imply conscious decision-making. Rather, it refers to the way individuals pursue their biosocial goals, and to the proximate and ultimate causation that impacted on one's life-history strategy. Encouraging patients to understand their individual life-history patterns through psychotherapy may eventually aid them to modify some of their behaviours. Individuals with 'fast' life-history strategies, for example, may benefit from 'slowing' down, which may have profound implications for how they interact with partners, children, and their own parents. Conversely, clients with 'slow' patterns may improve upon 'accelerating' their life-history strategy by being more open to new experiences, etc., though the concept of life-history theory has not explicitly been utilized in psychotherapy, but certainly will be in the future.

Individuals with 'fast' life-history strategies may benefit from 'slowing' down, which may have profound implications for how they interact with partners, children, and their own parents. Conversely, clients with 'slow' patterns may improve upon 'accelerating' their life-history strategy by being more open to new experiences, etc.

22.5 Sex differences in response to psychotherapy

Differences in the psychology of men and women may influence psychotherapy in many ways. For example, differences between the sexes exist regarding vulnerability to psychosocial stressors. Adverse life events, such as disruption of an emotionally intense relationship, or physical or sexual abuse, usually have greater impact on females. Conversely, males may be particularly susceptible to develop psychological distress due to actual or impending loss of social status. These differences may not only account for greater prevalence rates of depression, anxiety disorders, and PTSD in women, but also for differences in seeking therapeutic help, and in response to treatment (Glantz and Pearce 1989). Differences between men and women are deeply anchored in divergent adaptations of men and women to problems relating to the need to cooperate, to form close relationships with kin, to compete for mates, and to successfully reproduce (for details see Chapter 1). Typically, men are selected to compete intrasexually for access to women. Women, by contrast, are selected to invest more heavily in potential offspring, and, therefore, to carefully select suitable mates. Human females are highly cooperative breeders, a mechanism through which humans were able to shorten interbirth intervals considerably. Men, in contrast to women, face the problem of uncertain paternity, which has led to greater sexual jealousy in men (whereas emotional jealousy can also be intense in women; for details see Chapters 1 and 16).

Differences between the sexes exist regarding vulnerability to psychosocial stressors.

In psychotherapy, these divergent behavioural tendencies in men and women may manifest in differences in verbalization of emotional problems, response to emotional and social support, use of submissive behaviours, dysfunctional coping strategies such as drug or alcohol abuse, challenging the value of therapy, and feelings of being stigmatized by therapy (Rasgon et al. 2000). Men, for example, are more likely to conceal emotions and feelings of inferiority or vulnerability, whereas women may 'attach' to the therapist more easily compared to men. So it could be that women, even though they more often suffer severe trauma, including those that transgress important personal boundaries such as physical or sexual abuse, respond better to psychotherapy, because of women's greater openness and superior ability to verbalize and re-integrate negative emotions. In contrast, men may experience psychotherapeutic aid as a threat to social status and independence, which could explain men's greater reluctance to seek therapy (Troisi and McGuire 2000).

In psychotherapy, divergent behavioural tendencies in men and women may manifest in differences in verbalization of emotional problems, response to emotional and social support, use of submissive behaviours, dysfunctional coping strategies such as drug or alcohol abuse, challenging the value of therapy, and feelings of being stigmatized by therapy.

Taking these differences between the sexes seriously suggests that, depending on the nature of the disorder or psychological problem, women may be better therapists for women, and men may be better therapists for men. Acknowledging sex differences in behaviour may also be useful in special therapeutic settings such as couples therapy and other systemic approaches (Glantz and Moehl 2000).

Afterthought: are there side-effects of psychotherapy?

The question whether or not psychotherapeutic interventions can have adverse effects has received little attention. The matter is indeed hard to address empirically, because, unlike studies into psychopharmacology, double-blind placebo-controlled approaches are impracticable. Anecdotal reports suggest, however, that transgression of therapeutic rules and norms by the therapist can occur, if counter-transference is poorly controlled and the therapist fails to maintain therapeutic abstinence. In extreme cases this may include a sexual relationship between therapist and client. Psychotherapists acting that way probably disregard the special vulnerability of patients seeking attachment and a secure base, or even mistake a client's dysfunctional sexual advances for mature behaviour. Although no data exist, such violations of rules of conduct in psychotherapy on the side of the therapist are probably rare. In the strict sense, norm violations in therapy cannot be considered side-effects, because, by definition, side-effects occur despite proper application of treatment.

From an evolutionary point of view, which emphasizes the role of non-verbal communication between client and therapist, the classic settings of psychoanalysis may produce harmful effects in patients whose disorders require visual contact and exchange of supportive non-verbal signals, or patients whose condition may deteriorate if regressive tendencies induce overwhelming feelings of helplessness. Thus, in the treatment of patients with severe depression or personality disorders, for example, techniques such as 'free association' while the therapist is out of sight of the patient may have deleterious side-effects. Moreover, patients who are traumatized or have otherwise developed insecure attachment styles do probably not benefit from therapeutic neutrality. Instead, many patients require active encouragement, positive motivation, reassurance, and empathy (Gilbert 2009).

A disturbing finding is that patients with severe personality disorder may experience a substantial reduction of symptoms or even remission without therapy, and that spontaneous recovery rates may even be higher than in patients who received treatment. One speculative explanation that has been suggested is that patients with severe personality disorders who have deficits in mentalizing have difficulties in integrating interventions in insight-oriented psychotherapies, that is, interpretations of the patient's mental states offered by the therapist. In other words, dissonance between the patient's inner experience and the therapist's interpretation thereof may cause emotional turmoil and instability. Thus, premature explanations of unconscious material should be avoided in such patients (Bateman and Fonagy 2006).

Conversely, helping patients to understand own and others' mental states may be harmful if these patients misuse the ability to mentalize for deceptive and exploitative (selfish) purposes. Individuals with psychopathy usually have highly developed mentalizing skills; however, they fail to empathize with others. Improving mentalizing in psychopaths may therefore have a profoundly negative impact on interpersonal relationships in many ways. For example, skilful psychopathic mentalizers may better be able to anticipate and predict the behaviour of potential victims. Moreover, violent psychopaths in forensic custody with good mentalizing qualities may have the potential to convince therapists of their apparent progress in therapy.

Many more scenarios of possible side-effects of psychotherapy are conceivable, including false memories that can have deleterious effects on relationships (Linden and Schermuly-Haupt 2014). Future studies may be able to clarify some of the issues raised in the preceding paragraphs. It seems essential to consider both client and therapist variables, as well as factors relating to the specific psychotherapeutic technique that is offered to the client (Barlow 2010). In any event, all psychotherapeutic tools should be critically evaluated in terms of differential indication and possible contraindications.

Chapter 23

Psychotropic medication—insights from evolutionary medicine

Abstract

The therapeutic options for psychiatric disorders have been dramatically advanced by the development of medication for almost all conditions. However, personalized treatment approaches need to carefully consider costs (potential harm) and benefits. All psychotropic drugs have side-effects in relevant areas of life, including social play (stimulants), sexual attractiveness and experience of pleasure (antipsychotics), and reproduction (serotonin reuptake inhibitors). Conversely, many psychotropic substances have antimicrobial or antiparasitic properties. Finally, most psychotropic drugs have modest effects, with placebo effects of similar magnitude. In fact, placebo effects in the treatment of any medical condition need to be taken into account, as they can reduce sickness behaviour, impact on the immune system, and thus play a profound role in healing procedures across cultures.

Keywords

psychotropic medication, side-effects, placebo effects, antimicrobial, antiparasitic, healing

23.1 Introductory remarks to psychotropic medication

In the last few decades, the therapeutic options for psychiatric disorders have dramatically advanced with the development of medication for almost all conditions that were hitherto untreatable. For example, the introduction of antipsychotic drugs in the 1950s has greatly improved the lives of many with schizophrenia and other psychotic disorders. Similarly, the development of antidepressants in the late 1950s and early 1960s has profoundly progressed the treatment of depression and anxiety disorders. Aside from tricyclic antidepressants and the newer drugs such as SNRI, lithium treatment for bipolar disorder has become a success story for many people with recurrent affective disorders. Even more recently, drug treatment has become available for other psychiatric conditions, including ADHD, Alzheimer's disease, and substance dependence,

The therapeutic options for psychiatric disorders have dramatically advanced with the development of medication for almost all conditions that were hitherto untreatable.

which has helped many to cope with signs and symptoms, to lead independent lives longer, and to reduce the risk of relapse (Lieberman 2003).

Before pharmacological treatments became available, a large number of patients with psychiatric disorders were detained in asylums, often for years or even lifelong, sometimes forced to live under inhumane conditions. Kraepelin has provided us with a detailed description of life and 'therapy' in eighteenth-century asylums in a remarkable article on '100 years of psychiatry' (Kraepelin 1920).

The reformation of psychiatric treatment and the release of thousands of in-patients from mental hospitals from the 1970s onwards would possibly have never happened without the availability of psychopharmacological therapy for acute symptoms and relapse prevention (e.g. Newton et al. 2000).

However, drugs have side-effects, such that every personalized treatment approach needs to carefully consider costs (potential harm) and benefits to the patient. Psychopharmacological agents are no exception, and it should be emphasized that all psychopharmacological approaches are purely symptomatic, not causal. This chapter does not aim at recapitulating the pharmacodynamics of psychopharmacological substances, possible side-effects, and interactions, which have been dealt with in many comprehensive volumes (e.g. Stahl 2000). Instead, it focuses on insights from evolutionary psycho(patho)logy with regard to potential limitations and contraindications of some of the most commonly prescribed substances. This view does not denigrate psychopharmacological treatment altogether. Rather, this chapter intends to present some adverse effects of psychopharmacological substances that are often insufficiently considered, or even deemed irrelevant with regard to possible consequences for social interaction.

Drugs have side-effects, such that every personalized treatment approach needs to carefully consider costs (potential harm) and benefits to the patient.

23.2 **Stimulants**

A widely prescribed substance for ADHD is methylphenidate (MPH), which acts on dopaminergic and adrenergic pathways in agonistic ways by blocking the dopamine and noradrenaline transporters (Stahl 2000). While it is hotly debated whether or not ADHD has been overdiagnosed in recent years or whether or not the number of ADHD children has genuinely increased, the reality is that prescription figures have dramatically risen since 1995 with up to 20 percent of schoolboys receiving MPH to down-regulate impulsivity and hyperactivity (Frances 2013).

Animal studies have revealed that stimulants, when given in large dosages, produce stereotypic movements. Research in rats has demonstrated, however, that MPH also suppressed social play in a dose-dependent fashion.

Common side-effects of MPH are loss of appetite, weight loss, and increase of blood pressure, whereas tolerance and sensitization are uncommon. With regard to its effects on cognition, studies have shown that MPH improves attention and working memory in individuals with ADHD and healthy subjects. In contrast, there is a paucity of research into the effect of MPH on human social behaviour. Animal studies have revealed that stimulants, when given in large dosages, produce stereotypic movements (Ridley and Baker 1982). More recently, research in rats has demonstrated, however, that MPH also suppressed social play in a dose-dependent fashion. Young rats usually engage in rough-and-tumble play (Panksepp 1998), a behaviour that is blocked by the administration of MPH in a dose range of 0.3–3.0 mg per kg body weight, which is orally effective in the treatment of ADHD (Vanderschuren et al. 2008). In contrast, social exploration and locomotion were unaffected by MPH, yet the specific effect on social play pertained to both the initiation and the responsiveness to the initiation of rough-and-tumble play.

Similar effects have been demonstrated for atomoxetine, a noradrenaline reuptake inhibitor, but not for dopamine reuptake inhibitors, suggesting that the play-suppressing effect is modulated by noradrenaline (Vanderschuren et al. 2008). Although animal studies do not prove that identical effects can be expected in human subjects, the selective suppression of social play at therapeutic dosages suggests that this facet of behavioural suppression could play a role in human children receiving MPH. Social play is of eminent importance for children's social, physical, and intellectual development, making it imperative to scrutinize social play in children receiving MPH.

Social play is of eminent importance for children's social, physical, and intellectual development, making it imperative to scrutinize social play in children receiving MPH.

23.3 **Antipsychotics**

From the perspective of adverse effects, first-generation antipsychotic (FGA) substances are well known for their propensity to cause movement disorders (which is why they were called 'neuroleptics'), foremost acute dystonia, parkinsonism, and akathisia, and occasionally tardive dyskinesia. These side-effects arise from the dopamine-antagonizing properties of FGA. Ethologically speaking, akathisia resembles so-called displacement activities, indicating motivational ambivalence concerning flight or fight behaviour (Brüne et al. 1998).

Movement disorders caused by antipsychotics certainly contribute to stigmatization of patients, because abnormalities of gait, posture, or speech, especially when moderate to severe, can even be recognized by laypersons. Compared to FGA, newer or second-generation antipsychotics (SGA) cause movement disorders much less frequently. However, SGA are fraught with the problem of promoting metabolic syndromes, associated with weight gain, diabetes, and other medical conditions. Other side-effects of antipsychotics include skin manifestations (acne, hair loss, photosensibility and premature skin aging, hirsutism, pigmentation, and change in body odour), all of which contribute to undermining an individual's physical attractiveness (Seeman 2011). Evolutionary theory suggests that physical attractiveness is important for successful mating (see Chapter 1), and it seems that antipsychotics may alter the waist-to-hip ratio, body symmetry, etc. in negative ways.

Movement disorders caused by antipsychotics contribute to stigmatization of patients, because abnormalities of gait, posture, or speech, especially when moderate to severe, can even be recognized by laypersons. Other side-effects of antipsychotics include skin manifestations (acne, hair loss, photosensibility and premature skin aging, hirsutism, pigmentation, and change in body odour), all of which contribute to undermining an individual's physical attractiveness.

In light of hypotheses suggesting that schizophrenia could be associated with enhanced fluctuating asymmetry (see Chapter 8), antipsychotic treatment may actually worsen the situation. This underresearched issue is critical, not least because schizophrenia and related psychoses manifest in young people around the peak of fecundity (Paus et al. 2008).

Another critical issue associated with antipsychotic drug treatment concerns negative symptoms such as avolition, apathy, and anhedonia. Among these symptoms, social anhedonia, that is, the inability to appreciate social interaction as rewarding, has become a focus of specific interest, because the severity of social anhedonia contributes to poor social functioning and reduced quality of life in schizophrenia (Hooker et al. 2014). Antipsychotic medication, particularly FGA, can produce or enhance anhedonia through excessive blockade of dopaminergic pathways that are known to be involved in reward processing (Kirkpatrick 2014). In fact, there is currently no drug treatment available for social anhedonia or negative symptoms in general, rendering this issue a hitherto unmet need in psychosis therapy (Chue and Lalonde 2014).

Social anhedonia, that is, the inability to appreciate social interaction as rewarding, may be caused by antipsychotic medication. The severity of social anhedonia contributes to poor social functioning and reduced quality of life in schizophrenia.

23.4 Antidepressants

SSRI have been prescribed for depression, anxiety disorders, OCD, PTSD, binge-eating disorder, and other conditions. In some places, SSRI have even become lifestyle drugs to increase subjective well-being. Related to this, there has been a debate about the promotion of 'disease mongering', whereby illness boundaries are widened in unjustifiable ways, turning healthy individuals into patients (Moynihan and Henry 2006).

In any event, compared to tricyclic antidepressants, SSRI are often better tolerated, because they lack the typical anticholinergic side-effects of the former, including dry mouth, orthostatic dysregulation, and constipation. However, uncritical prescription of antidepressants is unwarranted due to several adverse effects, which, from an evolutionary psychological point of view, deserve special attention. Aside from reports suggesting that antidepressants have modest efficacy and may be superior to placebo only in severe (but not mild to moderate depression) depression, they can even be detrimental to brain function and promote apoptosis (cell death) and perhaps increase the risk of relapse in depression (Andrews et al. 2012). In addition, given the role of serotonin in regulating a large spectrum of body functions (see Chapter 2), it is unsurprising that elevation of serotonin levels impacts on many metabolic processes involved in maintaining homeostasis. So, there are widespread adverse effects of SSRI affecting the gut, cardiovascular system, and reproduction. With regard to the latter, tricyclic antidepressants and SSRI seem to impair sperm motility, volume, and morphology. They may also reduce sexual desire and arousal. SSRI delay ejaculation, an effect that has been used therapeutically in patients with social anxiety disorder and premature ejaculation (Tignol et al. 2006). Adverse effects of SSRI on human sexuality may also include a negative impact on attachment and romantic love (Fisher and Thomson 2006; Andrews et al. 2012), which may relate to research suggesting that SSRI have general effects on all emotions, that is, they may reduce not only negative emotions (desired effect), but also positive emotions and promote emotional withdrawal (Price et al. 2009).

SSRI have become lifestyle drugs to increase subjective well-being. Related to this, there has been a debate about the promotion of 'disease mongering', whereby illness boundaries are widened in unjustifiable ways, turning healthy individuals into patients.

Related to this, one of the most contentious issues in psychiatry concerns the question whether or not SSRI may increase the risk for suicidal behaviour. The evidence for this is mixed, though it would seem that SSRI may actually increase the risk for suicide in adolescents, but not in older populations (Andrews et al. 2012). While suicidal acts are generally rare in patients taking SSRI, a conservative stance would suggest carefully weighing benefits against potential costs of prescribing antidepressants.

Since DSM-5 has lowered the threshold for diagnosing depression in people suffering from grief (which, to some degree, overlaps with depression with regard to symptoms, including pain, preoccupation, loss of energy, guilt, and self-criticism), it is also a matter of controversy whether antidepressants are helpful or harmful in dealing with bereavement. This discussion is further pushed by reports suggesting that SSRI may cause emotional blunting and detachment (Price et al. 2009).

Antidepressants can be detrimental to brain function and promote apoptosis (cell death) and perhaps increase the risk of relapse in depression. Other adverse effects of SSRI affect the gut, cardiovascular system, and reproduction.

In essence, grief is part of humanness and an integral of our behavioural repertoire. It is unclear, though, if grief can be seen as an adaptation (akin to cough and fever) to the loss of a close relationship or as a by-product of attachment (Archer 1999; Nesse 2005). Archer (1999) has argued, for instance, that grief cannot be an adaptation, because it is associated with significant costs, including damage to the immune system and possibly premature death of the bereaving individual. Consistent with attachment theory and kinship theory (Hamilton 1964; Bowlby 1969) the severity of bereavement is associated with the degree of genetic relatedness to the deceased person. Conversely, grief may serve as a self-protective mechanism, similar to other negative emotions that incur costs, but are outweighed by their benefits as a defence (Nesse 2005). Schiefenhövel (2000) has described from a cross-cultural perspective how grief can be contained in ritual ceremonies, thereby providing social support for the grieving individual, which helps recuperate and integrate overwhelmingly strong emotions.

SSRI have general effects on all emotions; that is, they may reduce not only negative emotions (the desired effect), but also positive emotions and promote emotional withdrawal.

Grief may serve as a self-protective mechanism, similar to other negative emotions that incur costs but are outweighed by their benefits as a defence. Thus it may not be indicated to prescribe antidepressants for this condition.

That said, it is perhaps premature to unequivocally suggest abstaining from antidepressive drug treatment of bereavement. However, caution is warranted in regard to interfering with behaviour regulation systems by means of pharmacological treatment.

23.5 Stress, immunology, and pharmacophagy

In the preceding chapters, it has repetitively been discussed how psychopathology may interact with immune function. One possible mechanism involves the stress-dependent secretion of catecholamines (Freestone et al. 2008). Epinephrine and norepinephrine, for example, promote bacterial growth, whereas dopamine may, in addition, enhance the virulence of gram-negative and gram-positive bacteria (Roshchina 2010). Conversely, many bacteria have the potential to produce these substances in large quantities, which may interact with the host's behaviour in manifold ways (Roshchina 2010). Some algae species are able to deter sear urchins and snails by the secretion of dopamine. Other neurotransmitters such as acetylcholine play a role in the regulation of motility in unicellular organisms, whereas serotonin and histamine are involved in cellular aggregation. Depending on the concentration, these biomediators can act at the level of unicellular organisms as attractants or repellents (Roshchina 2010).

In plants, many of these agents impact on cell permeability and regulate growth, as well as fertilization. Moreover, serotonin and melatonin may serve as antioxidants. Over evolutionary time, eukaryotes 'co-opted' the function of biomediators for communication among neurons and other cells (Christophersen 1991). Since many unicellular organisms may have symbiotic as well as pathogenic (parasitic) relationships with their hosts, secretion of stress hormones may change the entire microbiotic environment, known as 'microbial endocrinology' (Freestone et al. 2008). Notably, plants have evolved strategies to shield themselves against micro-organisms. For example, many alkaloids inhibit the proliferation of bacteria, viruses, and fungi, while also being toxic for many insects and vertebrates (Roshchina 2010).

Many bacteria have the potential to produce catecholamines in large quantities to promote growth. Over evolutionary time, eukaryotes 'co-opted' the function of biomediators, such as catecholamines and acetylcholine, for communication among neurons and other cells. Secretion of stress hormones may change the entire microbiotic environment.

Animals, in turn, particularly herbivores, have evolved countermeasures against toxic plant products, including enzymatic degradation. In addition, the consumption of toxic plant products may serve the purpose to ingest antimicrobial, fungicidal, or antihelminthic substances, which may actually outweigh the risk of dangerous intoxication. This has been termed 'pharmacophagy', which is not specific for humans, but widespread among other animals, including non-human primates (Fabrega 1997). For example, several alkaloids such as caffeine, nicotine, and arecolin are antiparasitic when orally ingested (Sullivan and Hagen 2002; St John-Smith et al. 2013). As 'side-effects' these substances often act on the reward system and increase, for example, focused attention and endurance (St John-Smith et al. 2013).

Plants have evolved strategies to shield themselves against micro-organisms. In animals, the consumption of toxic plant products may serve the purpose to ingest antimicrobial, fungicidal, or antihelminthic substances. As 'side-effects' these substances often act on the reward system and increase focused attention and endurance.

In addition, many chemical substances that have been developed for therapeutic modification of the central nervous system function have antiparasitic properties, because they are structurally similar to toxic plant products (summarized in St John-Smith et al. 2013). For example, piperazine derivates, which include several anxiolytic, antidepressant, and antipsychotic substances, are antihelminthic, whereby the downside is that many novel 'designer drugs' are chemically also derivates of piperazine (St John-Smith et al. 2013).

Taken together, neurotransmitter systems are, by no means, just that. In addition to their direct action on the nervous system, these biomediators are involved in the regulation of microbiota–host interaction. Stress may destabilize the balance between beneficial (symbiotic) and detrimental (pathogenic) interaction. Deliberate ingestion of substances with psychotropic effects may, in the first place, have emerged from their utilization as antiparasitic toxins produced by plants (Sullivan et al. 2008). In other words, the psychotropic effect of these substances may be a by-product of the consumption of natural medicines. Conversely, the findings that substances with greater affinity to neurotransmitter receptors also have antiparasitic properties may underscore the view that evolution is a thrifty process that does not squander scarce resources.

Biomediators are involved in the regulation of microbiota–host interaction. Stress may destabilize the balance between beneficial (symbiotic) and detrimental (pathogenic) interaction.

Afterthought: mechanisms involved in the placebo effect

In medicine, the placebo effect has long been treated with ignorance and denial, at least as something that has no proper place in the treatment of medical conditions. In randomized placebo-controlled trials, the placebo effect has been negatively defined as 'noise' that needs to be distinguished from the 'signal' of efficacious medical treatment. In the most general vein, placebo effects include observations suggesting that larger number of pills work better than fewer, capsules better than tablets, intravenous administration better than oral, more expensive treatments better than cheaper ones, etc. (McQueen et al. 2013a, 2013b). Painkillers seem to be more effective than placebo, but only if given overtly, whereas covertly given substances such as the cholecystokinin antagonist proglumide are not superior to placebo (Benedetti et al. 1995).

Placebo effects appear to be related to patient variables such as expectations, motivation, conditioning, and personality factors and to therapist variables including communication style, compassion, and authority, as well as to patient–clinician interaction, that is, rapport, containment, and attachment. Reducing the placebo effect to the 'noise' in a signal-to-noise equation disregards, however, that placebo can be associated with spectacularly large effect sizes statistically, sometimes even larger than evidence-based treatments (termed the 'efficacy paradox'; McQueen and St John Smith 2012). Instead of discarding the placebo effect as being outside any scientific view on suffering, it seems warranted to ask questions such as why treatment success is apparently so dependent on irrational (and difficult to control) aspects of the human psyche and what evolutionary approaches can contribute to the understanding of the placebo effect.

From an evolutionary vantage point, it is striking to observe that healing rituals exist in virtually all known cultures, often tied to spiritual beliefs (Fabrega 1997, 2002), and that healing rituals can indeed be helpful in coping with illness (Schiefenhövel 1986). In fact, some scholars have argued that humans are particularly susceptible to 'medical disinformation' (i.e. placebo treatment) and take advantage of this susceptibility to see the world more optimistically than is justified by the evidence. Indirectly, by positively influencing one's mood, the prospects of finding a cure may indeed improve (Humphrey and Skoyles 2012).

Aside from defensive behaviour such as nausea, pain, and fever, sickness behaviour can be seen as an adaptive response to somatic illness. It involves a reduction of physical activity and drive, withdrawal, avoidance of certain foods, loss of appetite, and subjective feeling of low mood (Fabrega 1997). Sickness behaviour can be observed in non-human animals, and it helps save energy and avoids additional threats to the weakened and vulnerable organism. However, the expression of sickness behaviour is influenced by social contingencies such as mating opportunities and parental investment, which should down-regulate sickness behaviour as a survival strategy in favour of reproduction. Conversely, when changes of reproduction are low, organisms may tend to invest more in sickness behaviour, which may have implications for the understanding of depression and other psychiatric conditions in which immunological processes play a role (Lopes 2014).

In any event, from a psychological perspective, sickness behaviour emerges from biological dysfunction (disease), but also entails illness as a 'lived experience of distress' (Miller et al. 2009). The latter concerns an individual's attempt to integrate his or her subjective experience into something meaningful, which takes into account culture, social norms and values, as well as personal preferences and attitudes. Along similar lines, natural healing is different from technological and interpersonal healing. Natural healing involves somatic defence mechanisms against disease or injury; technological healing concerns any intervention that targets a specific sign or symptom, and can include prescription of medication or surgery. Interpersonal healing entails a relationship between healer and sufferer, often requiring participation of the patient.

Theoretically, placebo effects can occur in any one of these healing processes. However, interpersonal healing may be most susceptible to placebo effects, for example, if the ritual healing procedure is combined with some apotropaic extraction magic (Schiefenhövel 1986), thereby strengthening somatic defence mechanisms, rather than influencing the disease process itself (Nesse 2008). Whichever healing mode is employed, there is now increasing evidence to suggest that placebo effects impact on the autonomic nervous system, suggesting that the placebo effect does not necessarily require conscious reflection (Meissner 2011).

Much of the placebo effect can probably be traced back to attachment-related interpersonal factors that impact on the quality of therapeutic alliances. Decades ago, psychoanalytic schools have recognized the relevance of these processes, termed 'containment', 'attunement', or 'holding' (summarized in McQueen and St John-Smith 2012; McQueen et al. 2013). These considerations may explain why different psychotherapeutic interventions are practically indistinguishable with regard to efficacy, sometimes referred to as 'equivalence paradox' (McQueen et al. 2013a, 2013b). Put another way, in psychotherapy, specific intervention techniques explain less of the variance in outcome compared to non-specific aspects such as being in therapy. This seems to support the view suggesting that placebo mechanisms play an important role in psychotherapeutic treatment. However, it has been argued that many psychological interventions are different from mere placebo effects, because the former entail an 'alliance effect', induced by a deliberate medical alliance between a patient and a clinician (ideally involving shared decision-making), whereas the placebo effect involved a deliberate suggestion of clinical benefit (Verhulst et al. 2013). Thus, the quality of the patient–clinician relationship makes a significant contribution to the soothing of anxiety, which increases the success of healing and improves outcome (Meissner et al. 2011). These considerations suggest that it remains imperative—in light of an increasingly technicalized medicine—to safeguard medical care against anonymity, impersonality, and unfriendliness (McQueen et al. 2013a, 2013b).

Epilogue: why psychiatry and psychosomatic medicine need evolution

Much of what follows in this epilogue has been repetitively emphasized in preceding chapters. The most important issues—at least in my point of view—shall nevertheless be summarized, because I would like to envisage future psychiatry to be taken further as a pluralistic medical discipline that is thoroughly grounded in the framework of human biology.

Current diagnostic systems (the Diagnostic and Statistical Manual of Mental Disorders (DSM), 5th edition, and the forthcoming International Classification of Disorders (ICD), 11th edition) were conceptualized as largely atheoretical, purely descriptive frameworks to improve reliability and validity of the diagnostic process. In spite of the fact that these instruments have greatly facilitated communication between clinicians across divergent theoretical backgrounds, DSM and ICD are flawed by disregarding aetiological factors of psychiatric disorders, including idiographic material in favour of a nomothetic approach (Banzato 2004; Kramer 2014). Another unresolved problem is that current diagnostic manuals are insufficient in their ability to appreciate sex differences in the presentation of psychopathological signs and symptoms. DSM and ICD are also reductionist in that they constrain the richness of psychopathological signs and symptoms to a compilation of only the most conspicuous clinical symptomatology of disorders. The clinician is asked to make a diagnosis by choosing several signs and symptoms from a list that is neither exhaustive nor (in many instances) factor-analytically validated. Even though DSM and ICD are not designed that way, both manuals suggest the existence of nosological categories of psychiatric disorders. The inexperienced beginner may therefore be tempted to use either one as a surrogate textbook of psychiatry.

Similarly, contemporary psychiatry has put too much emphasis on structured interview technique, obviously at the expense of behavioural observation, and largely oblivious to the emotional content of communication (Richer 2014). Moreover, the current trend in psychiatry to conceptualize psychiatric disorders according to biological findings is one-sided, in that pathogenetic aspects are, by and large, reduced to abnormal brain functions, whereas aetiological issues of disorders usually comprise a conglomerate of hereditary (genetic) and acquired features that profoundly impact on individual life-history strategies.

This suggests that the suffix 'biological' to psychiatry appears greatly impoverished by equating 'biological' with findings from genetics, the activity of neurotransmitter systems, drug action, and perhaps brain imaging, while grossly neglecting the biology of evolved human social systems (i.e. the interpersonal dimension), with all their cognitive, emotional, and behavioural facets. In fact, it sometimes appears as if the term 'behaviour' (at least systematic behavioural observation) has been banished from the psychiatric literature, perhaps as a consequence of the fact that the value of a thorough psychiatric examination and description of psychopathology have been belittled, whereas the explanatory power of genetic findings has been inflated. For example, current research into psychiatric genetics greatly focuses on the impact of neurotrophins, only to discover that these factors are apparently not specific to any one particular disorder. Moreover, research in psychiatric genetics has surprisingly ignored many implications from evolutionary theory. For example, there is evidence to suggest that many alleles that predispose to the manifestation of psychiatric conditions have undergone positive selection in recent human history. While it is implausible to assume that such variation has occurred without biological meaning, psychiatric genetics is only beginning to acknowledge gene–environment correlation and interaction, and concepts such as 'differential susceptibility' (see Chapters 1 and 3).

Moreover, research and clinical practice are no longer equally covered by current diagnostic systems. While DSM and ICD draw lines between anxiety disorders and depression or between schizophrenia and bipolar affective disorder, respectively, research suggests that no natural boundaries between these disorders exist, in terms of neither genetics nor behaviour. Contrariwise, research itself is flawed by directing scientific enquiries along the lines of supposed 'disease entities'. A useful step in the right direction is certainly the description of endophenotypes (see Chapter 1), even though most biological markers are currently less useful for clinical purposes, and the available ones, such as the dexamethasone test, TRH test, and low CSF 5-HIAA in depression, are largely non-specific.

Accordingly, one of the most important purposes of this book is to draw attention to the fact that current psychiatry lacks a coherent theory of human behaviour. As predicted in the Epilogue of the first edition of this textbook, DSM-5 and ICD-11 will fail to address these problems (see also Stein et al. 2013).

It would seem that two things stand out that need to be addressed in the future: one refers to the fact that future conceptualizations of psychopathological conditions ought to more decisively eradicate categorical thinking in psychiatry and replace it by a dimensional approach, for which there is overwhelming empirical evidence. The second issue pertains to the necessary, radical, and unequivocal acknowledgement of two complementary and equally important historical processes that guide human experience and behaviour: one relates to the patient's individual, personal history; this should be standard in psychiatric examination. The other affects the evolved history of humans as a species; our psychological apparatus has been shaped by natural and sexual selection over aeons and this still determines how we experience, explore, and interact with our environment. In many respects, we strongly resemble other primates in our needs for attachment, security, gregariousness, social status, and trustworthy alliances with our fellow human beings. It ought to be part of the psychiatric examination to evaluate the possible function of cognitions, emotions, and behaviours in psychopathological conditions by extrapolating from the pathology to its physiological correlates. In other words, human behaviour, even in its most grotesque and distorted variations, has a function, or, at the very least, a physiological equivalent that can be examined in two ways: at the proximate level and at the ultimate level (Brüne et al. 2012).

One possible suggestion for future psychiatric manuals could be to reframe the multiaxial diagnostic system along the lines of the four 'W' questions proposed by Nikolaas Tinbergen (Nesse 2013; Brüne 2014b). These axial dimensions should include (1) a thorough description of current symptomatology (including behaviour), (2) examination of allelic variation of candidate genes and/or other biological markers, (3) assessment of early adverse events and other environmental risk factors, (4) evaluation of performance in achieving important biosocial goals, and (5) examination of the functional significance of psychopathological signs and symptoms by comparison with their evolved (adapted) equivalent. This would imply a paradigmatic shift; however, such a modified approach could help both to tailor individual treatment and to create a common ground for research into behavioural genetics, gene–environment correlations, animal models, psychotherapy, cross-cultural research, and neuropsychology of psychiatric disorders. Although no silver bullet exists, framing human psychopathological conditions along these lines utilizing life-history theory (e.g. Del Giudice 2014) may anchor psychiatry more thoroughly in evolutionary theory and neuroscience.

In terms of therapy, a most promising way to improve therapist–client interaction is to emphasize more strongly how minds interact—namely, by making inferences about one another's beliefs, goals, wishes, knowledge, and emotions. Patients' desires, needs, aims, and means to achieve important biosocial goals are not so much different from our own. Accordingly, it could be advisable to more often take the patient's perspective, or even to routinely include the attempt to see the situation with the patient's eyes, in both the diagnostic evaluation process and therapy.

Considering the evolutionary perspective in therapy can sometimes seem to be a perversion of what we believe is morally acceptable. For example, some psychopathological conditions can be interpreted as (unconscious) exploitative strategies of social systems and mental health services. Similarly, the romanticized view of mental health as a natural state of kindness and subjective well-being has been challenged by evolutionary theory; happiness has probably never been a target of selection (Nesse 2004); however, the pleasurable state of mind associated with happiness perhaps has been. Suffering—narrowly defined—can be regarded as an evolutionary by-product of self-awareness and conscious reflection upon one's own existence, or the empathic representation of another's illness. Moreover, psychiatric disorders cannot simply be defined as a combination of harmfulness to the individual and dysfunction of some psychological mechanism—this would leave out important contextual factors. The very same behaviour may be dysfunctional and harmful to the individual in one environment and entirely functional and beneficial in another. These differences in appreciating psychological distress in evolutionary perspective compared to standard psychiatric views largely arise from the relevance of examining functional significance; this is, however, necessary to improve therapy, for example, by making some of these unconscious processes accessible to patients' conscious reflections.

We, as therapists, want mental health for everybody, and rightly claim this as a moral imperative. Part of the story is that we empathize with others who are in need or suffer due to our evolved humaneness. This should also guide our therapeutic behaviour. However, as therapists we will never be able to eliminate psychological distress and mental illness. As long as humans exist, there will be conflict over social matters—resources, mates, alliances, and so forth. We nevertheless can encourage patients to change perspectives, perhaps sometimes to give up unrealistic goals. At present (and hopefully in the future), one cannot change an individual's genome, but environmental conditions, which indirectly influence epigenetic processes, such as gene methylation and gene expression, can be changed. Above all, we should do everything possible to create environments for our children that are worth living in. This, of course, includes the necessity to provide them with security, emotional warmth, and the possibility to explore the environment from a secure base. In other words, preventing psychiatric disorders is the best therapy. However, patients with psychiatric disorder often did not have the chance to grow up under favourable circumstances. Nevertheless, appreciating those environmental conditions to which humans have primarily adapted may greatly enrich treatment options for our fellow human beings.

References

Aase, H. & Sagvolden, T. (2006). Infrequent, but not frequent, reinforcers produce more variable responding and deficient sustained attention in young children with attention-deficit/hyperactivity disorder (ADHD). *J Child Psychol Psychiatry*, **47**, 457–71.

Abad-Rodriguez, J., Ledesma, M.D., Craessaerts, K., et al. (2004). Neuronal membrane cholesterol loss enhances amyloid peptide generation. *J Cell Biol*, **167**, 953–60.

Abecasis, G.R., Auton, A., Brooks, L.D., et al. (2012). An integrated map of genetic variation from 1,092 human genomes. *Nature*, **491**, 56–65.

Abed, R.T. (1998). The sexual competition hypothesis for eating disorders. *Br J Med Psychol*, **71**, 525–547.

Abed, R.T. (2000). Psychiatry and Darwinism. Time to reconsider? *Br J Psychiatry*, **177**, 1–3.

Abed, R.T. & Abbas, M.J. (2011). A reformulation of the social brain theory for schizophrenia: the case for out-group intolerance. *Perspect Biol Med*, **54**, 132–51.

Abed, R.T. & Abbas, M.J. (2014). Can the new epidemiology of schizophrenia help elucidate its causation? *Irish J Psychol Med*, **31**, 1–5.

Abed, R.T. & De Pauw, K.W. (1998). An evolutionary hypothesis for obsessive compulsive disorder: a ~psychological immune system? *Behav Neurol*, **11**, 245–50.

Abed, R., Mehta, S., Figueredo, A.J., et al. (2012). Eating disorders and intrasexual competition: testing an evolutionary hypothesis among young women. *Scientific World Journal*, **2012**, 1–8.

Abell, F. & Hare, D.J. (2005). An experimental investigation of the phenomenology of delusional beliefs in people with Asperger syndrome. *Autism*, **9**, 515–31.

Aboitiz, F. (1992). Mechanisms of adaptive evolution. Darwinism and Lamarckism restated. *Med Hypotheses*, **38**, 194–202.

Aboitiz, F., Morales, D., & Montiel, J. (2003). The evolutionary origin of the mammalian isocortex: towards an integrated developmental and functional approach. *Behav Brain Sci*, **26**, 535–52; discussion 552–85.

Abrams, K.M. & Robinson, G.E. (1998). Stalking. Part I: an overview of the problem. *Can J Psychiatry*, **43**, 473–76.

Abrams, M.P., Carleton, R.N., Taylor, S., & Asmundson, G.J. (2009). Human tonic immobility: measurement and correlates. *Depress Anxiety*, **26**, 550–56.

Abu-Akel, A. (1999). Impaired theory of mind in schizophrenia. *Pragmatics Cognition*, **7**, 247–82.

Abu-Akel, A. & Bailey, A.L. (2000). The possibility of different forms of theory of mind impairment in psychiatric and developmental disorders. *Psychol Med*, **30**, 735–38.

Addington, J., Saeedi, H., & Addington, D. (2006a). Influence of social perception and social knowledge on cognitive and social functioning in early psychosis. *Br J Psychiatry*, **189**, 373–78.

Addington, J., Saeedi, H., & Addington, D. (2006b). Facial affect recognition: a mediator between cognitive and social functioning in psychosis? *Schizophr Res*, **85**, 142–50.

Aderka, I.M., Weisman, O., Shahar, G., & Gilboa-Schechtman, E. (2009). The roles of the social rank and attachment systems in social anxiety. *Pers Individ Diff*, **47**, 284–88.

Adolphs, R. (1999). Social cognition and the human brain. *Trends Cogn Sci*, **3**, 469–79.

Adolphs, R. (2001). The neurobiology of social cognition. *Curr Opin Neurobiol*, **11**, 231–39.

Adolphs, R., Tranel, D., Damasio, H., & Damasio, A. (1994). Impaired recognition of emotion in facial expressions following bilateral damage to the human amygdala. *Nature*, **372**, 669–72.

Adolphs, R., Damasio, H., & Tranel, D. (2002). Neural systems for recognition of emotional prosody: a 3-D lesion study. *Emotion*, **2**, 23–51.

Agay, N., Kron, S., Carmel, Z., Mendlovic, S., & Levkovitz, Y. (2008). Ultimatum bargaining behavior of people affected by schizophrenia. *Psychiatry Res*, **157**, 39–46.

Ahluwalia, I.B., Mack, K.A., & Mokdad, A. (2004). Mental and physical distress and high-risk behaviors among reproductive-age women. *Obstet Gynecol*, **104**, 477–83.

Aiello, L.C. & Wheeler, P. (1995). The expensive-tissue hypothesis—the brain and the digestive-system in human and primate evolution. *Current Anthropol*, **36**, 199–221.

Ainsworth, M.D. & Bell, S.M. (1970). Attachment, exploration, and separation: illustrated by the behavior of one-year-olds in a strange situation. *Child Dev*, **41**, 49–67.

Akiskal, K.K. & Akiskal, H.S. (2005). The theoretical underpinnings of affective temperaments: implications for evolutionary foundations of bipolar disorder and human nature. *J Affect Disord*, **85**, 231–39.

Alcock, J. (2001). *The Triumph of Sociobiology*. Oxford University Press, Oxford.

Alegret, M., Junque, C., Valldeoriola, F., et al. (2001). Obsessive-compulsive symptoms in Parkinson's disease. *J Neurol Neurosurg Psychiatry*, **70**, 394–96.

Alexander, R.D. (1987). *The Biology of Moral Systems*. A. de Gruyter, Hawthorne, New York.

Allen, C. & Bekoff, M. (1994). Intentionality, social play, and definition. *Biol Philos*, **9**, 63–74.

Allen, J.P., Moore, C., Kuperminc, G., & Bell, K. (1998). Attachment and adolescent psychosocial functioning. *Child Development*, **69**, 1406–19.

Allen, J.S. & Sarich, V.M. (1988). Schizophrenia in an evolutionary perspective. *Perspectives Biol Med*, **32**, 132–53.

Allen, N.B. & Badcock, P.B. (2003). The social risk hypothesis of depressed mood: evolutionary, psychosocial, and neurobiological perspectives. *Psychol Bull*, **129**, 887–913.

Allen, N.B. & Gilbert, P. (2000). Social intelligence, deception, and psychopathology: a challenge for cognitive therapy? In: Gilbert, P. & Bailey, K.G. (eds) *Genes on the Couch. Explorations in Evolutionary Psychotherapy*. Brunner-Routledge, Hove.

Allison, A.C. (1954). Protection afforded by the sickle cell trait against subtertian malarial infection. *Br Med J*, **1**, 290–94.

Allman, J.M. (1999). *Evolving Brains*. Scientific American Library, New York. Distributed by W.H. Freeman and Co.

Allman, J. & Brothers, L. (1994). Neuropsychology—faces, fear and the amygdala. *Nature*, **372**, 613–14.

Allman, J.M., Hakeem, A., Erwin, J.M., Nimchinsky, E., & Hof, P. (2001). The anterior cingulate cortex. The evolution of an interface between emotion and cognition. *Ann N Y Acad Sci*, **935**, 107–17.

Allman, J.M., Tetreault, N.A., Hakeem, A.Y., et al. (2010). The von Economo neurons in frontoinsular and anterior cingulate cortex in great apes and humans. *Brain Struct Funct*, **214**, 495–517.

Allman, J.M., Tetreault, N.A., Hakeem, A.Y., et al. (2011). The von Economo neurons in the frontoinsular and anterior cingulate cortex. *Ann N Y Acad Sci*, **1225**, 59–71.

Almli, L.M., Fani, N., Smith, A.K., & Ressler, K.J. (2014). Genetic approaches to understanding post-traumatic stress disorder. *Int J Neuropsychopharmacol*, **17**, 355–70.

Altemus, M., Dhabhar, F.S., & Yang, R. (2006). Immune function in PTSD. *Ann N Y Acad Sci*, **1071**, 167–83.

Amad, A., Ramoz, N., Thomas, P., Jardri, R., & Gorwood, P. (2014). Genetics of borderline personality disorder: systematic review and proposal of an integrative model. *Neurosci Biobehav Rev*, 40C, 6–19.

Amaral, D.G. (2002). The primate amygdala and the neurobiology of social behavior: implications for understanding social anxiety. *Biol Psychiatry*, **51**, 11–17.

American Psychiatric Association (2013). *Diagnostic and Statistical Manual of Mental Disorders—DSM-5™ Handbook of Differential Diagnosis.* American Psychiatric Association, Arlington.

Amodio, M., Jost, J.T., Master, S.L., & Yee, C.M. (2007). Neurocognitive correlates of liberalism and conservatism. *Nat Neurosci,* **10**, 1246–47.

Anda, R.F., Felitti, V.J., Chapman, D.P., et al. (2001). Abused boys, battered mothers, and male involvement in teen pregnancy. *Pediatrics,* **107**, E19.

Anders, S., Tanaka, M., & Kinney, D.K. (2013). Depression as an evolutionary strategy for defense against infection. *Brain Behav Immun,* **31**, 9–22.

Anderson, C., John, O.P., Keltner, D., & Kring, A.M. (2001). Who attains social status? Effects of personality and physical attractiveness in social groups. *J Pers Soc Psychol,* **81**, 116–32.

Andersson, L., Sundstrom-Poromaa, I., Wulff, M., Astrom, M., & Bixo, M. (2004). Implications of antenatal depression and anxiety for obstetric outcome. *Obstet Gynecol,* **104**, 467–76.

Andreasen, N.C. (1997). Linking mind and brain in the study of mental illnesses: a project for a scientific psychopathology. *Science,* **275**, 1586–93.

Andrews, P.W. & Thomson, J.A. (2009). The bright side of being blue: depression as an adaptation for analyzing complex problems. *Psychological Rev,* **116**, 620–54.

Andrews, P.W. & Thomson, J.A. (2010). Depression's evolutionary roots. *Scientific American,* January, 56–61.

Andrews, P.W., Thomson, J.A., Jr, Amstadter, A., & Neale, M.C. (2012). Primum non nocere: an evolutionary analysis of whether antidepressants do more harm than good. *Front Psychol,* **3**, 1–19.

Angst, J. (1995). Epidemiology of the bipolar spectrum. *Encephale,* **21** (6), 37–42.

Anliker, B. & Muller, U. (2006). The functions of mammalian amyloid precursor protein and related amyloid precursor-like proteins. *Neurodegener Dis,* **3**, 239–46.

Annen, S., Roser, P., & Brüne, M. (2012). Nonverbal behavior during clinical interviews: similarities and dissimilarities among schizophrenia, mania, and depression. *J Nerv Ment Dis,* **200**, 26–32.

Antolin, M.F., Jenkins, K.P., Bergstrom, C.T., et al. (2012). Evolution and medicine in undergraduate education: a prescription for all biology students. *Evolution,* **66**, 1991–2006.

Arbib, M.A. (2005). From monkey-like action recognition to human language: an evolutionary framework for neurolinguistics. *Behav Brain Sci,* **28**, 105–24.

Arbib, M.A., Billard, A., Iacoboni, M., & Oztop, E. (2000). Synthetic brain imaging: grasping, mirror neurons and imitation. *Neural Netw,* **13**, 975–97.

Arce, M.D.G. & Sandler, T. (2005). Counterterrorism. A game-theoretic analysis. *J Conflict Resolution,* **49**, 183–200.

Archer, J. (1999). *The Nature of Grief.* Oxford University Press, New York.

Archer, J. (2013). Can evolutionary principles explain patterns of family violence? *Psychol Bull,* **139**, 403–40.

Arduino, P.J. & Gould, J.L. (1984). Is tonic immobility adaptive. *Animal Behav,* **32**, 921–23.

Arnsten, A.F.T. (2006). Stimulants: therapeutic actions in ADHD. *Neuropsychopharmacology,* **31**, 2376–83.

Artero, S., Touchon, J., Dupuy, A.M., Malafosse, A., & Ritchie, K. (2011). War exposure, 5-HTTLPR genotype and lifetime risk of depression. *Br J Psychiatry,* **199**, 43–48.

Ashwin, C., Baron-Cohen, S., Wheelwright, S., O'Riordan, M., & Bullmore, E.T. (2007). Differential activation of the amygdala and the 'social brain' during fearful face-processing in Asperger syndrome. *Neuropsychologia,* **45**, 2–14.

Asperger, H. (1944). Die autistischen Psychopathen im Kindesalter. *Archiv Psych Nervenkrankheiten,* **117**, 76–136.

Atran, S. (2003). Genesis of suicide terrorism. *Science,* **299**, 1534–39.

Aureli, F. & Waal, F.B.M.D. (2000). *Natural Conflict Resolution*. University of California Press, Berkeley.

Avis, J. & Harris, P.L. (1991). Belief-desire reasoning among Baka children—evidence for a universal conception of mind. *Child Development*, **62**, 460–67.

Axelrod, R. & Hamilton, W.D. (1981). The evolution of cooperation. *Science*, **211**, 1390–96.

Ayala, F.J. (1987). Sociobiology and ethics. 'Taking Darwin seriously'. By Michael Ruse. Essay review. *Hist Philos Life Sci*, **9**, 315–25.

Ayalew, M., Le-Niculescu, H., Levey, D.F., et al. (2012). Convergent functional genomics of schizophrenia: from comprehensive understanding to genetic risk prediction. *Mol Psychiatry*, **17**, 887–905.

Azevedo, F.A., Carvalho, L.R., Grinberg, L.T., et al. (2009). Equal numbers of neuronal and nonneuronal cells make the human brain an isometrically scaled-up primate brain. *J Comp Neurol*, **513**, 532–41.

Aziz-Zadeh, L., Koski, L., Zaidel, E., Mazziotta, J., & Iacoboni, M. (2006). Lateralization of the human mirror neuron system. *J Neurosci*, **26**, 2964–70.

Azmitia, E.C. (2010). Evolution of serotonin: sunlight to suicide. In: Müller, C.P. & Jacobs, B.L. (eds) *Handbook of the Behavioral Neurobiology of Serotonin*. Academic Press, Elsevier, London.

Babbitt, C.C., Fedrigo, O., Pfefferle, A.D., et al. (2010). Both noncoding and protein-coding RNAs contribute to gene expression evolution in the primate brain. *Genome Biol Evol*, **2**, 67–79.

Badcock, C.R. (1990). Is the Oedipus complex a Darwinian adaptation? *J Am Acad Psychoanal*, **18**, 368–77.

Badcock, C. & Crespi, B. (2006). Imbalanced genomic imprinting in brain development: an evolutionary basis for the aetiology of autism. *J Evol Biol*, **19**, 1007–32.

Badner, J.A. & Gershon, E.S. (2002). Meta-analysis of whole-genome linkage scans of bipolar disorder and schizophrenia. *Mol Psychiatry*, **7**, 405–11.

Bailer, U., Leisch, F., Meszaros, K., et al. (2002). Genome scan for susceptibility loci for schizophrenia and bipolar disorder. *Biol Psychiatry*, **52**, 40–52.

Bailey, J.M. (2000). How can psychological adaptations be heritable? *Novartis Found Symp*, **233**, 171–80; discussion 180–84.

Bailey, K.G. (2000). Evolution, kinship, and psychotherapy: promoting psychological health through human relationships. In: Gilbert, P. & Bailey, K.G. (eds) *Genes on the Couch. Explorations in Evolutionary Psychotherapy*. Brunner-Routledge, Hove.

Bailey, K.G. & Gilbert, P. (2000). Evolutionary psychotherapy: where to from here. In: Gilbert, P. & Bailey, K.G. (eds) *Genes on the Couch. Explorations in Evolutionary Psychotherapy*. Brunner-Routledge, Hove.

Bainton, R.J., Tsai, L.T.Y., Singh, C.M., et al. (2000). Dopamine modulates acute responses to cocaine, nicotine and ethanol in Drosophila. *Current Biol*, **10**, 187–94.

Baird, J., Stevenson, J.C., & Williams, D.C. (2000). The evolution of ADHD: a disorder of communication? *Q Rev Biol*, **75**, 17–35.

Baker, R.R. (1993). *Human Sperm Competition: Copulation, Masturbation, and Infertility*. Chapman & Hall, London.

Baker, R.R. & Bellis, M.A. (1995). *Human Sperm Competition: Copulation, Masturbation and Infidelity*. Chapman & Hall, London.

Bakermans-Kranenburg, M.J. & Van Ijzendoorn, M.H. (2013). Sniffing around oxytocin: review and meta-analyses of trials in healthy and clinical groups with implications for pharmacotherapy. *Transl Psychiatry*, **3**, e258.

Bakermans-Kranenburg, M.J. & Van Ijzendoorn, M.H. (2006). Gene–environment interaction of the dopamine D4 receptor (DRD4) and observed maternal insensitivity predicting externalizing behavior in preschoolers. *Dev Psychobiol*, **48**, 406–409.

Bakermans-Kranenburg, M.J. & Van Ijzendoorn, M.H. (2007). Research review: genetic vulnerability or differential susceptibility in child development: the case of attachment. *J Child Psychol Psych Allied Disciplines*, **48**, 1160–73.

Bakker, C., Gardner, R., Jr, Koliatsos, V., et al. (2002). The social brain: a unifying foundation for psychiatry. *Academic Psychiatry: The Journal of the American Association of Directors of Psychiatric Residency Training and the Association for Academic Psychiatry*, **26**, 219.

Ball, D. & Collier, D. (2005). Substance misuse. In: McGuffin, P., Owen, M.J., & Gottesman, I.I. (eds) *Psychiatric Genetics and Genomics*. Oxford University Press, Oxford.

Ball, EM., Young, D., Dotson, L.A., Brothers, L.T., & Robbins, D. (1994). Factors associated with dangerous behavior in forensic inpatients—results from a pilot-study. *Bull Am Acad Psychiatry Law*, **22**, 605–20.

Ballard, C., Gauthier, S., Corbett, A., et al. (2011). Alzheimer's disease. *Lancet*, **377**, 1019–31.

Balliet, D., Wu, J., & De Dreu, C.K. (2014). Ingroup favoritism in cooperation: a meta-analysis. *Psychol Bull*, **140**(6), 1556–81.

Bancroft, J. (2005). The endocrinology of sexual arousal. *J Endocrinol*, **186**, 411–27.

Bandelow, B., Spath, C., Tichauer, G.A., et al. (2002). Early traumatic life events, parental attitudes, family history, and birth risk factors in patients with panic disorder. *Comprehensive Psychiatry*, **43**, 269–78.

Banzato, C.E.M. (2004). Classification in psychiatry: the move towards ICD-11 and DSM-V. *Current Opinion Psychiatry*, **17**, 497–501.

Baptista, T., Aldana, E., Angeles, F., & Beaulieu, S. (2008). Evolution theory: an overview of its applications in psychiatry. *Psychopathology*, **41**, 17–27.

Bär, K.J., Greiner, W., Jochum, T., et al. (2004). The influence of major depression and its treatment on heart rate variability and pupillary light reflex parameters. *J Affect Disord*, **82**, 245–52.

Barkley, R.A., Edwards, G., Laneri, M., Fletcher, K., & Metevia, L. (2001). Executive functioning, temporal discounting, and sense of time in adolescents with attention deficit hyperactivity disorder (ADHD) and oppositional defiant disorder (ODD). *J Abnorm Child Psychol*, **29**, 541–56.

Barkow, J.H., Cosmides, L., & Tooby, J. (1992). *The Adapted Mind: Evolutionary Psychology and the Generation of Culture*. Oxford University Press, New York.

Barlow, D.H. (2010). Negative effects from psychological treatments: a perspective. *Am Psychol*, **65**, 13–20.

Barnes, L.L., Wilson, R.S., Bienias, J.L., et al. (2005). Sex differences in the clinical manifestations of Alzheimer disease pathology. *Arch Gen Psychiatry*, **62**, 685–91.

Baron-Cohen, S. (1988). Social and pragmatic deficits in autism: cognitive or affective? *J Autism Dev Disord*, **18**, 379–402.

Baron-Cohen, S. (1991). The theory of mind deficit in autism—how specific is it? *Br J Dev Psychol*, **9**, 301–14.

Baron-Cohen, S. (1995). *Mindblindness: An Essay on Autism and Theory of Mind*. MIT Press, Cambridge, Massachusetts.

Baron-Cohen, S., Leslie, A.M., & Frith, U. (1986). Mechanical, behavioral and intentional understanding of picture stories in autistic-children. *Br J Dev Psychol*, **4**, 113–25.

Baron-Cohen, S., Jolliffe, T., Mortimore, C., & Robertson, M. (1997). Another advanced test of theory of mind: evidence from very high functioning adults with autism or asperger syndrome. *J Child Psychol Psychiatry*, **38**, 813–22.

Baron-Cohen, S., O'Riordan, M., Stone, V., Jones, R., & Plaisted, K. (1999). Recognition of faux pas by normally developing children and children with Asperger syndrome or high-functioning autism. *J Autism Dev Disord*, **29**, 407–18.

Baron-Cohen, S., Wheelwright, S., Hill, J., Raste, Y., & Plumb, I. (2001). The 'Reading the Mind in the Eyes' Test revised version: a study with normal adults, and adults with Asperger syndrome or high-functioning autism. *J Child Psychol Psychiatry*, **42**, 241–51.

Baron-Cohen, S., Knickmeyer, R.C., & Belmonte, M.K. (2005). Sex differences in the brain: implications for explaining autism. *Science*, **310**, 819–23.

Barr, C.S., Newman, T.K., Lindell, S., et al. (2004). Interaction between serotonin transporter gene variation and rearing condition in alcohol preference and consumption in female primates. *Arch Gen Psychiatry*, **61**, 1146–52.

Barrett, L.W., Fletcher, S., & Wilton, S.D. (2012). Regulation of eukaryotic gene expression by the untranslated gene regions and other non-coding elements. *Cell Mol Life Sci*, **69**, 3613–34.

Bartels, A. & Zeki, S. (2000). The neural basis of romantic love. *Neuroreport*, **11**, 3829–34.

Bartz, J., Simeon, D., Hamilton, H., et al. (2011). Oxytocin can hinder trust and cooperation in borderline personality disorder. *Soc Cogn Affect Neurosci*, **6**, 556–63.

Bateman, A. & Fonagy, P. (2004). *Psychotherapy for Borderline Personality Disorder: Mentalization-Based Treatment*. Oxford University Press, Oxford.

Bateman, A. & Fonagy, P. (2006). *Mentalization-Based Treatment for Borderline Personality Disorder: A Practical Guide*. Oxford University Press, Oxford.

Bateson, M., Brilot, B., & Nettle, D. (2011). Anxiety: an evolutionary approach. *Can J Psychiatry*, **56**, 707–15.

Bateson, P. (1998). Genes, environment and the development of behavior. *Novartis Found Symp*, **213**, 160–70; discussion 170–75.

Bateson, P.P.G. & Hinde, R.A. (1976). *Growing Points in Ethology: Based on a Conference Sponsored by St. John's College and King's College, Cambridge*. Cambridge University Press, Cambridge.

Bauer, M. & Pfennig, A. (2005). Epidemiology of bipolar disorders. *Epilepsia*, **46** (Suppl 4), 8–13.

Beahrs, J.O. (1990). The evolution of post traumatic behavior: three hypotheses. *Dissociation*, **3**, 15–21.

Bebbington, P.E. (1998). Epidemiology of obsessive-compulsive disorder. *Br J Psychiatry Suppl*, **199**(35), 2–6.

Bebbington, P.E., Bhugra, D., Brugha, T., et al. (2004). Psychosis, victimisation and childhood disadvantage: evidence from the second British National Survey of Psychiatric Morbidity. *Br J Psychiatry*, **185**, 220–26.

Bechara, A., Damasio, A.R., Damasio, H., & Anderson, S.W. (1994). Insensitivity to future consequences following damage to human prefrontal cortex. *Cognition*, **50**, 7–15.

Bechara, A., Damasio, H., Tranel, D., & Damasio, A.R. (1997). Deciding advantageously before knowing the advantageous strategy. *Science*, **275**, 1293–95.

Bechara, A., Damasio, H., Tranel, D., & Anderson, S.W. (1998). Dissociation of working memory from decision making within the human prefrontal cortex. *J Neurosci*, **18**, 428–37.

Bechara, A., Damasio, H., & Damasio, A.R. (2000a). Emotion, decision making and the orbitofrontal cortex. *Cereb Cortex*, **10**, 295–307.

Bechara, A., Tranel, D., & Damasio, H. (2000b). Characterization of the decision-making deficit of patients with ventromedial prefrontal cortex lesions. *Brain*, **123** (Pt 11), 2189–202.

Bechara, A., Dolan, S., Denburg, N., et al. (2001). Decision-making deficits, linked to a dysfunctional ventromedial prefrontal cortex, revealed in alcohol and stimulant abusers. *Neuropsychologia*, **39**, 376–89.

Beck, A.T. (1964). Thinking and depression. II. Theory and therapy. *Arch Gen Psychiatry*, **10**, 561–71.

Beck, A.T. (1999). Cognitive aspects of personality disorders and their relation to syndromal disorders: a psychoevolutionary approach. In: Cloninger, C.R. (ed.) *Personality and Psychopathology*. American Psychiatric Press, Washington, DC.

Beer, D. (1992). The manifestations of insanity (Translation of Emil Kraepelin's 'Die Erscheinungsformen des Irreseins' 1920). *History Psychiatry*, **3**, 504–29.

Bell, D.C. (2001). Evolution of parental caregiving. *Pers Soc Psychol Rev*, **5**, 216–29.

Belsky, J. (1997). Theory testing, effect-size evaluation, and differential susceptibility to rearing influence: the case of mothering and attachment. *Child Dev*, **68**, 598–600.

Belsky, J. (1999). Modern evolutionary theory and patterns of attachment. In: Cassidy, J. & Shaver, P.R. (eds) *Handbook of Attachment. Theory, Research, and Clinical Applications*. Guilford Press, New York.

Belsky, J. & Beaver, K.M. (2011). Cumulative-genetic plasticity, parenting and adolescent self-regulation. *J Child Psychol Psychiatry*, **52**, 619–26.

Belsky, J. & Pluess, M. (2009). Beyond diathesis stress: differential susceptibility to environmental influences. *Psychol Bull*, **135**, 885–908.

Belsky, J., Steinberg, L., & Draper, P. (1991). Childhood experience, interpersonal development, and reproductive strategy: and evolutionary theory of socialization. *Child Dev*, **62**, 647–70.

Belsky, J., Campbell, S., Cohn, J.F., & Moore, G. (1996). Instability of infant–parent attachment security. *Dev Psychol*, **32**, 921–24.

Belsky, J., Jonassaint, C., Pluess, M., et al. (2009). Vulnerability genes or plasticity genes? *Mol Psychiatry*, **14**, 746–54.

Bemporad, J.R. (1991). Dementia praecox as a failure of neoteny. *Theor Med*, **12**, 45–51.

Ben-Dor, D.H., Laufer, N., Apter, A., Frisch, A., & Weizman, A. (2002). Heritability, genetics and association findings in anorexia nervosa. *Isr J Psychiatry Relat Sci*, **39**, 262–70.

Benecke, C. & Dammann, G. (2004). Nonverbales Verhalten von Patientinnen mit Borderline Persönlichkeitsstörung. In: Hermer, M. & Klinzing, H.G. (eds) *Nonverbale Prozesse in der Psychotherapie*. DGVT, Tübingen, pp. 261–72.

Benedetti, F., Amanzio, M., & Maggi, G. (1995). Potentiation of placebo analgesia by proglumide. *Lancet*, **346**, 1231.

Bennett, A.J., Lesch, K.P., Heils, A., et al. (2002). Early experience and serotonin transporter gene variation interact to influence primate CNS function. *Mol Psychiatry*, **7**, 118–22.

Bentall, R.P., Jackson, H.F., & Pilgrim, D. (1988). Abandoning the concept of 'schizophrenia': some implications of validity arguments for psychological research into psychotic phenomena. *Br J Clin Psychol*, **27** (Pt 4), 303–24.

Bernhardt, B.C. & Singer, T. (2012). The neural basis of empathy. *Annu Rev Neurosci*, **35**, 1–23.

Bernstein, D.P., Fink, L., Handelsman, L., et al. (1994). Initial reliability and validity of a new retrospective measure of child abuse and neglect. *Am J Psychiatry*, **151**, 1132–36.

Bernstein, E.M. & Putnam, F.W. (1986). Development, reliability, and validity of a dissociation scale. *J Nervous Mental Dis*, **174**, 727–35.

Berrettini, W.H. (2000a). Susceptibility loci for bipolar disorder: overlap with inherited vulnerability to schizophrenia. *Biol Psychiatry*, **47**, 245–51.

Berrettini, W.H. (2000b). Genetics of psychiatric disease. *Annu Rev Med*, **51**, 465–79.

Berrettini, W.H. (2001). Molecular linkage studies of bipolar disorders. *Bipolar Disorders*, **3**, 276–83.

Berry, K., Barrowclough, C., & Wearden, A. (2007). A review of the role of adult attachment style in psychosis: unexplored issues and questions for further research. *Clin Psychol Rev*, **27**, 458–75.

Bertram, L. & Tanzi, R.E. (2008). Thirty years of Alzheimer's disease genetics: the implications of systematic meta-analyses. *Nat Rev Neurosci*, **9**, 768–78.

Betzig, L. (1989). Causes of conjugal dissolution—a cross-cultural-study. *Current Anthropol*, **30**, 654–76.

Bezirganian, S., Cohen, P., & Brook, J.S. (1993). The impact of mother–child interaction on the development of borderline personality disorder. *Am J Psychiatry*, **150**, 1836–42.

Bibl, M., Mollenhauer, B., Lewczuk, P., et al. (2007). Validation of amyloid-beta peptides in CSF diagnosis of neurodegenerative dementias. *Mol Psychiatry*, **12**, 671–80.

Bickart, K.C., Wright, C.I., Dautoff, R.J., Dickerson, B.C., & Barrett, L.F. (2011). Amygdala volume and social network size in humans. *Nat Neurosci*, **14**, 163–64.

Biederman, J., Mick, E., Faraone, S.V., et al. (2002). Influence of gender on attention deficit hyperactivity disorder in children referred to a psychiatric clinic. *Am J Psychiatry*, **159**, 36–42.

Biederman, J., Faraone, S.V., Monuteaux, M.C., Bober, M., & Cadogen, E. (2004). Gender effects on attention-deficit/hyperactivity disorder in adults, revisited. *Biol Psychiatry*, **55**, 692–700.

Bielsky, I.F. & Young, L.J. (2004). Oxytocin, vasopressin, and social recognition in mammals. *Peptides*, **25**, 1565–74.

Bierer, L.M., Yehuda, R., Schmeidler, J., et al. (2003). Abuse and neglect in childhood: relationship to personality disorder diagnoses. *CNS Spectr*, **8**, 737–54.

Binder, E.B., Bradley, R.G., Liu, W., et al. (2008). Association of FKBP5 polymorphisms and childhood abuse with risk of posttraumatic stress disorder symptoms in adults. *JAMA*, **299**, 1291–305.

Birbaumer, N., Veit, R., Lotze, M., et al. (2005). Deficient fear conditioning in psychopathy: a functional magnetic resonance imaging study. *Arch Gen Psychiatry*, **62**, 799–805.

Birn, R.M., Shackman, A.J., Oler, J.A., et al. (2014). Extreme early-life anxiety is associated with an evolutionarily conserved reduction in the strength of intrinsic functional connectivity between the dorsolateral prefrontal cortex and the central nucleus of the amygdala. *Mol Psychiatry*, **19**, 853.

Bjorklund, D.F. (1997). The role of immaturity in human development. *Psychol Bull*, **122**, 153–69.

Bjorklund, D.F. & Kipp, K. (1996). Parental investment theory and gender differences in the evolution of inhibition mechanisms. *Psychol Bull*, **120**, 163–88.

Bjorklund, D.F. & Pellegrini, A.D. (2000). Child development and evolutionary psychology. *Child Development*, **71**, 1687–708.

Blair, H.T., Huynh, V.K., Vaz, V.T., et al. (2005). Unilateral storage of fear memories by the amygdala. *J Neurosci*, **25**, 4198–205.

Blair, R.J. (2001). Neurocognitive models of aggression, the antisocial personality disorders, and psychopathy. *J Neurol Neurosurg Psychiatry*, **71**, 727–31.

Bleuler, E. (1911). *Dementia praecox oder die Gruppe der Schizophrenien*. Deutike, Leipzig.

Blumberg, H.P., Stern, E., Ricketts, S., et al. (1999). Rostral and orbital prefrontal cortex dysfunction in the manic state of bipolar disorder. *Am J Psychiatry*, **156**, 1986–88.

Blurton Jones, N.G. (1972). *Ethological Studies of Child Behaviour*. University Press, Cambridge.

Boddaert, N. & Zilbovicius, M. (2002). Functional neuroimaging and childhood autism. *Pediatr Radiol*, **32**, 1–7.

Bodini, B., Iacoboni, M., & Lenzi, G.L. (2004). Acute stroke effects on emotions: an interpretation through the mirror system. *Curr Opin Neurol*, **17**, 55–60.

Bogin, B. (1999). Evolutionary perspective on human growth. *Annu Rev Anthropol*, **28**, 109–53.

Bogin, B. (2009). Childhood, adolescence, and longevity: a multilevel model of the evolution of reserve capacity in human life history. *Am J Hum Biol*, **21**, 567–77.

Boin, F., Zanardini, R., Pioli, R., et al. (2001). Association between -G308A tumor necrosis factor alpha gene polymorphism and schizophrenia. *Mol Psychiatry*, **6**, 79–82.

Bömmer, I. & Brüne, M. (2006). Social cognition in 'pure' delusional disorder. *Cogn Neuropsychiatry*, **11**, 493–503.

Boonstra, R. (2013). Reality as the leading cause of stress: rethinking the impact of chronic stress in nature. *Functional Ecol*, **27**, 11–23.

Boraska, V., Franklin, C.S., Floyd, J.A., et al. (2014). A genome-wide association study of anorexia nervosa. *Mol Psychiatry*, **19**, 1085–94.

Bord, L., Wheeler, J., Paek, M., et al. (2006). Primate disrupted-in-schizophrenia-1 (DISC1): high divergence of a gene for major mental illnesses in recent evolutionary history. *Neurosci Res*, **56**, 286–93.

Bos, E.H., Bouhuys, A.L., Geerts, E., Van Os, T.W., & Ormel, J. (2006). Lack of association between conversation partners' nonverbal behavior predicts recurrence of depression, independently of personality. *Psychiatry Res*, **142**, 79–88.

Bos, E.H., Bouhuys, A.L., Geerts, E., Van Os, T.W., & Ormel, J. (2007). Stressful life events as a link between problems in nonverbal communication and recurrence of depression. *J Affect Disord*, **97**, 161–69.

Bosacki, S. & Astington, J.W. (1999). Theory of mind in preadolescence: relations between social understanding and social competence. *Social Dev*, **8**, 237–55.

Botvinick, M., Nystrom, L.E., Fissell, K., Carter, C.S., & Cohen, J.D. (1999). Conflict monitoring versus selection-for-action in anterior cingulate cortex. *Nature*, **402**, 179–81.

Bouchard, T.J., Jr (1994). Genes, environment, and personality. *Science*, **264**, 1700–701.

Bouchard, T.J., Jr & Loehlin, J.C. (2001). Genes, evolution, and personality. *Behav Genet*, **31**, 243–73.

Bowlby, J. (1944). Forty-four juvenile thieves: their characters and home-life (II). *Int J Psychoanalysis*, **25**, 107–28.

Bowlby, J. (1953). Some pathological processes set in train by early mother–child separation. *J Mental Sci*, **99**, 265–72.

Bowlby, J. (1969). *Attachment and Loss*. Basic Books, New York.

Bowlby, J. (1973). *Attachment and Loss. Vol. 2. Separation: Anxiety and Anger*. Basic Books, New York.

Bowlby, J. (1980). *Attachment and Loss. Vol. 3. Loss*. Basic Books, New York.

Bowlby, J. (1991). Ethological light on psychoanalytical problems. In: Bateson, P. (ed.) *The Development and Integration of Behaviour: Essays in Honour of Robert Hinde*. Cambridge University Press, Cambridge.

Bowlby, J. (1997). *Attachment: Vol. 1 of the 'Attachment and loss' Trilogy*. Pimlico, London.

Bowler, D.M. (1992). Theory of mind in Asperger's syndrome. *J Child Psychol Psychiatry Allied Disciplines*, **33**, 877–93.

Boyce, W.T. & Ellis, B.J. (2005). Biological sensitivity to context: I. An evolutionary-developmental theory of the origins and functions of stress reactivity. *Dev Psychopathol*, **17**, 271–301.

Boyce, W.T., Chesney, M., Alkon, A., et al. (1995). Psychobiologic reactivity to stress and childhood respiratory illnesses: results of two prospective studies. *Psychosom Med*, **57**, 411–22.

Boyd, R., Gintis, H., Bowles, S., & Richerson, P.J. (2003). The evolution of altruistic punishment. *Proc Natl Acad Sci USA*, **100**, 3531–35.

Bracha, H.S. (2004). Freeze, flight, fight, fright, faint: adaptationist perspectives on the acute stress response spectrum. *CNS Spectr*, **9**, 679–85.

Bradley, R., Schwartz, A.C., & Kaslow, N.J. (2005). Posttraumatic stress disorder symptoms among low-income, African American women with a history of intimate partner violence and suicidal behaviors: self-esteem, social support, and religious coping. *J Trauma Stress*, **18**, 685–96.

Bradshaw, G.A., Capaldo, T., Lindner, L., & Grow, G. (2008). Building an inner sanctuary: complex PTSD in chimpanzees. *J Trauma Dissociation*, **9**, 9–34.

Bradshaw, J.L. (1997). *Human Evolution: A Neuropsychological Perspective*. Psychology Press, Hove.

Bradshaw, J.L. & Sheppard, D.M. (2000). The neurodevelopmental frontostriatal disorders: evolutionary adaptiveness and anomalous lateralization. *Brain Lang*, **73**, 297–320.

Brady, K.T., Killeen, T.K., Brewerton, T., & Lucerini, S. (2000). Comorbidity of psychiatric disorders and posttraumatic stress disorder. *J Clin Psychiatry*, **61** (Suppl 7), 22–32.

Braff, D.L., Freedman, R., Schork, N.J., & Gottesman, I. (2007). Deconstructing schizophrenia: an overview of the use of endophenotypes in order to understand a complex disorder. *Schizophr Bull*, **33**, 21–32.

Brähler, C., Harper, J., & Gilbert, P. (2013). Compassion focused group therapy for recovery after psychosis. In: Steel, C. (ed.) *Cognitive Behaviour Therapy for Schizophrenia: Evidence-Based Interventions and Future Directions.* John Wiley, New York.

Brambilla, P., Barale, F., Caverzasi, E., & Soares, J.C. (2002). Anatomical MRI findings in mood and anxiety disorders. *Epidemiol Psichiatr Soc,* **11**, 88–99.

Brandt, H., Hauert, C., & Sigmund, K. (2006). Punishing and abstaining for public goods. *Proc Natl Acad Sci USA,* **103**, 495–97.

Brannigan, C.R. & Humphries, D.A. (1974). Human non-verbal behaviour, a means of communication. In: Blurton Jones, N.G. (ed.) *Ethological Studies of Child Behaviour.* Cambridge University Press, Cambridge.

Brasil-Neto, J.P., Pascual-Leone, A., Valls-Sole, J., Cohen, L.G., & Hallett, M. (1992). Focal transcranial magnetic stimulation and response bias in a forced-choice task. *J Neurol Neurosurg Psychiatry,* **55**, 964–66.

Brass, M. & Heyes, C. (2005). Imitation: is cognitive neuroscience solving the correspondence problem? *Trends Cogn Sci,* **9**, 489–95.

Braza, F. (2004). Human prenatal investment affected by maternal age and parity. *Human Ecol,* **32**, 163–75.

Breiter, H.C., Rauch, S.L., Kwong, K.K., et al. (1996). Functional magnetic resonance imaging of symptom provocation in obsessive-compulsive disorder. *Arch Gen Psychiatry,* **53**, 595–606.

Brekke, J.S., Prindle, C., Bae, S.W., & Long, J.D. (2001). Risks for individuals with schizophrenia who are living in the community. *Psychiatr Serv,* **52**, 1358–66.

Brekke, J., Kay, D.D., Lee, K.S., & Green, M.F. (2005). Biosocial pathways to functional outcome in schizophrenia. *Schizophr Res,* **80**, 213–25.

Bremner, J.D. (1999). Does stress damage the brain? *Biol Psychiatry,* **45**, 797–805.

Brennan, P.A., Pargas, R., Walker, E.F., et al. (2008). Maternal depression and infant cortisol: influences of timing, comorbidity and treatment. *J Child Psychol Psychiatry,* **49**, 1099–107.

Brent, E., Rios, P., Happe, F., & Charman, T. (2004). Performance of children with autism spectrum disorder on advanced theory of mind tasks. *Autism,* **8**, 283–99.

Brewer, D.D., Potterat, J.J., Garrett, S.B., et al. (2000). Prostitution and the sex discrepancy in reported number of sexual partners. *Proc Natl Acad Sci USA,* **97**, 12385–88.

Brewerton, T.D. (2007). Eating disorders, trauma, and comorbidity: focus on PTSD. *Eat Disord,* **15**, 285–304.

Brockington, I.F. (1996). *Motherhood and Mental Health.* Oxford University Press, Oxford.

Broder, A. & Hohmann, N. (2003). Variations in risk, taking behavior over the menstrual cycle—An improved replication. *Evol Human Behav,* **24**, 391–98.

Brody, G.H., Yu, T., Chen, Y.F., et al. (2013). Supportive family environments, genes that confer sensitivity, and allostatic load among rural African American emerging adults: a prospective analysis. *J Fam Psychol,* **27**, 22–29.

Brody, J.F. (2001). Evolutionary recasting: ADHD, mania and its variants. *J Affect Disord,* **65**, 197–215.

Bronikowski, A.M., Altmann, J., Brockman, D.K., et al. (2011). Aging in the natural world: comparative data reveal similar mortality patterns across primates. *Science,* **331**, 1325–28.

Brookman, F. & Nolan, J. (2006). The dark figure of infanticide in England and Wales—complexities of diagnosis. *J Interpers Violence,* **21**, 869–89.

Brothers, L. (1989). A biological perspective on empathy. *Am J Psychiatry,* **146**, 10–19.

Brothers, L. (1990a). The neural basis of primate social communication. *Motivation Emotion,* **14**, 81–91.

Brothers, L. (1990b). The social brain: a project for integrating primate behavior and neurophysiology in a new domain. *Concepts Neurosci,* **1**, 27–51.

Brothers, L., Ring, B., & Kling, A. (1990). Response of neurons in the macaque amygdala to complex social-stimuli. *Behav Brain Res*, **41**, 199–213.

Brower, M.C. & Price, B.H. (2001). Neuropsychiatry of frontal lobe dysfunction in violent and criminal behaviour: a critical review. *J Neurol Neurosurg Psychiatry*, **71**, 720–26.

Brown, E.C. & Brüne, M. (2012). The role of prediction in social neuroscience. *Front Hum Neurosci*, **6**, 147.

Brown, E.C. & Brüne, M. (2014). Reward in the mirror neuron system, social context, and the implications on psychopathology. *Behav Brain Sci*, **37**, 196–97.

Brown, E.C., Wiersema, J.R., Pourtois, G., & Brüne, M. (2013). Modulation of motor cortex activity when observing rewarding and punishing actions. *Neuropsychologia*, **51**, 52–58.

Brown, E.C., Tas, C., Kuzu, D., et al. (2014). Social approach and avoidance behaviour for negative emotions is modulated by endogenous oxytocin and paranoia in schizophrenia. *Psychiatry Res*, **219**, 436–42.

Brown, G.W. (2002). Social roles, context and evolution in the origins of depression. *J Health Soc Behav*, **43**, 255–76.

Bruckner, T.A., Catalano, R., & Ahern, J. (2010). Male fetal loss in the U.S. following the terrorist attacks of September 11, 2001. *BMC Public Health*, **10**, 273.

Brüne, M. (2000). Neoteny, psychiatric disorders and the social brain hypothesis. *Anthropology Med*, **7**, 301–18.

Brüne, M. (2001a). De Clerambault's syndrome (erotomania) in an evolutionary perspective. *Evolution Human Behav*, **22**, 409–15.

Brüne, M. (2001b). Evolutionary fallacies of Nazi psychiatry—implications for current research. *Perspect Biol Med*, **44**, 426–33.

Brüne, M. (2002). Toward an integration of interpersonal and biological processes: evolutionary psychiatry as an empirically testable framework for psychiatric research. *Psychiatry*, **65**, 48–57.

Brüne, M. (2003a). Erotomanic stalking in evolutionary perspective. *Behav Sci Law*, **21**, 83–88.

Brüne, M. (2003b). Social cognition and behaviour in schizophrenia. In: Brüne, M., Ribbert, H., & Schiefenhövel, W. (eds) *The Social Brain: Evolution and Pathology*. John Wiley, Chichester.

Brüne, M. (2003c). Erotomania revisited: clues of its origin from evolutionary theory. In: Shohov, S.P. (ed.) *Advances in Psychology Research*. Nova Science, New York.

Brüne, M. (2004). Schizophrenia—an evolutionary enigma? *Neurosci Biobehav Rev*, **28**, 41–53.

Brüne, M. (2005). 'Theory of mind' in schizophrenia: a review of the literature. *Schizophr Bull*, **31**, 21–42.

Brüne, M. (2006). The evolutionary psychology of obsessive-compulsive disorder: the role of cognitive metarepresentation. *Perspect Biol Med*, **49**, 317–29.

Brüne, M. (2007). On human self-domestication, psychiatry, and eugenics. *Philos Ethics Humanit Med*, **2**, 21.

Brüne, M. (2012). Does the oxytocin receptor (OXTR) polymorphism (rs2254298) confer 'vulnerability' for psychopathology or 'differential susceptibility'? Insights from evolution. *BMC Med*, **10**, 38.

Brüne, M. (2014a). Life history theory as organizing principle of psychiatric disorders: Implications and prospects exemplified by borderline personality disorder. A commentary on Marco del Giudice's article 'An evolutionary life history framework for psychopathology'. *Psycholog Inquiry*, **25**, 311–21.

Brüne, M. (2014b). On aims and methods of psychiatry. A reminiscence of 50 years of Tinbergen's famous questions about the biology of behavior. *BMC Psychiatry*, **14**, 364.

Brüne, M. & Brüne-Cohrs, U. (2006). Theory of mind—evolution, ontogeny, brain mechanisms and psychopathology. *Neurosci Biobehav Rev*, **30**, 437–55.

Brüne, M. & Hochberg, Z. (2013). Evolutionary medicine—the quest for a better understanding of health, disease and prevention. *BMC Med*, **11**, 116.

Brüne, M. & Mulcahy, E. (2003). Exaptation, cooptation and the evolution of human cognition. *Evol Cognition*, **9**, 25–30.

Brüne, M., Bräunig, P., & Schiefenhövel, W. (1998). Ethological remarks on diagnosis and therapy of neuroleptic-induced akathisia. *Nervenheilkunde*, **17**, 401–406.

Brüne, M., Ribbert, H., & Schiefenhövel, W. (2003). *The Social Brain: Evolution and Pathology*. Wiley, Chichester.

Brüne, M., Brüne-Cohrs, U., & McGrew, W.C. (2004). Psychiatric treatment for great apes? *Science*, **306**, 2039.

Brüne, M., Brüne-Cohrs, U., McGrew, W.C., & Preuschoft, S. (2006). Psychopathology in great apes: concepts, treatment options and possible homologies to human psychiatric disorders. *Neurosci Biobehav Rev*, **30**, 1246–59.

Brüne, M., Sonntag, C., Abdel-Hamid, M., et al. (2008). Nonverbal behavior during standardized interviews in patients with schizophrenia spectrum disorders. *J Nerv Ment Dis*, **196**, 282–88.

Brüne, M., Schöbel, A., Karau, R., et al. (2010). Von Economo neuron density in the anterior cingulate cortex is reduced in early onset schizophrenia. *Acta Neuropathol*, **119**, 771–78.

Brüne, M., Schöbel, A., Karau, R., et al. (2011). Neuroanatomical correlates of suicide in psychosis: the possible role of von Economo neurons. *PLoS One*, **6**, e20936.

Brüne, M., Belsky, J., Fabrega, H., et al. (2012). The crisis of psychiatry—insights and prospects from evolutionary theory. *World Psychiatry*, **11**, 55–57.

Brüne, M., Ebert, A., Kolb, M., et al. (2013). Oxytocin influences avoidant reactions to social threat in adults with borderline personality disorder. *Human Psychopharmacol*, **28**, 552–61.

Brüne, M., Kolb, M., Ebert, A., Roser, P., & Edel, M.A. (2015). Nonverbal communication of patients with borderline personality disorder during clinical interviews: a double-blind placebo-controlled study using intranasal oxytocin. *J Nervous Mental Dis*, **203**, 107–11.

Brunnstrom, H.R. & Englund, E.M. (2009). Cause of death in patients with dementia disorders. *Eur J Neurol*, **16**, 488–92.

Buccino, G., Solodkin, A., & Small, S.L. (2006). Functions of the mirror neuron system: implications for neurorehabilitation. *Cogn Behav Neurol*, **19**, 55–63.

Buchheim, A., George, C., Liebl, V., Moser, A., & Benecke, C. (2007). Affective facial behavior of borderline patients during the Adult Attachment Projective. *Z Psychosom Med Psychother*, **53**, 339–54.

Buckholtz, J.W., Sust, S., Tan, H.Y., et al. (2007). fMRI evidence for functional epistasis between COMT and RGS4. *Mol Psychiatry*, **12**, 893–95, 885.

Buitelaar, J.K. & Van Der Wees, M. (1997). Are deficits in the decoding of affective cues and in mentalizing abilities independent? *J Autism Dev Disord*, **27**, 539–56.

Buitelaar, J.K., Van Der Wees, M., Swaab-Barneveld, H., & Van Der Gaag, R.J. (1999a). Verbal memory and performance IQ predict theory of mind and emotion recognition ability in children with autistic spectrum disorders and in psychiatric control children. *J Child Psychol Psychiatry*, **40**, 869–81.

Buitelaar, J.K., Van Der Wees, M., Swaab-Barneveld, H., & Van Der Gaag, R.J. (1999b). Theory of mind and emotion-recognition functioning in autistic spectrum disorders and in psychiatric control and normal children. *Dev Psychopathol*, **11**, 39–58.

Bulik, C. M., Sullivan, P. F., Fear, J. L., et al. (1999). Fertility and reproduction in women with anorexia nervosa: a controlled study. *J Clin Psychiatry*, **60**, 130–35; quiz 135–37.

Bulik, C.M., Prescott, C.A., & Kendler, K.S. (2001). Features of childhood sexual abuse and the development of psychiatric and substance use disorders. *Br J Psychiatry*, **179**, 444–49.

Bullmore, E. & Sporns, O. (2012). The economy of brain network organization. *Nat Rev Neurosci*, **13**, 336–49.

Burges Watson, I.P., Wilson, G., & Hornsby, H. (1992). War neurosis and associated physical condition: a statistical analysis. *Irish J Psychol Med*, **9**, 30–36.

Burges Watson, I.P., Brüne, M., & Bradley, A.J. (submitted). Systemic aspects of trauma and stress-related disorders: Insights from molecular evolution.

Burgess, R.G. & Macdonald, K.B. (2005). *Evolutionary Perspectives on Human Development*. Sage Publications, Thousand Oaks, California.

Burnham, T.C. (2007). High-testosterone men reject low ultimatum game offers. *Proc Biol Sci*, **274**, 2327–30.

Burns, J.K. (2004). An evolutionary theory of schizophrenia: cortical connectivity, metarepresentation, and the social brain. *Behav Brain Sci*, **27**, 831–55; discussion 855–85.

Burns, J. (2007). *The Descent of Madness: Evolutionary Origins of Psychosis and the Social Brain*. Routledge, London.

Burt, S.A., McGue, M., Demarte, J.A., Krueger, R.F., & Iacono, W.G. (2006). Timing of menarche and the origins of conduct disorder. *Arch Gen Psychiatry*, **63**, 890–96.

Burton-Bradley, B.G. (1979). The future of psychiatry in Papua New Guinea. *Aust N Z J Psychiatry*, **13**, 321–26.

Burton-Bradley, B.G. (1990). The mental health systems of Papua New Guinea and their modernization. *P N G Med J*, **33**, 51–54.

Busatto, G.F., Zamignani, D.R., Buchpiguel, C.A., et al. (2000). A voxel-based investigation of regional cerebral blood flow abnormalities in obsessive-compulsive disorder using single photon emission computed tomography (SPECT). *Psychiatry Res*, **99**, 15–27.

Buss, D.M. (1988a). The evolution of human intrasexual competition: tactics of mate attraction. *J Pers Soc Psychol*, **54**, 616–28.

Buss, D.M. (1988b). From vigilance to violence—tactics of mate retention in American undergraduates. *Ethol Sociobiol*, **9**, 291–317.

Buss, D.M. (1989). Sex-differences in human mate preferences—evolutionary hypothesis tested in 37 cultures. *Behav Brain Sci*, **12**, 1–14.

Buss, D.M. (1995). Evolutionary psychology—a new paradigm for psychological science. *Psycholog Inquiry*, **6**, 1–30.

Buss, D.M. (1998). Sexual strategies theory: Historical origins and current status. *J Sex Res*, **35**, 19–31.

Buss, D.M. (1999). *Evolutionary Psychology: The New Science of the Mind*. Allyn and Bacon, Boston.

Buss, D.M. (2000a). Desires in human mating. *Ann N Y Acad Sci*, **907**, 39–49.

Buss, D.M. (2000b). *The Dangerous Passion: Why Jealousy Is as Necessary as Love and Sex*. Free Press, New York.

Buss, D.M. & Schmitt, D.P. (1993). Sexual strategies theory: an evolutionary perspective on human mating. *Psychol Rev*, **100**, 204–32.

Buss, D.M. & Shackelford, T.K. (1997). From vigilance to violence: mate retention tactics in married couples. *J Pers Soc Psychol*, **72**, 346–61.

Buss, D.M., Abbott, M., Angleitner, A., et al. (1990). International preferences in selecting mates—a study of 37 cultures. *J Cross-Cult Psychol*, **21**, 5–47.

Buss, D.M., Shackelford, T.K., & Leblanc, G.J. (2000). Number of children desired and preferred spousal age difference: context-specific mate preference patterns across 37 cultures. *Evol Human Behav*, **21**, 323–31.

Buster, J.E. (2013). Managing female sexual dysfunction. *Fertil Steril*, **100**, 905–15.

Buston, P.M. & Emlen, S.T. (2003). Cognitive processes underlying human mate choice: the relationship between self-perception and mate preference in Western society. *Proc Natl Acad Sci USA*, **100**, 8805–10.

Butter, C.M. & Snyder, D.R. (1972). Alterations in aversive and aggressive behaviors following orbital frontal lesions in rhesus monkeys. *Acta Neurobiol Exp (Wars)*, **32**, 525–65.

Butti, C. & Hof, P.R. (2010). The insular cortex: a comparative perspective. *Brain Structure Function*, **214**, 477–93.

Buunk, B.P., Dijkstra, P., Kenrick, D.T., & Warntjes, A. (2001). Age preferences for mates as related to gender, own age, and involvement level. *Evol Human Behav*, **22**, 241–50.

Buxbaum, L J., Kyle, K.M., & Menon, R. (2005). On beyond mirror neurons: Internal representations subserving imitation and recognition of skilled object-related actions in humans. *Cognitive Brain Res*, **25**, 226–39.

Buydens-Branchey, L., Branchey, M., Hudson, J., & Fergeson, P. (2000). Low HDL cholesterol, aggression and altered central serotonergic activity. *Psychiatry Res*, **93**, 93–102.

Byars, S.G., Ewbank, D., Govindaraju, D.R., & Stearns, S.C. (2010). Natural selection in a contemporary human population. *Proc Natl Acad Sci USA*, **107**, 1787–92.

Byrne, R.W. (1995). *The Thinking Ape: Evolutionary Origins of Intelligence*. Oxford University Press, Oxford.

Byrne, R.W. & Whiten, A. (1988). *Machiavellian Intelligence: Social Expertise and the Evolution of Intellect in Monkeys, Apes, and Humans*. Clarendon Press, Oxford University Press, Oxford.

Byrne, R.W. & Whiten, A. (1992). Cognitive evolution in primates—evidence from tactical deception. *Man*, **27**, 609–27.

Caceres, M., Lachuer, J., Zapala, M.A., et al. (2003). Elevated gene expression levels distinguish human from non-human primate brains. *Proc Natl Acad Sci USA*, **100**, 13030–35.

Cachelin, F.M., Rebeck, R.M., Chung, G.H., & Pelayo, E. (2002). Does ethnicity influence body-size preference? A comparison of body image and body size. *Obes Res*, **10**, 158–66.

Caldwell, H.K., Stephens, S.L., & Young, W.S., 3rd (2009). Oxytocin as a natural antipsychotic: a study using oxytocin knockout mice. *Mol Psychiatry*, **14**, 190–96.

Caldwell, W., McInnis, O.A., McQuaid, R.J., et al. (2013). The role of the Val66Met polymorphism of the brain derived neurotrophic factor gene in coping strategies relevant to depressive symptoms. *PLoS One*, **8**, e65547.

Call, J. (2001). Chimpanzee social cognition. *Trends Cogn Sci*, **5**, 388–93.

Callies, I.T., Machleidt, W., Ziegenbein, M., & Haltenhof, H. (2007). Suizidalität im Kulturenvergleich. *Fortschritte Neurol Psychiatrie*, **75**, 653–64.

Calogeras, R.C. (1973). 'Emic' and 'etic' research strategies for psychoanalysis. *Bull Menninger Clin*, **37**, 598–614.

Calvin, W.H. (1987). The brain as a Darwin machine. *Nature*, **330**, 33–34.

Camerer, C. (2003a). *Behavioral Game Theory: Experiments in Strategic Interaction*. Russell Sage Foundation, Princeton University Press, New York.

Camerer, C.F. (2003b). Psychology and economics. Strategizing in the brain. *Science*, **300**, 1673–75.

Camerer, C.F. (2003c). Behavioural studies of strategic thinking in games. *Trends Cogn Sci*, **7**, 225–31.

Campbell, B.G. (1972). *Sexual Selection and the Descent of Man, 1871–1971*. Aldine, Chicago.

Campos, L.D., Otta, E., & Siqueira, J.D. (2002). Sex differences in mate selection strategies: content analyses and responses to personal advertisements in Brazil. *Evol Human Behav*, **23**, 395–406.

Canli, T. & Lesch, K.P. (2007). Long story short: the serotonin transporter in emotion regulation and social cognition. *Nat Neurosci*, **10**, 1103–109.

Cannon, M., Caspi, A., Moffitt, T.E., et al. (2002). Evidence for early-childhood, pan-developmental impairment specific to schizophreniform disorder: results from a longitudinal birth cohort. *Arch Gen Psychiatry*, **59**, 449–56.

Cantor, C. (2005). Evolution and Posttraumatic Stress: Disorders of Vigilance and Defence. Hove, Routledge.

Cantor, C. (2009). Post-traumatic stress disorder: evolutionary perspectives. *Aust N Z J Psychiatry*, **43**, 1038–48.

Cantor, C. & Price, J. (2007). Traumatic entrapment, appeasement and complex post-traumatic stress disorder: evolutionary perspectives of hostage reactions, domestic abuse and the Stockholm syndrome. *Aust N Z J Psychiatry*, **41**, 377–84.

Capitanio, J.P. (2004). Personality factors between and within species. In: Thierry, B., Singh, M., & Kaumanns, W. (eds) *Macaque Societies*. Cambridge University Press, Cambridge.

Cardno, A. & McGuffin, P. (2005). Quantitative genetics. In: McGuffin, P., Owen, M.J., & Gottesman, I. (eds) *Psychiatric Genetics and Genomics*. Oxford University Press, Oxford.

Carlsson, R., Nyman, H., Ganse, G., & Cullberg, J. (2006). Neuropsychological functions predict 1- and 3-year outcome in first-episode psychosis. *Acta Psychiatr Scand*, **113**, 102–11.

Carpendale, J.I. & Lewis, C. (2004). Constructing an understanding of mind: the development of children's social understanding within social interaction. *Behav Brain Sci*, **27**, 79–96; discussion 96–151.

Carroll, S.B. (2003). Genetics and the making of *Homo sapiens*. *Nature*, **422**, 849–57.

Carstensen, L.L. & Lockenhoff, C.E. (2003). Aging, emotion, and evolution: the bigger picture. *Ann N Y Acad Sci*, **1000**, 152–79.

Carter, A.S., Garrity-Rokous, F.E., Chazan-Cohen, R., Little, C., & Briggs-Gowan, M.J. (2001). Maternal depression and comorbidity: predicting early parenting, attachment security, and toddler social-emotional problems and competencies. *J Am Acad Child Adolesc Psychiatry*, **40**, 18–26.

Carter, M. & Watts, C.A. (1971). Possible biological advantages among schizophrenics' relatives. *Br J Psychiatry*, **118**, 453–60.

Cartwright, J. (2000). *Evolution and Human Behavior: Darwinian Perspectives on Human Nature*. MIT Press, Cambridge, Massachusetts.

Carvalho Fernando, S., Beblo, T., Schlosser, N., et al. (2012). Associations of childhood trauma with hypothalamic-pituitary-adrenal function in borderline personality disorder and major depression. *Psychoneuroendocrinology*, **37**, 1659–68.

Carver, C.S. & White, T.L. (1994). Behavioral-inhibition, behavioral activation, and affective responses to impending reward and punishment—the BIS BAS scales. *J Pers Soc Psychol*, **67**, 319–33.

Cason, T.N., Saijo, T., & Yamato, T. (2002). Voluntary participation and spite in public good provision experiments: an international comparison. *Experiment Econ*, **5**, 133–53.

Caspi, A., McClay, J., Moffitt, T.E., et al. (2002). Role of genotype in the cycle of violence in maltreated children. *Science*, **297**, 851–54.

Caspi, A., Sugden, K., Moffitt, T.E., et al. (2003). Influence of life stress on depression: moderation by a polymorphism in the 5-HTT gene. *Science*, **301**, 386–89.

Cassidy, J. & Shaver, P.R. (1999). *Handbook of Attachment: Theory, Research, and Clinical Applications*. Guilford Press, New York.

Cassin, S.E. & Von Ranson, K.M. (2005). Personality and eating disorders: a decade in review. *Clin Psychol Rev*, **25**, 895–916.

Cattaneo, L., Fabbri-Destro, M., Boria, S., et al. (2007). Impairment of actions chains in autism and its possible role in intention understanding. *Proc Natl Acad Sci USA*, **104**, 17825–30.

Cavalcanti-Ribeiro, P., Andrade-Nascimento, M., Morais-De-Jesus, M., et al. (2012). Post-traumatic stress disorder as a comorbidity: impact on disease outcomes. *Expert Rev Neurother,* **12**, 1023–37.

Cecil, C.A., Lysenko, L.J., Jaffee, S. R., et al. (2014). Environmental risk, oxytocin receptor gene (OXTR) methylation and youth callous-unemotional traits: a 13-year longitudinal study. *Mol Psychiatry,* **19**, 1071–77.

Cerling, T.E., Wynn, J.G., Andanje, S.A., et al. (2011). Woody cover and hominin environments in the past 6 million years. *Nature,* **476**, 51–56.

Chakrabarti, B. & Baron-Cohen, S. (2011). Variation in the human cannabinoid receptor CNR1 gene modulates gaze duration for happy faces. *Mol Autism,* **2**, 10.

Chance, M.R.A. (ed.) (1988). *Social Fabrics of the Mind.* Lawrence Erlbaum, Hove.

Charlton, B.G. (1995). Cognitive neuropsychiatry and the future of diagnosis: a 'PC' model of the mind. *Br J Psychiatry,* **167**, 149–53; discussion 153–58.

Charlton, B.G. (1997). The inequity of inequality: egalitarian instincts and evolutionary psychology. *J Health Psychol,* **2**, 413–25.

Charlton, B. (2000). *Psychiatry and the Human Condition.* Radcliffe Medical, Abingdon.

Charney, D.S. (2003). Neuroanatomical circuits modulating fear and anxiety behaviors. *Acta Psychiatr Scand Suppl,* **2003**(417), 38–50.

Charnov, E.L. & Berrigan, D. (1993). Why do female primates have such long lifespans and so few babies? or life in the slow lane. *Evol Anthropol,* **1**, 191–94.

Charuvastra, A. & Cloitre, M. (2008). Social bonds and posttraumatic stress disorder. *Annu Rev Psychol,* **59**, 301–28.

Chavanne, T.J. & Gallup, G.G. (1998). Variation in risk taking behavior among female college students as a function of the menstrual cycle. *Evol Human Behav,* **19**, 27–32.

Chen, C.S., Burton, M., Greenberger, E., & Dmitrieva, J. (1999). Population migration and the variation of dopamine D4 receptor (DRD4) allele frequencies around the globe. *Evol Human Behav,* **20**, 309–24.

Chiao, J.Y. & Blizinsky, K. D. (2010). Culture–gene coevolution of individualism–collectivism and the serotonin transporter gene. *Proc Biol Sci,* **277**, 529–37.

Chiarlone, A., Bellocchio, L., Blazquez, C., et al. (2014). A restricted population of CB1 cannabinoid receptors with neuroprotective activity. *Proc Natl Acad Sci USA,* **111**, 8257–62.

Chiavetto, L.B., Boin, F., Zanardini, R., et al. (2002). Association between promoter polymorphic haplotypes of interleukin-10 gene and schizophrenia. *Biol Psychiatry,* **51**, 480–84.

Chioqueta, A.P. & Stiles, T.C. (2004). Assessing suicide risk in cluster C personality disorders. *Crisis J Crisis Intervention Suicide Prev,* **25**, 128–33.

Chong, T.T., Cunnington, R., Williams, M.A., Kanwisher, N., & Mattingley, J.B. (2008). fMRI adaptation reveals mirror neurons in human inferior parietal cortex. *Curr Biol,* **18**, 1576–80.

Christensen, B.K. & Bilder, R.M. (2000). Dual cytoarchitectonic trends: an evolutionary model of frontal lobe functioning and its application to psychopathology. *Can J Psychiatry,* **45**, 247–56.

Christophersen, C. (1991). Evolution in molecular structure and adaptive variance in metabolism. *Comp Biochem Physiol B,* **98**, 427–32.

Chua, P., Krams, M., Toni, I., Passingham, R., & Dolan, R. (1999). A functional anatomy of anticipatory anxiety. *Neuroimage,* **9**, 563–71.

Chue, P. & Lalonde, J.K. (2014). Addressing the unmet needs of patients with persistent negative symptoms of schizophrenia: emerging pharmacological treatment options. *Neuropsychiatric Dis Treat,* **10**, 777–89.

Cicchetti, D., Rogosch, F.A., Hecht, K.F., Crick, N.R., & Hetzel, S. (2014). Moderation of maltreatment effects on childhood borderline personality symptoms by gender and oxytocin receptor and FK506 binding protein 5 genes. *Dev Psychopathol*, **26**, 831–49.

Cikara, M., Bruneau, E.G., & Saxe, R.R. (2011). Us and them: intergroup failures of empathy. *Curr Directions Psychol Sci*, **20**, 149–53.

Clark, D.M. (1999). Anxiety disorders: why they persist and how to treat them. *Behav Res Therapy*, **37** (Suppl 1), S5–27.

Clark, L.A., Kochanska, G., & Ready, R. (2000). Mothers' personality and its interaction with child temperament as predictors of parenting behavior. *J Pers Soc Psychol*, **79**, 274–85.

Clarke, A.S. & Boinski, S. (1995). Temperament in nonhuman-primates. *Am J Primatol*, **37**, 103–25.

Cloninger, C.R. (1987). Neurogenetic adaptive mechanisms in alcoholism. *Science*, **236**, 410–16.

Cloninger, C.R. (1999). *Personality and Psychopathology*. American Psychiatric Press, Washington, DC.

Cloninger, C.R. (2000). Biology of personality dimensions. *Curr Opin Psychiatry*, **13**, 611–16.

Cloninger, C.R., Svrakic, D.M., & Przybeck, T.R. (1993). A psychobiological model of temperament and character. *Arch Gen Psychiatry*, **50**, 975–90.

Cohen, D.L. & Belsky, J. (2008). Individual differences in female mate preferences as a function of attachment and hypothetical ecological conditions. *J Evol Psychol*, **6**, 25–42.

Cohen, L.J., McGeoch, P.G., Gans, S.W., et al. (2002). Childhood sexual history of 20 male pedophiles vs. 24 male healthy control subjects. *J Nerv Ment Dis*, **190**, 757–66.

Comings, D.E. & Blum, K. (2000). Reward deficiency syndrome: genetic aspects of behavioral disorders. *Prog Brain Res*, **126**, 325–41.

Conejero-Goldberg, C., Gomar, J.J., Bobes-Bascaran, T., et al. (2014). APOE2 enhances neuroprotection against Alzheimer's disease through multiple molecular mechanisms. *Mol Psychiatry*, **19**, 1243–50.

Coop, G., Pickrell, J.K., Novembre, J., et al. (2009). The role of geography in human adaptation. *PLoS Genet*, **5**, e1000500.

Coplan, J.D., Andrews, M.W., Rosenblum, L.A., et al. (1996). Persistent elevations of cerebrospinal fluid concentrations of corticotropin-releasing factor in adult nonhuman primates exposed to early-life stressors: implications for the pathophysiology of mood and anxiety disorders. *Proc Natl Acad Sci USA*, **93**, 1619–23.

Corballis, M.C. (1997). The genetics and evolution of handedness. *Psychol Rev*, **104**, 714–27.

Corballis, M.C. (2003). From mouth to hand: gesture, speech, and the evolution of right-handedness. *Behav Brain Sci*, **26**, 199–208; discussion 208–60.

Cordain, L., Eaton, S.B., Sebastian, A., et al. (2005). Origins and evolution of the Western diet: health implications for the 21st century. *Am J Clin Nutr*, **81**, 341–54.

Corwyn, R.F. & Bradley, R.H. (1999). Determinants of paternal and maternal investment in children. *Infant Ment Health J*, **20**, 238–56.

Coryell, W.H. (2006). Clinical assessment of suicide risk in depressive disorder. *CNS Spectr*, **11**, 455–61.

Coryell, W. & Schlesser, M. (2001). The dexamethasone suppression test and suicide prediction. *Am J Psychiatry*, **158**, 748–53.

Cosmides, L. (1989). The logic of social exchange: has natural selection shaped how humans reason? Studies with the Wason selection task. *Cognition*, **31**, 187–276.

Cosmides, L. & Tooby, J. (1994). Beyond intuition and instinct blindness: toward an evolutionarily rigorous cognitive science. *Cognition*, **50**, 41–77.

Cosmides, L. & Tooby, J. (1997). Dissecting the computational architecture of social inference mechanisms. *Ciba Found Symp*, **208**, 132–56; discussion 156–61.

Cosmides, L. & Tooby, J. (1999). Toward an evolutionary taxonomy of treatable conditions. *J Abnorm Psychol*, **108**, 453–64.

Cosmides, L., Tooby, J., & Barkow, J.H. (1992). Introduction: evolutionary psychology and conceptual integration. In: Barkow, J.H., Cosmides, L., & Tooby, J. (eds) *The Adapted Mind*. Oxford University Press, Oxford.

Costello, E.J., Keeler, G.P., & Angold, A. (2001). Poverty, race/ethnicity, and psychiatric disorder: a study of rural children. *Am J Public Health*, **91**, 1494–98.

Cowan, W.M., Kopnisky, K.L., & Hyman, S.E. (2002). The human genome project and its impact on psychiatry. *Annu Rev Neurosci*, **25**, 1–50.

Craddock, N. & Jones, I. (2001). Molecular genetics of bipolar disorder. *Br J Psychiatry*, **178**, S128–33.

Craddock, N., O'Donovan, M.C., & Owen, M.J. (2006). Genes for schizophrenia and bipolar disorder? Implications for psychiatric nosology. *Schizophr Bull*, **32**, 9–16.

Craig, A.D. (2003). Interoception: the sense of the physiological condition of the body. *Curr Opin Neurobiol*, **13**, 500–505.

Crebbin, K., Mitford, E., Paxton, R., & Turkington, D. (2008). First-episode psychosis: an epidemiological survey comparing psychotic depression with schizophrenia. *J Affect Disord*, **105**, 117–24.

Crespi, B. & Badcock, C. (2008). Psychosis and autism as diametrical disorders of the social brain. *Behav Brain Sci*, **31**, 241–320.

Crespi, B., Summers, K., & Dorus, S. (2007). Adaptive evolution of genes underlying schizophrenia. *Proc Biol Sci*, **274**, 2801–10.

Crespi, B., Foster, K., & Ubeda, F. (2014). First principles of Hamiltonian medicine. *Philos Trans R Soc Lond B Biol Sci*, **369**, 20130366.

Crichton-Browne, J. (1879). On the weight of the brain and its component parts in the insane. *Brain*, **2**, 42–67.

Critchley, H.D., Daly, E.M., Bullmore, E.T., et al. (2000). The functional neuroanatomy of social behaviour—changes in cerebral blood flow when people with autistic disorder process facial expressions. *Brain*, **123**, 2203–12.

Crow, T.J. (1988). Sex chromosomes and psychosis. The case for a pseudoautosomal locus. *Br J Psychiatry*, **153**, 675–83.

Crow, T.J. (1990). The continuum of psychosis and its genetic origins. The sixty-fifth Maudsley lecture. *Br J Psychiatry*, **156**, 788–97.

Crow, T.J. (1991). The origins of psychosis and 'The Descent of Man'. *Br J Psychiatry Suppl*, **159**(14), 76–82.

Crow, T.J. (1995a). Constraints on concepts of pathogenesis. Language and the speciation process as the key to the etiology of schizophrenia. *Arch Gen Psychiatry*, **52**, 1011–14; discussion 1019–24.

Crow, T.J. (1995b). A Darwinian approach to the origins of psychosis. *Br J Psychiatry*, **167**, 12–25.

Crow, T.J. (1995c). A theory of the evolutionary origins of psychosis. *Eur Neuropsychopharmacol*, **1997** (5 Suppl), 59–63.

Crow, T.J. (1997a). Is schizophrenia the price that Homo sapiens pays for language? *Schizophr Res*, **28**, 127–41.

Crow, T.J. (1997b). Schizophrenia as failure of hemispheric dominance for language. *Trends Neurosci*, **20**, 339–43.

Crow, T.J. (1997c). Temporolimbic or transcallosal connections: where is the primary lesion in schizophrenia and what is its nature? *Schizophr Bull*, **23**, 521–23.

Crow, T.J. (1998a). Nuclear schizophrenic symptoms as a window on the relationship between thought and speech. *Br J Psychiatry*, **173**, 303–309.

Crow, T.J. (1998b). From Kraepelin to Kretschmer leavened by Schneider: the transition from categories of psychosis to dimensions of variation intrinsic to *Homo sapiens*. *Arch Gen Psychiatry*, **55**, 502–504.

Crow, T.J. (1998c). Schizophrenia as a transcallosal misconnection syndrome. *Schizophr Res*, **30**, 111–14.

Crow, T.J. (1999). Commentary on Annett, Yeo et al., Klar, Saugstad and Orr: cerebral asymmetry, language and psychosis—the case for a *Homo sapiens*-specific sex-linked gene for brain growth. *Schizophr Res*, **39**, 219–31.

Crow, T.J. (2002). *The Speciation of Modern* Homo sapiens. Oxford University Press, Oxford.

Crow, T.J., Done, D.J., & Sacker, A. (1995). Childhood precursors of psychosis as clues to its evolutionary origins. *Eur Arch Psychiatry Clin Neurosci*, **245**, 61–69.

Crow, T.J., Done, D.J., & Sacker, A. (1996). Cerebral lateralization is delayed in children who later develop schizophrenia. *Schizophr Res*, **22**, 181–85.

Cryan, J.F. & Dinan, T.G. (2012). Mind-altering microorganisms: the impact of the gut microbiota on brain and behaviour. *Nat Rev Neurosci*, **13**, 701–12.

Cummings, J.L. & Cunningham, K. (1992). Obsessive-compulsive disorder in Huntington's disease. *Biol Psychiatry*, **31**, 263–70.

Cutting, J. & Murphy, D. (1990). Impaired ability of schizophrenics, relative to manics or depressives, to appreciate social knowledge about their culture. *Br J Psychiatry*, **157**, 355–58.

Daly, M. & Wilson, M. (1988). Evolutionary social psychology and family homicide. *Science*, **242**, 519–24.

Daly, M. & Wilson, M.I. (1999). Human evolutionary psychology and animal behaviour. *Anim Behav*, **57**, 509–19.

Daly, M., Wilson, M., & Weghorst, S.J. (1982). Male sexual jealousy. *Ethol Sociobiol*, **3**, 11–27.

Damasio, A.R. (1994). *Descartes' Error: Emotion, Reason, and the Human Brain*. Putnam, New York.

Damasio, A.R. (1995). Toward a neurobiology of emotion and feeling: operational concepts and hypotheses. *Neuroscientist*, **1**, 19–25.

Damasio, A.R. (1996). The somatic marker hypothesis and the possible functions of the prefrontal cortex. *Philos Trans R Soc Lond B Biol Sci*, **351**, 1413–20.

Damasio, A. & Carvalho, G.B. (2013). The nature of feelings: evolutionary and neurobiological origins. *Nat Rev Neurosci*, **14**, 143–52.

Danese, A. & Tan, M. (2014). Childhood maltreatment and obesity: systematic review and meta-analysis. *Mol Psychiatry*, **19**, 544–54.

Dannlowski, U., Stuhrmann, A., Beutelmann, V., et al. (2012). Limbic scars: long-term consequences of childhood maltreatment revealed by functional and structural magnetic resonance imaging. *Biol Psychiatry*, **71**, 286–93.

Darwin, C. (1859). *On the Origin of Species by Means of Natural Selection*. J. Murray, London.

Darwin, C. (1871). *The Descent of Man and Selection in Relation to Sex*. Printed for the Limited Editions Club at the Griffin Press, Adelaide.

Darwin, C. (1872). *The Expression of Emotions in Man and Animals*. J. Murray, London.

Davidson, J.R. (2000). Pharmacotherapy of posttraumatic stress disorder: treatment options, long-term follow-up, and predictors of outcome. *J Clin Psychiatry*, **61** (Suppl 5), 52–56; discussion 57–59.

Davidson, R.J. (2002). Anxiety and affective style: role of prefrontal cortex and amygdala. *Biol Psychiatry*, **51**, 68–80.

Dawkins, R. (1976). *The Selfish Gene*. Oxford University Press, New York.

Dawkins, R. (1982). *The Extended Phenotype*. Oxford University Press, Oxford.

Dawkins, R. (1986). *The Blind Watchmaker*. Norton, New York.

Dawkins, R. & Krebs, J.R. (1979). Arms races between and within species. *Proc R Soc Lond B Biol Sci*, **205**, 489–511.

De Beer, G. (1958). *Embryos and Ancestors*. Clarendon Press, Oxford.

De Bellis, M.D., Keshavan, M.S., Beers, S.R., et al. (2001). Sex differences in brain maturation during childhood and adolescence. *Cereb Cortex*, **11**, 552–57.

De Catanzaro, D. (1995). Reproductive status, family interactions, and suicidal ideation: surveys of the general public and high-risk groups. *Ethol Sociobiol*, **16**, 385–94.

De Clérambault, G.G. (1942). Les psychoses passionelles. *Oevre Psychiatrique. Presses Univ Fr*, **331**, 337–39, 357, 408.

De Dreu, C.K., Shalvi, S., Greer, L.L., Van Kleef, G.A., & Handgraaf, M.J. (2012). Oxytocin motivates non-cooperation in intergroup conflict to protect vulnerable in-group members. *PLoS One*, **7**, e46751.

De Quervain, D.J., Fischbacher, U., Treyer, V., et al. (2004). The neural basis of altruistic punishment. *Science*, **305**, 1254–58.

De Shazer, S. (1985). *Keys to Solution in Brief Therapy*. W.W. Norton, New York.

De Souza, A.A., Baiao, V.B., & Otta, E. (2003). Perception of men's personal qualities and prospect of employment as a function of facial hair. *Psychol Rep*, **92**, 201–208.

Deacon, T.W. (1990a). Fallacies of progression in theories of brain-size evolution. *Int J Primatol*, **11**, 193–236.

Deacon, T.W. (1990b). Problems of ontogeny and phylogeny in brain-size evolution. *Int J Primatol*, **11**, 237–82.

Decety, J. & Chaminade, T. (2005). The neurophysiology of imitation and intersubjectivity. In: Hurley, S. & Chater, N. (eds) *Perspectives on Imitation. Vol. 1. Mechanisms of Imitation and Imitation in Animals*. MIT Press, Cambridge, Massachusetts.

Deckert, J., Catalano, M., Syagailo, Y.V., et al. (1999). Excess of high activity monoamine oxidase A gene promoter alleles in female patients with panic disorder. *Hum Mol Genet*, **8**, 621–24.

Del Ben, K. & Fremouw, W. (2002). Stalking: developing an empirical typology to classify stalkers. *J Forensic Sci*, **47**, 152–58.

Del Giudice, M. (2014). An evolutionary life history framework for psychopathology. *Psychol Inquiry*, **25**, 261–300.

Del Giudice, M., Angeleri, R., Brizio, A., & Elena, M.R. (2010). The evolution of autistic-like and schizotypal traits: a sexual selection hypothesis. *Front Psychol*, **1**, 41.

Del Giudice, M., Booth, T., & Irwing, P. (2012). The distance between Mars and Venus: measuring global sex differences in personality. *PLoS One*, **7**, e29265.

Delisi, L.E. (1997). Gender and age at onset of schizophrenia. *Br J Psychiatry*, **171**, 188.

Delisi, L.E. (2001). Speech disorder in schizophrenia: review of the literature and exploration of its relation to the uniquely human capacity for language. *Schizophr Bull*, **27**, 481–96.

Delisi, L.E., Shaw, S., Sherrington, R., et al. (2000). Failure to establish linkage on the X chromosome in 301 families with schizophrenia or schizoaffective disorder. *Am J Med Genet*, **96**, 335–41.

Delvecchio, E., Di Riso, D., Salcuni, S., Lis, A., & George, C. (2014). Anorexia and attachment: dysregulated defense and pathological mourning. *Front Psychol*, **5**, 1218.

Demoulin, S. & De Dreu, C.K.W. (2010). Introduction: Negotiation in intergroup conflict. *Group Processes Intergroup Relations*, **13**, 675–83.

Den Boer, J.A. (2000). Social anxiety disorder/social phobia: epidemiology, diagnosis, neurobiology, and treatment. *Compr Psychiatry*, **41**, 405–15.

Dennett, D.C. (1983). Intentional systems in cognitive ethology—the panglossian paradigm defended. *Behav Brain Sci*, **6**, 343–55.

Dennett, D.C. (1984). *Elbow Room: The Varieties of Free Will Worth Wanting*. MIT Press, Cambridge, Massachusetts.

Dennett, D.C. (1995). *Darwin's Dangerous Idea: Evolution and the Meanings of Life*. Simon & Schuster, New York.

Dennett, D.C. (2003). *Freedom Evolves*. Viking, New York.

Deussing, J.M. & Wurst, W. (2007). Amygdala and neocortex: common origins and shared mechanisms. *Nat Neurosci*, **10**, 1081–82.

Devinsky, O., Morrell, M.J., & Vogt, B.A. (1995). Contributions of anterior cingulate cortex to behaviour. *Brain*, **118** (Pt 1), 279–306.

Diamond, J.M. (1988). Tay-Sachs carriers and tuberculosis resistance—reply. *Nature*, **331**, 666.

Diamond, J. (2012). *The World Until Yesterday*. Viking Press, New York.

Dickerson, S.S., Gruenewald, T.L., & Kemeny, M.E. (2004). When the social self is threatened: shame, physiology, and health. *J Pers*, **72**, 1191–216.

Dimic, S., Wildgrube, C., McCabe, R., et al. (2010). Non-verbal behaviour of patients with schizophrenia in medical consultations—a comparison with depressed patients and association with symptom levels. *Psychopathology*, **43**, 216–22.

Ding, Y.C., Chi, H.C., Grady, D.L., et al. (2002). Evidence of positive selection acting at the human dopamine receptor D4 gene locus. *Proc Natl Acad Sci USA*, **99**, 309–14.

Distel, M.A., Middeldorp, C.M., Trull, T.J., et al. (2011). Life events and borderline personality features: the influence of gene–environment interaction and gene–environment correlation. *Psychol Med*, **41**, 849–60.

Dixon, A.K. (1986). Ethological aspects of psychiatry. *Schweiz Arch Neurol Psychiatr*, **137**, 151–63.

Dixon, A.K. (1998). Ethological strategies for defence in animals and humans: their role in some psychiatric disorders. *Br J Med Psychol*, **71** (Pt 4), 417–45.

Dixon, A.K., Fisch, H.U., Huber, C., & Walser, A. (1989). Ethological studies in animals and man, their use in psychiatry. *Pharmacopsychiatry*, **22** (Suppl 1), 44–50.

Doi, N., Hoshi, Y., Itokawa, M., et al. (2009). Persistence criteria for susceptibility genes for schizophrenia: a discussion from an evolutionary viewpoint. *PLoS One*, **4**, e7799.

Dolan, M. & Davies, G. (2006). Psychopathy and institutional outcome in patients with schizophrenia in forensic settings in the UK. *Schizophr Res*, **81**, 277–81.

Dolan, M. & Park, I. (2002). The neuropsychology of antisocial personality disorder. *Psychol Med*, **32**, 417–27.

Dolan, R.J. (1999). On the neurology of morals. *Nat Neurosci*, **2**, 927–29.

Dölen, G., Darvishzadeh, A., Huang, K.W. & Malenka, R.C. (2013). Social reward requires coordinated activity of nucleus accumbens oxytocin and serotonin. *Nature*, **501**, 179–84.

Domes, G., Heinrichs, M., Michel, A., Berger, C., & Herpertz, S.C. (2007). Oxytocin improves 'mind-reading' in humans. *Biol Psychiatry*, **61**, 731–33.

Donahoe, J.W. (2002). Behavior analysis and neuroscience. *Behav Processes*, **57**, 241–59.

Donaldson, Z.R. & Young, L.J. (2008). Oxytocin, vasopressin, and the neurogenetics of sociality. *Science*, **322**, 900–904.

Donnelly, S.L., Wolpert, C.M., Menold, M.M., et al. (2000). Female with autistic disorder and monosomy X (Turner syndrome): parent-of-origin effect of the X chromosome. *Am J Med Genet*, **96**, 312–16.

Dorban, P.T. (1979). Women who kill their children. *Br J Psychiatry*, **134**, 560–71.

Downing, L.J., Caprio, T.V., & Lyness, J.M. (2013). Geriatric psychiatry review: differential diagnosis and treatment of the 3 D's—delirium, dementia, and depression. *Curr Psychiatry Rep*, **15**, 365.

Dozier, M., Stovall, K.C., & Albus, K.E. (1999). Attachment and psychopathology in adulthood. In: Cassidy, J. & Shaver, P.R. (eds) *Handbook of Attachment. Theory, Research, and Clinical Applications.* Guilford Press, New York.

Driessen, M., Herrmann, J., Stahl, K., et al. (2000). Magnetic resonance imaging volumes of the hippocampus and the amygdala in women with borderline personality disorder and early traumatization. *Arch Gen Psychiatry*, **57**, 1115–22.

Drigotas, S.M. & Barta, W. (2001). The cheating heart: scientific explorations of infidelity. *Curr Directions Psychol Sci*, **10**, 177–80.

Drotar, D. (1991). The family context of nonorganic failure-to-thrive. *Am J Orthopsychiatry*, **61**, 23–34.

Dube, S.R., Anda, R.F., Felitti, V.J., et al. (2001). Childhood abuse, household dysfunction, and the risk of attempted suicide throughout the life span: findings from the Adverse Childhood Experiences Study. *JAMA*, **286**, 3089–96.

Dubrovsky, B. (2002). Evolutionary psychiatry. Adaptationist and nonadaptationist conceptualizations. *Prog Neuropsychopharmacol Biol Psychiatry*, **26**, 1–19.

Duchaine, B., Cosmides, L., & Tooby, J. (2001). Evolutionary psychology and the brain. *Curr Opin Neurobiol*, **11**, 225–30.

Dudley, R. (2000). Evolutionary origins of human alcoholism in primate frugivory. *Q Rev Biol*, **75**, 3–15.

Dudley, R. (2002). Fermenting fruit and the historical ecology of ethanol ingestion: is alcoholism in modern humans an evolutionary hangover? *Addiction*, **97**, 381–88.

Dumais, A., Lesage, A.D., Boyer, R., et al. (2005). Psychiatric risk factors for motor vehicle fatalities in young men. *Can J Psychiatry*, **50**, 838–44.

Dunbar, R.I.M. (1995). Neocortex size and group-size in primates—a test of the hypothesis. *J Human Evol*, **28**, 287–96.

Dunbar, R.I.M. (1998). The social brain hypothesis. *Evol Anthropol*, **6**, 178–90.

Dunbar, R. (2003a). Evolution of the social brain. *Science*, **302**, 1160–61.

Dunbar, R.I.M. (2003b). The social brain: mind, language, and society in evolutionary perspective. *Annu Rev Anthropol*, **32**, 163–81.

Dunbar, R.I. & Shultz, S. (2007a). Evolution in the social brain. *Science*, **317**, 1344–47.

Dunbar, R.I. & Shultz, S. (2007b). Understanding primate brain evolution. *Philos Trans R Soc Lond B Biol Sci*, **362**, 649–58.

Dunn, J. (1993). Psychic conflict and the external world in Freud's theory of the instinctual drives in light of his adherence to Darwin. *Int J Psychoanal*, **74** (Pt 2), 231–40.

Dunne, F.J. & Schipperheijn, J.A. (2000). Stalking (obsessive pursuit). *Hospital Med*, **61**, 31–32.

Dvash, J., Gilam, G., Ben-Ze'ev, A., Hendler, T., & Shamay-Tsoory, S.G. (2010). The envious brain: the neural basis of social comparison. *Hum Brain Mapp*, **31**, 1741–50.

Dyck, M.J., Ferguson, K., & Shochet, I.M. (2001). Do autism spectrum disorders differ from each other and from non-spectrum disorders on emotion recognition tests? *Eur Child Adolesc Psychiatry*, **10**, 105–16.

Eaton, S.B., Konner, M.J., & Cordain, L. (2010). Diet-dependent acid load, Paleolithic [corrected] nutrition, and evolutionary health promotion. *Am J Clin Nutr*, **91**, 295–97.

Ebert, A., Kolb, M., Heller, J., et al. (2013). Modulation of interpersonal trust in borderline personality disorder by intranasal oxytocin and childhood trauma. *Soc Neurosci*, **8**, 305–13.

Ebstein, R.P., Israel, S., Chew, S.H., Zhong, S., & Knafo, A. (2010). Genetics of human social behavior. *Neuron*, **65**, 831–44.

Eckel, C.C. & Grossman, P.J. (2001). Chivalry and solidarity in ultimatum games. *Econ Inquiry*, **39**, 171–88.

Ege, M.J., Strachan, D.P., Cookson, W.O., et al. (2011). Gene–environment interaction for childhood asthma and exposure to farming in Central Europe. *J Allergy Clin Immunol*, **127**, 138–44, 144 e1–4.

Eggers, H.M. & Blakemore, C. (1978). Physiological basis of anisometropic amblyopia. *Science*, **201**, 264–67.

Ehnvall, A., Parker, G., Hadzi-Pavlovic, D., & Malhi, G. (2008). Perception of rejecting and neglectful parenting in childhood relates to lifetime suicide attempts for females—but not for males. *Acta Psychiatr Scand*, **117**, 50–56.

Ehrlich, P.R. (2000). *Human Natures: Genes, Cultures, and the Human Prospect*. Island Press for Shearwater Books, Washington, DC.

Eibl-Eibesfeldt, I. (1995). *Die Biologie Menschlichen Verhaltens. Grundriss der Humanethologie*. Piper, Zürich.

Eisenberg, D.T., Campbell, B., Gray, P.B., & Sorenson, M.D. (2008). Dopamine receptor genetic polymorphisms and body composition in undernourished pastoralists: an exploration of nutrition indices among nomadic and recently settled Ariaal men of northern Kenya. *BMC Evol Biol*, **8**, 173.

Eisenberger, N.I. (2012). The pain of social disconnection: examining the shared neural underpinnings of physical and social pain. *Nat Rev Neurosci*, **13**, 421–34.

Eissler, R. (ed.) (1945). *The Psychoanalytic Study of the Child*. International Universities Press, New York.

Ekman, P. (1982). *Emotion in the Human Face*. Cambridge University Press, Cambridge.

Ekman, P. (2003). *Emotions Revealed. Understanding Faces and Feelings*. Weidenfeld and Nicolson, London.

El-Kamary, S.S., Higman, S.M., Fuddy, L., et al. (2004). Hawaii's healthy start home visiting program: determinants and impact of rapid repeat birth. *Pediatrics*, **114**, e317–26.

Eley, T.C., Collier, D., & McGuffin, P. (2005). Anxiety and eating disorders. In: McGuffin, P., Owen, M.J., & Gottesman, I. (eds) *Psychiatric Genetics and Genomics*. Oxford University Press, Oxford.

Elliott, R., Vollm, B., Drury, A., et al. (2006). Co-operation with another player in a financially rewarded guessing game activates regions implicated in theory of mind. *Soc Neurosci*, **1**, 385–95.

Ellis, B.J. & Del Giudice, M. (2014). Beyond allostatic load: rethinking the role of stress in regulating human development. *Dev Psychopathol*, **26**, 1–20.

Ellis, B.J. & Symons, D. (1990). Sex-differences in sexual fantasy—an evolutionary psychological approach. *J Sex Res*, **27**, 527–55.

Ellis, B.J., McFadyen-Ketchum, S., Dodge, K.A., Pettit, G.S., & Bates, J.E. (1999). Quality of early family relationships and individual differences in the timing of pubertal maturation in girls: a longitudinal test of an evolutionary model. *J Pers Soc Psychol*, **77**, 387–401.

Ellis, B.J., Boyce, W.T., Belsky, J., Bakermans-Kranenburg, M.J., & Van Ijzendoorn, M.H. (2011a). Differential susceptibility to the environment: an evolutionary—neurodevelopmental theory. *Dev Psychopathol*, **23**, 7–28.

Ellis, B.J., Shirtcliff, E.A., Boyce, W.T., Deardorff, J., & Essex, M.J. (2011b). Quality of early family relationships and the timing and tempo of puberty: effects depend on biological sensitivity to context. *Dev Psychopathol*, **23**, 85–99.

Ellsworth, P.C., Carlsmith, J.M., & Henson, A. (1972). The stare as a stimulus to flight in human subjects: a series of field experiments. *J Pers Soc Psychol*, **21**, 302–11.

Elphick, M.R. & Egertova, M. (2001). The neurobiology and evolution of cannabinoid signalling. *Philos Trans R Soc Lond Ser B-Biol Sci*, **356**, 381–408.

Emery, N.J., Clayton, N.S., & Frith, C.D. (2007). Introduction. Social intelligence: from brain to culture. *Philos Trans R Soc Lond Ser B-Biol Sci*, **362**, 485–88.

Emlen, S.T. (1995). An evolutionary theory of the family. *Proc Natl Acad Sci USA*, **92**, 8092–99.

Enard, W., Przeworski, M., Fisher, S.E., et al. (2002). Molecular evolution of FOXP2, a gene involved in speech and language. *Nature*, **418**, 869–72.

Engel, G.L. (1977). The need for a new medical model: a challenge for biomedicine. *Science*, **196**, 129–36.

Enoch, M.A. (2006). Genetic and environmental influences on the development of alcoholism: resilience vs. risk. *Ann N Y Acad Sci*, **1094**, 193–201.

Enquist, M. & Arak, A. (1993). Selection of exaggerated male traits by female aesthetic senses. *Nature*, **361**, 446–48.

Erickson, M.T. (2000). The evolution of incest avoidance: Oedipus and the psychopathologies of kinship. In: Gilbert, P. & Bailey, K.G. (eds) *Genes on the Couch. Explorations in Evolutionary Psychotherapy*. Brunner-Routledge, Hove.

Erickson, M.T. (2006). Nature disrupted: evolution, kinship and child sexual abuse. *Clin Neuropsychiatry*, **3**, 110–20.

Erlenmeyer-Kimling, L. (1968). Mortality rates in the offspring of schizophrenic parents and a physiological advantage hypothesis. *Nature*, **220**, 798–800.

Eronen, M., Angermeyer, M.C., & Schulze, B. (1998). The psychiatric epidemiology of violent behaviour. *Soc Psychiatry Psychiatr Epidemiol*, **33** (Suppl 1), S13–23.

Esquirol, J.E.D. (1805/1980). *Des Passions. Considérées comme Causes Symptômes et Moyen Curatifs d'alienation Mentale*. Les Deux Mondes, Paris.

Estes, L.S. & Tidwell, R. (2002). Sexually abused children's behaviours: impact of gender and mother's experience of intra- and extra-familial sexual abuse. *Fam Pract*, **19**, 36–44.

Etkin, A. & Wager, T.D. (2007). Functional neuroimaging of anxiety: a meta-analysis of emotional processing in PTSD, social anxiety disorder, and specific phobia. *Am J Psychiatry*, **164**, 1476–88.

Etkin, A., Pittenger, C., Polan, H.J., & Kandel, E.R. (2005). Toward a neurobiology of psychotherapy: basic science and clinical applications. *J Neuropsychiatry Clin Neurosci*, **17**, 145–58.

Evans, D.A., Bennett, D.A., Wilson, R.S., et al. (2003). Incidence of Alzheimer disease in a biracial urban community: relation to apolipoprotein E allele status. *Arch Neurol*, **60**, 185–89.

Evans, P.D., Anderson, J.R., Vallender, E.J., Choi, S.S., & Lahn, B.T. (2004). Reconstructing the evolutionary history of microcephalin, a gene controlling human brain size. Hum Mol Genet, **13**, 1139–45.

Evrard, H.C., Forro, T., & Logothetis, N.K. (2012). Von Economo neurons in the anterior insula of the macaque monkey. *Neuron*, **74**, 482–89.

Ewbank, D.C. (2002). Mortality differences by APOE genotype estimated from demographic synthesis. *Genetic Epidemiol*, **22**, 146–55.

Ewbank, D.C. (2004). The APOE gene and differences in life expectancy in Europe. *J Gerontol A Biol Sci Med Sci*, **59**, 16–20.

Eyring, W.E., 3rd & Sobelman, S. (1996). Narcissism and birth order. *Psychol Rep*, **78**, 403–406.

Eysenck, H. J. & Martin, I. (1987). *Theoretical Foundations of Behavior Therapy*. Plenum Press, New York.

Fabrega, H., Jr. (1990). The concept of somatization as a cultural and historical product of Western medicine. *Psychosom Med*, **52**, 653–72.

Fabrega, H., Jr. (1994). International systems of diagnosis in psychiatry. *J Nerv Ment Dis*, **182**, 256–63.

Fabrega, H., Jr. (1997). Earliest phases in the evolution of sickness and healing. *Med Anthropol Q*, **11**, 26–55.

Fabrega, H. (2002). *Origins of Psychopathology: The Phylogenetic and Cultural Basis of Mental Illness*. Rutgers University Press, New Brunswick.

Fabrega, H., Jr. (2006). Why psychiatric conditions are special: an evolutionary and cross-cultural perspective. *Perspect Biol Med*, **49**, 586–601.

Fabrega, H., Jr. (2007). How psychiatric conditions were made. *Psychiatry*, **70**, 130–53.

Faer, L.M., Hendriks, A., Abed, R.T., & Figueredo, A.J. (2005). The evolutionary psychology of eating disorders: female competition for mates or for status? *Psychol Psychother*, **78**, 397–417.

Fagundo, A.B., De La Torre, R., Jimenez-Murcia, S., et al. (2012). Executive functions profile in extreme eating/weight conditions: from anorexia nervosa to obesity. *PLoS One*, **7**, e43382.

Fahim, C., Stip, E., Mancini-Marie, A., et al. (2004). Negative socio-emotional resonance in schizophrenia: a functional magnetic resonance imaging hypothesis. *Med Hypotheses*, **63**, 467–75.

Fajardo, C., Escobar, M.I., Buritica, E., et al. (2008). Von Economo neurons are present in the dorsolateral (dysgranular) prefrontal cortex of humans. *Neurosci Lett*, **435**, 215–18.

Fanous, A.H., Neale, M.C., Gardner, C.O., et al. (2007). Significant correlation in linkage signals from genome-wide scans of schizophrenia and schizotypy. *Mol Psychiatry*, **12**, 958–65.

Faravelli, C., Giugni, A., Salvatori, S., & Ricca, V. (2004). Psychopathology after rape. *Am J Psychiatry*, **161**, 1483–85.

Fardilha, M., Vieira, S.I., Barros, A., et al. (2007). Differential distribution of Alzheimer's amyloid precursor protein family variants in human sperm. *Ann N Y Acad Sci*, **1096**, 196–206.

Farrer, L.A., Friedland, R.P., Bowirrat, A., et al. (2003). Genetic and environmental epidemiology of Alzheimer's disease in arabs residing in Israel. *J Mol Neurosci*, **20**, 207–12.

Fatemi, S.H., Reutiman, T.J., Folsom, T.D., et al. (2008). Maternal infection leads to abnormal gene regulation and brain atrophy in mouse offspring: implications for genesis of neurodevelopmental disorders. *Schizophr Res*, **99**, 56–70.

Fava, M. & Rosenbaum, J. F. (1999). Anger attacks in patients with depression. *J Clin Psychiatry*, **60** (Suppl 15), 21–24.

Favaro, A., Zanetti, T., Tenconi, E., et al. (2005). The relationship between temperament and impulsive behaviors in eating disordered subjects. *Eat Disord*, **13**, 61–70.

Favaro, A., Tenconi, E., & Santonastaso, P. (2006). Perinatal factors and the risk of developing anorexia nervosa and bulimia nervosa. *Arch Gen Psychiatry*, **63**, 82–88.

Fazel, S. & Danesh, J. (2002). Serious mental disorder in 23000 prisoners: a systematic review of 62 surveys. *Lancet*, **359**, 545–50.

Fear, C.F. & Healy, D. (1997). Probabilistic reasoning in obsessive-compulsive and delusional disorders. *Psychol Med*, **27**, 199–208.

Feder, A., Nestler, E.J., & Charney, D.S. (2009). Psychobiology and molecular genetics of resilience. *Nat Rev Neurosci*, **10**, 446–57.

Feeney, B.C. & Collins, N.L. (2001). Predictors of caregiving in adult intimate relationships: an attachment theoretical perspective. *J Pers Soc Psychol*, **80**, 972–94.

Fehm, H.L., Kern, W., & Peters, A. (2006). The selfish brain: competition for energy resources. *Prog Brain Res*, **153**, 129–40.

Fehr, E. & Fischbacher, U. (2004a). Social norms and human cooperation. *Trends Cogn Sci*, **8**, 185–90.

Fehr, E. & Fischbacher, U. (2004b). Third-party punishment and social norms. *Evol Human Behav*, **25**, 63–87.

Fehr, E. & Gachter, S. (2002). Altruistic punishment in humans. *Nature*, **415**, 137–40.

Fehr, E. & Rockenbach, B. (2004). Human altruism: economic, neural, and evolutionary perspectives. *Curr Opin Neurobiol*, **14**, 784–90.

Feierman, J.R. (1987). The ethology of psychiatric populations—an introduction. *Ethol Sociobiol*, **8**, S1–8.

Feierman, J.R. (1994). A testable hypothesis about schizophrenia generated by evolutionary-theory. *Ethol Sociobiol*, **15**, 263–82.

Feierman, J.R. (2006). The ethology of psychiatric populations II: Darwinian neuro-psychiatry. *Clin Neuropsychiatry*, **3**, 87–109.

Feierman, J.R. & Feierman, L.A. (2000). Paraphilias. In: Szuchman, L.T. & Muscarella, F. (eds) *Psychological Perspectives on Human Sexuality*. John Wiley, New York.

Feifel, D., Macdonald, K., Nguyen, A., et al. (2010). Adjunctive intranasal oxytocin reduces symptoms in schizophrenia patients. *Biol Psychiatry*, **68**, 678–80.

Feinberg, I. (1983). Schizophrenia—caused by a fault in programmed synaptic elimination during adolescence. *J Psychiatric Res*, **17**, 319–34.

Feinberg, M.E., Button, T.M., Neiderhiser, J.M., Reiss, D., & Hetherington, E.M. (2007). Parenting and adolescent antisocial behavior and depression: evidence of genotype x parenting environment interaction. *Arch Gen Psychiatry*, **64**, 457–65.

Feldman, M., Mallouh, K., & Lewis, D.O. (1986). Filicidal abuse in the histories of 15 condemned murderers. *Bull Am Acad Psychiatry Law*, **14**, 345–52.

Feldman, R. (2012). Oxytocin and social affiliation in humans. *Hormones Behav*, **61**, 380–91.

Feldman, R., Gordon, I., Schneiderman, I., Weisman, O., & Zagoory-Sharon, O. (2010). Natural variations in maternal and paternal care are associated with systematic changes in oxytocin following parent-infant contact. *Psychoneuroendocrinology*, **35**, 1133–41.

Feldman, R., Rosenthal, Z., & Eidelman, A.I. (2014). Maternal-preterm skin-to-skin contact enhances child physiologic organization and cognitive control across the first 10 years of life. *Biol Psychiatry*, **75**, 56–64.

Ferdowsian, H. & Merskin, D. (2012). Parallels in sources of trauma, pain, distress, and suffering in humans and nonhuman animals. *J Trauma Dissociation*, **13**, 448–68.

Finch, C. (2007). *The Biology of Human Longevity: Inflammation, Nutrition, and Aging in the Evolution of Life Spans*. Academic Press, Burlington, Massachusetts.

Finch, C.E. (2010). Evolution in health and medicine Sackler colloquium: evolution of the human lifespan and diseases of aging: roles of infection, inflammation, and nutrition. *Proc Natl Acad Sci USA*, **107** (Suppl 1), 1718–24.

Finch, C.E. & Sapolsky, R.M. (1999). The evolution of Alzheimer disease, the reproductive schedule, and apoE isoforms. *Neurobiol Aging*, **20**, 407–28.

Finch, C.E. & Stanford, C.B. (2004). Meat-adaptive genes and the evolution of slower aging in humans. *Q Rev Biol*, **79**, 3–50.

Fine, R., Zhang, J., & Stevens, H.E. (2014). Prenatal stress and inhibitory neuron systems: implications for neuropsychiatric disorders. *Mol Psychiatry*, **19**, 641–51.

Finlay, B.L., Darlington, R.B., & Nicastro, N. (2001). Developmental structure in brain evolution. *Behav Brain Sci*, **24**, 263–78; discussion 278–308.

Finzi-Dottan, R., Manor, I., & Tyano, S. (2006). ADHD, temperament, and parental style as predictors of the child's attachment patterns. *Child Psychiatry Hum Dev*, **37**, 103–14.

Fischer-Shofty, M., Brüne, M., Ebert, A., et al. (2013). Improving social perception in schizophrenia: the role of oxytocin. *Schizophrenia Res*, **146**, 357–62.

Fisher, H.E., Aron, A., Mashek, D., Li, H., & Brown, L.L. (2002). Defining the brain systems of lust, romantic attraction, and attachment. *Arch Sex Behav*, **31**, 413–19.

Fisher, H.W., & Thomson, J.A. (2006). Lust romance and attachment:Do the side-effects of serotonin-enhancing antidepressants jeopardize romantic love, marriage, and fertility? In: Platek, SM, Keenan, JP, Shackelford, TK (eds) Evolutionary cognitive neuroscience. Cambridge MA, MIT Press, pp. 245–283.

Fisher, P.L. & Wells, A. (2005). Experimental modification of beliefs in obsessive-compulsive disorder: a test of the metacognitive model. *Behav Res Therapy*, **43**, 821–29.

Fisher, R.A. (1915). The evolution of sexual preference. *Eugen Rev*, **7**, 184–92.

Fisher, R.A. (1958). *The Genetical Theory of Natural Selection*. Dover Publications, New York.

Fiske, A.P. & Haslam, N. (1997). Is obsessive-compulsive disorder a pathology of the human disposition to perform socially meaningful rituals? Evidence of similar content. *J Nerv Ment Dis*, **185**, 211–22.

Fitch, W.T. (2000). The evolution of speech: a comparative review. *Trends Cogn Sci*, **4**, 258–67.

Flannelly, K.J., Koenig, H.G., Galek, K., & Ellison, C.G. (2007). Beliefs, mental health, and evolutionary threat assessment systems in the brain. *J Nerv Ment Dis*, **195**, 996–1003.

Flavell, J.H. (1999). Cognitive development: children's knowledge about the mind. *Annu Rev Psychol*, **50**, 21–45.

Fleisher, A., Grundman, M., Jack, C.R., Jr, et al. (2005). Sex, apolipoprotein E epsilon 4 status, and hippocampal volume in mild cognitive impairment. *Arch Neurol*, **62**, 953–57.

Flinn, M.V. (1997). Culture and the evolution of social learning. *Evol Human Behav*, **18**, 23–67.

Flinn, M.V. & England, B.G. (1997). Social economics of childhood glucocorticoid stress response and health. *Am J Phys Anthropol*, **102**, 33–53.

Flint, J. & Munafo, M. (2014). Schizophrenia: genesis of a complex disease. *Nature*, **511**, 412–13.

Fodor, J.A. (1983). *The Modularity of Mind: An Essay on Faculty Psychology*. MIT Press, Cambridge, Massachusetts.

Foley, R. (1996). The adaptive legacy of human evolution: a search for the environment of evolutionary adaptedness. *Evol Anthropol*, **4**, 194–203.

Fombonne, E. (1999). The epidemiology of autism: a review. *Psychol Med*, **29**, 769–86.

Fonagy, P. (1991). Thinking about thinking: some clinical and theoretical considerations in the treatment of a borderline patient. *Int J Psychoanal*, **72** (Pt 4), 639–56.

Fonagy, P. (1999). Psychoanalytic theory from the viewpoint of attachment theory and research. In: Cassidy, J. & Shaver, P.R. (eds) *Handbook of Attachment. Theory, Research, and Clinical Applications*. Guilford Press, New York.

Fonagy, P. (2000). Attachment and borderline personality disorder. *J Am Psychoanal Assoc*, **48**, 1129–46; discussion 1175–87.

Fontenelle, L.F. & Hasler, G. (2008). The analytical epidemiology of obsessive-compulsive disorder: risk factors and correlates. *Prog Neuropsychopharmacol Biol Psychiatry*, **32**, 1–15.

Fontenot, M.B., Kaplan, J.R., Manuck, S.B., Arango, V., & Mann, J.J. (1995). Long-term effects of chronic social stress on serotonergic indices in the prefrontal cortex of adult male cynomolgus macaques. *Brain Res*, **705**, 105–108.

Förstl, H. (ed.) (2006). *Theory of Mind*. Springer, Heidelberg.

Fossati, A., Donati, D., Donini, M., et al. (2001). Temperament, character, and attachment patterns in borderline personality disorder. *J Pers Disord*, **15**, 390–402.

Frances, A. (2013). The past, present and future of psychiatric diagnosis. *World Psychiatry*, **12**, 111–12.

Frankel, M., Cummings, J.L., Robertson, M.M., et al. (1986). Obsessions and compulsions in Gilles de la Tourette's syndrome. *Neurology*, **36**, 378–82.

Franko, D.L. & Keel, P.K. (2006). Suicidality in eating disorders: occurrence, correlates, and clinical implications. *Clin Psychol Rev*, **26**, 769–82.

Freeman, D. & Garety, P.A. (2003). Connecting neurosis and psychosis: the direct influence of emotion on delusions and hallucinations. *Behav Res Ther*, **41**, 923–47.

Freestone, P.P., Sandrini, S.M., Haigh, R.D., & Lyte, M. (2008). Microbial endocrinology: how stress influences susceptibility to infection. *Trends Microbiol*, **16**, 55–64.

Friedman, M.J. (2000). What might the psychobiology of posttraumatic stress disorder teach us about future approaches to pharmacotherapy? *J Clin Psychiatry*, **61** (Suppl 7), 44–51.

Friedman, S.H., Horwitz, S.M., & Resnick, P.J. (2005). Child murder by mothers: a critical analysis of the current state of knowledge and a research agenda. *Am J Psychiatry*, **162**, 1578–87.

Friesen, W.V. & Ekman, P. (1984). EMFACS-7: Emotional Facial Action Coding System (Version 7). (Version 7) Unpublished. University of California at San Francisco.

Frith, C.D. (1992). *The Cognitive Neuropsychology of Schizophrenia*. Lawrence Erlbaum Associates, Hove.

Frith, C.D. & Frith, U. (1999). Interacting minds—a biological basis. *Science*, **286**, 1692–95.

Frith, C.D., Blakemore, S., & Wolpert, D.M. (2000). Explaining the symptoms of schizophrenia: abnormalities in the awareness of action. *Brain Res Brain Res Rev*, **31**, 357–63.

Frith, U. & De Vignemont, F. (2005). Egocentrism, allocentrism, and Asperger syndrome. *Conscious Cogn*, **14**, 719–38.

Frith, U. & Frith, C. (2001). The biological basis of social interaction. *Curr Directions Psycholog Sci*, **10**, 151–55.

Frith, U. & Frith, C.D. (2003). Development and neurophysiology of mentalizing. *Philos Trans R Soc Lond B Biol Sci*, **358**, 459–73.

Fullerton, S.M., Clark, A.G., Weiss, K.M., et al. (2000). Apolipoprotein E variation at the sequence haplotype level: implications for the origin and maintenance of a major human polymorphism. *Am J Human Genet*, **67**, 881–900.

Fusar-Poli, P., Crippa, J.A., Bhattacharyya, S., et al. (2009). Distinct effects of {delta}9-tetrahydrocannabinol and cannabidiol on neural activation during emotional processing. *Arch Gen Psychiatry*, **66**, 95–105.

Fuster, J.M. (1997). *The Prefrontal Cortex: Anatomy, Physiology, and Neuropsychology of the Frontal Lobe*. Lippincott-Raven, Philadelphia.

Fuster, J.M. (2001). The prefrontal cortex—an update: time is of the essence. *Neuron*, **30**, 319–33.

Gaebel, W. (1989). Visuomotor behavior in schizophrenia. *Pharmacopsychiatry*, **22** (Suppl 1), 29–34.

Gaebel, W. & Wolwer, W. (2004). Facial expressivity in the course of schizophrenia and depression. *Eur Arch Psychiatry Clin Neurosci*, **254**, 335–42.

Gaher, R., Hofman, N.L., Simons, J., & Hunsaker, R. (2013). Emotion regulation deficits as mediators between trauma exposure and borderline symptoms. *Cogn Ther Res*, **37**, 466–75.

Galdikas, B.M. & Wood, J.W. (1990). Birth spacing patterns in humans and apes. *Am J Phys Anthropol*, **83**, 185–91.

Gallese, V. & Goldman, A. (1998). Mirror neurons and the simulation theory of mind-reading. *Trends Cogn Sci*, **2**, 493–501.

Galvin, M., Shekhar, A., Simon, J., et al. (1991). Low dopamine-beta-hydroxylase: a biological sequela of abuse and neglect? *Psychiatry Res*, **39**, 1–11.

Gangadhar, B.N., Panner Selvan, C., Subbakrishna, D.K., & Janakiramaiah, N. (2002). Age-at-onset and schizophrenia: reversed gender effect. *Acta Psychiatr Scand*, **105**, 317–19.

Gangestad, S.W. & Simpson, J.A. (1990). Toward an evolutionary history of female sociosexual variation. *J Pers*, **58**, 69–96.

Gannon, P.J., Holloway, R.L., Broadfield, D.C., & Braun, A.R. (1998). Asymmetry of chimpanzee planum temporale: humanlike pattern of Wernicke's brain language area homolog. *Science*, **279**, 220–22.

Garakani, A., Martinez, J.M., Aaronson, C.J., et al. (2009). Effect of medication and psychotherapy on heart rate variability in panic disorder. *Depress Anxiety*, **26**, 251–58.

Garcia, J. (1996). The Darwinian status of mind. *J Behav Ther Exp Psychiatry*, **27**, 347–50.

Garcia-Campayo, J., Fayed, N., Serrano-Blanco, A., & Roca, M. (2009). Brain dysfunction behind functional symptoms: neuroimaging and somatoform, conversive, and dissociative disorders. *Curr Opin Psychiatry*, **22**, 224–31.

Gardner, R., Jr (1982). Mechanisms in manic-depressive disorder: an evolutionary model. *Arch Gen Psychiatry*, **39**, 1436–41.

Gardner, R., Jr (1997). Sociophysiology as the basic science of psychiatry. *Theoret Med*, **18**, 335–56.

Gardner, R., Jr (2001). Evolutionary perspectives on stress and affective disorder. *Semin Clin Neuropsychiatry*, **6**, 32–42.

Garver, D.L., Holcomb, J., Mapua, F.M., Wilson, R., & Barnes, B. (2001). Schizophrenia spectrum disorders: an autosomal-wide scan in multiplex pedigrees. *Schizophr Res*, **52**, 145–60.

Gascon, E., Lynch, K., Ruan, H., et al. (2014). Alterations in microRNA-124 and AMPA receptors contribute to social behavioral deficits in frontotemporal dementia. *Nat Med*, **20**, 1444–51.

Gatward, N. (2007). Anorexia nervosa: an evolutionary puzzle. *Eur Eat Disord Rev*, **15**, 1–12.

Gaulin, S.J. (1997). Cross-cultural patterns and the search for evolved psychological mechanisms. *Ciba Found Symp*, **208**, 195–207, discussion 207–11.

Gaulin, S.J. & Robbins, C.J. (1991). Trivers-Willard effect in contemporary North American society. *Am J Phys Anthropol*, **85**, 61–69.

Geerts, E. & Bouhuys, N. (1998). Multi-level prediction of short-term outcome of depression: non-verbal interpersonal processes, cognitions and personality traits. *Psychiatry Res*, **79**, 59–72.

Geerts, E. & Brüne, M. (2009). Ethological approaches to psychiatric disorders: focus on depression and schizophrenia. *Aust N Z J Psychiatry*, **43**, 1007–15.

Geerts, E., Bouhuys, N., & Van Den Hoofdakker, R.H. (1996). Nonverbal attunement between depressed patients and an interviewer predicts subsequent improvement. *J Affect Disord*, **40**, 15–21.

Geerts, E., Van Os, T., Ormel, J., & Bouhuys, N. (2006). Nonverbal behavioral similarity between patients with depression in remission and interviewers in relation to satisfaction and recurrence of depression. *Depress Anxiety*, **23**, 200–209.

Geher, G. & Miller, G.F. (2008). *Mating Intelligence: Sex, Relationships, and the Mind's Reproductive System*. Lawrence Erlbaum, New York.

Gerdes, L.U., Gerdes, C., Hansen, P.S., Klausen, I.C., & Faergeman, O. (1996). Are men carrying the apolipoprotein epsilon 4- or epsilon 2 allele less fertile than epsilon 3 epsilon 3 genotypes? *Hum Genet*, **98**, 239–42.

Gerlach, G., Herpertz, S., & Löber, S. (2015). Personality traits and obesity: a systematic review. *Obesity Rev*, **16**, 32–63.

Gianotti, L., Lanfranco, F., Ramunni, J., et al. (2002). GH/IGF-I axis in anorexia nervosa. *Eat Weight Disord*, **7**, 94–105.

Gibbins, C. & Weiss, M. (2007). Clinical recommendations in current practice guidelines for diagnosis and treatment of ADHD in adults. *Curr Psychiatry Rep*, **9**, 420–26.

Giedd, J.N. (2004). Structural magnetic resonance imaging of the adolescent brain. *Ann N Y Acad Sci*, **1021**, 77–85.

Giesen-Bloo, J., Van Dyck, R., Spinhoven, P., et al. (2006). Outpatient psychotherapy for borderline personality disorder: randomized trial of schema-focused therapy vs transference-focused psychotherapy. *Arch Gen Psychiatry*, **63**, 649–58.

Gigerenzer, G. (1996). The psychology of good judgment: frequency formats and simple algorithms. *Med Decis Making*, **16**, 273–80.

Gilbert, P. (1998). Evolutionary psychopathology: why isn't the mind designed better than it is? *Br J Med Psychol*, **71** (Pt 4), 353–73.

Gilbert, P. (2000). Social mentalities: internal 'social' conflict and the role of inner warmth and compassion in cognitive therapy. In: Gilbert, P. & Bailey, K.G. (eds) *Genes on the Couch. Explorations in Evolutionary Psychotherapy*. Brunner-Routledge, Hove.

Gilbert, P. (2001). Evolutionary approaches to psychopathology: the role of natural defences. *Aust N Z J Psychiatry*, **35**, 17–27.

Gilbert, P. (2006). Old and new ideas on the evolution of mind and psychotherapy. *Clin Neuropsychiatry*, **3**, 139–53.

Gilbert, P. (2009). Introducing compassion-focused therapy. *Adv Psychiatric Treatm*, **15**, 199–208.

Gilbert, P. (2010). Compassion-focused therapy. In: Dryden, W. (ed.) *The CBT Distinctive Features Series*. Routledge, London.

Gilbert, P. (2013). An evolutionary and compassion focused approach to dissociation. In: Kennedy, F., Kennerley, H., & Pearson, D. (eds) *Cognitive Behavioural Approaches to the Understanding and Treatment of Dissociation*. Routledge, London.

Gilbert, P. (2014). The origins and nature of compassion focused therapy. *Br J Clin Psychol*, **53**, 6–41.

Gilbert, P. & Bailey, K.G. (eds) (2000). *Genes on the Couch. Explorations in Evolutionary Psychotherapy*. Brunner-Routledge, Hove.

Gilbert, P., Bailey, K.G., & McGuire, M.T. (2000). Evolutionary psychotherapy: principles and outline. In: Gilbert, P. & Bailey, K.G. (eds) *Genes on the Couch. Explorations in Evolutionary Psychotherapy*. Brunner-Routledge, Hove.

Gilbert, P., Allan, S., Brough, S., Melley, S., & Miles, J.N. (2002). Relationship of anhedonia and anxiety to social rank, defeat and entrapment. *J Affect Disord*, **71**, 141–51.

Gilbert, P., Gilbert, J., & Irons, C. (2004). Life events, entrapments and arrested anger in depression. *J Affect Disord*, **79**, 149–60.

Gilman, S.E., Kawachi, I., Fitzmaurice, G.M., & Buka, S.L. (2002). Socioeconomic status in childhood and the lifetime risk of major depression. *Int J Epidemiol*, **31**, 359–67.

Glantz, K. & Moehl, M.B. (2000). Reluctant males: evolutionary perspectives on male psychology in couples therapy. In: Gilbert, P. & Bailey, K.G. (eds) *Genes on the Couch. Explorations in Evolutionary Psychotherapy*. Brunner-Routledge, Hove.

Glantz, K. & Pearce, J.K. (1989). *Exiles from Eden: Psychotherapy from an Evolutionary Perspective*. Norton, New York.

Glas, G. (2004). Philosophical aspects of neurobiological research on anxiety and anxiety disorders. *Curr Opin Psychiatry*, **17**, 457–64.

Glass, D.J. (2012). Evolutionary clinical psychology, broadly construed: perspectives on absessive-compulsive disorder. *J Soc Evol Cult Psychol*, **6**, 292–308.

Glass, D.J. & Arnold, S.E. (2012). Some evolutionary perspectives on Alzheimer's disease pathogenesis and pathology. *Alzheimers Dementia*, **8**, 343–51.

Glover, H., Lader, W., & Walker-O'Keefe, J. (1995). Vulnerability scale scores in female inpatients diagnosed with self-injurious behaviour, dissociative identity disorder, and major depression. *Psychol Rep*, 77, 987–93.

Goddard, A.W., Mason, G.F., Appel, M., et al. (2004). Impaired GABA neuronal response to acute benzodiazepine administration in panic disorder. *Am J Psychiatry*, **161**, 2186–93.

Goldberg, R.L., Mann, L.S., Wise, T.N., & Segall, E.A. (1985). Parental qualities as perceived by borderline personality disorders. *Hillside J Clin Psychiatry*, **7**, 134–40.

Goldman, J.S., Farmer, J.M., Van Deerlin, V.M., et al. (2004). Frontotemporal dementia: genetics and genetic counseling dilemmas. *Neurologist*, **10**, 227–34.

Goldstein, J.M., Seidman, L.J., O'Brien, L.M., et al. (2002). Impact of normal sexual dimorphisms on sex differences in structural brain abnormalities in schizophrenia assessed by magnetic resonance imaging. *Arch Gen Psychiatry*, **59**, 154–64.

Golomb, B.A., Stattin, H., & Mednick, S. (2000). Low cholesterol and violent crime. *J Psychiatr Res*, **34**, 301–309.

Gonzalez-Liencres, C., Shamay-Tsoory, S.G., & Brüne, M. (2013). Towards a neuroscience of empathy: ontogeny, phylogeny, brain mechanisms, context and psychopathology. *Neurosci Biobehav Rev*, **37**, 1537–48.

Goodman, A. (1997). Organic unity theory: an integrative mind-body theory for psychiatry. *Theor Med*, **18**, 357–78.

Gorwood, P., Bouvard, M., Mouren-Simeoni, M.C., Kipman, A., & Ades, J. (1998). Genetics and anorexia nervosa: a review of candidate genes. *Psychiatr Genet*, **8**, 1–12.

Gorwood, P., Kipman, A., & Foulon, C. (2003). The human genetics of anorexia nervosa. *Eur J Pharmacol*, **480**, 163–70.

Gos, T., Becker, K., Bock, J., et al. (2006). Early neonatal and postweaning social emotional deprivation interferes with the maturation of serotonergic and tyrosine hydroxylase-immunoreactive afferent fiber systems in the rodent nucleus accumbens, hippocampus and amygdala. *Neuroscience*, **140**, 811–21.

Gosling, S.D. (2001). From mice to men: what can we learn about personality from animal research? *Psychol Bull*, **127**, 45–86.

Gosling, S.D., Lilienfeld, S.O., & Marino, L. (2003). Personality. In: Mastrepieri, D. (ed.) *Primate Psychology*. Harvard University Press, Cambridge Massachusetts.

Gould, S.J. (1982). Darwinism and the expansion of evolutionary theory. *Science*, **216**, 380–87.

Gould, S.J. & Lewontin, R.C. (1979). The spandrels of San Marco and the Panglossian paradigm: a critique of the adaptationist programme. *Proc R Soc Lond B Biol Sci*, **205**, 581–98.

Gowaty, P.A. (1995). False criticisms of sociobiology and behavioral ecology—genetic determinism, untestability, and inappropriate comparisons. *Politics Life Sci*, **14**, 174–80.

Graeber, M.B. & Muller, U. (2003). Dementia with Lewy bodies: disease concept and genetics. *Neurogenetics*, **4**, 157–62.

Graham, Y.P., Heim, C., Goodman, S.H., Miller, A.H., & Nemeroff, C.B. (1999). The effects of neonatal stress on brain development: implications for psychopathology. *Dev Psychopathol*, **11**, 545–65.

Grant, B.F., Hasin, D.S., Stinson, F.S., et al. (2004). Prevalence, correlates, and disability of personality disorders in the United States: results from the national epidemiologic survey on alcohol and related conditions. *J Clin Psychiatry*, **65**, 948–58.

Grant, E.C. (1968). An ethological description of non-verbal behaviour during interviews. *Br J Med Psychol*, **41**, 177–84.

Grant, E.C. (1969). Human facial expression. *Man*, **4**, 523–36.

Grant, K.A., Shively, C.A., Nader, M.A., et al. (1998). Effect of social status on striatal dopamine D-2 receptor binding characteristics in cynomolgus monkeys assessed with positron emission tomography. *Synapse*, **29**, 80–83.

Green, M.J. & Phillips, M.L. (2004). Social threat perception and the evolution of paranoia. *Neurosci Biobehav Rev*, **28**, 333–42.

Greenberg, M.T. (1999). Attachment and psychopathology in childhood. In: Cassidy, J. & Shaver, P.R. (eds) *Handbook of Attachment. Theory, Research, and Clinical Applications*. Guilford Press, New York.

Greenfield, P.M., Keller, H., Fuligni, A., & Maynard, A. (2003). Cultural pathways through universal development. *Annu Rev Psychol*, **54**, 461–90.

Greenspan, N.S. (2013). Clinical consequences of human evolution shaped by cultural trends. *Evol Med Public Health*, **2013**, 24–26.

Gregory, C., Lough, S., Stone, V., et al. (2002). Theory of mind in patients with frontal variant frontotemporal dementia and Alzheimer's disease: theoretical and practical implications. *Brain*, **125**, 752–64.

Griesinger, W. (1965). *Mental Pathology and Therapeutics*. Hafner, New York.

Grippo, A.J., Lamb, D.G., Carter, C.S., & Porges, S.W. (2007). Social isolation disrupts autonomic regulation of the heart and influences negative affective behaviors. *Biol Psychiatry*, **62**, 1162–70.

Grube, M. (2006). Towards an empirically based validation of intuitive diagnostic: Rumke's 'praecox feeling' across the schizophrenia spectrum: preliminary results. *Psychopathology*, **39**, 209–17.

Gruhle, U.H., Jung, W.R., Mayer-Gross, W., & Müller, M. (eds) (1964). *Psychiatrie der Gegenwart*. Springer, Berlin.

Grupe, D.W. & Nitschke, J.B. (2013). Uncertainty and anticipation in anxiety: an integrated neurobiological and psychological perspective. *Nat Rev Neurosci*, **14**, 488–501.

Guo, J., Simmons, W.K., Herscovitch, P., Martin, A., & Hall, K.D. (2014). Striatal dopamine D2-like receptor correlation patterns with human obesity and opportunistic eating behavior. *Mol Psychiatry*, **19**, 1078–84.

Gur, R.C., Gunning-Dixon, F., Bilker, W.B., & Gur, R.E. (2002). Sex differences in temporo-limbic and frontal brain volumes of healthy adults. *Cereb Cortex*, **12**, 998–1003.

Guth, W., Schmittberger, R., & Schwarze, B. (1982). An Experimental-Analysis of Ultimatum Bargaining. *J Econ Behav Organiz*, **3**, 367–88.

Guy, W. & Ban, T.A. (eds) (1982). *The AMDP-System: Manual for the Assessment and Documentation of Psychopathology*. Springer, Berlin.

Guzder, J., Paris, J., Zelkowitz, P., & Feldman, R. (1999). Psychological risk factors for borderline pathology in school-age children. *J Am Acad Child Adolesc Psychiatry*, **38**, 206–12.

Guze, S.B. (1993). Genetics of Briquet's syndrome and somatization disorder. A review of family, adoption, and twin studies. *Ann Clin Psychiatry*, **5**, 225–30.

Hafner, H. & Maurer, K. (2006). Early detection of schizophrenia: current evidence and future perspectives. *World Psychiatry*, **5**, 130–38.

Hagen, E.H. (1999). The functions of postpartum depression. *Evol Human Behav*, **20**, 325–59.

Hagen, E.H. (2011). Evolutionary theories of depression: a critical review. *Can J Psychiatry*, **56**, 716–26.

Hagen, E.H., Watson, P.J., & Hammerstein, P. (2008). Gestures of despair and hope: a view on deliberate self-harm from economics and evolutionary biology. *Biol Theory*, **3**, 123–38.

Haggard, P. (2005). Conscious intention and motor cognition. *Trends Cogn Sci*, **9**, 290–95.

Haggard, P. (2008). Human volition: towards a neuroscience of will. *Nat Rev Neurosci*, **9**, 934–46.

Haig, D. (1993). Genetic conflicts in human-pregnancy. *Q R Biol*, **68**, 495–532.

Haig, D. (2010). Colloquium papers: transfers and transitions: parent–offspring conflict, genomic imprinting, and the evolution of human life history. *Proc Natl Acad Sci USA*, **107** (Suppl 1), 1731–35.

Haig, D. (2014). Troubled sleep: night waking, breastfeeding and parent–offspring conflict. *Evol Med Public Health*, **2014**, 32–39.

Hall, W. (2002). Taking Darwin seriously: more than telling just so stories. *Addiction*, **97**, 472–73.

Hamilton, C.E. (2000). Continuity and discontinuity of attachment from infancy through adolescence. *Child Development*, **71**, 690–94.

Hamilton, W.D. (1964). Genetical evolution of social behaviour. I and II. *J Theoret Biol*, **7**, 1–52.

Hammen, C., Bower, J.E., & Cole, S.W. (2014). Oxytocin receptor gene variation and differential susceptibility to family environment in predicting youth borderline symptoms. *J Pers Disord*, 1–16.

Hammerstein, P. & Leimar, O. (2006). Cooperating for direct fitness benefits. *J Evol Biol*, **19**, 1400–402; discussion 1426–36.

Hammock, E.A. (2015). Developmental perspectives on oxytocin and vasopressin. *Neuropsychopharmacology*, **40**, 24–42.

Hammock, E.A. & Young, L.J. (2006). Oxytocin, vasopressin and pair bonding: implications for autism. *Philos Trans R Soc Lond B Biol Sci*, **361**, 2187–98.

Hand, I. (1998). Out-patient, multi-modal behaviour therapy for obsessive-compulsive disorder. *Br J Psychiatry Suppl*, **1998**(35), 45–52.

Hanna, J.L. (1995). The power of dance: health and healing. *J Altern Complement Med*, **1**, 323–31.

Hanson, D.R. & Gottesman, I. (2005). Theories of schizophrenia: a genetic-inflammatory-vascular synthesis. *BMC Med Genet*, **6**, 7.

Happé, F.G. (1993). Communicative competence and theory of mind in autism: a test of relevance theory. *Cognition*, **48**, 101–19.

Happé, F. & Loth, E. (2002). 'Theory of mind' and tracking speakers' intentions. *Mind Lang*, **17**, 24–36.

Happé, F., Ronald, A., & Plomin, R. (2006). Time to give up on a single explanation for autism. *Nat Neurosci*, **9**, 1218–20.

Harari, H., Shamay-Tsoory, S.G., Ravid, M., & Levkovitz, Y. (2010). Double dissociation between cognitive and affective empathy in borderline personality disorder. *Psychiatry Res*, **175**, 277–79.

Hardan, A.Y., Muddasani, S., Vemulapalli, M., Keshavan, M.S., & Minshew, N.J. (2006). An MRI study of increased cortical thickness in autism. *Am J Psychiatry*, **163**, 1290–92.

Hare, R.D. (1996). Psychopathy and antisocial personality disorder: a case of diagnostic confusion. *Psychiatric Times*, **13**, 39–40.

Harlow, H.F. & Zimmermann, R.R. (1959). Affectional responses in the infant monkey; orphaned baby monkeys develop a strong and persistent attachment to inanimate surrogate mothers. *Science*, **130**, 421–32.

Harlow, H.F., Dodsworth, R.O., & Harlow, M.K. (1965). Total social isolation in monkeys. *Proc Natl Acad Sci USA*, **54**, 90–97.

Harmon, R.B., Rosner, R., & Owens, H. (1995). Obsessional harassment and erotomania in a criminal court population. *J Forensic Sci*, **40**, 188–96.

Harrigan, J.A. & Taing, K.T. (1997). Fooled by a smile: Detecting anxiety in others. *J Nonverbal Behav*, **21**, 203–21.

Harrison, P.J. (1995). S182: from worm sperm to Alzheimer's disease. *Lancet*, **346**, 388.

Hartge, P. (2009). Genetics of reproductive lifespan. *Nat Genet*, **41**, 637–38.

Hashimoto, K., Koizumi, H., Nakazato, M., Shimizu, E., & Iyo, M. (2005). Role of brain-derived neurotrophic factor in eating disorders: recent findings and its pathophysiological implications. *Prog Neuropsychopharmacol Biol Psychiatry*, **29**, 499–504.

Hauert, C., Holmes, M., & Doebeli, M. (2006). Evolutionary games and population dynamics: maintenance of cooperation in public goods games. *Proc Biol Sci*, **273**, 2565–70.

Haveman, R., Wolfe, B., & Spaulding, J. (1991). Childhood events and circumstances influencing high school completion. *Demography*, **28**, 133–57.

Hawes, D.J., Brennan, J., & Dadds, M.R. (2009). Cortisol, callous-unemotional traits, and pathways to antisocial behavior. *Curr Opin Psychiatry*, **22**, 357–62.

Hawton, K., Harriss, L., & Zahl, D. (2006). Deaths from all causes in a long-term follow-up study of 11,583 deliberate self-harm patients. *Psychol Med*, **36**, 397–405.

Hecker, E. (1871). Die Hebephrenie. *Archiv Patholog Anat (Berl)*, **52**, 394–429.

Heide, K.M. & Solomon, E.P. (2006). Biology, childhood trauma, and murder: rethinking justice. *Int J Law Psychiatry*, **29**, 220–33.

Heim, C., Newport, D.J., Bonsall, R., Miller, A.H., & Nemeroff, C.B. (2001). Altered pituitary-adrenal axis responses to provocative challenge tests in adult survivors of childhood abuse. *Am J Psychiatry*, **158**, 575–81.

Heim, C., Young, L. J., Newport, D. J., et al. (2009). Lower CSF oxytocin concentrations in women with a history of childhood abuse. *Mol Psychiatry*, **14**, 954–58.

Heinz, A. & Smolka, M.N. (2006). The effects of catechol O-methyltransferase genotype on brain activation elicited by affective stimuli and cognitive tasks. *Rev Neurosci*, **17**, 359–67.

Heinz, A., Goldman, D., Gallinat, J., Schumann, G., & Puls, I. (2004). Pharmacogenetic insights to monoaminergic dysfunction in alcohol dependence. *Psychopharmacology (Berl)*, **174**, 561–70.

Heiser, M., Iacoboni, M., Maeda, F., Marcus, J., & Mazziotta, J.C. (2003). The essential role of Broca's area in imitation. *Eur J Neurosci*, **17**, 1123–28.

Heisler, L.K., Pronchuk, N., Nonogaki, K., et al. (2007). Serotonin activates the hypothalamic-pituitary-adrenal axis via serotonin 2C receptor stimulation. *J Neurosci*, **27**, 6956–64.

Hell, D. (1993). *Ethologie der Depression: Familientherapeutische Möglichkeiten*. Fischer, Stuttgart.

Helmchen, H., Henn, F., Lauter, H., & Sartorius, N. (eds.) (1999). *Psychiatrie der Gegenwart*. Springer, Berlin.

Hembree, E.A. & Foa, E.B. (2000). Posttraumatic stress disorder: psychological factors and psychosocial interventions. *J Clin Psychiatry*, **61** (Suppl 7), 33–39.

Hendrie, H.C. (1998). Epidemiology of dementia and Alzheimer's disease. *Am J Geriatr Psychiatry*, **6**, S3–18.

Herbert, W. (1982). The Evolution of child abuse. *Science News*, **122**, 24–26.

Herculano-Houzel, S. (2009). The human brain in numbers: a linearly scaled-up primate brain. *Front Hum Neurosci*, **3**, 31.

Herholz, K. (1996). Neuroimaging in anorexia nervosa. *Psychiatry Res*, **62**, 105–10.

Herrenkohl, T.I., Maguin, E., Hill, K.G., et al. (2000). Developmental risk factors for youth violence. *J Adolesc Health*, **26**, 176–86.

Herz, J. & Chen, Y. (2006). Reelin, lipoprotein receptors and synaptic plasticity. *Nat Rev Neurosci*, **7**, 850–59.

Heyes, C.M. (1998). Theory of mind in nonhuman primates. *Behav Brain Sci*, **21**, 101–14; discussion 115–48.

Hidalgo, R.B. & Davidson, J.R. (2000). Posttraumatic stress disorder: epidemiology and health-related considerations. *J Clin Psychiatry*, **61** (Suppl 7), 5–13.

Hildebrand, M., De Ruiter, C., & De Vogel, V. (2004). Psychopathy and sexual deviance in treated rapists: association with sexual and nonsexual recidivism. *Sex Abuse*, **16**, 1–24.

Hill, A., Habermann, N., Klusmann, D., Berner, W., & Briken, P. (2008). Criminal recidivism in sexual homicide perpetrators. *Int J Offender Ther Comp Criminol*, **52**, 5–20.

Hill, D. (1974). Non-verbal behaviour in mental illness. *Br J Psychiatry*, **124**, 221–30.

Hill, E.M. & Newlin, D.B. (2002). Evolutionary approaches to addiction: introduction. *Addiction*, **97**, 375–79.

Hill, K.R., Walker, R.S., Bozicevic, M., et al. (2011). Co-residence patterns in hunter-gatherer societies show unique human social structure. *Science*, **331**, 1286–89.

Hillbrand, M., Waite, B.M., Miller, D.S., Spitz, R.T., & Lingswiler, V.M. (2000). Serum cholesterol concentrations and mood states in violent psychiatric patients: an experience sampling study. *J Behav Med*, **23**, 519–29.

Hills, A.L., Cox, B.J., McWilliams, L.A., & Sareen, J. (2005). Suicide attempts and externalizing psychopathology in a nationally representative sample. *Compr Psychiatry*, **46**, 334–39.

Hinde, R.A. & Bateson, P.P.G. (1991). *The Development and Integration of Behaviour: Essays in Honour of Robert Hinde*. Cambridge University Press, Cambridge.

Hinshaw, S.P. (2003). Impulsivity, emotion regulation, and developmental psychopathology: specificity versus generality of linkages. *Ann N Y Acad Sci*, **1008**, 149–59.

Hiraiwa-Hasegawa, M. (2000). The sight of the peacock's tail makes me sick: the early arguments on sexual selection. *J Biosci*, **25**, 11–18.

Hitti, F.L. & Siegelbaum, S.A. (2014). The hippocampal CA2 region is essential for social memory. *Nature*, **508**, 88–92.

Hochberg, Z. & Belsky, J. (2013). Evo-devo of human adolescence: beyond disease models of early puberty. *BMC Med*, **11**, 113.

Hodges, J.R. & Miller, B. (2001). The classification, genetics and neuropathology of frontotemporal dementia. Introduction to the special topic papers: Part I. *Neurocase*, **7**, 31–35.

Hodgins, S., Kratzer, L., & McNeil, T.F. (2001). Obstetric complications, parenting, and risk of criminal behavior. *Arch Gen Psychiatry*, **58**, 746–52.

Hof, P.R., Nimchinsky, E.A., Perl, D.P., & Erwin, J.M. (2001). An unusual population of pyramidal neurons in the anterior cingulate cortex of hominids contains the calcium-binding protein calretinin. *Neurosci Lett*, **307**, 139–42.

Hofer, A., Benecke, C., Edlinger, M., et al. (2009). Facial emotion recognition and its relationship to symptomatic, subjective, and functional outcomes in outpatients with chronic schizophrenia. *Eur Psychiatry*, **24**, 27–32.

Hoff, P. (1998). Emil Kraepelin and forensic psychiatry. *Int J Law Psychiatry*, **21**, 343–53.

Hofman, M.A. (2001). Evolution and complexity of the human brain: some organizing principles. In: Roth, G. & Wullimann, M.F. (eds) *Brain Evolution and Cognition*. Wiley, New York.

Holden, C. & Mace, R. (1999). Sexual dimorphism in stature and women's work: a phylogenetic cross-cultural analysis. *Am J Phys Anthropol*, **110**, 27–45.

Hollander, E., Bartz, J., Chaplin, W., et al. (2007). Oxytocin increases retention of social cognition in autism. *Biol Psychiatry*, **61**, 498–503.

Holmes, J. (1993). Attachment theory: a biological basis for psychotherapy? *Br J Psychiatry*, **163**, 430–38.

Holroyd, S. & Baroncohen, S. (1993). How far can people with autism go in developing a theory of mind. *J Autism Dev Disord*, **23**, 379–85.

Holt-Lunstad, J., Smith, T.B., & Layton, J.B. (2010). Social relationships and mortality risk: a meta-analytic review. *PLoS Med*, **7**, e1000316.

Homberg, J.R. & Lesch, K.P. (2011). Looking on the bright side of serotonin transporter gene variation. *Biol Psychiatry*, **69**, 513–19.

Hooker, C.I., Benson, T.L., Gyurak, A., et al. (2014). Neural activity to positive expressions predicts daily experience of schizophrenia-spectrum symptoms in adults with high social anhedonia. *J Abnorm Psychol*, **123**, 190–204.

Hopkins, W.D. & Rilling, J.K. (2000). A comparative MRI study of the relationship between neuroanatomical asymmetry and interhemispheric connectivity in primates: implication for the evolution of functional asymmetries. *Behav Neurosci*, **114**, 739–48.

Hopkins, W.D., Marino, L., Rilling, J.K., & MacGregor, L.A. (1998). Planum temporale asymmetries in great apes as revealed by magnetic resonance imaging (MRI). *Neuroreport*, **9**, 2913–18.

Horrobin, D.F. (1999). Lipid metabolism, human evolution and schizophrenia. *Prostaglandins Leukot Essent Fatty Acids*, **60**, 431–37.

Horsthemke, B. (2009). Of wolves and men: the role of paternal child care in the evolution of genomic imprinting. *Eur J Hum Genet*, **17**, 273–74.

Horwath, E. & Weissman, M.M. (2000). The epidemiology and cross-national presentation of obsessive-compulsive disorder. *Psychiatr Clin N Am*, **23**, 493–507.

Houck, C.D., Nugent, N.R., Lescano, C.M., Peters, A., & Brown, L.K. (2010). Sexual abuse and sexual risk behavior: beyond the impact of psychiatric problems. *J Pediatr Psychol*, **35**, 473–83.

Howard, L.M., Thornicroft, G., Salmon, M., & Appleby, L. (2004). Predictors of parenting outcome in women with psychotic disorders discharged from mother and baby units. *Acta Psychiatr Scand*, **110**, 347–55.

Hoy, J.A., Hatton, C., & Hare, D. (2004). Weak central coherence: a cross-domain phenomenon specific to autism? *Autism*, **8**, 267–81.

Hrdy, S.B. (2000). *Mother Nature*. Vintage, London.

Hrdy, S.B., Tanson, C., & Van Schaik, C.P. (1994). Infanticide: let's not throw out the bay with the bath water. *Evol Anthropol*, **3**, 151–54.

Huffaker, S.J., Chen, J., Nicodemus, K.K., et al. (2009). A primate-specific, brain isoform of KCNH2 affects cortical physiology, cognition, neuronal repolarization and risk of schizophrenia. *Nat Med*, **15**, 509–18.

Hughes, C. & Ensor, R. (2006). Behavioural problems in 2-year-olds: links with individual differences in theory of mind, executive function and harsh parenting. *J Child Psychol Psychiatry*, **47**, 488–97.

Humphrey, N.K. (1976). The social function of intellect. In: Bateson, P.P.G. & Hinde, R.A. (eds) *Growing Points in Ethology*. Cambridge University Press, Cambridge.

Humphrey, N. & Skoyles, J. (2012). The evolutionary psychology of healing: a human success story. *Curr Biol*, **22**, R695–98.

Humphreys, K.L. & Zeanah, C.H. (2015). Deviations from the expectable environment in early childhood and emerging psychopathology. *Neuropsychopharmacology*, **40**, 154–70.

Hung, C.C., Chen, Y.H., Tsai, M.T., & Chen, C.H. (2001). Systematic search for mutations in the human tissue inhibitor of metalloproteinases-3 (TIMP-3) gene on chromosome 22 and association study with schizophrenia. *Am J Med Genet*, **105**, 275–78.

Hurley, S. & Chater, N. (eds.) (2005). *Perspectives on Imitation: From Neuroscience to Social Science. Volume 1: Mechanisms of Imitation and Imitation in Animals*. MIT Press, Cambridge, Massachusetts.

Huxley, J., Mayr, E., Osmond, H., & Hoffer, A. (1964). Schizophrenia as a genetic morphism. *Nature*, **204**, 220–21.

Hyman, S.E. (2009). How adversity gets under the skin. *Nat Neurosci*, **12**, 241–43.

Iacoboni, M. (2005). Neural mechanisms of imitation. *Curr Opin Neurobiol*, **15**, 632–37.

Iacoboni, M. & Dapretto, M. (2006). The mirror neuron system and the consequences of its dysfunction. *Nat Rev Neurosci*, **7**, 942–51.

Ineichen, B. (2000). The epidemiology of dementia in Africa: a review. *Soc Sci Med*, **50**, 1673–77.

Insel, T.R. (1988). Obsessive-compulsive disorder: a neuroethological perspective. *Psychopharmacol Bull*, **24**, 365–69.

Insel, T. R. (1997). A neurobiological basis of social attachment. *Am J Psychiatry*, **154**, 726–35.

Insel, T.R. (2002). Social anxiety: from laboratory studies to clinical practice. *Biol Psychiatry*, **51**, 1–3.

Insel, T.R. (2003). Is social attachment an addictive disorder? *Physiol Behav*, **79**, 351–57.

Insel, T.R. & Fernald, R.D. (2004). How the brain processes social information: searching for the social brain. *Annu Rev Neurosci*, **27**, 697–722.

Jabbi, M., Korf, J., Kema, I.P., et al. (2007). Convergent genetic modulation of the endocrine stress response involves polymorphic variations of 5-HTT, COMT and MAOA. *Mol Psychiatry*, **12**, 483–90.

Jablensky, A. (2000). Epidemiology of schizophrenia: the global burden of disease and disability. *Eur Arch Psychiatry Clin Neurosci*, **250**, 274–85.

Jablensky, A. (2006). Subtyping schizophrenia: implications for genetic research. *Mol Psychiatry*, **11**, 815–36.

Jablensky, A. & Cole, S.W. (1997). Is the earlier age at onset of schizophrenia in males a confounded finding? Results from a cross-cultural investigation. *Br J Psychiatry*, **170**, 234–40.

Jackson, J.H. (1884). The Croonian lectures on evolution and dissolution of the nervous system. *Br Med J*, **1**, 703–707.

Jacob, C.P., Muller, J., Schmidt, M., et al. (2005). Cluster B personality disorders are associated with allelic variation of monoamine oxidase A activity. *Neuropsychopharmacology*, **30**, 1711–18.

Jacob, S., Brune, C.W., Carter, C.S., et al. (2007). Association of the oxytocin receptor gene (OXTR) in Caucasian children and adolescents with autism. *Neurosci Lett*, **417**, 6–9.

Jankord, R. & Herman, J.P. (2008). Limbic regulation of hypothalamo-pituitary-adrenocortical function during acute and chronic stress. *Ann N Y Acad Sci*, **1148**, 64–73.

Janssen, I., Krabbendam, L., Bak, M., et al. (2003). Childhood abuse as a risk factor for psychotic experiences. *Schizophr Res*, **60**, 40–40.

Jarskog, L.F. (2006). Apoptosis in schizophrenia: pathophysiologic and therapeutic considerations. *Curr Opin Psychiatry*, **19**, 307–12.

Jarvelainen, J., Schurmann, M., & Hari, R. (2004). Activation of the human primary motor cortex during observation of tool use. *Neuroimage*, **23**, 187–92.

Jarvik, L.F. & Deckard, B.S. (1977). Odyssean personality—survival advantage for carriers of genes predisposing to schizophrenia. *Neuropsychobiology*, **3**, 179–91.

Jasienska, G. (2009). Reproduction and lifespan: trade-offs, overall energy budgets, intergenerational costs, and costs neglected by research. *Am J Hum Biol*, **21**, 524–32.

Jennen-Steinmetz, C., Loffler, W., & Häfner, H. (1997). Demography and age of onset of schizophrenia. *Br J Psychiatry*, **170**, 485–86.

Jensen, P.S., Mrazek, D., Knapp, P.K., et al. (1997). Evolution and revolution in child psychiatry: ADHD as a disorder of adaptation. *J Am Acad Child Adolesc Psychiatry*, **36**, 1672–79; discussion 1679–81.

Jerison, H.J. (2001). The evolution of neural and behavioral complexity. In: Roth, G. & Wullimann, M.F. (eds) *Brain Evolution and Cognition*. Wiley, New York.

Jimerson, D.C. & Wolfe, B.E. (2004). Neuropeptides in eating disorders. *CNS Spectr*, **9**, 516–22.

Joffe, T.H. (1997). Social pressures have selected for an extended juvenile period in primates. *J Hum Evol*, **32**, 593–605.

Johnson, J.G., Cohen, P., Kasen, S., Smailes, E., & Brook, J.S. (2001). Association of maladaptive parental behavior with psychiatric disorder among parents and their offspring. *Arch Gen Psychiatry*, **58**, 453–60.

Johnson, R.J., Ross, M.W., Taylor, W.C., et al. (2006). Prevalence of childhood sexual abuse among incarcerated males in county jail. *Child Abuse Negl*, **30**, 75–86.

Joiner, T.E., Pettit, J.W., Walker, R.L., et al. (2002). Perceived burdensomeness and suicidality: two studies on the suicide notes of those attempting and those completing suicide. *J Soc Clin Psychol*, **21**, 531–45.

Joiner, T.E., Brown, J.S., & Wingate, L.R. (2005). The psychology and neurobiology of suicidal behavior. *Annu Rev Psychol*, **56**, 287–314.

Jolly, A. (1966). Lemur social behavior and primate intelligence. *Science*, **153**, 501–506.

Jones, I.H. (1971). Ethology and psychiatry. *Aust N Z J Psychiatry*, **5**, 258–63.

Jones, I. & Blackshaw, J.K. (2000). An evolutionary approach to psychiatry. *Aust N Z J Psychiatry*, **34**, 8–13.

Jones, I.H. & Daniels, B.A. (1996). An ethological approach to self-injury. *Br J Psychiatry*, **169**, 263–67.

Jones, I.H. & Pansa, M. (1979). Some nonverbal aspects of depression and schizophrenia occurring during the interview. *J Nerv Ment Dis*, **167**, 402–409.

Jones, I., Kent, L., & Craddock, N. (2005). Genetics of affective disorders. In: McGuffin, P., Owen, M.J., & Gottesman, I. (eds) *Psychiatric Genetics and Genomics*. Oxford University Press, Oxford.

Jones, N.B. (1986). Bushman birth spacing—a test for optimal interbirth intervals. *Ethol Sociobiol*, **7**, 91–105.

Jones, P.A. (2012). Functions of DNA methylation: islands, start sites, gene bodies and beyond. *Nat Rev Genet*, **13**, 484–92.

Jones, R. (2012). Neurogenetics: mapping gene expression in the human brain. *Nat Rev Neurosci*, **13**, 737.

Jones, S., Martin, R.D., & Pilbeam, D.R. (1992). *The Cambridge Encyclopedia of Human Evolution*. Cambridge University Press, Cambridge.

Jovev, M., Green, M., Chanen, A., et al. (2012). Attentional processes and responding to affective faces in youth with borderline personality features. *Psychiatry Res*, **199**, 44–50.

Juckel, G., Hegerl, U., Giegling, I., et al. (2008). Association of 5-HT1B receptor polymorphisms with the loudness dependence of auditory evoked potentials in a community-based sample of healthy volunteers. *Am J Med Genet Part B-Neuropsychiatr Genet*, 147B, 454–58.

Jung, R.E. (2014). Evolution, creativity, intelligence, and madness: 'here be dragons'. *Front Psychol*, **5**, 784.

Just, M.A., Cherkassky, V.L., Keller, T.A., Kana, R.K., & Minshew, N.J. (2007). Functional and anatomical cortical underconnectivity in autism: evidence from an FMRI study of an executive function task and corpus callosum morphometry. *Cereb Cortex*, **17**, 951–61.

Kaessmann, H. & Paabo, S. (2002). The genetical history of humans and the great apes. *J Intern Med*, **251**, 1–18.

Kagel, J.H. & Roth, A.E. (1995). *The Handbook of Experimental Economics.*, Princeton University Press, Princeton.

Kahlbaum, K.L. (1874/1973). *Die Katatonie oder das Spannungsirresein. Eine klinische Form Psychischer Krankheit* (English translation: *Catatonia: The Tension Insanity*). Hirschwald, Berlin.

Kahn, J.P. (2013). *Angst. Origins of Anxiety and Depression.* Oxford University Press, Oxford.

Kalhbaum, K.L. (1963). *Die Gruppirung der Psychischen Krankheiten und die Eintheilung der Seelenstörungen.* Kafemann, Danzig.

Kalsi, G., Curtis, D., Brynjolfsson, J., et al. (1995). Investigation by linkage analysis of the XY pseudoautosomal region in the genetic susceptibility to schizophrenia. *Br J Psychiatry*, **167**, 390–93.

Kamali, M., Oquendo, M.A., & Mann, J.J. (2001). Understanding the neurobiology of suicidal behavior. *Depress Anxiety*, **14**, 164–76.

Kanazawa, S. (2001). Why father absence might precipitate early menarche—the role of polygyny. *Evol Human Behav*, **22**, 329–34.

Kandel, E. R. (1998). A new intellectual framework for psychiatry. *Am J Psychiatry*, **155**, 457–69.

Kanner, L. (1972). *Child Psychiatry.* C.C. Thomas, Springfield.

Kaplan, G.A., Turrell, G., Lynch, J.W., et al. (2001). Childhood socioeconomic position and cognitive function in adulthood. *Int J Epidemiol*, **30**, 256–63.

Kaplan, J.R., Shively, C.A., Fontenot, M.B., et al. (1994). Demonstration of an association among dietary cholesterol, central serotonergic activity, and social behavior in monkeys. *Psychosom Med*, **56**, 479–84.

Kappas, A. (1997). The fascination with faces: are they windows to our soul? *J Nonverbal Behav*, **21**, 157–61.

Kapur, S. (2003). Psychosis as a state of aberrant salience: a framework linking biology, phenomenology, and pharmacology in schizophrenia. *Am J Psychiatry*, **160**, 13–23.

Karlsson, E.K., Kwiatkowski, D.P., & Sabeti, P.C. (2014). Natural selection and infectious disease in human populations. *Nat Rev Genet*, **15**, 379–93.

Karlsson, J.L. (1968). Genealogic studies of schizophrenia. In: Rosenthal, D. & Kety, S.S. (eds) *The Transmission of Schizophrenia.* Pergamon Press, London.

Katz, D.B. & Steinmetz, J.E. (2002). Psychological functions of the cerebellum. *Behav Cogn Neurosci Rev*, **1**, 229–41.

Katzman, M.A., Hermans, K.M., Van Hoeken, D., & Hoek, H.W. (2004). Not your 'typical island woman': anorexia nervosa is reported only in subcultures in Curacao. *Cult Med Psychiatry*, **28**, 463–92.

Kaye, W.H., Bulik, C.M., Thornton, L., Barbarich, N., & Masters, K. (2004). Comorbidity of anxiety disorders with anorexia and bulimia nervosa. *Am J Psychiatry*, **161**, 2215–21.

Keane, T.M., Marshall, A.D., & Taft, C.T. (2006). Posttraumatic stress disorder: etiology, epidemiology, and treatment outcome. *Annu Rev Clin Psychol*, **2**, 161–97.

Keet, C.M. (2003). Towards a resolution of terrorism using game theory. Coalitions, negotiations and audience costs. MA Thesis. Department of Government and Society, University of Limerick, Limerick.

Keller, H. (1998). Die Rolle der Eltern für die Interaktionsregulation in der frühen Kindheit. *Vierteljahresschr Heilpädagogik Nachbargebiete*, **67**, 1–11.

Keller, H., Lohaus, A., Kuensemueller, P., et al. (2004). The bio-culture of parenting: evidence from five cultural communities. *Parenting-Sci Pract*, **4**, 25–50.

Keller, M.C. & Miller, G. (2006). Resolving the paradox of common, harmful, heritable mental disorders: which evolutionary genetic models work best? *Behav Brain Sci*, **29**, 385–404; discussion 405–52.

Keller, M.C. & Nesse, R.M. (2006). The evolutionary significance of depressive symptoms: different adverse situations lead to different depressive symptom patterns. *J Pers Soc Psychol*, **91**, 316–30.

Keller, T.A., Kana, R.K., & Just, M.A. (2007). A developmental study of the structural integrity of white matter in autism. *Neuroreport*, **18**, 23–27.

Kellett, J.M. (1973). Evolutionary theory for the dichotomy of the functional psychoses. *Lancet*, **1**, 860–63.

Kelley, M.E., Van Kammen, D.P., & Allen, D.N. (1999). Empirical validation of primary negative symptoms: independence from effects of medication and psychosis. *Am J Psychiatry*, **156**, 406–11.

Kellogg, S.H. & Young, J.E. (2006). Schema therapy for borderline personality disorder. *J Clin Psychol*, **62**, 445–58.

Kelly, A. C., Zuroff, D. C., Leybman, M. J. & Gilbert, P. (2012). Social safeness, received social support, and maladjustment: testing a tripartite model of affect regulation. *Cogn Ther Res*, **36**, 815–26.

Kelly, Y.J., Nazroo, J.Y., McMunn, A., Boreham, R., & Marmot, M. (2001). Birthweight and behavioural problems in children: a modifiable effect? *Int J Epidemiol*, **30**, 88–94.

Kempermann, G. (2012). New neurons for 'survival of the fittest'. *Nat Rev Neurosci*, **13**, 727–36.

Kennedy, D.P., Glascher, J., Tyszka, J.M., & Adolphs, R. (2009). Personal space regulation by the human amygdala. *Nat Neurosci*, **12**, 1226–27.

Kenrick, D.T. & Li, N. (2000). The Darwin is in the details. *Am Psychol*, **55**, 1060–61.

Kéri, S. (2009). Genes for psychosis and creativity: a promoter polymorphism of the neuregulin 1 gene is related to creativity in people with high intellectual achievement. *Psychol Sci*, **20**, 1070–73.

Kerwin, R.W. & Arranz, M.J. (2005). Psychopharmacogenetics. In: McGuffin, P., Owen, M. J., & Gottesman, I. (eds) *Psychiatric Genetics and Genomics*. Oxford University Press, Oxford.

Keski-Rahkonen, A., Hoek, H.W., Susser, E.S., et al. (2007). Epidemiology and course of anorexia nervosa in the community. *Am J Psychiatry*, **164**, 1259–65.

Kessler, R.C., Keller, M.B., & Wittchen, H.U. (2001). The epidemiology of generalized anxiety disorder. *Psychiatr Clin N Am*, **24**, 19–39.

Kessler, R.C., Andrade, L.H., Bijl, R.V., et al. (2002). The effects of co-morbidity on the onset and persistence of generalized anxiety disorder in the ICPE surveys. International Consortium in Psychiatric Epidemiology. *Psychol Med*, **32**, 1213–25.

Kety, S.S., Wender, P.H., Jacobsen, B., et al. (1994). Mental illness in the biological and adoptive relatives of schizophrenic adoptees. Replication of the Copenhagen Study in the rest of Denmark. *Arch Gen Psychiatry*, **51**, 442–55.

Keverne, E.B. & Curley, J.P. (2008). Epigenetics, brain evolution and behaviour. *Front Neuroendocrinol*, **29**, 398–412.

Khaitovich, P., Hellmann, I., Enard, W., et al. (2005). Parallel patterns of evolution in the genomes and transcriptomes of humans and chimpanzees. *Science*, **309**, 1850–54.

Khaitovich, P., Lockstone, H.E., Wayland, M.T., et al. (2008). Metabolic changes in schizophrenia and human brain evolution. *Genome Biol*, **9**, R124.

Khashan, A.S., Abel, K.M., McNamee, R., et al. (2008). Higher risk of offspring schizophrenia following antenatal maternal exposure to severe adverse life events. *Arch Gen Psychiatry*, **65**, 146–52.

Kidd, T., Hamer, M., & Steptoe, A. (2011). Examining the association between adult attachment style and cortisol responses to acute stress. *Psychoneuroendocrinology*, **36**, 771–79.

Kienast, T., Hariri, A.R., Schlagenhauf, F., et al. (2008). Dopamine in amygdala gates limbic processing of aversive stimuli in humans. *Nat Neurosci*, **11**, 1381–82.

Kienlen, K.K., Birmingham, D.L., Solberg, K.B., O'Regan, J.T., & Meloy, J.R. (1997). A comparative study of psychotic and nonpsychotic stalking. *J Am Acad Psychiatry Law*, **25**, 317–34.

Kilpinen, H., Ylisaukko-Oja, T., Hennah, W., et al. (2008). Association of DISC1 with autism and Asperger syndrome. *Mol Psychiatry*, **13**, 187–96.

Kim, H.S., Wadekar, R.V., Takenaka, O., et al. (1999). SINE-R.C2 (a Homo sapiens specific retroposon) is homologous to CDNA from postmortem brain in schizophrenia and to two loci in the Xq21.3/Yp block linked to handedness and psychosis. *Am J Med Genet*, **88**, 560–66.

Kim-Cohen, J., Moffitt, T.E., Taylor, A., Pawlby, S.J., & Caspi, A. (2005). Maternal depression and children's antisocial behavior: nature and nurture effects. *Arch Gen Psychiatry*, **62**, 173–81.

King-Casas, B., Sharp, C., Lomax-Bream, L., et al. (2008). The rupture and repair of cooperation in borderline personality disorder. *Science*, **321**, 806–10.

Kingsberg, S.A. & Rezaee, R.L. (2013). Hypoactive sexual desire in women. *Menopause*, **20**, 1284–300.

Kinzey, W.G., American Anthropological Association Meeting, & American Association of Physical Anthropologists (1987). *The Evolution of Human Behavior: Primate Models*. State University of New York Press, Albany.

Kirkpatrick, B. (2014). Developing concepts in negative symptoms: primary vs secondary and apathy vs expression. *J Clin Psychiatry*, **75** (Suppl 1), 3–7.

Kirkwood, T.B. & Rose, M.R. (1991). Evolution of senescence: late survival sacrificed for reproduction. *Philos Trans R Soc Lond B Biol Sci*, **332**, 15–24.

Kishida, K.T., King-Casas, B., & Montague, P.R. (2010). Neuroeconomic approaches to mental disorders. *Neuron*, **67**, 543–54.

Kleinknecht, E. & Beike, D.R. (2004). How knowing and doing inform an autobiography: Relations among preschoolers' theory of mind, narrative, and event memory skills. *Appl Cogn Psychol*, **18**, 745–64.

Kleinstäuber, M., Witthoft, M., Steffanowski, A., et al. (2014). Pharmacological interventions for somatoform disorders in adults. *Cochrane Database Syst Rev*, **11**, CD010628.

Klugmann, M., Goepfrich, A., Friemel, C.M., & Schneider, M. (2011). AAV-mediated overexpression of the cb1 receptor in the mpfc of adult rats alters cognitive flexibility, social behavior, and emotional reactivity. *Front Behav Neurosci*, **5**, 37.

Klüver, H. & Bucy, P. C. (1937). 'Psychic blindness' and other symptoms following bilateral temporal lobectomy in rhesus monkeys. *Am J Physiol*, **119**, 352–53.

Knoch, D., Pascual-Leone, A., Meyer, K., Treyer, V., & Fehr, E. (2006). Diminishing reciprocal fairness by disrupting the right prefrontal cortex. *Science*, **314**, 829–32.

Knutson, B. (2004). Behavior. Sweet revenge? *Science*, **305**, 1246–47.

Knutson, B. & Cooper, J.C. (2005). Functional magnetic resonance imaging of reward prediction. *Curr Opin Neurol*, **18**, 411–17.

Knutson, B., Adams, C.M., Fong, G.W., & Hommer, D. (2001). Anticipation of increasing monetary reward selectively recruits nucleus accumbens. *J Neurosci*, **21**, RC159.

Kobak, R. (1999). The emotional dynamics of disruptions in attachment relationships: implications for theory, research, and clinical intervention. In: Cassidy, J. & Shaver, P.R. (eds) *Handbook of Attachment. Theory, Research, and Clinical Applications*. Guilford Press, New York.

Koenigs, M. & Tranel, D. (2007). Irrational economic decision-making after ventromedial prefrontal damage: evidence from the Ultimatum Game. *J Neurosci*, **27**, 951–56.

Kofman, O. (2002). The role of prenatal stress in the etiology of developmental behavioural disorders. *Neurosci Biobehav Rev*, **26**, 457–70.

Kohler, E., Keysers, C., Umilta, M.A., et al. (2002). Hearing sounds, understanding actions: action representation in mirror neurons. *Science*, **297**, 846–48.

Kohls, G., Herpertz-Dahlmann, B., & Konrad, K. (2009). Hyperresponsiveness to social rewards in children and adolescents with attention-deficit/hyperactivity disorder (ADHD). *Behav Brain Funct*, **5**, 20.

Kondo, H., Saleem, K.S., & Price, J.L. (2003). Differential connections of the temporal pole with the orbital and medial prefrontal networks in macaque monkeys. *J Comp Neurol*, **465**, 499–523.

Konner, M. (1977). Child development in an evolutionary context. *Science*, **196**, 1310–11.

Koo, M.S., Dickey, C.C., Park, H.J., et al. (2006). Smaller neocortical gray matter and larger sulcal cerebrospinal fluid volumes in neuroleptic-naive women with schizotypal personality disorder. *Arch Gen Psychiatry*, **63**, 1090–100.

Koochmeshgi, J., Hosseini-Mazinani, S.M., Morteza Seifati, S., Hosein-Pur-Nobari, N., & Teimoori-Toolabi, L. (2004). Apolipoprotein E genotype and age at menopause. *Ann N Y Acad Sci*, **1019**, 564–67.

Korzan, W.J. & Summers, C.H. (2007). Behavioral diversity and neurochemical plasticity: selection of stress coping strategies that define social status. *Brain Behav Evol*, **70**, 257–66.

Kosik, K.S. (2000). The long reach of evolution and development. Effects on the Alzheimer brain. *Ann N Y Acad Sci*, **924**, 76–80.

Kottler, M.J. (1980). Darwin, Wallace, and the origin of sexual dimorphism. *Proc Am Philos Soc*, **124**, 203–26.

Koubaa, S., Hallstrom, T., Lindholm, C., & Hirschberg, A.L. (2005). Pregnancy and neonatal outcomes in women with eating disorders. *Obstet Gynecol*, **105**, 255–60.

Kourtzi, Z. & Kanwisher, N. (2000). Activation in human MT/MST by static images with implied motion. *J Cogn Neurosci*, **12**, 48–55.

Koyama, T., Miyake, Y., & Kurita, H. (2007). Parental ages at birth of children with pervasive developmental disorders are higher than those of children in the general population. *Psychiatry Clin Neurosci*, **61**, 200–202.

Kraemer, G.W. (1997). Psychobiology of early social attachment in rhesus monkeys. Clinical implications. *Ann N Y Acad Sci*, **807**, 401–18.

Kraemer, G.W. & McKinney, W.T. (1985). Social separation increases alcohol consumption in rhesus monkeys. *Psychopharmacology (Berl)*, **86**, 182–89.

Kraepelin, E. (1880). *Die Abschaffung des Strafmaßes. Ein Vorschlag zur Reform der Heutigen Rechtspflege*. F. Enke, Stuttgart.

Kraepelin, E. (1920). Die Erscheinungsformen des Irreseins. *Z Ges Neurol Psychiatr*, **62**, 1–29.

Kramer, D.A. (2014). DSM-5, NIMH, and the dark cave of reductionism in twenty-first century psychiatry. *AACAP NEWS*, January/February, 18–19.

Kramer, D.A. & McKinney, W.T., Jr (1979). The overlapping territories of psychiatry and ethology. *J Nerv Ment Dis*, **167**, 3–22.

Kramer, K.L. (2008). Early sexual maturity among Pume foragers of Venezuela: fitness implications of teen motherhood. *Am J Phys Anthropol*, **136**, 338–50.

Krause, R., Steimer, E., Sanger-Alt, C., & Wagner, G. (1989). Facial expression of schizophrenic patients and their interaction partners. *Psychiatry*, **52**, 1–12.

Krebs, J.R. & Davies, N.B. (1993). *An Introduction to Behavioural Ecology*. Blackwell Scientific Publications, Oxford.

Kretschmer, E. (1960). *Hysteria, Reflex, and Instinct*. Philosophical Library, New York.

Krimer, L.S., Hyde, T.M., Herman, M.M., & Saunders, R.C. (1997). The entorhinal cortex: an examination of cyto- and myeloarchitectonic organization in humans. *Cereb Cortex*, **7**, 722–31.

Kringelbach, M.L. (2005). The human orbitofrontal cortex: linking reward to hedonic experience. *Nat Rev Neurosci*, **6**, 691–702.

Kroenke, K. (2007). Efficacy of treatment for somatoform disorders: a review of randomized controlled trials. *Psychosom Med*, **69**, 881–88.

Kroes, R.A., Panksepp, J., Burgdorf, J., Otto, N.J., & Moskal, J.R. (2006). Modeling depression: social dominance-submission gene expression patterns in rat neocortex. *Neuroscience*, **137**, 37–49.

Krueger, R.B. & Kaplan, M.S. (2001). The paraphilic and hypersexual disorders: an overview. *J Psychiatr Pract*, **7**, 391–403.

Krysinska, K. & Lester, D. (2010). Post-traumatic stress disorder and suicide risk: a systematic review. *Arch Suicide Res*, **14**, 1–23.

Krysinska, K., Heller, T.S., & De Leo, D. (2006). Suicide and deliberate self-harm in personality disorders. *Curr Opin Psychiatry*, **19**, 95–101.

Krysko, K.M. & Rutherford, M.D. (2009). A threat-detection advantage in those with autism spectrum disorders. *Brain and Cognition*, **69**, 472–80.

Kuhar, M.J. (2002). Social rank and vulnerability to drug abuse. *Nat Neurosci*, **5**, 88–90.

Kukull, W.A. & Bowen, J.D. (2002). Dementia epidemiology. *Med Clin N Am*, **86**, 573–90.

Kumm, J. & Feldman, M.W. (1997). Gene-culture coevolution and sex ratios: II. Sex-chromosomal distorters and cultural preferences for offspring sex. *Theor Popul Biol*, **52**, 1–15.

Kumm, J., Laland, K.N., & Feldman, M.W. (1994). Gene-culture coevolution and sex ratios: the effects of infanticide, sex-selective abortion, sex selection, and sex-biased parental investment on the evolution of sex ratios. *Theor Popul Biol*, **46**, 249–78.

Kundakovic, M. & Champagne, F.A. (2015). Early-life experience, epigenetics, and the developing brain. *Neuropsychopharmacology*, **40**, 141–53.

Kurt, J.L. (1995). Stalking as a variant of domestic violence. *Bull Am Acad Psychiatry Law*, **23**, 219–30.

Kuttner, R.E. & Lorincz, A.B. (1966). Schizophrenia and evolution. *Eugen Q*, **13**, 355–56.

Kuttner, R.E., Lorincz, A.B., & Swan, D.A. (1967). The schizophrenia gene and social evolution. *Psychol Rep*, **20**, 407–12.

Köhler, W. (1921). *Intelligenzprüfungen an Menschenaffen*. Julius Springer, Berlin.

Ladygina-Kots, N.N., Waal, F.B.M.D., Vekker, B., & Center, Y.R.P.R. (2002). *Infant Chimpanzee and Human Child: A Classic 1935 Comparative Study of Ape Emotions and Intelligence*. Oxford University Press, Oxford.

Lahiri, D.K., Rogers, J.T., Greig, N.H., & Sambamurti, K. (2004). Rationale for the development of cholinesterase inhibitors as anti-Alzheimer agents. *Curr Pharm Des*, **10**, 3111–19.

Lalovic, A., Merkens, L., Russell, L., et al. (2004). Cholesterol metabolism and suicidality in Smith-Lemli-Opitz syndrome carriers. *Am J Psychiatry*, **161**, 2123–26.

Lam, K.S., Aman, M.G., & Arnold, L.E. (2006). Neurochemical correlates of autistic disorder: a review of the literature. *Res Dev Disabil*, **27**, 254–89.

Lambert, M.J. (2004). *Bergin and Garfield's Handbook of Psychotherapy and Behavior Change*. Wiley, New York.

Lampert, A. & Friedman, A. (1992). Sex differences in vulnerability and maladjustment as a function of parental investment: an evolutionary approach. *Soc Biol*, **39**, 65–81.

Landa, A., Peterson, B.S., & Fallon, B.A. (2012). Somatoform pain: a developmental theory and translational research review. *Psychosom Med*, **74**, 717–27.

Lane, L.W. & Luchins, D.J. (1988). Evolutionary approaches to psychiatry and problems of method. *Compr Psychiatry*, **29**, 598–603.

Lang, S., Af Klinteberg, B., & Alm, P.O. (2002). Adult psychopathy and violent behavior in males with early neglect and abuse. *Acta Psychiatr Scand Suppl*, **2002** (412), 93–100.

Lang, U.E., Bajbouj, M., Sander, T., & Gallinat, J. (2007). Gender-dependent association of the functional catechol-O-methyltransferase Val158Met genotype with sensation seeking personality trait. *Neuropsychopharmacology*, **32**, 1950–55.

Langdon, R. & Coltheart, M. (2001). Visual perspective-taking and schizotypy: evidence for a simulation-based account of mentalizing in normal adults. *Cognition*, **82**, 1–26.

Langdon, R., Michie, P.T., Ward, P.B., et al. (1997). Defective self and/or other mentalising in schizophrenia: a cognitive neuropsychological approach. *Cogn Neuropsychiatry*, **2**, 167–93.

Langdon, R., Corner, T., McLaren, J., Coltheart, M., & Ward, P.B. (2006). Attentional orienting triggered by gaze in schizophrenia. *Neuropsychologia*, **44**, 417–29.

Laucht, M., Skowronek, M.H., Becker, K., et al. (2007). Interacting effects of the dopamine transporter gene and psychosocial adversity on attention-deficit/hyperactivity disorder symptoms among 15-year-olds from a high-risk community sample. *Arch Gen Psychiatry*, **64**, 585–90.

Laursen, T.M., Munk-Olsen, T., Nordentoft, M., & Bo Mortensen, P. (2007). A comparison of selected risk factors for unipolar depressive disorder, bipolar affective disorder, schizoaffective disorder, and schizophrenia from a danish population-based cohort. *J Clin Psychiatry*, **68**, 1673–81.

Laval, S.H., Dann, J.C., Butler, R.J., et al. (1998). Evidence for linkage to psychosis and cerebral asymmetry (relative hand skill) on the X chromosome. *Am J Med Genet*, **81**, 420–27.

Leach, H., Groves, C., O'Connor, T., Pearson, O., & Zeder, M. (2003). Human domestication reconsidered. *Curr Anthropol*, **44**, 349–68.

Leckman, J.F. & Herman, A.E. (2002). Maternal behavior and developmental psychopathology. *Biol Psychiatry*, **51**, 27–43.

Leckman, J.F. & Mayes, L.C. (1999). Preoccupations and behaviors associated with romantic and parental love. Perspectives on the origin of obsessive-compulsive disorder. *Child Adolesc Psychiatr Clin N Am*, **8**, 635–65.

Lederbogen, F., Kirsch, P., Haddad, L., et al. (2011). City living and urban upbringing affect neural social stress processing in humans. *Nature*, **474**, 498–501.

Ledoux, J.E. (1996). *The Emotional Brain: The Mysterious Underpinnings of Emotional Life*. Simon & Schuster, New York.

Ledyard, J. (1995). Public goods: a survey of experimental research. In: Roth, K. (ed.) *The Handbook of Experimental Economics*. Princeton University Press, Princeton.

Lee, A.L., Ogle, W.O., & Sapolsky, R.M. (2002a). Stress and depression: possible links to neuron death in the hippocampus. *Bipolar Disord*, **4**, 117–28.

Lee, H.J. & Kwon, S.M. (2003). Two different types of obsession: autogenous obsessions and reactive obsessions. *Behav Res Ther*, **41**, 11–29.

Lee, H.J., Kim, Z.S., & Kwon, S.M. (2005a). Thought disorder in patients with obsessive-compulsive disorder. *J Clin Psychol*, **61**, 401–13.

Lee, J.K., Jackson, H.J., Pattison, P., & Ward, T. (2002b). Developmental risk factors for sexual offending. *Child Abuse Negl*, **26**, 73–92.

Lee, R., Geracioti, T.D., Jr, Kasckow, J.W., & Coccaro, E.F. (2005b). Childhood trauma and personality disorder: positive correlation with adult CSF corticotropin-releasing factor concentrations. *Am J Psychiatry*, **162**, 995–97.

Lemaire, V., Koehl, M., Le Moal, M., & Abrous, D.N. (2000). Prenatal stress produces learning deficits associated with an inhibition of neurogenesis in the hippocampus. *Proc Natl Acad Sci USA*, **97**, 11032–37.

Lende, D.H. (2008). Evolution and modern behavioral problems, the case of addiction. In: Trevathan, W.R., Smith, E.O., & McKenna, J.J. (eds) *Evolutionary Medicine and Health*. Oxford University Press, Oxford.

Lende, D.H. & Smith, E.O. (2002). Evolution meets biopsychosociality: an analysis of addictive behavior. *Addiction*, **97**, 447–58.

Lendon, C.L., Ashall, F., & Goate, A.M. (1997). Exploring the etiology of Alzheimer disease using molecular genetics. *JAMA*, **277**, 825–31.

Lenzenweger, M.F., Lane, M.C., Loranger, A.W., & Kessler, R.C. (2007). DSM-IV personality disorders in the National Comorbidity Survey Replication. *Biol Psychiatry*, **62**, 553–64.

Leonhardt, H., Tillmann, B., Töndury, G., & Zilles, K. (eds) (1987). *Anatomie des Menschen. Band III. Nervensystem und Sinnesorgane*. Thieme, Stuttgart.

Lepage, M., Ghaffar, O., Nyberg, L,. & Tulving, E. (2000). Prefrontal cortex and episodic memory retrieval mode. *Proc Natl Acad Sci USA*, **97**, 506–11.

Leppanen, J.M. & Nelson, C.A. (2009). Tuning the developing brain to social signals of emotions. *Nat Rev Neurosci*, **10**, 37–47.

Lerner, J.S. & Keltner, D. (2001). Fear, anger, and risk. *J Pers Soc Psychol*, **81**, 146–59.

Lesch, K.P. (2004). Gene–environment interaction and the genetics of depression. *J Psychiatry Neurosci*, **29**, 174–84.

Leslie, A.M. (1987). Pretense and representation—the origins of Theory of Mind. *Psycholog Rev*, **94**, 412–26.

Leslie, K.R., Johnson-Frey, S. H. & Grafton, S. T. (2004). Functional imaging of face and hand imitation: towards a motor theory of empathy. *Neuroimage*, **21**, 601–607.

Leung, A. & Chue, P. (2000). Sex differences in schizophrenia, a review of the literature. *Acta Psychiatr Scand*, **101**, 3–38.

Levav, I., Lipshitz, I., Novikov, I., et al. (2007). Cancer risk among parents and siblings of patients with schizophrenia. *Br J Psychiatry*, **190**, 156–61.

Levitt, P. (2003). Structural and functional maturation of the developing primate brain. *J Pediatrics*, **143**, S35–45.

Levy, S. & Strausberg, R. L. (2008). Human genetics: Individual genomes diversify. *Nature*, **456**, 49–51.

Lewis, C.M., Levinson, D.F., Wise, L.H., et al. (2003). Genome scan meta-analysis of schizophrenia and bipolar disorder, part II: Schizophrenia. *Am J Human Genet*, **73**, 34–48.

Lewis, D.A. & Levitt, P. (2002). Schizophrenia as a disorder of neurodevelopment. *Annu Rev Neurosci*, **25**, 409–32.

Libet, B., Gleason, C.A., Wright, E.W., & Pearl, D.K. (1983). Time of conscious intention to act in relation to onset of cerebral activity (readiness-potential). The unconscious initiation of a freely voluntary act. *Brain*, **106** (Pt 3), 623–42.

Liddell, M.B., Williams, J., & Owen, M.J. (2005). The dementias. In: McGuffin, P., Owen, M. J., & Gottesman, I.I. (eds) *Psychiatric Genetics and Genomics*. Oxford University Press, Oxford.

Liddle, B. & Nettle, D. (2006). Higher-order theory of mind and social competence in school-age children. *J Cult Evol Psychol*, **4**, 231–44.

Lieberman, J.A. (2003). History of the use of antidepressants in primary care. *J Clin Psychiatry*, **5**, 6–10.

Lieberman, J.A., Stroup, T.S., McEvoy, J.P., et al. (2005). Effectiveness of antipsychotic drugs in patients with chronic schizophrenia. *N Engl J Med*, **353**, 1209–23.

Lilienfeld, S.O. & Marino, L. (1999). Essentialism revisited: evolutionary theory and the concept of mental disorder. *J Abnorm Psychol*, **108**, 400–11.

Lilienfeld, S.O., Gershon, J., Duke, M., Marino, L., & De Waal, F.B. (1999). A preliminary investigation of the construct of psychopathic personality (psychopathy) in chimpanzees (Pan troglodytes). *J Comp Psychol*, **113**, 365–75.

Lim, M.M. & Young, L.J. (2006). Neuropeptidergic regulation of affiliative behavior and social bonding in animals. *Hormones Behav*, **50**, 506–17.

Limer, K.L., Nicholl, B.I., Thomson, W., & McBeth, J. (2008). Exploring the genetic susceptibility of chronic widespread pain: the tender points in genetic association studies. *Rheumatology (Oxford)*, **47**, 572–77.

Linden, M. & Schermuly-Haupt, M.L. (2014). Definition, assessment and rate of psychotherapy side effects. *World Psychiatry*, **13**, 306–309.

Linehan, M. (1993). *Cognitive-Behavioral Treatment of Borderline Personality Disorder*. Guilford Press, New York.

Liotti, G. (2000). Disorganized attachment, models of borderline states and evolutionary psychotherapy. In: Gilbert, P. & Bailey, K.G. (eds) *Genes on the Couch. Explorations in Evolutionary Psychotherapy*. Brunner-Routledge, Hove.

Littlefield, C.H. & Lumsden, C.J. (1987). Gene culture coevolution and the strategies of psychiatric healing. *Ethol Sociobiol*, **8**, S151–63.

Littlefield, C.H. & Rushton, J.P. (1986). When a child dies—the sociobiology of bereavement. *J Pers Soc Psychol*, **51**, 797–802.

Liu, J.H., Raine, A., Venables, P.H., & Mednick, S.A. (2004). Malnutrition at age 3 years and externalizing behavior problems at ages 8, 11, and 17 years. *Am J Psychiatry*, **161**, 2005–13.

Lochner, C. & Stein, D.J. (2001). Gender in obsessive-compulsive disorder and obsessive-compulsive spectrum disorders. *Arch Women's Mental Health*, **4**, 19–26.

Lopes, M. & Santos-Victor, J. (2005). Visual learning by imitation with motor representations. *IEEE Trans Syst Man Cybern B Cybern*, **35**, 438–49.

Lopes, P.C. (2014). When is it socially acceptable to feel sick? *Proc Biol Sci*, **281**, 20140218.

Lopez, L.M., Harris, S.E., Luciano, M., et al. (2012). Evolutionary conserved longevity genes and human cognitive abilities in elderly cohorts. *Eur J Hum Genet*, **20**, 341–47.

Lopez-Larson, M.P., Delbello, M. P., Zimmerman, M.E., Schwiers, M.L., & Strakowski, S.M. (2002). Regional prefrontal gray and white matter abnormalities in bipolar disorder. *Biol Psychiatry*, **52**, 93–100.

Lorenz, K. (1943). Die angeborenen Formen möglicher Erfahrung. *Z Tierpsychol*, **5**, 94–125.

Lorenz, K. (1973). *Die Rückseite des Spiegels; Versuch einer Naturgeschichte Menschlichen Erkennens*. R. Piper, München.

Lough, S., Kipps, C.M., Treise, C., et al. (2006). Social reasoning, emotion and empathy in frontotemporal dementia. *Neuropsychologia*, **44**, 950–58.

Lubman, D.I., Yücel, M., & Pantelis, C. (2004). Addiction, a condition of compulsive behaviour? Neuroimaging and neuropsychological evidence of inhibitory dysregulation. *Addiction*, **99**, 1491–502.

Luhrman, T.M. (2000). *Of Two Minds: The Growing Disorder in American Psychiatry.* Alfred A. Knopf, New York.

Lutenbacher, M. (2002). Relationships between psychosocial factors and abusive parenting attitudes in low-income single mothers. *Nurs Res*, **51**, 158–67.

Luykx, J.J., Bakker, S.C., Van Geloven, N., et al. (2013). Seasonal variation of serotonin turnover in human cerebrospinal fluid, depressive symptoms and the role of the 5-HTTLPR. *Transl Psychiatry*, **3**, e311.

Lycett, J.E. & Dunbar, R.I. (1999). Abortion rates reflect the optimization of parental investment strategies. *Proc Biol Sci*, **266**, 2355–58.

Lynch, W.J., Roth, M.E., & Carroll, M.E. (2002). Biological basis of sex differences in drug abuse: preclinical and clinical studies. *Psychopharmacology (Berl)*, **164**, 121–37.

Lyons, D.M., Yang, C., Mobley, B.W., Nickerson, J.T., & Schatzberg, A.F. (2000). Early environmental regulation of glucocorticoid feedback sensitivity in young adult monkeys. *J Neuroendocrinol*, **12**, 723–28.

MacArthur, R.H. & Wilson, E.O. (1967). *The Theory of Island Biogeography*. Princeton University Press, Princeton.

Maccoby, E.E. (1991). Different reproductive strategies in males and females. *Child Dev*, **62**, 676–81; discussion 682–85.

Macdonald, R. (2000). Time to talk about rape. *BMJ*, **321**, 1034–35.

Mace, R. (1998). The coevolution of human fertility and wealth inheritance strategies. *Philos Trans R Soc Lond B Biol Sci*, **353**, 389–97.

Mace, R. (2000). Evolutionary ecology of human life history. *Anim Behav*, **59**, 1–10.

Mace, R. & Sear, R. (1997). Birth interval and the sex of children in a traditional African population: an evolutionary analysis. *J Biosoc Sci*, **29**, 499–507.

Macintosh, K. & Dissanayake, C. (2006). A comparative study of the spontaneous social interactions of children with high-functioning autism and children with Asperger's disorder. *Autism*, **10**, 199–220.

MacLean, P.D. (1990). *The Triune Brain in Evolution: Role in Paleocerebral Functions*. Plenum Press, New York.

MacLeod, C.E., Zilles, K., Schleicher, A., Rilling, J.K., & Gibson, K.R. (2003). Expansion of the neocerebellum in Hominoidea. *J Human Evol*, **44**, 401–29.

Maddox, J. (1997). Schizophrenia—the price of language? *Nature*, **388**, 424–25.

Maestripieri, D. (ed.) (2003). *Primate Psychology*. Harvard University Press, Cambridge, Massachusetts.

Maestripieri, D. & Carroll, K.A. (1998). Child abuse and neglect: usefulness of the animal data. *Psychol Bull*, **123**, 211–23.

Mahley, R.W. & Rall, S. C. (1999). Is epsilon 4 the ancestral human apoE allele? *Neurobiol Aging*, **20**, 429–30.

Maina, G., Vaschetto, P., Ziero, S., Di Lorenzo, R., & Bogetto, F. (2001). Post-partum as a specific risk factor for the onset of obsessive-compulsive disorder: clinical-controlled study. *Epidemiol Psichiatr Soc*, **10**, 90–95.

Manning, J.T. (2002). *Digit Ratio: A Pointer to Fertility, Behavior, and Health*. Rutgers University Press, New Brunswick.

Manstead, A.S.R., Fischer, A.H., & Jakobs, E.B. (1999). The social and emotional functions of facial displays. In: Philippot, P., Feldman, R.S., & Coats, E.J. (eds) *The Social Context of Nonverbal Behavior*. Cambridge University Press, Cambridge.

Markow, T.A. (1994). *Developmental Instability: Its Origins and Evolutionary Implications. Proceedings of the International Conference on Developmental Instabilbity, its Origins and Evolutionary Implications, Tempe, Arizona, 14–15 June 1993*. Kluwer Academic, Dordrecht.

Markow, T.A. & Gottesman, I.I. (1994). Behavioral phenodeviance: a Lernersque conjecture. In: Markow, T.A. (ed.) *Developmental Instability: Its Origins and Evolutionary Implications*. Kluwer Academic, Dordrecht.

Marks, I.M. (1986). Genetics of fear and anxiety disorders. *Br J Psychiatry*, **149**, 406–18.

Marks, I.M. (1987). Behavioral aspects of panic disorder. *Am J Psychiatry*, **144**, 1160–65.

Marks, I.M. & Nesse, R.M. (1994). Fear and fitness—an evolutionary analysis of anxiety disorders. *Ethol Sociobiol*, **15**, 247–61.

Marks, J. (1992). Chromosomal evolution in primates. In: Jones, S., Martin, R., & Pilbeam, D. (eds) *The Cambridge Encyclopedia of Human Evolution*. Cambridge University Press, Cambridge.

Marmorstein, N.R., Malone, S.M., & Iacono, W.G. (2004). Psychiatric disorders among offspring of depressed mothers: Associations with paternal psychopathology. *Am J Psychiatry*, **161**, 1588–94.

Martin, G.M. (1997). Genetics and the pathobiology of ageing. *Philos Trans R Soc Lond B Biol Sci*, **352**, 1773–80.

Martin, G.M. (2002). The evolutionary substrate of aging. *Arch Neurol*, **59**, 1702–705.

Martinowich, K., Manji, H., & Lu, B. (2007). New insights into BDNF function in depression and anxiety. *Nat Neurosci*, **10**, 1089–93.

Martins, S.S., Tavares, H., Da Silva Lobo, D.S., Galetti, A.M., & Gentil, V. (2004). Pathological gambling, gender, and risk-taking behaviors. *Addict Behav*, **29**, 1231–35.

Marvin, R.S. & Britner, P.A. (1999). Normative development: the ontogeny of attachment. In: Cassidy, J. & Shaver, P.R. (eds) *Handbook of Attachment. Theory, Research, and Clinical Applications*. Guilford Press, New York.

Marx, J. (1996). Dissecting how presinilins function—and malfunction. *Science*, **274**, 1838–40.

Matsunaga, S. (2009). Junk DNA promotes sex chromosome evolution. *Heredity (Edinb)*, **102**, 525–26.

Matthews, L.J. & Butler, P.M. (2011). Novelty-seeking DRD4 polymorphisms are associated with human migration distance out-of-Africa after controlling for neutral population gene structure. *Am J Phys Anthropol*, **145**, 382–89.

Maudsley, H. (1867). *The Physiology and Pathology of the Mind*. Appleton, New York.

Maynard-Smith, J. (1998). *Evolutionary Genetics*. Oxford University Press, Oxford.

Mayr, E. (1974). Behavior programs and evolutionary strategies. *Am Scientist*, **62**, 650–59.

Mayr, E. (1977). Darwin and natural selection. *Am Scientist*, **65**, 321–27.

Mayr, E. (2001). *What Evolution Is*. Basic Books, New York.

McCall, G.J. & Resick, P.A. (2003). A pilot study of PTSD symptoms among Kalahari Bushmen. *J Trauma Stress*, **16**, 445–50.

McCann, J.T. (1998). Subtypes of stalking (obsessional following) in adolescents. *J Adolesc*, **21**, 667–75.

McCracken, J.T., McGough, J., Shah, B., et al. (2002). Risperidone in children with autism and serious behavioral problems. *N Engl J Med*, **347**, 314–21.

McCrae, R.R. & Costa, P.T., Jr (1987). Validation of the five-factor model of personality across instruments and observers. *J Pers Soc Psychol*, **52**, 81–90.

McCullough, M.E., Kurzban, R., & Tabak, B.A. (2013). Cognitive systems for revenge and forgiveness. *Behav Brain Sci*, **36**, 1–15.

McEwen, B.S. (2002). Sex, stress and the hippocampus: allostasis, allostatic load and the aging process. *Neurobiol Aging*, **23**, 921–39.

McGirr, A., Paris, J., Lesage, A., Renaud, J., & Turecki, G. (2007). Risk factors for suicide completion in borderline personality disorder: a case-control study of cluster B comorbidity and impulsive aggression. *J Clin Psychiatry*, **68**, 721–29.

McGlashan, T.H. (2006). At issue: is natural selection rendering schizophrenia less severe? *Schizophr Bull*, **32**, 428–29.

McGlashan, T.H. & Hoffman, R.E. (2000). Schizophrenia as a disorder of developmentally reduced synaptic connectivity. *Arch Gen Psychiatry*, **57**, 637–48.

McGough, J.J., Smalley, S.L., McCracken, J.T., et al. (2005). Psychiatric comorbidity in adult attention deficit hyperactivity disorder: findings from multiplex families. *Am J Psychiatry*, **162**, 1621–27.

McGowan, P.O., Sasaki, A., D'alessio, A.C., et al. (2009). Epigenetic regulation of the glucocorticoid receptor in human brain associates with childhood abuse. *Nat Neurosci*, **12**, 342–48.

McGrath, J.J. (2006). Variations in the incidence of schizophrenia: data versus dogma. *Schizophr Bull*, **32**, 195–97.

McGrew, W.C. (1981). Social and cognitive capabilities of nonhuman-primates—lessons from the wild to captivity. *Int J Study Animal Problems*, **2**, 138–49.

McGrew, W.C., Marchant, L.F., & Nishida, T. (1996). *Great Ape Societies*. Cambridge University Press, Cambridge.

McGuffin, P., Owen, M.J., & Gottesman, I.I. (eds) (2005). *Psychiatric Genetics and Genomics*. Oxford University Press, Oxford.

McGuire, M.T. (1988). On the possibility of ethological explanations of psychiatric disorders. *Acta Psychiatr Scand Suppl*, **341**, 7–22.

McGuire, M.T. & Polsky, R.H. (1979). Behavioral changes in hospitalized acute schizophrenics. An ethological perspective. *J Nerv Ment Dis*, **167**, 651–57.

McGuire, M.T. & Polsky, R.H. (1983). Sociospatial behavioral relationships among hospitalized psychiatric patients. *Psychiatry Res*, **8**, 225–36.

McGuire, M.T. & Troisi, A. (1987). General-theory and methods.1. Physiological regulation, deregulation and psychiatric-disorders. *Ethol Sociobiol*, **8**, S9–25.

McGuire, M.T. & Troisi, A. (1998). *Darwinian Psychiatry*. Oxford University Press, New York.

McGuire, M.T. & Troisi, A. (2006a). Steps toward an evolutionary-based theory of psychotherapy—I. *Clin Neuropsychiatry*, **3**, 162–69.

McGuire, M.T. & Troisi, A. (2006b). Steps toward an evolutionary-based theory of psychotherapy—II. *Clin Neuropsychiatry*, **3**, 170–74.

McGuire, M.T., Essock-Vitale, S.M., & Polsky, R.H. (1981). Psychiatric disorders in the context of evolutionary biology. An ethological model of behavioral changes associated with psychiatric disorders. *J Nerv Ment Dis*, **169**, 687–704.

McKinney, M.L. & McNamara, K. (1991). *Heterochrony: The Evolution of Ontogeny*. Plenum Press, New York.

McKinney, W.T., Gardner, R., Barlow, G.W., & McGuire, M.T. (1994). Conceptual basis of animal-models in psychiatry—a conference summary. *Ethol Sociobiol*, **15**, 369–82.

McLean, C.Y., Reno, P.L., Pollen, A.A., et al. (2011). Human-specific loss of regulatory DNA and the evolution of human-specific traits. *Nature*, **471**, 216–19.

McMackin, R.A., Leisen, M.B., Cusack, J.F., Lafratta, J., & Litwin, P. (2002). The relationship of trauma exposure to sex offending behavior among male juvenile offenders. *J Child Sex Abus*, **11**, 25–40.

McNamara, P., Durso, R., & Harris, E. (2007). 'Machiavellianism' and frontal dysfunction: evidence from Parkinson's disease. *Cogn Neuropsychiatry*, **12**, 285–300.

McQueen, D. & St John-Smith, P. (2012). Placebo effects: a new paradigm and relevance to psychiatry. *Int Psychiatry*, **9**, 1–3.

McQueen, D., Cohen, S., St John-Smith, P., & Rampes, H. (2013a). Rethinking placebo in psychiatry: the range of placebo effects. *Adv Psychiatr Treatm*, **19**, 162–70.

McQueen, D., Cohen, S., St John-Smith, P., & Rampes, H. (2013b). Rethinking placebo in psychiatry: how and why placebo effects occur. *Adv Psychiatr Treatm*, **19**, 171–80.

Mealey, L. (1995). The sociobiology of sociopathy—an integrated evolutionary model. *Behav Brain Sci*, **18**, 523–41.

Mealey, L. (2002). Anorexia: a 'dis-ease' of low, low fertility. In: Rodgers, J.L. & Kohler, H.P. (eds) *The Biodemography of Human Reproduction and Fertility*. Kluwer Academic, New York.

Meaney, M.J. (2001). Maternal care, gene expression, and the transmission of individual differences in stress reactivity across generations. *Annu Rev Neurosci*, **24**, 1161–92.

Meares, R., Stevenson, J., & Gordon, E. (1999). A Jacksonian and biopsychosocial hypothesis concerning borderline and related phenomena. *Aust N Z J Psychiatry*, **33**, 831–40.

Medicus, G. (1987). An ethological perspective on psychiatry—theory and practice.4. toward an etho-psychology—a phylogenetic tree of behavioral capabilities proposed as a common basis for communication between current theories in psychology and psychiatry. *Ethol Sociobiol*, **8**, S131–50.

Medicus, G. (1995). Ethological aspects of aggression. On the biological foundation of psychotherapy and psychiatry. *Evol Cogn*, **1**, 54–63.

Mehta, D. & Binder, E.B. (2012). Gene × environment vulnerability factors for PTSD: the HPA-axis. *Neuropharmacology*, **62**, 654–62.

Meissner, K. (2011). The placebo effect and the autonomic nervous system: evidence for an intimate relationship. *Philos Trans R Soc Lond B Biol Sci*, **366**, 1808–17.

Meissner, K., Kohls, N., & Colloca, L. (2011). Introduction to placebo effects in medicine: mechanisms and clinical implications. *Philos Trans R Soc Lond B Biol Sci*, **366**, 1783–89.

Mekel-Bobrov, N., Gilbert, S.L., Evans, P. D., et al. (2005). Ongoing adaptive evolution of ASPM, a brain size determinant in Homo sapiens. *Science*, **309**, 1720–22.

Meloy, J.R. (1989). Unrequited love and the wish to kill. Diagnosis and treatment of borderline erotomania. *Bull Menninger Clin*, **53**, 477–92.

Meloy, J.R. (1999). Stalking. An old behavior, a new crime. *Psychiatr Clin N Am*, **22**, 85–99.

Meltzoff, A.N. & Moore, M.K. (1977). Imitation of facial and manual gestures by human neonates. *Science*, **198**, 75–78.

Menzies, R.P. (1994). Male erotomania and dangerousness. *Br J Psychiatry*, **165**, 554–55.

Merai, A., Diamant, I., Bibi, A., Brosh, Y., & Zakin, G. (2009). Personality characteristics of 'self-martyrs'/'suicide bombers' and organizers of suicide attacks. *Terrorism Political Violence*, **22**, 87–101.

Mesquita, S.C., Shuhama, R., Osorio, F.L., et al. (2011). The response of social anxiety disorder patients to threat scenarios differs from that of healthy controls. *Braz J Med Biol Res*, **44**, 1261–68.

Meyer-Lindenberg, A., Domes, G., Kirsch, P., & Heinrichs, M. (2011). Oxytocin and vasopressin in the human brain: social neuropeptides for translational medicine. *Nat Rev Neurosci*, **12**, 524–38.

Middleton, W. (2004). Dissociative disorders: a personal 'work in progress'. *Australas Psychiatry*, **12**, 245–52.

Mikach, S.M. & Bailey, J.M. (1999). What distinguishes women with unusually high numbers of sex partners? *Evol Human Behav*, **20**, 141–50.

Mikulincer, M. & Shaver, P.R. (2001). Attachment theory and intergroup bias: evidence that priming the secure base schema attenuates negative reactions to out-groups. *J Pers Soc Psychol*, **81**, 97–115.

Milad, M.R. & Rauch, S.L. (2007). The role of the orbitofrontal cortex in anxiety disorders. *Ann NY Acad Sci*, **1121**, 546–61.

Milgram, N. & Toubiana, Y. (1999). Academic anxiety, academic procrastination, and parental involvement in students and their parents. *Br J Educ Psychol*, **69**, 345–61.

Millar, T.P. (1987). Schizophrenia: an etiological speculation. *Perspect Biol Med*, **30**, 597–607.

Miller, B.L. & Cummings, J.L. (1999). *The Human Frontal Lobes: Functions and Disorders*. Guilford Press, New York.

Miller, E.K. & Cohen, J.D. (2001). An integrative theory of prefrontal cortex function. *Annu Rev Neurosci*, **24**, 167–202.

Miller, F.G., Colloca, L., & Kaptchuk, T.J. (2009). The placebo effect: illness and interpersonal healing. *Perspect Biol Med*, **52**, 518–39.

Miller, T.W., Nigg, J.T., & Faraone, S.V. (2007). Axis I and II comorbidity in adults with ADHD. *J Abnormal Psychol*, **116**, 519–28.

Mineka, S. (1987). A primate model of phobic fears. In: Eysenck, H.J. & Martin, I. (eds) *Theoretical Foundations of Behaviour Therapy*. Plenum Press, New York.

Minzenberg, M.J., Fan, J., New, A.S., Tang, C.Y., & Siever, L.J. (2008). Frontolimbic structural changes in borderline personality disorder. *J Psychiatr Res*, **42**, 727–33.

Mitchell, R.L. & Crow, T.J. (2005). Right hemisphere language functions and schizophrenia: the forgotten hemisphere? *Brain*, **128**, 963–78.

Mizrahi, R., Bagby, R.M., Zipursky, R.B., & Kapur, S. (2005). How antipsychotics work: the patients' perspective. *Prog Neuropsychopharmacol Biol Psychiatry*, **29**, 859–64.

Mizrahi, R., Kiang, M., Mamo, D.C., et al. (2006). The selective effect of antipsychotics on the different dimensions of the experience of psychosis in schizophrenia spectrum disorders. *Schizophr Res*, **88**, 111–18.

Mizuno, A., Villalobos, M.E., Davies, M.M., Dahl, B.C., & Muller, R.A. (2006). Partially enhanced thalamocortical functional connectivity in autism. *Brain Res*, **1104**, 160–74.

Modestin, J., Ebner, G., Junghan, M., & Erni, T. (1996). Dissociative experiences and dissociative disorders in acute psychiatric inpatients. *Compr Psychiatry*, **37**, 355–61.

Modestin, J., Oberson, B., & Erni, T. (1998). Identity disturbance in personality disorders. *Compr Psychiatry*, **39**, 352–57.

Moller A.P. & Thornhill, R. (1998). Male parental care, differential parental investment by females and sexual selection. *Anim Behav*, **55**, 1507–15.

Monroe, S.M. & Simons, A.D. (1991). Diathesis-stress theories in the context of life stress research: implications for the depressive disorders. *Psychol Bull*, **110**, 406–25.

Montagu, A. (1989). *Growing Young*. Bergin & Garvey, Granby, Massachusetts.

Morehead, D. (1999). Oedipus, Darwin, and Freud: one big, happy family? *Psychoanal Q*, **68**, 347–75.

Morgan, B.E., Horn, A.R., & Bergman, N.J. (2011). Should neonates sleep alone? *Biol Psychiatry*, **70**, 817–25.

Morgan, D., Grant, K.A., Gage, H.D., et al. (2002). Social dominance in monkeys: dopamine D2 receptors and cocaine self-administration. *Nat Neurosci*, **5**, 169–74.

Morgane, P.J. & Mokler, D J. (2006). The limbic brain: continuing resolution. *Neurosci Biobehav Rev*, **30**, 119–25.

Morrison, J.H. & Hof, P.R. (1997). Life and death of neurons in the aging brain. *Science*, **278**, 412–19.

Moskowitz, A.K. (2004). 'Scared stiff': catatonia as an evolutionary-based fear response. *Psychol Rev*, **111**, 984–1002.

Moss, H.B., Lynch, K.G., Hardie, T.L., & Baron, D.A. (2002). Family functioning and peer affiliation in children of fathers with antisocial personality disorder and substance dependence: associations with problem behaviors. *Am J Psychiatry*, **159**, 607–14.

Moulding, R., Kyrios, M., Doron, G., & Nedeljkovic, M. (2007). Autogenous and reactive obsessions: further evidence for a two-factor model of obsessions. *J Anxiety Disord*, **21**, 677–90.

Moynihan, R. & Henry, D. (2006). The fight against disease mongering: generating knowledge for action. *PLoS Med*, **3**, e191.

Moynihan, R. & Smith, R. (2002). Too much medicine? *BMJ*, **324**, 859–60.

Muhle, R., Trentacoste, S.V., & Rapin, I. (2004). The genetics of autism. *Pediatrics*, **113**, e472–86.

Mullen, P.E. & Pathe, M. (1994a). The pathological extensions of love. *Br J Psychiatry*, **165**, 614–23.

Mullen, P.E. & Pathe, M. (1994b). Stalking and the pathologies of love. *Aust N Z J Psychiatry*, **28**, 469–77.

Mullen, P.E., Pathe, M., Purcell, R., & Stuart, G.W. (1999). Study of stalkers. *Am J Psychiatry*, **156**, 1244–49.

Mullen, P.E., Pathe, M., & Purcell, R. (2001). Stalking: new constructions of human behaviour. *Aust N Z J Psychiatry*, **35**, 9–16.

Müller, C.P. & Jacobs, B.L. (eds) (2010). *Handbook of the Behavioral Neurobiology of Serotonin*. Academic Press, London.

Murgatroyd, C., Patchev, A.V., Wu, Y., et al. (2009). Dynamic DNA methylation programs persistent adverse effects of early-life stress. *Nat Neurosci*, **12**, 1559–66.

Murphy, H.B.M. (1982). *Comparative Psychiatry: The International and Intercultural Distribution of Mental Illness*. Springer, Berlin.

Murray, R.M. (1994). Neurodevelopmental schizophrenia: the rediscovery of dementia praecox. *Br J Psychiatry Suppl*, **1994** (25), 6–12.

Muscarella, F., Fink, B., Grammer, K., & Kirk-Smith, M. (2001). Homosexual orientation in males: evolutionary and ethological aspects. *Neuro Endocrinol Lett*, **22**, 393–400.

Myers, A.J., Gibbs, J.R., Webster, J.A., et al. (2007). A survey of genetic human cortical gene expression. *Nat Genet*, **39**, 1494–99.

Myers, B.J. (1984). Mother–infant bonding—the status of this critical-period hypothesis. *Dev Rev*, **4**, 240–74.

Myers, S.G. & Wells, A. (2005). Obsessive-compulsive symptoms: the contribution of metacognitions and responsibility. *J Anxiety Disord*, **19**, 806–17.

Mysore, A., Parks, R.W., Lee, K.H., et al. (2007). Neurocognitive basis of insight in schizophrenia. *Br J Psychiatry*, **190**, 529–30.

Narr, K., Thompson, P., Sharma, T., et al. (2001). Three-dimensional mapping of gyral shape and cortical surface asymmetries in schizophrenia: gender effects. *Am J Psychiatry*, **158**, 244–55.

National Research Council (US) Committee on the Earth System Context for Hominin Evolution. (2010). Understanding Climate's Influence on Human Evolution. The National Academies Press. Washington D.C.

Naudts, K. & Hodgins, S. (2006a). Schizophrenia and violence: a search for neurobiological correlates. *Curr Opin Psychiatry*, **19**, 533–38.

Naudts, K. & Hodgins, S. (2006b). Neurobiological correlates of violent behavior among persons with schizophrenia. *Schizophr Bull*, **32**, 562–72.

Navarrete, A., Van Schaik, C. P. & Isler, K. (2011). Energetics and the evolution of human brain size. *Nature*, **480**, 91-U252.

Navarro-Mateu, F., Escamez, T., Koenen, K.C., Alonso, J., & Sanchez-Meca, J. (2013). Meta-analyses of the 5-HTTLPR polymorphisms and post-traumatic stress disorder. *PLoS One*, **8**, e66227.

Neel, J.V. (1962). Diabetes mellitus: a 'thrifty' genotype rendered detrimental by 'progress'? *Am J Human Genet*, **14**, 353–62.

Nelson, E.C., Heath, A.C., Madden, P.A., et al. (2002). Association between self-reported childhood sexual abuse and adverse psychosocial outcomes: results from a twin study. *Arch Gen Psychiatry*, **59**, 139–45.

Nelson, E.C., Agrawal, A., Pergadia, M.L., et al. (2009). Association of childhood trauma exposure and GABRA2 polymorphisms with risk of posttraumatic stress disorder in adults. *Mol Psychiatry*, **14**, 234–35.

Nelson, E.E. & Winslow, J.T. (2009). Non-human primates: model animals for developmental psychopathology. *Neuropsychopharmacology*, **34**, 90–105.

Nelson, T. J. & Alkon, D. L. (2005). Oxidation of cholesterol by amyloid precursor protein and beta-amyloid peptide. *J Biol Chem*, **280**, 7377–87.

Nesse, R.M. (1988). Life table tests of evolutionary theories of senescence. *Exp Gerontol*, **23**, 445–53.

Nesse, R.M. (1994). An evolutionary perspective on substance-abuse. *Ethol Sociobiol*, **15**, 339–48.

Nesse, R. (1998). Emotional disorders in evolutionary perspective. *Br J Med Psychol*, **71** (Pt 4), 397–415.

Nesse, R.M. (2000). Is depression an adaptation? *Arch Gen Psychiatry*, **57**, 14–20.

Nesse, R.M. (2001). The smoke detector principle. Natural selection and the regulation of defensive responses. *Ann N Y Acad Sci*, **935**, 75–85.

Nesse, R.M. (2004). Natural selection and the elusiveness of happiness. *Philos Trans R Soc Lond B Biol Sci*, **359**, 1333–47.

Nesse, R. M. (2005). *An Evolutionary Framework for the Understanding of Grief.* Springer, New York.

Nesse, R.M. (2007). Runaway social selection for displays of partner value and altruism. *Biological Theory*, **2**, 143–55.

Nesse, R.M. (2008). What evolutionary biology offers public health. *Bull World Health Organ*, **86**, 83.

Nesse, R.M. (2009). Evolution at 150: time for truly biological psychiatry. *Br J Psychiatry*, **195**, 471–72.

Nesse, R.M. (2011). Ten questions for evolutionary studies of disease vulnerability. *Evol Applic*, **4**, 264–77.

Nesse, R.M. (2013). Tinbergen's four questions, organized: a response to Bateson and Laland. *Trends Ecol Evol*, **28**, 681–82.

Nesse, R.M. & Berridge, K.C. (1997). Psychoactive drug use in evolutionary perspective. *Science*, **278**, 63–66.

Nesse, R.M. & Jackson, E.D. (2006). Evolution: psychiatric nosology's missing biological foundation. *Clin Neuropsychiatry*, **3**, 121–31.

Nesse, R.M. & Lloyd, A.T. (1992). The evolution of psychodynamic mechanisms. In: Barkow, J.H., Cosmides, L., & Tooby, J. (eds) *The Adapted Mind. Evolutionary Psychology and the Generation of Culture*. Oxford University Press, Oxford.

Nesse, R.M. & Stearns, S.C. (2008). The great opportunity: Evolutionary applications to medicine and public health. *Evol Appl*, **1**, 28–48.

Nesse, R.M. & Stein, D.J. (2012). Towards a genuinely medical model for psychiatric nosology. *BMC Med*, **10**, 5.

Nesse, R.M. & Williams, G.C. (1994). *Why We Get Sick: The New Science of Darwinian Medicine*. Times Books, New York.

Nesse, R.M., Stearns, S.C., & Omenn, G.S. (2006). Medicine needs evolution. *Science*, **311**, 1071.

Nesse, R.M., Bergstrom, C.T., Ellison, P.T., et al. (2010). Evolution in health and medicine Sackler colloquium: Making evolutionary biology a basic science for medicine. *Proc Natl Acad Sci USA*, **107** (Suppl 1), 1800–807.

Nettle, D. (2004). Evolutionary origins of depression: a review and reformulation. *J Affect Disord*, **81**, 91–102.

Nettle, D. (2014). What the future held: childhood psychosocial adversity is associated with health deterioration through adulthood in a cohort of British women. *Peer J PrePrints*, **1**.

Nettle, D., Coall, D.A., & Dickins, T.E. (2011). Early-life conditions and age at first pregnancy in British women. *Proc Biol Sci*, **278**, 1721–27.

New, A.S., Hazlett, E.A., Buchsbaum, M.S., et al. (2007). Amygdala-prefrontal disconnection in borderline personality disorder. *Neuropsychopharmacology*, **32**, 1629–40.

Newton, L., Rosen, A., Tennant, C., et al. (2000). Deinstitutionalisation for long-term mental illness: an ethnographic study. *Aust N Z J Psychiatry*, **34**, 484–90.

Nichols, K.A. & Champnes, B.G. (1971). Eye gaze and GSR. *J Exp Social Psychol*, **7**, 623–26.

Nieuwenhuys, R. (2012). The insular cortex: a review. *Prog Brain Res*, **195**, 123–63.

Nijenhuis, E.R., Van Der Hart, O., Kruger, K., & Steele, K. (2004). Somatoform dissociation, reported abuse and animal defence-like reactions. *Aust N Z J Psychiatry*, **38**, 678–86.

Nilsson, P.M., Nyberg, P., & Ostergren, P.O. (2001). Increased susceptibility to stress at a psychological assessment of stress tolerance is associated with impaired fetal growth. *Int J Epidemiol*, **30**, 75–80.

Nimchinsky, E.A., Gilissen, E., Allman, J.M., et al. (1999). A neuronal morphologic type unique to humans and great apes. *Proc Natl Acad Sci USA*, **96**, 5268–73.

Noble, W. & Davidson, I. (1996). *Human Evolution, Language, and Mind: A Psychological and Archaeological Inquiry*. Cambridge University Press, Cambridge.

Noftle, E.E. & Shaver, P.R. (2006). Attachment dimensions and the big five personality traits: associations and comparative ability to predict relationship quality. *J Res Pers*, **40**, 179–208.

Northcutt, R.G. (2001). Changing views of brain evolution. *Brain Res Bull*, **55**, 663–74.

Northoff, G. (2002a). What catatonia can tell us about 'top-down modulation': a neuropsychiatric hypothesis. *Behav Brain Sci*, **25**, 555–77; discussion 578–604.

Northoff, G. (2002b). Catatonia and neuroleptic malignant syndrome: psychopathology and pathophysiology. *J Neural Transm*, **109**, 1453–67.

Northoff, G., Bermpohl, F., Schoeneich, F., & Boeker, H. (2007). How does our brain constitute defense mechanisms? First-person neuroscience and psychoanalysis. *Psychother Psychosom*, **76**, 141–53.

Nöth, W. (1994). *Origins of Semiosis: Sign Evolution in Nature and Culture*. Mouton de Gruyter, Berlin.

Nowak, M.A. (2006). Five rules for the evolution of cooperation. *Science*, **314**, 1560–63.

Nowak, M. & Sigmund, K. (1993). A strategy of win-stay, lose-shift that outperforms tit-for-tat in the Prisoner's Dilemma game. *Nature*, **364**, 56–58.

Nowak, M.A. & Sigmund, K. (1998). Evolution of indirect reciprocity by image scoring. *Nature*, **393**, 573–77.

Nurnberg, H.G., Keith, S.J., & Paxton, D.M. (1997). Consideration of the relevance of ethological animal models for human repetitive behavioral spectrum disorders. *Biol Psychiatry*, **41**, 226–29.

Nye, C.L., Zucker, R.A., & Fitzgerald, H.E. (1999). Early family-based intervention in the path to alcohol problems: rationale and relationship between treatment process characteristics and child and parenting outcomes. *J Stud Alcohol Suppl*, **13**, 10–21.

Oberman, L.M., Hubbard, E.M., McCleery, J.P., et al. (2005). EEG evidence for mirror neuron dysfunction in autism spectrum disorders. *Cogn Brain Res*, **24**, 190–98.

O'Bleness, M., Searles, V.B., Varki, A., Gagneux, P., & Sikela, J.M. (2012). Evolution of genetic and genomic features unique to the human lineage. *Nat Rev Genet*, **13**, 853–66.

O'Connor, L.E., Berry, J.W., Weiss, J., & Gilbert, P. (2002). Guilt, fear, submission, and empathy in depression. *J Affect Disord*, **71**, 19–27.

O'Donovan, M.C. & Owen, M.J. (2005). Basic molecular genetics. In: McGuffin, P., Owen, M.J., & Gottesman, I.I. (eds) *Psychiatric Genetics and Genomics*. Oxford University Press, Oxford.

O'Dwyer, A.M. & Marks, I. (2000). Obsessive-compulsive disorder and delusions revisited. *Br J Psychiatry*, **176**, 281–84.

Okuda, J., Fujii, T., Yamadori, A., et al. (1998). Participation of the prefrontal cortices in prospective memory: evidence from a PET study in humans. *Neurosci Lett*, **253**, 127–30.

Olds, D.L. (2002). Prenatal and infancy home visiting by nurses: from randomized trials to community replication. *Prevention Sci*, **3**, 153–72.

Olds, D.L., Eckenrode, J., Henderson, C.R., Jr., et al. (1997). Long-term effects of home visitation on maternal life course and child abuse and neglect. Fifteen-year follow-up of a randomized trial. *JAMA*, **278**, 637–43.

Olson, J.M., Vernon, P.A., Harris, J.A., & Jang, K.L. (2001). The heritability of attitudes: a study of twins. *J Pers Soc Psychol*, **80**, 845–60.

Olsson, A. & Phelps, E.A. (2007). Social learning of fear. *Nat Neurosci*, **10**, 1095–102.

Olver, M.E. & Wong, S.C. (2006). Psychopathy, sexual deviance, and recidivism among sex offenders. *Sex Abuse*, **18**, 65–82.

O'Riordan M,A. (2004). Superior visual search in adults with autism. *Autism*, **8**, 229–48.

Ostermann, S., Herbsleb, M., Schulz, S., et al. (2013). Exercise reveals the interrelation of physical fitness, inflammatory response, psychopathology, and autonomic function in patients with schizophrenia. *Schizophr Bull*, **39**, 1139–49.

Ostrov, J.M. (2006). Deception and subtypes of aggression during early childhood. *J Exp Child Psychol*, **93**, 322–36.

Osuch, E.A., Noll, J.G., & Putnam, F.W. (1999). The motivations for self-injury in psychiatric inpatients. *Psychiatry*, **62**, 334–46.

Otta, E., Queiroz, R.D.S., Campos, L.D.S., Da Silva, M.W.D., & Silveira, M.T. (1999). Age differences between spouses in a Brazilian marriage sample. *Evol Human Behav*, **20**, 99–103.

Ottaviani, E. (2011). Evolution of immune-neuroendocrine integration from an ecological immunology perspective. *Cell Tissue Res*, **344**, 213–15.

Otto, M.W., Pollack, M.H., Maki, K.M., et al. (2001). Childhood history of anxiety disorders among adults with social phobia: rates, correlates, and comparisons with patients with panic disorder. *Depress Anxiety*, **14**, 209–13.

Overpeck, M.D., Brenner, R.A., Trumble, A.C., Trifiletti, L.B., & Berendes, H.W. (1998). Risk factors for infant homicide in the United States. *N Engl J Med*, **339**, 1211–16.

Owen, M.J., & Gottesman, I.I. (eds) *Psychiatric Genetics and Genomics*. Oxford University Press, Oxford.

Owen, M.J., Craddock, N., & Jablensky, A. (2007). The genetic deconstruction of psychosis. *Schizophr Bull*, **33**, 905–11.

Owens, D., Horrocks, J., & House, A. (2002). Fatal and non-fatal repetition of self-harm. Systematic review. *Br J Psychiatry*, **181**, 193–99.

Owens, D.C., Johnstone, E.C., Miller, P., Macmillan, J.F., & Crow, T.J. (2010). Duration of untreated illness and outcome in schizophrenia: test of predictions in relation to relapse risk. *Br J Psychiatry*, **196**, 296–301.

Oyama, O., Paltoo, C., & Greengold, J. (2007). Somatoform disorders. *Am Fam Physician*, **76**, 1333–38.

Pagnoni, G., Zink, C.F., Montague, P.R., & Berns, G.S. (2002). Activity in human ventral striatum locked to errors of reward prediction. *Nat Neurosci*, **5**, 97–98.

Pally, R. (2002). The neurobiology of borderline personality disorder: the synergy of 'nature and nurture'. *J Psychiatr Pract*, **8**, 133–42.

Panksepp, J. (1998). *Affective Neuroscience: The Foundations of Human and Animal Emotions*. Oxford University Press, New York.

Panksepp, J. (2005). Affective consciousness: core emotional feelings in animals and humans. *Conscious Cogn*, **14**, 30–80.

Panksepp, J. (2006). Emotional endophenotypes in evolutionary psychiatry. *Prog Neuropsychopharmacol Biol Psychiatry*, **30**, 774–84.

Panksepp, J.B. & Huber, R. (2004). Ethological analyses of crayfish behavior: a new invertebrate system for measuring the rewarding properties of psychostimulants. *Behav Brain Res*, **153**, 171–80.

Panksepp, J. & Panksepp, J. B. (2000). The seven sins of evolutionary psychology. *Evol Cogn*, **6**, 108–31.

Panksepp, J., Knutson, B., & Burgdorf, J. (2002). The role of brain emotional systems in addictions: a neuro-evolutionary perspective and new 'self-report' animal model. *Addiction*, **97**, 459–69.

Paradise, J.E. (2001). Current concepts in preventing sexual abuse. *Curr Opin Pediatr*, **13**, 402–407.

Paris, J. (1997). Antisocial and borderline personality disorders: two separate diagnoses or two aspects of the same psychopathology? *Compr Psychiatry*, **38**, 237–42.

Paris, J. (2004). Gender differences in personality traits and disorders. *Curr Psychiatry Rep*, **6**, 71–74.

Parker, G. (1982). Re-searching the schizophrenogenic mother. *J Nerv Ment Dis*, **170**, 452–62.

Patel, D.R., Phillips, E.L., & Pratt, H.D. (1998). Eating disorders. *Indian J Pediatr*, **65**, 487–94.

Pato, M.T., Schindler, K.M., & Pato, C.N. (2001). The genetics of obsessive-compulsive disorder. *Curr Psychiatry Rep*, **3**, 163–68.

Paulk, D. (2000). In your practice. Recognizing child abuse and neglect. *JAAPA*, **13**, 65–66, 69–74.

Pauls, D.L. & Alsobrook, J.P., 2nd (1999). The inheritance of obsessive-compulsive disorder. *Child Adolesc Psychiatr Clin N Am*, **8**, 481–96, viii.

Pauls, D.L., Abramovitch, A., Rauch, S.L., & Geller, D.A. (2014). Obsessive-compulsive disorder: an integrative genetic and neurobiological perspective. *Nat Rev Neurosci*, **15**, 410–24.

Paus, T. (2001). Primate anterior cingulate cortex: where motor control, drive and cognition interface. *Nat Rev Neurosci*, **2**, 417–24.

Paus, T., Tomaiuolo, F., Otaky, N., et al. (1996). Human cingulate and paracingulate sulci: pattern, variability, asymmetry, and probabilistic map. *Cereb Cortex*, **6**, 207–14.

Paus, T., Keshavan, M., & Giedd, J.N. (2008). Why do many psychiatric disorders emerge during adolescence? *Nat Rev Neurosci*, **9**, 947–57.

Pearce, J.M. (2004). Richard Morton: origins of anorexia nervosa. *Eur Neurol*, **52**, 191–92.

Pearce, J.W. & Pezzot-Pearce, T.D. (2001). Psychotherapeutic approaches to children in foster care: guidance from attachment theory. *Child Psychiatry Hum Dev*, **32**, 19–44.

Pearlson, G.D. & Folley, B.S. (2008). Schizophrenia, psychiatric genetics, and Darwinian psychiatry: an evolutionary framework. *Schizophr Bull*, **34**, 722–33.

Pearlstein, T. (2000). Antidepressant treatment of posttraumatic stress disorder. *J Clin Psychiatry*, **61** (Suppl 7), 40–43.

Pedersen, C.A., Smedley, K.L., Leserman, J., et al. (2013). Intranasal oxytocin blocks alcohol withdrawal in human subjects. *Alcohol Clin Exper Res*, **37**, 484–89.

Pedersen, J., Schelde, J.T., Hannibal, E., et al. (1988). An ethological description of depression. *Acta Psychiatr Scand*, **78**, 320–30.

Pelphrey, K.A., Morris, J.P., & McCarthy, G. (2005). Neural basis of eye gaze processing deficits in autism. *Brain*, **128**, 1038–48.

Pereira, V.M., Arias-Carrion, O., Machado, S., Nardi, A.E., & Silva, A.C. (2013). Sex therapy for female sexual dysfunction. *Int Arch Med*, **6**, 37.

Perner, J. (1991). *Understanding the Representational Mind.* MIT Press, Cambridge, Massachusetts.

Perner, J. & Wimmer, H. (1985). John thinks that mary thinks that—attribution of 2nd-order beliefs by 5-year-old to 10-year-old children. *J Exper Child Psychol*, **39**, 437–71.

Perner, J., Frith, U., Leslie, A.M., & Leekam, S.R. (1989). Exploration of the autistic child's theory of mind: knowledge, belief, and communication. *Child Dev*, **60**, 688–700.

Perris, C., Jacobsson, L., Lindstrom, H., Von Knorring, L., & Perris, H. (1980). Development of a new inventory assessing memories of parental rearing behaviour. *Acta Psychiatr Scand*, **61**, 265–74.

Perroud, N., Dayer, A., Piguet, C., et al. (2014a). Childhood maltreatment and methylation of the glucocorticoid receptor gene NR3C1 in bipolar disorder. *Br J Psychiatry*, **204**, 30–35.

Perroud, N., Rutembesa, E., Paoloni-Giacobino, A., et al. (2014b). The Tutsi genocide and transgenerational transmission of maternal stress: epigenetics and biology of the HPA axis. *World J Biol Psychiatry*, **15**, 334–45.

Peters, J. (2014). The role of genomic imprinting in biology and disease: an expanding view. *Nat Rev Genet*, **15**, 517–30.

Petrovic, P., Kalisch, R., Singer, T., & Dolan, R.J. (2008). Oxytocin attenuates affective evaluations of conditioned faces and amygdala activity. *J Neurosci*, **28**, 6607–15.

Pfefferbaum, A., Mathalon, D.H., Sullivan, E.V., et al. (1994). A quantitative magnetic resonance imaging study of changes in brain morphology from infancy to late adulthood. *Arch Neurol*, **51**, 874–87.

Pfeifer, K. (2000). Mechanisms of genomic imprinting. *Am J Human Genet*, **67**, 777–87.

Pfeiffer, W.M. (1994). *Transkulturelle Psychiatrie*. Thieme, Stuttgart.

Philippot, P., Feldman, R.S., & Coats, E.J. (1999). *The Social Context of Nonverbal Behavior*. Cambridge University Press, Cambridge.

Philipsen, A. (2006). Differential diagnosis and comorbidity of attention-deficit/hyperactivity disorder (ADHD) and borderline personality disorder (BPD) in adults. *Eur Arch Psychiatry Clin Neurosci*, **256** (Suppl 1), i42–46.

Pilling, S., Bebbington, P., Kuipers, E., et al. (2002). Psychological treatments in schizophrenia: II. Meta-analyses of randomized controlled trials of social skills training and cognitive remediation. *Psychol Med*, **32**, 783–91.

Pillmann, F. (2001). Social rank and depression—an example of 'evolutionary psychopathology'. *Fortschr Neurol Psychiatr*, **69**, 268–77.

Pineda, J.A. (2005). The functional significance of mu rhythms: translating 'seeing' and 'hearing' into 'doing'. *Brain Res Brain Res Rev*, **50**, 57–68.

Pinel, P. (1806). *A Treatise on Insanity, in Which Are Contained the Principles of a New and More Practical Nosology of Maniacal Disorders*. W. Todd, Sheffield.

Pitman, R.K. (1989). Animal models of compulsive behavior. *Biol Psychiatry*, **26**, 189–98.

Pitman, R.K., Kolb, B., Orr, S.P., et al. (1987a). Ethological methods and empirical-studies on the utility of ethological data in psychiatric research—the example of facial behavior in schizophrenia. *Ethol Sociobiol*, **8**, S111–16.

Pitman, R.K., Kolb, B., Orr, S.P., & Singh, M.M. (1987b). Ethological study of facial behavior in nonparanoid and paranoid schizophrenic patients. *Am J Psychiatry*, **144**, 99–102.

Pitman, R.K., Sanders, K.M., Zusman, R.M., et al. (2002). Pilot study of secondary prevention of posttraumatic stress disorder with propranolol. *Biol Psychiatry*, **51**, 189–92.

Pitman, R.K., Rasmusson, A.M., Koenen, K.C., et al. (2012). Biological studies of post-traumatic stress disorder. *Nat Rev Neurosci*, **13**, 769–87.

Pliszka, S. (2007). Practice parameter for the assessment and treatment of children and adolescents with attention-deficit/hyperactivity disorder. *J Am Acad Child Adolesc Psychiatry*, **46**, 894–921.

Ploeger, A. & Galis, F. (2011). Evolutionary approaches to autism- an overview and integration. *Mcgill J Med*, **13**, 38.

Plomin, R., Owen, M.J., & McGuffin, P. (1994). The genetic basis of complex human behaviors. *Science*, **264**, 1733–39.

Plomin, R., Happé, F., & Caspi, A. (2005). Personality and cognitive abilities. In: McGuffin, P., Owen, M.J., & Gottesman, I.I. (eds) *Psychiatric Genetics and Genomics*. Oxford University Press, Oxford.

Ploog, D. (1964). Verhaltensforschung und Psychiatrie. In: Gruhle, U.H., Jung, W.R., Mayer-Gross, W., & Müller, M. (eds) *Psychiatrie der Gegenwart*. Springer, Berlin.

Ploog, D. (1988). An outline of human neuroethology. *Hum Neurobiol*, **6**, 227–38.

Ploog, D. (1989). Zur Evolution des Bewusstseins. In: Pöppel, E. (ed.) *Gehirn und Bewusstsein*. VHC Verlagsgesellschaft, Weinheim.

Ploog, D. (1999). Evolutionsbiologie der Emotionen. In: Helmchen, H., Henn, F., Lauter, H., & Sartorius, N. (eds) *Psychiatrie der Gegenwart*. Springer, Berlin.

Ploog, D.W. & Pirke, K.M. (1987). Psychobiology of anorexia nervosa. *Psychol Med*, **17**, 843–59.

Polanczyk, G., Caspi, A., Williams, B., et al. (2009). Protective effect of CRHR1 gene variants on the development of adult depression following childhood maltreatment: replication and extension. *Arch Gen Psychiatry*, **66**, 978–85.

Polimeni, J. & Reiss, J.P. (2002). How shamanism and group selection may reveal the origins of schizophrenia. *Med Hypotheses*, **58**, 244–48.

Polimeni, J. & Reiss, J.P. (2003). Evolutionary perspectives on schizophrenia. *Can J Psychiatry*, **48**, 34–39.

Polimeni, J., Reiss, J.P., & Sareen, J. (2005). Could obsessive-compulsive disorder have originated as a group-selected adaptive trait in traditional societies? *Med Hypotheses*, **65**, 655–64.

Pollard, K.S., Salama, S.R., King, B., (2006). Forces shaping the fastest evolving regions in the human genome. *PLoS Genet*, **2**, e168.

Polsky, R. & McGuire, M.T. (1979). An ethological analysis of manic-depressive disorder. *J Nerv Ment Dis*, **167**, 56–65.

Polsky, R.H. & McGuire, M.T. (1981). Social ethology of acute psychiatric patients. The influence of sex, hospital environment, and spatial proximity. *J Nerv Ment Dis*, **169**, 28–36.

Ponnet, K.S., Roeyers, H., Buysse, A., De Clercq, A., & Van Der Heyden, E. (2004). Advanced mind-reading in adults with Asperger syndrome. *Autism*, **8**, 249–66.

Ponseti, J., Granert, O., Van Eimeren, T., et al. (2014). Human face processing is tuned to sexual age preferences. *Biol Lett*, **10**, 20140200.

Pooley, E.C., Fineberg, N., & Harrison, P. J. (2007). The met(158) allele of catechol-O-methyltransferase (COMT) is associated with obsessive-compulsive disorder in men: case-control study and meta-analysis. *Mol Psychiatry*, **12**, 556–61.

Poortinga, Y.H. & Van Hemert, D.A. (2001). Personality and culture: demarcating between the common and the unique. *J Pers*, **69**, 1033–60.

Pope, S.K., Shue, V.M., & Beck, C. (2003). Will a healthy lifestyle help prevent Alzheimer's disease? *Annu Rev Public Health*, **24**, 111–32.

Pöppel, E. (ed.) (1989). *Gehirn und Bewusstsein*. VHC Verlagsgesellschaft, Weinheim.

Porges, S.W. (1992). Vagal tone: a physiologic marker of stress vulnerability. *Pediatrics*, **90**, 498–504.

Porges, S.W. (1995). Orienting in a defensive world: mammalian modifications of our evolutionary heritage. A polyvagal theory. *Psychophysiology*, **32**, 301–18.

Porges, S.W. (2007). The polyvagal perspective. *Biol Psychol*, **74**, 116–43.

Porges, S.W. (2009). The polyvagal theory: new insights into adaptive reactions of the autonomic nervous system. *Cleve Clin J Med*, **76** (Suppl 2), S86–90.

Post, F. (1994). Creativity and psychopathology. A study of 291 world-famous men. *Br J Psychiatry*, **165**, 22–34.

Potash, J.B., Willour, V.L., Chiu, Y.F., et al. (2001). The familial aggregation of psychotic symptoms in bipolar disorder pedigrees. *Am J Psychiatry*, **158**, 1258–64.

Povinelli, D.J. (1993). Reconstructing the evolution of mind. *Am Psychol*, **48**, 493–509.

Powers, K.E. & Heatherton, T.F. (2012). Characterizing socially avoidant and affiliative responses to social exclusion. *Front Integr Neurosci*, **6**, 46.

Premack, D. & Woodruff, G. (1978). Does the chimpanzee have a Theory of Mind? *Behav Brain Sci*, **1**, 515–26.

Preston, S.D. (2013). The origins of altruism in offspring care. *Psychol Bull*, **139**, 1305–41.

Preston, S.D., Hofelich, A.J., & Stansfield, R.B. (2013). The ethology of empathy: a taxonomy of real-world targets of need and their effect on observers. *Front Hum Neurosci*, **7**, 1–13.

Preter, M. & Klein, D.F. (2008). Panic, suffocation false alarms, separation anxiety and endogenous opioids. *Prog Neuropsychopharmacol Biol Psychiatry*, **32**, 603–12.

Preti, A. (2011). Animal model and neurobiology of suicide. *Prog Neuropsychopharmacol Biol Psychiatry*, **35**, 818–30.

Preti, A. & Wilson, D.R. (2011). Schizophrenia, cancer and obstetric complications in an evolutionary perspective-an empirically based hypothesis. *Psychiatry Investig*, **8**, 77–88.

Preuschoft, S. (2000). Primate faces and facial expressions. *Social Res*, **67**, 245–71.

Preuschoft, S. & Preuschoft, H. (1994). Primate nonverbal communication: our communicatory heritage. In: Nöth, W. (ed.) *Origins of Semiosis*. Mouton de Gruyter, Berlin.

Preuschoft, S. & Van Schaik, C.P. (2000). Dominance and communication: conflict management in various social settings. In: Aureli, F. & De Waal, F.B.M. (eds) *Natural Conflict Resolution*. University of California Press, Berkeley.

Price, J. (1998a). The adaptive function of mood change. *Br J Med Psychol*, **71** (Pt 4), 465–77.

Price, J.S. (1998b). Evolution of schizotypy. *Br J Psychiatry*, **173**, 183.

Price, J.S. (2013). An evolutionary perspective on anxiety and anxiety disorders. In: Durbano, F. (ed.) *New Insights into Anxiety Disorders*. InTech, Rijeka.

Price, J.S. & Sloman, L. (1984). The evolutionary model of psychiatric disorder. *Arch Gen Psychiatry*, **41**, 211.

Price, J.S. & Wilson, D.R. (2011). *Male Philopatry, Female Entrapment, and Sex Difference in the Incidence of Depressive Illness.* University of Athens Press, Athens.

Price, J., Cole, V., & Goodwin, G.M. (2009). Emotional side-effects of selective serotonin reuptake inhibitors: qualitative study. *Br J Psychiatry*, **195**, 211–17.

Price, J.S., Gardner, R., & Erickson, M. (2004). Can depression, anxiety and somatization be understood as appeasement displays? *J Affect Disord*, **79**, 1–11.

Price, J.S., Gardner, R.J., Wilson, D.R., et al. (2007). Territory, rank and mental health: the history of an idea. *Evol Psychol*, **5**, 531–54.

Pridmore, S., Brüne, M., Ahmadi, J., & Dale, J. (2008). Echopraxia in schizophrenia: possible mechanisms. *Aust N Z J Psychiatry*, **42**, 565–71.

Priebe, S., Matanov, A., Jankovic Gavrilovic, J., et al. (2009). Consequences of untreated posttraumatic stress disorder following war in former Yugoslavia: morbidity, subjective quality of life, and care costs. *Croat Med J*, **50**, 465–75.

Priel, B. & Besser, A. (2000). Adult attachment styles, early relationships, antenatal attachment, and perceptions of infant temperament: a study of first-time mothers. *Personal Relationships*, **7**, 291–310.

Pujol, J., Soriano-Mas, C., Alonso, P., et al. (2004). Mapping structural brain alterations in obsessive-compulsive disorder. *Arch Gen Psychiatry*, **61**, 720–30.

Putkonen, H., Komulainen, E.J., Virkkunen, M., Eronen, M., & Lonnqvist, J. (2003). Risk of repeat offending among violent female offenders with psychotic and personality disorders. *Am J Psychiatry*, **160**, 947–51.

Quartz, S.R. (1999). The constructivist brain. *Trend Cogn Sci*, **3**, 48–57.

Quinn, J.J., Hitchcott, P.K., Umeda, E.A., Arnold, A.P., & Taylor, J.R. (2007). Sex chromosome coemplement regulates habit formation. *Nat Neurosci*, **10**, 1398–400.

Rademakers, R., Cruts, M., & Van Broeckhoven, C. (2003). Genetics of early-onset Alzheimer dementia. *ScientificWorldJournal*, **3**, 497–519.

Rai, R.S. & Mitchell, P. (2004). Five-year-old children's difficulty with false belief when the sought entity is a person. *J Exper Child Psychol*, **89**, 112–26.

Raison, C.L. & Miller, A.H. (2013). The evolutionary significance of depression in pathogen host defense (PATHOS-D). *Mol Psychiatry*, **18**, 15–37.

Rakic, P., Bourgeois, J.P., Eckenhoff, M.F., Zecevic, N., & Goldman-Rakic, P.S. (1986). Concurrent overproduction of synapses in diverse regions of the primate cerebral cortex. *Science*, **232**, 232–35.

Raleigh, M.J., McGuire, M.T., Brammer, G.L., & Yuwiler, A. (1984). Social and environmental influences on blood serotonin concentrations in monkeys. *Arch Gen Psychiatry*, **41**, 405–10.

Raleigh, M.J., Brammer, G.L., McGuire, M.T., & Yuwiler, A. (1985). Dominant social status facilitates the behavioral effects of serotonergic agonists. *Brain Res*, **348**, 274–82.

Raleigh, M.J., McGuire, M.T., Brammer, G.L., Pollack, D.B., & Yuwiler, A. (1991). Serotonergic mechanisms promote dominance acquisition in adult male vervet monkeys. *Brain Res*, **559**, 181–90.

Ramseyer, F. & Tschacher, W. (2014). Nonverbal synchrony of head- and body-movement in psychotherapy: different signals have different associations with outcome. *Front Psychol*, **5**, 979.

Randall, P.L. (1983). Schizophrenia, abnormal connection, and brain evolution. *Med Hypotheses*, **10**, 247–80.

Randall, P.L. (1998). Schizophrenia as a consequence of brain evolution. *Schizophr Res*, **30**, 143–48.

Rapoport, S.I. (1990). Integrated phylogeny of the primate brain, with special reference to humans and their diseases. *Brain Res Rev*, **15**, 267–94.

Rapoport, J.L. & Fiske, A. (1998). The new biology of obsessive-compulsive disorder: implications for evolutionary psychology. *Perspect Biol Med*, **41**, 159–75.

Rasgon, N., McGuire, M.T., & Troisi, A. (2000). Gender and psychotherapy: an evolutionary perspective. In: Gilbert, P. & Bailey, K.G. (eds) *Genes on the Couch. Explorations in Evolutionary Psychotherapy*. Brunner-Routledge, Hove.

Rasmussen, P. & Gillberg, C. (2000). Natural outcome of ADHD with developmental coordination disorder at age 22 years: a controlled, longitudinal, community-based study. *J Am Acad Child Adolesc Psychiatry*, **39**, 1424–31.

Ratner, R.K. & Miller, D.T. (2001). The norm of self-interest and its effects on social action. *J Pers Soc Psychol*, **81**, 5–16.

Redon, R., Ishikawa, S., Fitch, K.R., et al. (2006). Global variation in copy number in the human genome. *Nature*, **444**, 444–54.

Reiches, M.W., Ellison, P.T., Lipson, S.F., et al. (2009). Pooled energy budget and human life history. *Am J Hum Biol*, **21**, 421–29.

Reif, A., Rosler, M., Freitag, C.M., et al. (2007). Nature and nurture predispose to violent behavior: serotonergic genes and adverse childhood environment. *Neuropsychopharmacology*, **32**, 2375–83.

Reist, C., Ozdemir, V., Wang, E., et al. (2007). Novelty seeking and the dopamine D4 receptor gene (DRD4) revisited in Asians: haplotype characterization and relevance of the 2-repeat allele. *Am J Med Genet B Neuropsychiatr Genet*, **144**B, 453–57.

Renou, J., De Luca, V., Zai, C.C., et al. (2007). Multiple variants of the DRD3, but not BDNF gene, influence age-at-onset of schizophrenia. *Mol Psychiatry*, **12**, 1058–60.

Ressler, K.J., Mercer, K.B., Bradley, B., et al. (2011). Post-traumatic stress disorder is associated with PACAP and the PAC1 receptor. *Nature*, **470**, 492–97.

Ribases, M., Gratacos, M., Fernandez-Aranda, F., et al. (2004). Association of BDNF with anorexia, bulimia and age of onset of weight loss in six European populations. *Hum Mol Genet*, **13**, 1205–12.

Ribeiro, J.D. & Joiner, T.E. (2009). The interpersonal-psychological theory of suicidal behavior: current status and future directions. *J Clin Psychol*, **65**, 1291–99.

Richer, J. (2014). 'Disordered' behaviour. Alternatives to DSM-5 from an ethological perspective. *Hum Ethol Bull*, **29**, 27–55.

Richter, P., Scheurer, H., Barnett, W., & Krober, H.L. (1996). Forecasting recidivism in delinquency by intelligence and related constructs. *Med Sci Law*, **36**, 337–42.

Rickert, V.I., Wiemann, C.M., Vaughan, R.D., & White, J.W. (2004). Rates and risk factors for sexual violence among an ethnically diverse sample of adolescents. *Arch Pediatr Adolesc Med*, **158**, 1132–39.

Ridley, M. (2004). *Evolution*. Oxford University Press, Oxford.

Ridley, R.M. & Baker, H.F. (1982). Stereotypy in monkeys and humans. *Psychol Med*, **12**, 61–72.

Rief, W., Hennings, A., Riemer, S., & Euteneuer, F. (2010). Psychobiological differences between depression and somatization. *J Psychosom Res*, **68**, 495–502.

Riemenschneider, M., Mahmoodzadeh, S., Eisele, T., et al. (2004). Association analysis of genes involved in cholesterol metabolism located within the linkage region on chromosome 10 and Alzheimer's disease. *Neurobiol Aging*, **25**, 1305–308.

Rilling, J.K. & Insel, T.R. (1998). Evolution of the cerebellum in primates: differences in relative volume among monkeys, apes and humans. *Brain Behav Evol*, **52**, 308–14.

Rilling, J.K. & Insel, T.R. (1999a). The primate neocortex in comparative perspective using magnetic resonance imaging. *J Hum Evol*, **37**, 191–223.

Rilling, J.K. & Insel, T.R. (1999b). Differential expansion of neural projection systems in primate brain evolution. *Neuroreport*, **10**, 1453–59.

Rilling, J.K. & Seligman, R.A. (2002). A quantitative morphometric comparative analysis of the primate temporal lobe. *J Hum Evol*, **42**, 505–33.

Rilling, J.K., Sanfey, A.G., Aronson, J.A., Nystrom, L.E., & Cohen, J.D. (2004). The neural correlates of theory of mind within interpersonal interactions. *Neuroimage*, **22**, 1694–703.

Rilling, J.K., Goldsmith, D.R., Glenn, A.L., et al. (2008). The neural correlates of the affective response to unreciprocated cooperation. *Neuropsychologia*, **46**, 1256–66.

Ringer, J.M., Buchanan, E.E., Olesek, K., & Lysaker, P.H. (2014). Anxious and avoidant attachment styles and indicators of recovery in schizophrenia: associations with self-esteem and hope. *Psychol Psychother*, **87**, 209–21.

Rinn, W.E. (1984). The neuropsychology of facial expression: a review of the neurological and psychological mechanisms for producing facial expressions. *Psychol Bull*, **95**, 52–77.

Rison, R.A. (1998). Schizophrenia and N-methyl-D-aspartate receptors: evolutionary adaptations from malfunctioning molecules? *Neuropsychiatry Neuropsychol Behav Neurol*, **11**, 236–40.

Ritter, L.M., Meador-Woodruff, J.H., & Dalack, G.W. (2004). Neurocognitive measures of prefrontal cortical dysfunction in schizophrenia. *Schizophr Res*, **68**, 65–73.

Ritvo, L.B. (1974). The impact of Darwin on Freud. *Psychoanal Q*, **43**, 177–92.

Rizzolatti, G. & Arbib, M.A. (1998). Language within our grasp. *Trends Neurosci*, **21**, 188–94.

Rizzolatti, G. & Craighero, L. (2004). The mirror-neuron system. *Annu Rev Neurosci*, **27**, 169–92.

Rizzolatti, G., Fogassi, L., & Gallese, V. (2002). Motor and cognitive functions of the ventral premotor cortex. *Curr Opin Neurobiol*, **12**, 149–54.

Robbins, T.W. & Everitt, B.J. (1999). Drug addiction: bad habits add up. *Nature*, **398**, 567–70.

Roberts, S.C., Cobey, KD., Klapilova, K., & Havlicek, J. (2014). Oral contraception and romantic relationships—from the lab to the real world. *Hum Ethol Bull*, **29**, 4–13.

Robertson, S.A. (2010). Immune regulation of conception and embryo implantation-all about quality control? *J Reprod Immunol*, **85**, 51–57.

Rockliff, H., Karl, A., McEwan, K., et al. (2011). Effects of intranasal oxytocin on 'compassion focused imagery'. *Emotion*, **11**, 1388–96.

Rodgers, J.L. & Kohler, H.-P. (2003). *The Biodemography of Human Reproduction and Fertility*. Kluwer, Boston.

Roelcke, V. (1997). Biologizing social facts: an early 20th century debate on Kraepelin's concepts of culture, neurasthenia, and degeneration. *Cult Med Psychiatry*, **21**, 383–403.

Roeyers, H., Buysse, A., Ponnet, K., & Pichal, B. (2001). Advancing advanced mind-reading tests: empathic accuracy in adults with a pervasive developmental disorder. *J Child Psychol Psychiatry*, **42**, 271–78.

Roff, D.A. (2007). Contributions of genomics to life-history theory. *Nat Rev Genet*, **8**, 116–25.

Rohde, P. (2001). The relevance of hierarchies, territories, defeat for depression in humans: hypotheses and clinical predictions. *J Affect Disord*, **65**, 221–30.

Rook, G.a.W. (2009). *The Hygiene Hypothesis and Darwinian Medicine*. Birkhäuser, Basel.

Rook, G.a.W. & Lowry, C.A. (2009). The hygiene hypothesis and affective and anxiety disorders. In: Rook, G.a.W. (ed.) *The Hygiene Hypothesis and Darwinian Medicine*. Birkhäuser, Basel.

Roser, P., Gallinat, J., Weinberg, G., et al. (2009). Psychomotor performance in relation to acute oral administration of Delta9-tetrahydrocannabinol and standardized cannabis extract in healthy human subjects. *Eur Arch Psychiatry Clin Neurosci*, **259**, 284–92.

Roshchina, V.V. (2010). Evolutionary considerations of neurotransmitters in microbial, plant, and animal cells. In: Lyte M. & Freestone, P.P.E. (eds). *Microbial Endocrinology, Interkingdom Signaling in Infectious Disease and Health*. Springer, Berlin, pp. 17–52.

Ross, H.E., Freeman, S.M., Spiegel, L.L., et al. (2009). Variation in oxytocin receptor density in the nucleus accumbens has differential effects on affiliative behaviors in monogamous and polygamous voles. *J Neurosci*, **29**, 1312–18.

Rossano, M.J. (2003). *Evolutionary Psychology. The Science of Human Behavior and Evolution*. Wiley, Hoboken.

Roth, G. (2001). The evolution of consciousness. In: Roth, G. & Wullimann, M.F. (eds) *Brain Evolution and Cognition*. Wiley, New York.

Roth, G. (2006). Über objective und subjective Willensfreiheit. In: Förstl, H. (ed.) *Theory of Mind*. Springer, Heidelberg.

Roth, G. & Wullimann, M.F. (eds) (2001). *Brain Evolution and Cognition*. Wiley, New York.

Rottenberg, J. (2014). *The Depths. The Evolutionary Origins of the Depression Epidemic*. Basic Books, New York.

Rowe, R., Maughan, B., & Eley, T.C. (2006). Links between antisocial behavior and depressed mood: the role of life events and attributional style. *J Abnorm Child Psychol*, **34**, 293–302.

Rowland, A.S., Lesesne, C.A., & Abramowitz, A.J. (2002). The epidemiology of attention-deficit/ hyperactivity disorder(ADHD): a public health view. *Ment Retard Dev Disab Res Rev*, **8**, 162–70.

Roy, A., Hu, X.Z., Janal, M.N., & Goldman, D. (2007). Interaction between childhood trauma and serotonin transporter gene variation in suicide. *Neuropsychopharmacology*, **32**, 2046–52.

Rubin, L.H., Carter, C.S., Drogos, L., et al. (2010). Peripheral oxytocin is associated with reduced symptom severity in schizophrenia. *Schizophr Res*, **124**, 13–21.

Ruby, P. & Decety, J. (2001). Effect of subjective perspective taking during simulation of action: a PET investigation of agency. *Nat Neurosci*, **4**, 546–50.

Ruchkin, V.V., Koposov, R.A., Eisemann, M., & Hagglof, B. (2001). Conduct problems in Russian adolescents: the role of personality and parental rearing. *Eur Child Adolesc Psychiatry*, **10**, 19–27.

Ruchkin, V.V., Schwab-Stone, M., Koposov, R., Vermeiren, R., & Steiner, H. (2002). Violence exposure, posttraumatic stress, and personality in juvenile delinquents. *J Am Acad Child Adolesc Psychiatry*, **41**, 322–29.

Rucklidge, J.J., Brown, D.L., Crawford, S., & Kaplan, B.J. (2006). Retrospective reports of childhood trauma in adults with ADHD. *J Atten Disord*, **9**, 631–41.

Ruiz, A., Blanco, R., Santander, J., & Miranda, E. (2000). Relationship between sex differences in onset of schizophrenia and puberty. *J Psychiatr Res*, **34**, 349–53.

Rümke, H.C. (1941). Das Kernsyndrom der Schizophrenie und das 'Praecox Gefühl'. *Zentrabl ges Neurol Psychiat*, **102**, 168–69.

Rüsch, N., Schulz, D., Valerius, G., et al. (2011). Disgust and implicit self-concept in women with borderline personality disorder and posttraumatic stress disorder. *Eur Arch Psychiatry Clin Neurosci*, **261**, 369–76.

Russell, J., Mauthner, N., Sharpe, S., & Tidswell, T. (1991). The windows task as a measure of strategic deception in preschoolers and autistic subjects. *Br J Dev Psychol*, **9**, 331–49.

Russo, S.J., Murrough, J.W., Han, M.H., Charney, D.S., & Nestler, E.J. (2012). Neurobiology of resilience. *Nat Neurosci*, **15**, 1475–84.

Rust, J. & Smith, A. (2006). How should the effectiveness of Social Stories to modify the behaviour of children on the autistic spectrum be tested? Lessons from the literature. *Autism*, **10**, 125–38.

Rutberg, A.T. (1983). The evolution of monogamy in primates. *J Theoret Biol*, **104**, 93–112.

Ryan, T.J. & Grant, S.G. (2009). The origin and evolution of synapses. *Nat Rev Neurosci*, **10**, 701–12.

Saah, T. (2005). The evolutionary origins and significance of drug addiction. *Harm Reduct J*, **2**, 8.

Sadeh, A., Rubin, S.S., & Berman, E. (1993). Parental and relationship representations and experiences of depression in college students. *J Pers Assess*, **60**, 192–204.

Sagvolden, T., Johansen, E.B., Aase, H., & Russell, V.A. (2005). A dynamic developmental theory of attention-deficit/hyperactivity disorder (ADHD) predominantly hyperactive/impulsive and combined subtypes. *Behav Brain Sci*, **28**, 397–419; discussion 419–68.

Saha, S., Chant, D.C., Welham, J.L., & McGrath, J.J. (2006). The incidence and prevalence of schizophrenia varies with latitude. *Acta Psychiatr Scand*, **114**, 36–39.

Saint-Cyr, J.A., Taylor, A.E., & Nicholson, K. (1995). Behavior and the basal ganglia. In: Weiner, W.J. & Lang, A.E. (eds) *Behavioral Neurology of Movement Disorders. Advances in Neurology*. Raven Press, New York.

Sally, D. & Hill, E. (2006). The development of interpersonal strategy: autism, theory-of-mind, cooperation and fairness. *J Econ Psychol*, **27**, 73–97.

Salvatore, G., Dimaggio, G., & Lysaker, P.H. (2007). An intersubjective perspective on negative symptoms of schizophrenia: implications of simulation theory. *Cogn Neuropsychiatry*, **12**, 144–64.

Samuel, D.B. & Gore, W.L. (2012). Maladaptive variants of conscientiousness and agreeableness. *J Pers*, **80**, 1669–96.

San Jose, C., Braza, F., & Casanova, X. (1997). Reproductive status of mothers affects sex-biased parental investment in humans. *Percept Mot Skills*, **85**, 917–18.

Sanchez, M.M., Alagbe, O., Felger, J.C., et al. (2007). Activated p38 MAPK is associated with decreased CSF 5-HIAA and increased maternal rejection during infancy in rhesus monkeys. *Mol Psychiatry*, **12**, 895–97.

Sanders, A.R., Duan, J., Levinson, D.F., et al. (2008). No significant association of 14 candidate genes with schizophrenia in a large European ancestry sample: Implications for psychiatric genetics. *Am J Psychiatry*, **165**, 497–506.

Sanfey, A.G. (2007). Social decision-making: insights from game theory and neuroscience. *Science*, **318**, 598–602.

Sanfey, A.G., Rilling, J.K., Aronson, J.A., Nystrom, L.E., & Cohen, J.D. (2003). The neural basis of economic decision-making in the Ultimatum Game. *Science*, **300**, 1755–58.

Sanjuan, J. (1999). Evolutionary theories of schizophrenia. *Actas Esp Psiquiatr*, **27**, 390–97.

Sanjuan, J., Tolosa, A., Gonzalez, J.C., et al. (2006). Association between FOXP2 polymorphisms and schizophrenia with auditory hallucinations. *Psychiatr Genet*, **16**, 67–72.

Sansone, R.A. & Sansone, L.A. (2007). Childhood trauma, borderline personality, and eating disorders: a developmental cascade. *Eat Disord*, **15**, 333–46.

Santillo, A.F., Nilsson, C., & Englund, E. (2013). Von Economo neurones are selectively targeted in frontotemporal dementia. *Neuropathol Appl Neurobiol*, **39**, 572–79.

Santos, M., Uppal, N., Butti, C., Wicinski, B., Schmeidler, J., Giannakopoulos, P., Heinsen, H., Schmitz, C., & Hof, PR. (2011). Von Economo neurons in autism: a stereologic study of the frontoinsular cortex in children. *Brain Res*, **1380**, 206–17.

Sapolsky, R.M. & Finch, C.E. (2000). Alzheimer's disease and some speculations about the evolution of its modifiers. *Ann N Y Acad Sci*, **924**, 99–103.

Sapolsky, R.M., Romero, L.M., & Munck, A.U. (2000). How do glucocorticoids influence stress responses? Integrating permissive, suppressive, stimulatory, and preparative actions. *Endocr Rev*, **21**, 55–89.

Sar, V., Akyuz, G., Kundakci, T., Kiziltan, E., & Dogan, O. (2004). Childhood trauma, dissociation, and psychiatric comorbidity in patients with conversion disorder. *Am J Psychiatry*, **161**, 2271–76.

Sarfati, Y. & Hardy-Bayle, M.C. (1999). How do people with schizophrenia explain the behaviour of others? A study of theory of mind and its relationship to thought and speech disorganization in schizophrenia. *Psychol Med*, **29**, 613–20.

Saugstad, L.F. (1989). Age at puberty and mental illness. Towards a neurodevelopmental aetiology of Kraepelin's endogenous psychoses. *Br J Psychiatry*, **155**, 536–44.

Saugstad, L.F. (1998). Cerebral lateralisation and rate of maturation. *Int J Psychophysiol*, **28**, 37–62.

Saugstad, L.F. (1999). A lack of cerebral lateralization in schizophrenia is within the normal variation in brain maturation but indicates late, slow maturation. *Schizophr Res*, **39**, 183–96.

Savitz, J.B., Van Der Merwe, L., Newman, T.K., et al. (2008). The relationship between childhood abuse and dissociation. Is it influenced by catechol-O-methyltransferase (COMT) activity? *Int J Neuropsychopharmacol*, **11**, 149–61.

Saxe, R. (2006). Uniquely human social cognition. *Curr Opin Neurobiol*, **16**, 235–39.

Saxe, R. & Kanwisher, N. (2003). People thinking about thinking people. The role of the temporo-parietal junction in 'theory of mind'. *Neuroimage*, **19**, 1835–42.

Saxe, R., Carey, S., & Kanwisher, N. (2004). Understanding other minds: linking developmental psychology and functional neuroimaging. *Annu Rev Psychol*, **55**, 87–124.

Saxena, S. & Rauch, S.L. (2000). Functional neuroimaging and the neuroanatomy of obsessive-compulsive disorder. *Psychiatr Clin N Am*, **23**, 563–86.

Saxena, S., Brody, A.L., Maidment, K.M., et al. (1999). Localized orbitofrontal and subcortical metabolic changes and predictors of response to paroxetine treatment in obsessive-compulsive disorder. *Neuropsychopharmacology*, **21**, 683–93.

Scahill, L. & Schwab-Stone, M. (2000). Epidemiology of ADHD in school-age children. *Child Adolesc Psychiatr Clin N Am*, **9**, 541–55, vii.

Schaffner, K.F. (2001). Nature and nurture. *Curr Opin Psychiatry*, **14**, 485–90.

Schelde, J.T.M. (1998). Major depression: behavioral markers of depression and recovery. *J Nerv Ment Dis*, **186**, 133–40.

Schelde, J.T.M. (2000). Schizophrenic, depressed, and nonpsychiatric medical patients—an ethologically based comparison. *J Nerv Ment Dis*, **188**, 377–80.

Schelde, J.T., Pedersen, J., Hannibal, E., et al. (1988). An ethological analysis of depression: comparison between ethological recording and Hamilton rating of five endogenously depressed patients. *Acta Psychiatr Scand*, **78**, 331–40.

Schelde, T. (1994). Ethological research in psychiatry. *Ethol Sociobiol*, **15**, 349–68.

Schelde, T. & Hertz, M. (1994). Ethology and psychotherapy. *Ethol Sociobiol*, **15**, 383–92.

Schellenberg, G.D., Dawson, G., Sung, Y.J., et al. (2006). Evidence for multiple loci from a genome scan of autism kindreds. *Mol Psychiatry*, **11**, 1049–60

Scheres, A. & Sanfey, A.G. (2006). Individual differences in decision making: drive and reward responsiveness affect strategic bargaining in economic games. *Behav Brain Funct*, **2**, 35.

Schiefenhövel, W. (1986). Extraktionszauber. Domäne der Heilkundigen. *Curare*, S5, 353–72.

Schiefenhövel, W. (1994). Trust—an ethological and etymological view. In: Hof, H., Kummer, H., & Weingart, P. (eds) *Recht und Verhalten. Verhaltensgrundlagen des Rechts—zum Beispiel Vertrauen*. Nomos, Baden-Baden, pp. 225–33.

Schiefenhövel, W. (1995). Perception, expression, and social function of pain: a human ethological view. *Sci Context*, **8**, 31–46.

Schiefenhövel, W. (2000). Suffering without meaning? Illness, pain and death. Development of evolutionary medicine. *Gesundheitswesen*, **62**, S3–8.

Schiefenhövel, W. (2002). Evolutionary and transcultural perspectives in psychiatry. Grief and depression. *Nervenheilkunde*, **21**, 119–26.

Schiltz, K., Witzel, J., Northoff, G., et al. (2007). Brain pathology in pedophilic offenders: evidence of volume reduction in the right amygdala and related diencephalic structures. *Arch Gen Psychiatry*, **64**, 737–46.

Schizophrenia Working Group of the Psychiatric Genomics Consortium (2014). Biological insights from 108 schizophrenia-associated genetic loci. *Nature*, **511**, 421–27.

Schlesinger, D., Grinberg, L.T., Alba, J.G., et al. (2013). African ancestry protects against Alzheimer's disease-related neuropathology. *Mol Psychiatry*, **18**, 79–85.

Schmahmann, J.D., Weilburg, J.B., & Sherman, J.C. (2007). The neuropsychiatry of the cerebellum—insights from the clinic. *Cerebellum*, **6**, 254–67.

Schmidt, K.L. & Cohn, J.F. (2001). Human facial expressions as adaptations: evolutionary questions in facial expression research. *Am J Phys Anthropol*, **2001** (Suppl 33), 3–24.

Schmitt, D.P. & Buss, D.M. (2001). Human mate poaching: tactics and tempations for infiltrating existing mateships. *J Pers Soc Psychol*, **80**, 894–917.

Schmitt, D.P., Alcalay, L., Allik, J., et al. (2004). Patterns and universals of mate poaching across 53 nations: the effects of sex, culture, and personality on romantically attracting another person's partner. *J Pers Soc Psychol*, **86**, 560–84.

Schneider, B., Wetterling, T., Sargk, D., et al. (2006). Axis I disorders and personality disorders as risk factors for suicide. *Eur Arch Psychiatry Clin Neurosci*, **256**, 17–27.

Scholl, B.J. & Leslie, A.M. (1999). Modularity, development and 'theory of mind'. *Mind Lang*, **14**, 131–53.

Schore, A.N. (2002). Dysregulation of the right brain: a fundamental mechanism of traumatic attachment and the psychopathogenesis of posttraumatic stress disorder. *Aust N Z J Psychiatry*, **36**, 9–30.

Schuiling, G.A. (2000). Pre-eclampsia: a parent-offspring conflict. *J Psychosom Obstet Gynaecol*, **21**, 179–82.

Schultz, W., Tremblay, L., & Hollerman, J.R. (2000). Reward processing in primate orbitofrontal cortex and basal ganglia. *Cereb Cortex*, **10**, 272–84.

Schwartz, B.L. & Evans, S. (2001). Episodic memory in primates. *Am J Primatol*, **55**, 71–85.

Seamans, J.K. & Yang, C.R. (2004). The principal features and mechanisms of dopamine modulation in the prefrontal cortex. *Prog Neurobiol*, **74**, 1–58.

Sebastiani, P., Sun, F.X., Andersen, S.L., et al. (2013). Families enriched for exceptional longevity also have increased health-span: findings from the long life family study. *Front Public Health*, **1**, 38.

Sedler, M.J. (1985). The legacy of Ewald Hecker—a new translation of 'Die Hebephrenie'. *Am J Psychiatry*, **142**, 1265–71.

Seedat, S., Stein, D.J., & Carey, P.D. (2005). Post-traumatic stress disorder in women: epidemiological and treatment issues. *CNS Drugs*, **19**, 411–27.

Seeger, G., Schloss, P., Schmidt, M.H., Ruter-Jungfleisch, A., & Henn, F.A. (2004). Gene–environment interaction in hyperkinetic conduct disorder (HD + CD) as indicated by season of birth variations in dopamine receptor (DRD4) gene polymorphism. *Neurosci Lett*, **366**, 282–86.

Seeman, M.V. (2011). Antipsychotics and physical attractiveness. *Clin Schizophr Relat Psychoses*, **5**, 142–46.

Segal, N.L. & Bouchard, T.J., Jr (1993). Grief intensity following the loss of a twin and other relatives: test of kinship genetic hypotheses. *Hum Biol*, **65**, 87–105.

Segalowitz, S.J. & Davies, P.L. (2004). Charting the maturation of the frontal lobe: an electrophysiological strategy. *Brain Cogn*, **55**, 116–33.

Sei, Y., Ren-Patterson, R., Li, Z., et al. (2007). Neuregulin1-induced cell migration is impaired in schizophrenia: association with neuregulin1 and catechol-o-methyltransferase gene polymorphisms. *Mol Psychiatry*, **12**, 946–57.

Seiferth, N.Y., Pauly, K., Kellermann, T., et al. (2009). Neuronal correlates of facial emotion discrimination in early onset schizophrenia. *Neuropsychopharmacology*, **34**, 477–87.

Selten, J.P. & Cantor-Graae, E. (2005). Social defeat: risk factor for schizophrenia? *Br J Psychiatry*, **187**, 101–102.

Semendeferi, K. & Damasio, H. (2000). The brain and its main anatomical subdivisions in living hominoids using magnetic resonance imaging. *J Hum Evol*, **38**, 317–32.

Semendeferi, K., Damasio, H., Frank, R., & Van Hoesen, G.W. (1997). The evolution of the frontal lobes: a volumetric analysis based on three-dimensional reconstructions of magnetic resonance scans of human and ape brains. *J Hum Evol*, **32**, 375–88.

Semendeferi, K., Armstrong, E., Schleicher, A., Zilles, K., & Van Hoesen, G.W. (1998). Limbic frontal cortex in hominoids: a comparative study of area 13. *Am J Phys Anthropol*, **106**, 129–55.

Semendeferi, K., Armstrong, E., Schleicher, A., Zilles, K., & Van Hoesen, G.W. (2001). Prefrontal cortex in humans and apes: a comparative study of area 10. *Am J Phys Anthropol*, **114**, 224–41.

Semendeferi, K., Lu, A., Schenker, N., & Damasio, H. (2002). Humans and great apes share a large frontal cortex. *Nat Neurosci*, **5**, 272–76.

Sen, S., Burmeister, M., & Ghosh, D. (2004). Meta-analysis of the association between a serotonin transporter promoter polymorphism (5-HTTLPR) and anxiety-related personality traits. *Am J Med Genet B Neuropsychiatr Genet*, 127B, 85–89.

Sergi, M.J., Rassovsky, Y., Nuechterlein, K.H., & Green, M.F. (2006). Social perception as a mediator of the influence of early visual processing on functional status in schizophrenia. *Am J Psychiatry*, **163**, 448–54.

Sery, O., Didden, W., Mikes, V., et al. (2006). The association between high-activity COMT allele and alcoholism. *Neuro Endocrinol Lett*, **27**, 231–35.

Seymour, B., Singer, T., & Dolan, R. (2007). The neurobiology of punishment. *Nat Rev Neurosci*, **8**, 300–11.

Shachnow, J., Clarkin, J., Dipalma, C.S., et al. (1997). Biparental psychopathology and borderline personality disorder. *Psychiatry*, **60**, 171–81.

Shackelford, T.K. (2003). Preventing, correcting, and anticipating female infidelity. *Evol Cogn*, **9**, 90–96.

Shackelford, T.K. & Buss, D.M. (1997). Cues to infidelity. *Pers Soc Psychol Bull*, **23**, 1034–45.

Shackelford, T.K., Leblanc, G.J., Weekes-Shackelford, V.A., et al. (2002). Psychological adaptation to human sperm competition. *Evol Hum Behav*, **23**, 123–38.

Shahar, G. (2001). Maternal personality and distress as predictors of child neglect. *J Res Pers*, **35**, 537–45.

Sham, P. & McGuffin, P. (2005). Linkage and association. In: McGuffin, P., Owen, M.J., & Gottesman, I.I. (eds) *Psychiatric Genetics and Genomics*. Oxford University Press, Oxford.

Shamay-Tsoory, S.G., Abu-Akel, A., Palgi, S., et al. (2013). Giving peace a chance: oxytocin increases empathy to pain in the context of the Israeli–Palestinian conflict. *Psychoneuroendocrinology*, **38**, 3139–44.

Shaner, A., Miller, G., & Mintz, J. (2004). Schizophrenia as one extreme of a sexually selected fitness indicator. *Schizophr Res*, **70**, 101–109.

Shaner, A., Miller, G., & Mintz, J. (2007). Evidence of a latitudinal gradient in the age at onset of schizophrenia. *Schizophr Res*, **94**, 58–63.

Shaner, A., Miller, G., & Mintz, J. (2008a). Mental disorders as catastrophic failures of mating intelligence. In: Geher, G. & Miller, G. (eds) *Mating Intelligence. Sex, Relationships, and the Mind's Reproductive System*. Lawrence Erlbaum, Hillsdale.

Shaner, A., Miller, G., & Mintz, J. (2008b). Autism as the low-fitness extreme of a parentally selected fitness indicator. *Hum Nat*, **19**, 389–413.

Sharma, B.R. (2007). Sudden infant death syndrome: a subject of medicolegal research. *Am J Forensic Med Pathol*, **28**, 69–72.

Sharma, M.P. & Manjula, M. (2013). Behavioural and psychological management of somatic symptom disorders: an overview. *Int Rev Psychiatry*, **25**, 116–24.

Shaver, P.R. & Mikulincer, M. (2005). Attachment theory and research: resurrection of the psychodynamic approach to personality. *J Res Pers*, **39**, 22–45.

Sheets, V.L., Fredendall, L.L., & Claypool, H.M. (1997). Jealousy evocation, partner reassurance, and relationship stability: An exploration of the potential benefits of jealousy. *Evol Hum Behav*, **18**, 387–402.

Shelley-Tremblay, J.F. & Rosen, L.A. (1996). Attention deficit hyperactivity disorder: an evolutionary perspective. *J Genet Psychol*, **157**, 443–53.

Sheppard, B., Chavira, D., Azzam, A., et al. (2010). ADHD prevalence and association with hoarding behaviors in childhood-onset OCD. *Depress Anxiety*, **27**, 667–74.

Shiloh, R., Schwartz, B., Weizman, A., & Radwan, M. (1995). Catatonia as an unusual presentation of posttraumatic stress disorder. *Psychopathology*, **28**, 285–90.

Shin, L.M., Wright, C.I., Cannistraro, P.A., et al. (2005). A functional magnetic resonance imaging study of amygdala and medial prefrontal cortex responses to overtly presented fearful faces in posttraumatic stress disorder. *Arch Gen Psychiatry*, **62**, 273–81.

Shohov, S.P. (ed.) (2003). *Advances in Psychology Research*. Nova Science, New York.

Shoji, M., Kawarabayashi, T., Harigaya, Y., et al. (1990). Alzheimer amyloid beta-protein precursor in sperm development. *Am J Pathol*, **137**, 1027–32.

Siebner, H.R., Willoch, F., Peller, M., et al. (1998). Imaging brain activation induced by long trains of repetitive transcranial magnetic stimulation. *Neuroreport*, **9**, 943–48.

Siegal, M. & Varley, R. (2002). Neural systems involved in 'theory of mind'. *Nat Rev Neurosci*, **3**, 463–71.

Simhandl, C., Konig, B., & Amann, B.L. (2014). A prospective 4-year naturalistic follow-up of treatment and outcome of 300 bipolar I and II patients. *J Clin Psychiatry*, **75**, 254–62; quiz 263.

Simon, A.E., Cattapan-Ludewig, K., Zmilacher, S., et al. (2007). Cognitive functioning in the schizophrenia prodrome. *Schizophr Bull*, **33**, 761–71.

Simon, R.I. & Gold, L.H. (2010). *The American Psychiatric Publishing Textbook of Forensic Psychiatry*. American Psychiatric Publishing, Arlington.

Simpson, J.A. (1999). Attachment theory in modern evolutionary perspectives. In: Cassidy, J. & Shaver, P.R. (eds) *Handbook of Attachment. Theory, Research, and Clinical Applications*. Guilford Press, New York.

Singer, T., Seymour, B., O'Doherty, J., et al. (2004). Empathy for pain involves the affective but not sensory components of pain. *Science*, **303**, 1157–62.

Singer, T., Seymour, B., O'Doherty, J.P., et al. (2006). Empathic neural responses are modulated by the perceived fairness of others. *Nature*, **439**, 466–69.

Skodol, A.E. & Bender, D.S. (2003). Why are women diagnosed borderline more than men? *Psychiatr Q*, **74**, 349–60.

Skuse, D.H. (2000). Imprinting, the X-chromosome, and the male brain: explaining sex differences in the liability to autism. *Pediatr Res*, **47**, 9–16.

Skuse, D.H., James, R.S., Bishop, D.V., et al. (1997). Evidence from Turner's syndrome of an imprinted X-linked locus affecting cognitive function. *Nature*, **387**, 705–708.

Slap, G., Goodman, E., & Huang, B. (2001). Adoption as a risk factor for attempted suicide during adolescence. *Pediatrics*, **108**, E30.

Sloman, L. (2008). A new comprehensive evolutionary model of depression and anxiety. *J Affect Disord*, **106**, 219–28.

Smith, J.M. (2000). *The Units of Selection*. Novartis Foundation Symposium, Basel.

Snitz, B.E., Macdonald, A., 3rd, Cohen, J.D., et al. (2005). Lateral and medial hypofrontality in first-episode schizophrenia: functional activity in a medication-naive state and effects of short-term atypical antipsychotic treatment. *Am J Psychiatry*, **162**, 2322–29.

Snowden, J.S., Neary, D., & Mann, D.M. (2002). Frontotemporal dementia. *Br J Psychiatry*, **180**, 140–43.

Snyder, A.W. & Thomas, M. (1997). Autistic artists give clues to cognition. *Perception*, **26**, 93–96.

Soares, J.C., Kochunov, P., Monkul, E.S., et al. (2005). Structural brain changes in bipolar disorder using deformation field morphometry. *Neuroreport*, **16**, 541–44.

Solantaus-Simula, T., Punamaki, R.L., & Beardslee, W.R. (2002). Children's responses to low parental mood. I: Balancing between active empathy, overinvolvement, indifference, and avoidance. *J Am Acad Child Adolesc Psychiatry*, **41**, 278–86.

Solnick, S.J. (2001). Gender differences in the ultimatum game. *Econ Inq*, **39**, 189–200.

Somashekar, B., Jainer, A., & Wuntakal, B. (2013). Psychopharmacotherapy of somatic symptoms disorders. *Int Rev Psychiatry*, **25**, 107–15.

Somel, M., Liu, X.L., & Khaitovich, P. (2013). Human brain evolution: transcripts, metabolites and their regulators. *Nat Rev Neurosci*, **14**, 112–27.

Sommer, M., Hajak, G., Dohnel, K., et al. (2006). Integration of emotion and cognition in patients with psychopathy. *Prog Brain Res*, **156**, 457–66.

Sourander, A., Klomek, A.B., Niemela, S., et al. (2009). Childhood predictors of completed and severe suicide attempts: findings from the Finnish 1981 Birth Cohort Study. *Arch Gen Psychiatry*, **66**, 398–406.

Spauwen, J., Krabbendam, L., Lieb, R., Wittchen, H.U., & Van Os, J. (2004). Early maternal stress and health behaviours and offspring expression of psychosis in adolescence. *Acta Psychiatr Scand*, **110**, 356–64.

Spencer-Booth, Y. & Hinde, R.A. (1971). Effects of brief separations from mothers during infancy on behaviour of rhesus monkeys 6–24 months later. *J Child Psychol Psychiatry*, **12**, 157–72.

Sperber, D. & Wilson, D. (2002). Pragmatics, modularity and mind-reading. *Mind Lang*, **17**, 3–23.

Spinelli, M.G. (2004). Maternal infanticide associated with mental illness: prevention and the promise of saved lives. *Am J Psychiatry*, **161**, 1548–57.

Spitz, R.A. (1945). Hospitalism. An inquiry into the genesis of psychiatric conditions in early childhood. In: Eissler, R. (ed.) *The Psychoanalytic Study of the Child*. International Universities Press, New York.

Spitzer, M., Fischbacher, U., Herrnberger, B., Gron, G., & Fehr, E. (2007). The neural signature of social norm compliance. *Neuron*, **56**, 185–96. Spitzer, R.L. & Wakefield, J.C. (1999). DSM-IV diagnostic criterion for clinical significance: does it help solve the false positives problem? *Am J Psychiatry*, **156**, 1856–64.

Spitzer, R.L. (1999). Harmful dysfunction and the DSM definition of mental disorder. *J Abnorm Psychol*, **108**, 430–32.

Sprock, J., Blashfield, R.K., & Smith, B. (1990). Gender weighting of DSM-III-R personality disorder criteria. *Am J Psychiatry*, **147**, 586–90.

Squire, L.R. & Kandel, E.R. (1999). *Memory: From Mind to Molecules*. Scientific American Library, New York.

St John-Smith, P., McQueen, D., Edwards, L., & Schifano, F. (2013). Classical and novel psychoactive substances: rethinking drug misuse from an evolutionary psychiatric perspective. *Hum Psychopharmacol*, **28**, 394–401.

Stadtland, C. & Nedopil, N. (2005). Psychiatric disorders and the prognosis for criminal recidivism. *Nervenarzt*, **76**, 1402–11.

Stahl, S.M. (2000). *Essential Psychopharmacology: Neuroscientific Basis and Practical Application*. Cambridge University Press, Cambridge.

Stearns, S.C. (1992). *The Evolution of Life Histories*. Oxford University Press, Oxford.

Stearns, S.C., Byars, S.G., Govindaraju, D.R., & Ewbank, D. (2010a). Measuring selection in contemporary human populations. *Nat Rev Genet*, **11**, 611–22.

Stearns, S.C., Nesse, R.M., Govindaraju, D.R., & Ellison, P.T. (2010b). Evolution in health and medicine Sackler colloquium: Evolutionary perspectives on health and medicine. *Proc Natl Acad Sci USA*, **107** (Suppl 1), 1691–95.

Stefan, M.D. & Murray, R.M. (1997). Schizophrenia: developmental disturbance of brain and mind? *Acta Paediatr Suppl*, **422**, 112–16.

Stein, D.J. & Bouwer, C. (1997). A neuro-evolutionary approach to the anxiety disorders. *J Anxiety Disord*, **11**, 409–29.

Stein, D.J. & Muller, J. (2008). Cognitive-affective neuroscience of somatization disorder and functional somatic syndromes: reconceptualizing the triad of depression-anxiety-somatic symptoms. *CNS Spectr*, **13**, 379–84.

Stein, D.J., Ono, Y., Tajima, O., & Muller, J.E. (2004). The social anxiety disorder spectrum. *J Clin Psychiatry*, **65** (Suppl 14), 27–33; quiz 34–36.

Stein, D.J., Lund, C., & Nesse, R.M. (2013). Classification systems in psychiatry: diagnosis and global mental health in the era of DSM-5 and ICD-11. *Curr Opin Psychiatry*, **26**, 493–97.

Stein, M.B. (2011). Psychiatry: a molecular shield from trauma. *Nature*, **470**, 468–69.

Stein, M.B., Schork, N.J., & Gelernter, J. (2008). Gene-by-environment (serotonin transporter and childhood maltreatment) interaction for anxiety sensitivity, an intermediate phenotype for anxiety disorders. *Neuropsychopharmacology*, **33**, 312–19.

Steinert, C., Hofmann, M., Kruse, J., & Leichsenring, F. (2014). Relapse rates after psychotherapy for depression—stable long-term effects? A meta-analysis. *J Affect Disord*, **168**, 107–18.

Stepp, S.D., Whalen, D.J., Pilkonis, P.A., Hipwell, A.E., & Levine, M.D. (2012). Children of mothers with borderline personality disorder: identifying parenting behaviors as potential targets for intervention. *Personal Disord*, **3**, 76–91.

Stevens, A. (2000). Jungian analysis and evolutionary psychotherapy: an integrative approach. In: Gilbert, P. & Bailey, K.G. (eds) *Genes on the Couch. Explorations in Evolutionary Psychotherapy*. Brunner-Routledge, Hove.

Stevens, A. & Price, J. (1996). *Evolutionary Psychiatry. A New Beginning*. Routledge, New York.

Stevenson, J.C. & Williams, D.C. (2000). Parental investment, self-control, and sex differences in the expression of ADHD. *Hum Nat Interdisc Biosoc Persp*, **11**, 405–22.

Stoffers, J.M., Vollm, B.A., Rucker, G., et al. (2012). Psychological therapies for people with borderline personality disorder. *Cochrane Database Syst Rev*, **8**, CD005652.

Stone, M.H. (2006). Management of borderline personality disorder: a review of psychotherapeutic approaches. *World Psychiatry*, **5**, 15–20.

Stone, M.H., Steinmeyer, E., Dreher, J., & Krischer, M. (2005). Infanticide in female forensic patients: the view from the evolutionary standpoint. *J Psychiatr Pract*, **11**, 35–45.

Stoppel, C., Bielau, H., Bogerts, B., & Northoff, G. (2006). Neurobiological basis of depressive disorders. *Fortschr Neurol Psychiatr*, **74**, 696–705.

Stotland, N.L. (2011). Psychiatric aspects of induced abortion. *J Nerv Ment Dis*, **199**, 568–70.

Strickland, P.L., Deakin, J.F., Percival, C., et al. (2002). Bio-social origins of depression in the community. Interactions between social adversity, cortisol and serotonin neurotransmission. *Br J Psychiatry*, **180**, 168–73.

Ströhle, A., Stoy, M., Wrase, J., et al. (2008). Reward anticipation and outcomes in adult males with attention-deficit/hyperactivity disorder. *Neuroimage*, **39**, 966–72.

Suddendorf, T. (2013). *The Gap: The Science of What Separates us from Other Animals*. Basic Books, New York.

Suddendorf, T. & Corballis, M.C. (1997). Mental time travel and the evolution of the human mind. *Genet Soc Gen Psychol Monogr*, **123**, 133–67.

Suddendorf, T. & Corballis, M.C. (2007). The evolution of foresight: what is mental time travel, and is it unique to humans? *Behav Brain Sci*, **30**, 299–313; discussion 313–51.

Suddendorf, T. & Whiten, A. (2001). Mental evolution and development: evidence for secondary representation in children, great ages, and other animals. *Psychol Bull*, **127**, 629–50.

Sugiyama, L.S., Tooby, J., & Cosmides, L. (2002). Cross-cultural evidence of cognitive adaptations for social exchange among the Shiwiar of Ecuadorian Amazonia. *Proc Natl Acad Sci USA*, **99**, 11537–42.

Sullivan, R.J. & Hagen, E.H. (2002). Psychotropic substance-seeking: evolutionary pathology or adaptation? *Addiction*, **97**, 389–400.

Sullivan, R.J., Hagen, E.H., & Hammerstein, P. (2008). Revealing the paradox of drug reward in human evolution. *Proc Biol Sci*, **275**, 1231–41.

Sulloway, F.J. (1986). Freud and biology: the hidden legacy. *Acta Psychiatr Belg*, **86**, 760–88.

Summers, C.H. & Winberg, S. (2006). Interactions between the neural regulation of stress and aggression. *J Exp Biol*, **209**, 4581–89.

Suomi, S.J. (2003). Gene–environment interactions and the neurobiology of social conflict. *Ann N Y Acad Sci*, **1008**, 132–39.

Suomi, S.J. (2006). Risk, resilience, and gene × environment interactions in rhesus monkeys. *Annal N Y Acad Sci*, **1094**, 52–62.

Surbey, M.K. (1998). Parent and offspring strategies in the transition at adolescence. *Hum Nat Interdiscip Biosoc Persp*, **9**, 67–94.

Swain, J.E., Tasgin, E., Mayes, L.C., et al. (2008). Maternal brain response to own baby-cry is affected by cesarean section delivery. *J Child Psychol Psychiatry*, **49**, 1042–52.

Swartz, J.R., Miller, B.L., Lesser, I.M., et al. (1997). Behavioral phenomenology in Alzheimer's disease, frontotemporal dementia, and late-life depression: a retrospective analysis. *J Geriatr Psychiatry Neurol*, **10**, 67–74.

Swedo, S.E., Rapoport, J.L., Cheslow, D.L., et al. (1989a). High prevalence of obsessive-compulsive symptoms in patients with Sydenham's chorea. *Am J Psychiatry*, **146**, 246–49.

Swedo, S.E., Rapoport, J.L., Leonard, H., Lenane, M., & Cheslow, D. (1989b). Obsessive-compulsive disorder in children and adolescents. Clinical phenomenology of 70 consecutive cases. *Arch Gen Psychiatry*, **46**, 335–41.

Symons, D. (1979). *The Evolution of Human Sexuality*. Oxford University Press, New York.

Synofzik, M., Vosgerau, G., & Newen, A. (2008). Beyond the comparator model: a multifactorial two-step account of agency. *Conscious Cogn*, **17**, 219–39.

Szechtman, H., Sulis, W., & Eilam, D. (1998). Quinpirole induces compulsive checking behavior in rats: a potential animal model of obsessive-compulsive disorder (OCD). *Behav Neurosci*, **112**, 1475–85.

Szuchmann, L.T. & Muscarella, F. (eds) (2000). *Psychological Perspectives on Human Sexuality*. John Wiley, New York.

Tabibnia, G., Satpute, A.B., & Lieberman, M.D. (2008). The sunny side of fairness: preference for fairness activates reward circuitry (and disregarding unfairness activates self-control circuitry). *Psychol Sci*, **19**, 339–47.

Talge, N.M., Neal, C., & Glover, V. (2007). Antenatal maternal stress and long-term effects on child neurodevelopment: how and why? *J Child Psychol Psychiatry*, **48**, 245–61.

Tancredi, L.R. & Volkow, N.D. (1992). A theory of the mind/brain dichotomy with special reference to the contribution of positron emission tomography. *Perspect Biol Med*, **35**, 549–71.

Tandon, K. & McGuffin, P. (2002). The genetic basis for psychiatric illness in man. *Eur J Neurosci*, **16**, 403–407.

Tautz, D. & Domazet-Loso, T. (2011). The evolutionary origin of orphan genes. *Nat Rev Genet*, **12**, 692–702.

Taylor, P.A. & Glenn, N.D. (1976). Utility of education and attractiveness for females status attainment through marriage. *Am Sociolog Rev*, **41**, 484–98.

Taylor, P.J., Gooding, P.A., Wood, A.M., et al. (2010). Defeat and entrapment in schizophrenia: the relationship with suicidal ideation and positive psychotic symptoms. *Psychiatry Res*, **178**, 244–48.

Taylor, P.J., Gooding, P., Wood, A.M., & Tarrier, N. (2011). The role of defeat and entrapment in depression, anxiety, and suicide. *Psychol Bull*, **137**, 391–420.

Taylor, S.E., Way, B.M., Welch, W.T., et al. (2006). Early family environment, current adversity, the serotonin transporter promoter polymorphism, and depressive symptomatology. *Biol Psychiatry*, **60**, 671–76.

Teicher, M.H., Andersen, S.L., Polcari, A., et al. (2003). The neurobiological consequences of early stress and childhood maltreatment. *Neurosci Biobehav Rev*, **27**, 33–44.

Teicher, M.H., Anderson, C.M., & Polcari, A. (2012). Childhood maltreatment is associated with reduced volume in the hippocampal subfields CA3, dentate gyrus, and subiculum. *Proc Natl Acad Sci USA*, **109**, E563–72.

Temrin, H., Buchmayer, S., & Enquist, M. (2000). Step-parents and infanticide: new data contradict evolutionary predictions. *Proc Biol Sci*, **267**, 943–45.

Thapar, A. & Scourfield, J. (2005). Childhood disorders. In: McGuffin, P., Owen, M.J., & Gottesman, I.I. (eds) *Psychiatric Genetics and Genomics*. Oxford University Press, Oxford.

Thapar, A., Langley, K., Asherson, P., & Gill, M. (2007). Gene–environment interplay in attention-deficit hyperactivity disorder and the importance of a developmental perspective. *Br J Psychiatry*, **190**, 1–3.

Thierry, B., Mewa, S., & Kaumanns, W. (2004). *Macaque Societies: A Model for the Study of Social Organization*. Cambridge University Press, Cambridge.

Thoeringer, C.K., Binder, E.B., Salyakina, D., et al. (2007). Association of a Met88Val diazepam binding inhibitor (DBI) gene polymorphism and anxiety disorders with panic attacks. *J Psychiatr Res*, **41**, 579–84.

Thornhill, R. & Palmer, C.T. (2000). *A Natural History of Rape: Biological Bases of Sexual Coercion*. MIT Press, Cambridge, Massachusetts.

Thornton, D. (2006). Age and sexual recidivism: a variable connection. *Sex Abuse*, **18**, 123–35.

Tienari, P., Lahti, I., Sorri, A., et al. (1987). The Finnish adoptive family study of schizophrenia. *J Psychiatr Res*, **21**, 437–45.

Tienari, P., Wynne, L.C., Moring, J., et al. (2000). Finnish adoptive family study: sample selection and adoptee DSM-III-R diagnoses. *Acta Psychiatr Scand*, **101**, 433–43.

Tienari, P., Wynne, L.C., Laksy, K., et al. (2003). Genetic boundaries of the schizophrenia spectrum: evidence from the Finnish Adoptive Family Study of Schizophrenia. *Am J Psychiatry*, **160**, 1587–94.

Tienari, P., Wynne, L.C., Sorri, A., et al. (2004). Genotype–environment interaction in schizophrenia-spectrum disorder. Long-term follow-up study of Finnish adoptees. *Br J Psychiatry*, **184**, 216–22.

Tignol, J., Martin-Guehl, C., Aouizerate, B., Grabot, D., & Auriacombe, M. (2006). Social phobia and premature ejaculation: a case-control study. *Depress Anxiety*, **23**, 153–57.

Timpe, K. (2006). *Free Will*. Internet Encyclopedia of Philosophy, <http://www.iep.utm.edu>.

Tinbergen, N. (1952). Derived activities; their causation, biological significance, origin, and emancipation during evolution. *Q Rev Biol*, **27**, 1–32.

Tinbergen, N. (2005). On aims and methods of ethology (reprinted from Z Tierpsychol, 20, 410, 1963). *Animal Biol*, **55**, 297–321.

Tinbergen, E.A. & Tinbergen, N. (1972). *Early Childhood Autism: An Ethological Approach*. Parey, Berlin.

Tiraboschi, P., Hansen, L.A., Masliah, E., et al. (2004). Impact of APOE genotype on neuropathologic and neurochemical markers of Alzheimer disease. *Neurology*, **62**, 1977–83.

Tirupati, S., Padmavati, R., Thara, R., & McCreadie, R.G. (2007). Insight and psychopathology in never-treated schizophrenia. *Compr Psychiatry*, **48**, 264–68.

Toga, A.W., Thompson, P.M., Mori, S., Amunts, K., & Zilles, K. (2006). Towards multimodal atlases of the human brain. *Nat Rev Neurosci*, **7**, 952–66.

Tomasello, M. & Call, J. (1997). *Primate Cognition*. Oxford University Press, New York.

Tomasello, M., Call, J., & Hare, B. (2003). Chimpanzees understand psychological states—the question is which ones and to what extent. *Trends Cogn Sci*, **7**, 153–56.

Tomasello, M. & Vaish, A. (2013). Origins of human cooperation and morality. *Annu Rev Psychol*, **64**, 231–55.

Tomotake, M. & Ohmori, T. (2002). Personality profiles in patients with eating disorders. *J Med Invest*, **49**, 87–96.

Tooby, J. & Cosmides, L. (1990). The past explains the present—emotional adaptations and the structure of ancestral environments. *Ethol Sociobiol*, **11**, 375–424.

Tooby, J. & Devore, I. (1987). The reconstruction of hominid behavioral evolution through strategic modelling. In: Kinzey, W. (ed.) *The Evolution of Human Behavior: Primate Models*. Suny Press, Albany.

Tooke, W. & Camire, L. (1991). Patterns of deception in intersexual and intrasexual mating strategies. *Ethol Sociobiol*, **12**, 345–64.

Torrey, E.F. (2007). Schizophrenia and the inferior parietal lobule. *Schizophr Res*, **97**, 215–25.

Torrey, E.F., Torrey, B.B., & Burton-Bradley, B.G. (1974). The epidemiology of schizophrenia in Papua New Guinea. *Am J Psychiatry*, **131**, 567–73.

Toth, M. (2015). Mechanisms of non-genetic inheritance and psychiatric disorders. *Neuropsychopharmacology*, **40**, 129–40.

Townsend, E. (2007). Suicide terrorists: are they suicidal? *Suicide Life Threat Behav*, **37**, 35–49.

Travis, R. & Kohli, V. (1995). The birth order factor: ordinal position, social strata, and educational achievement. *J Soc Psychol*, **135**, 499–507.

Tremeau, F., Malaspina, D., Duval, F., et al. (2005). Facial expressiveness in patients with schizophrenia compared to depressed patients and nonpatient comparison subjects. *Am J Psychiatry*, **162**, 92–101.

Trezza, V., Damsteegt, R., Manduca, A., et al. (2012). Endocannabinoids in amygdala and nucleus accumbens mediate social play reward in adolescent rats. *J Neurosci*, **32**, 14899–908.

Trivers, R. (1972). Parental investment and sexual selection. In: Campbell, B. (ed.) *Sexual Selection and the Descent of Man*. Aldine-Atherton, Chicago.

Trivers, R.L. (1971). Evolution of reciprocal altruism. *Q Rev Biol*, **46**, 35–57.

Trivers, R.L. (1974). Parent–offspring conflict. *Am Zoologist*, **14**, 249–64.

Trivers, R. (2000). The elements of a scientific theory of self-deception. *Annal N Y Acad Sci*, **907**, 114–31.

Trivers, R.L. & Hare, H. (1976). Haplodiploidy and evolution of social insects. *Science*, **191**, 249–63.

Trivers, R. L. & Willard, D. E. (1973). Natural selection of parental ability to vary the sex ratio of offspring. *Science*, **179**, 90–92.

Troisi, A. (1999). Ethological research in clinical psychiatry: the study of nonverbal behavior during interviews. *Neurosci Biobehav Rev*, **23**, 905–13.

Troisi, A. (2001). Gender differences in vulnerability to social stress: a Darwinian perspective. *Physiol Behav*, **73**, 443–49.

Troisi, A. (2002). Displacement activities as a behavioral measure of stress in nonhuman primates and human subjects. *Stress*, **5**, 47–54.

Troisi, A. (2003). Psychopathology. In: Mastrepieri, D. (ed.) *Primate Psychology*. Harvard University Press, Cambridge, Massachusetts.

Troisi, A. (2005). The concept of alternative strategies and its relevance to psychiatry and clinical psychology. *Neurosci Biobehav Rev*, **29**, 159–68.

Troisi, A. (2009). Cholesterol in coronary heart disease and psychiatric disorders: same or opposite effects on morbidity risk? *Neurosci Biobehav Rev*, **33**, 125–32.

Troisi, A. (2012). Mental health and well-being: clinical applications of Darwinian psychiatry. In: Roberts, S.C. (ed.) *Applied Evolutionary Psychology*. Oxford University Press, Oxford.

Troisi, A. (2014). Functional classification of psychiatric disorders: a luminous future? *Psycholog Inq*, **25**, 1–4.

Troisi, A. & McGuire M.T. (1990). Deception in somatizing disorders. In: Stefanis, C.N., Rabavilas, A.D., & Soldatos, C.R. (eds) *Psychiatry: A World Perspective*. Elsevier, New York, pp. 973–78.

Troisi, A. & McGuire, M.T. (2000). Psychotherapy in the context of Darwinian psychiatry. In: Gilbert, P. & Bailey, K.G. (eds) *Genes on the Couch. Explorations in Evolutionary Psychotherapy*. Brunner-Routledge, Hove.

Troisi, A., Pasini, A., Bersani, G., Grispini, A., & Ciani, N. (1989). Ethological predictors of amitriptyline response in depressed outpatients. *J Affect Disord*, **17**, 129–36.

Troisi, A., Pasini, A., Bersani, G., Grispini, A., & Ciani, N. (1990). Ethological assessment of the DSM-III subtyping of unipolar depression. *Acta Psychiatr Scand*, **81**, 560–64.

Troisi, A., Spalletta, G., & Pasini, A. (1998). Non-verbal behaviour deficits in schizophrenia: an ethological study of drug-free patients. *Acta Psychiatr Scand*, **97**, 109–15.

Troisi, A., Di Lorenzo, G., Alcini, S., et al. (2006). Body dissatisfaction in women with eating disorders: relationship to early separation anxiety and insecure attachment. *Psychosom Med*, **68**, 449–53.

Troisi, A., Pompili, E., Binello, L., & Sterpone, A. (2007). Facial expressivity during the clinical interview as a predictor functional disability in schizophrenia. a pilot study. *Prog Neuropsychopharmacol Biol Psychiatry*, **31**, 475–81.

Troop, N.A. & Hiskey, S. (2013). Social defeat and PTSD symptoms following trauma. *Br J Clin Psychol*, **52**, 365–79.

Tsankova, N., Renthal, W., Kumar, A., & Nestler, E.J. (2007). Epigenetic regulation in psychiatric disorders. *Nat Rev Neurosci*, **8**, 355–67.

Tuite, M.F. & Stansfield, I. (1994). Translation—knowing when to stop. *Nature*, **372**, 614–15.

Turecki, G. (2014). The molecular bases of the suicidal brain. *Nat Rev Neurosci*, **15**, 802–16.

Uchimura, Y. (1956). Imu, a psychoreactive manifestation in Ainu women. *Nervenarzt*, **27**, 535–40.

Uher, J. (2008). Comparative personality research: methodological approaches. *Eur J Pers*, **22**, 427–55.

Uher, J. & Asendorpf, J.B. (2008). Personality assessment in the Great Apes: comparing ecologically valid behavior measures, behavior ratings, and adjective ratings. *J Res Pers*, **42**, 821–38.

Uher, R. & McGuffin, P. (2008). The moderation by the serotonin transporter gene of environmental adversity in the aetiology of mental illness: review and methodological analysis. *Mol Psychiatry*, **13**, 131–46.

Umekage, T., Tochigi, M., Marui, T., et al. (2003). Serotonin transporter-linked promoter region polymorphism and personality traits in a Japanese population. *Neurosci Lett*, **337**, 13–16.

Umilta, M.A., Kohler, E., Gallese, V., et al. (2001). I know what you are doing. a neurophysiological study. *Neuron*, **31**, 155–65.

Vallortigara, G. & Rogers, L.J. (2005). Survival with an asymmetrical brain: advantages and disadvantages of cerebral lateralization. *Behav Brain Sci*, **28**, 575–89; discussion 589–633.

Van Den Bergh, B. & Dewitte, S. (2006). Digit ratio (2D:4D) moderates the impact of sexual cues on men's decisions in ultimatum games. *Proc Biol Sci*, **273**, 2091–95.

Van Den Bergh, B.R. & Marcoen, A. (2004). High antenatal maternal anxiety is related to ADHD symptoms, externalizing problems, and anxiety in 8- and 9-year-olds. *Child Dev*, **75**, 1085–97.

Van Der Hart, O., Nijenhuis, E., Steele, K., & Brown, D. (2004). Trauma-related dissociation: conceptual clarity lost and found. *Aust N Z J Psychiatry*, **38**, 906–14.

Van Der Kolk, B.A. (2001). The psychobiology and psychopharmacology of PTSD. *Hum Psychopharmacol*, **16**, S49–64.

Vanderschuren, L.J., Trezza, V., Griffioen-Roose, S., et al. (2008). Methylphenidate disrupts social play behavior in adolescent rats. *Neuropsychopharmacology*, **33**, 2946–56.

Vanderwolf, C.H. (1998). Brain, behavior, and mind: what do we know and what can we know? *Neurosci Biobehav Rev*, **22**, 125–42.

Van Dessel, N., Den Boeft, M., Van Der Wouden, J.C., et al. (2014). Non-pharmacological interventions for somatoform disorders and medically unexplained physical symptoms (MUPS) in adults. *Cochrane Database Syst Rev*, **11**, CD011142.

Van Ijzendoorn, M.H. & Sagi, A. (1999). Cross-cultural patterns of attachment: universal and contextual dimensions. In: Cassidy, J. & Shaver, P.R. (eds) *Handbook of Attachment. Theory, Research, and Clinical Applications*. Guilford Press, New York.

Van Ijzendoorn, M.H., Rutgers, A.H., Bakermans-Kranenburg, M.J., et al. (2007). Parental sensitivity and attachment in children with autism spectrum disorder: comparison with children with mental retardation, with language delays, and with typical development. *Child Dev*, **78**, 597–608.

Van Ijzendoorn, M.H., Bakermans-Kranenburg, M.J., & Mesman, J. (2008). Dopamine system genes associated with parenting in the context of daily hassles. *Gene Brain Behav*, **7**, 403–10.

Van Ijzendoorn, M.H., Belsky, J., & Bakermans-Kranenburg, M.J. (2012). Serotonin transporter genotype 5HTTLPR as a marker of differential susceptibility? A meta-analysis of child and adolescent gene-by-environment studies. *Transl Psychiatry*, **2**, e147.

Van Os, J., Verdoux, H., Maurice-Tison, S., et al. (1999). Self-reported psychosis-like symptoms and the continuum of psychosis. *Soc Psychiatry Psychiatr Epidemiol*, **34**, 459–63.

Van Os, J., Hanssen, M., Bijl, R.V., & Ravelli, A. (2000). Strauss (1969) revisited: a psychosis continuum in the general population? *Schizophr Res*, **45**, 11–20.

Van Praag, H.M. (1988). Biological psychiatry audited. *J Nerv Ment Dis*, **176**, 195–99.

Van Voorhees, E. & Scarpa, A. (2004). The effects of child maltreatment on the hypothalamic-pituitary-adrenal axis. *Trauma Violence Abuse*, **5**, 333–52.

Varga, S. (2013). Vulnerability to psychosis, I-thou intersubjectivity and the praecox-feeling. *Phenomenol Cogn Sci*, **12**, 131–143.

Varki, A. & Altheide, T.K. (2005). Comparing the human and chimpanzee genomes: searching for needles in a haystack. *Genome Res*, **15**, 1746–58.

Vella, G., Aragona, M., & Alliani, D. (2000). The complexity of psychiatric comorbidity: a conceptual and methodological discussion. *Psychopathology*, **33**, 25–30.

Verdoux, H. & Van Os, J. (2002). Psychotic symptoms in non-clinical populations and the continuum of psychosis. *Schizophr Res*, **54**, 59–65.

Verhulst, J., Kramer, D., Swann, A.C., Hale-Richlen, B., & Beahrs, J. (2013). The medical alliance: from placebo response to alliance effect. *J Nerv Ment Dis*, **201**, 546–52.

Vermetten, E. & Lanius, R.A. (2012). Biological and clinical framework for posttraumatic stress disorder. In: Schlaepfer, T.E. & Nemeroff, C.B. (eds) *Handbook of Clinical Neurology*. Elsevier, Amsterdam.

Vicentic, A., Francis, D., Moffett, M., et al. (2006). Maternal separation alters serotonergic transporter densities and serotonergic 1A receptors in rat brain. *Neuroscience*, **140**, 355–65.

Viding, E. (2004). Annotation: understanding the development of psychopathy. *J Child Psychol Psychiatry*, **45**, 1329–37.

Vidovic, V., Juresa, V., Begovac, I., Mahnik, M., & Tocilj, G. (2005). Perceived family cohesion, adaptability and communication in eating disorders. *Eur Eat Disord Rev*, **13**, 19–28.

Villalobos, M.E., Mizuno, A., Dahl, B.C., Kemmotsu, N., & Muller, R.A. (2005). Reduced functional connectivity between V1 and inferior frontal cortex associated with visuomotor performance in autism. *Neuroimage*, **25**, 916–925.

Vogeley, K., Bussfeld, P., Newen, A., et al. (2001). Mind reading: neural mechanisms of theory of mind and self-perspective. *Neuroimage*, **14**, 170–81.

Voland, E. (1998). Evolutionary ecology of human reproduction. *Annu Rev Anthropol*, **27**, 347–74.

Voland, E. & Dunbar, R.I. (1995). Resource competition and reproduction: the relationship between economic and parental strategies in the Krummhorn population (1720–1874). *Hum Nat*, **6**, 33–49.

Voland, E. & Voland, R. (1989). Evolutionary biology and psychiatry—the case of anorexia-nervosa. *Ethol Sociobiol*, **10**, 223–40.

Volavka, J., Bilder, R., & Nolan, K. (2004). Catecholamines and aggression: the role of COMT and MAO polymorphisms. *Ann N Y Acad Sci*, **1036**, 393–98.

Völker, K.A., Spitzer, C., Limberg, A., et al. (2009). Executive dysfunctions in female patients with borderline personality disorder with regard to impulsiveness and depression. *Psychother Psychosom Med Psychol*, **59**, 264–72.

Vollm, B., Richardson, P., Stirling, J., et al. (2004). Neurobiological substrates of antisocial and borderline personality disorder: preliminary results of a functional fMRI study. *Crim Behav Ment Health*, **14**, 39–54.

Vollm, B., Richardson, P., McKie, S., et al. (2007). Neuronal correlates of reward and loss in Cluster B personality disorders: a functional magnetic resonance imaging study. *Psychiatry Res*, **156**, 151–67.

Von Economo, C. (1926). Eine neue Art Spezialzellen des Lobus cinguli nad Lobus insulae. *Z Ges Neurol Psychiatr*, **100**, 706–712.

Von Helversen, B., Wilke, A., Johnson, T., Schmid, G., & Klapp, B. (2011). Performance benefits of depression: sequential decision making in a healthy sample and a clinically depressed sample. *J Abnorm Psychol*, **120**, 962–68.

Von Hippel, W. & Trivers, R. (2011). The evolution and psychology of self-deception. *Behav Brain Sci*, **34**, 1–16; discussion 16–56.

Von Klitzing, K., Simoni, H., & Burgin, D. (1999). Child development and early triadic relationships. *Int J Psychoanal*, **80** (Pt 1), 71–89.

Vrba, E.S. (1998). Multiphasic growth models and the evolution of prolonged growth exemplified by human brain evolution. *J Theor Biol*, **190**, 227–39.

Waal, F.B.M.D. (1989). *Chimpanzee Politics: Power and Sex Among Apes*. Johns Hopkins University Press, Baltimore.

Waal, F.B.M.D. (1996). *Good Natured: The Origins of Right and Wrong in Humans and Other Animals*. Harvard University Press, Cambridge, Massachusetts.

Waal, F.B.M.D. & Lanting, F. (1997). *Bonobo: The Forgotten Ape*. University of California Press, Berkeley.

Waddell, C. (1998). Creativity and mental illness: is there a link? *Can J Psychiatry*, **43**, 166–72.

Wahlbeck, K., Osmond, C., Forsen, T., Barker, D.J., & Eriksson, J.G. (2001). Associations between childhood living circumstances and schizophrenia: a population-based cohort study. *Acta Psychiatr Scand*, **104**, 356–60.

Wahlberg, K.E., Wynne, L.C., Oja, H., et al. (1997). Gene–environment interaction in vulnerability to schizophrenia: findings from the Finnish Adoptive Family Study of Schizophrenia. *Am J Psychiatry*, **154**, 355–62.

Wakefield, J.C. (1999). Evolutionary versus prototype analyses of the concept of disorder. *J Abnorm Psychol*, **108**, 374–99.

Walker, R.S., Hill, K.R., Flinn, M.V., & Ellsworth, R.M. (2011). Evolutionary history of hunter-gatherer marriage practices. *PLoS One*, **6**, e19066.

Walker, S.C. & McGlone, F.P. (2013). The social brain: neurobiological basis of affiliative behaviours and psychological well-being. *Neuropeptides*, **47**, 379–93.

Wallace, B., Cesarini, D., Lichtenstein, P., & Johannesson, M. (2007). Heritability of ultimatum game responder behavior. *Proc Natl Acad Sci USA*, **104**, 15631–34.

Wallbott, H.G. (1998). Bodily expression of emotion. *Eur J Soc Psychol*, **28**, 879–96.

Waller, G., Corstorphine, E., & Mountford, V. (2007). The role of emotional abuse in the eating disorders: implications for treatment. *Eat Disord*, **15**, 317–31.

Wallwiener, C.W., Wallwiener, L.M., Seeger, H., et al. (2010). Prevalence of sexual dysfunction and impact of contraception in female German medical students. *J Sex Med*, **7**, 2139–48.

Walmsley, T. (2003). Crichton-Browne's biological psychiatry. *Psychiatr Bull*, **27**, 20–22.

Walsh, E., Buchanan, A., & Fahy, T. (2002). Violence and schizophrenia: examining the evidence. *Br J Psychiatry*, **180**, 490–95.

Walsh, E., Gilvarry, C., Samele, C., et al. (2004). Predicting violence in schizophrenia: a prospective study. *Schizophr Res*, **67**, 247–52.

Walter, H., Adenzato, M., Ciaramidaro, A., et al. (2004). Understanding intentions in social interaction: the role of the anterior paracingulate cortex. *J Cogn Neurosci*, **16**, 1854–63.

Walters, J.T. & Owen, M.J. (2007). Endophenotypes in psychiatric genetics. *Mol Psychiatry*, **12**, 886–90.

Wampold, B. (2001). *The Great Psychotherapy Debate: Models, Methods, and Findings*. Lawrence Erlbaum, Mahwah.

Wang, E., Ding, Y.C., Flodman, P., et al. (2004). The genetic architecture of selection at the human dopamine receptor D4 (DRD4) gene locus. *Am J Hum Genet*, **74**, 931–44.

Ward, A., Ramsay, R., Turnbull, S., et al. (2001). Attachment in anorexia nervosa: a transgenerational perspective. *Br J Med Psychol*, **74**, 497–505.

Warneken, F. & Tomasello, M. (2006). Altruistic helping in human infants and young chimpanzees. *Science*, **311**, 1301–303.

Warneken, F., Hare, B., Melis, A.P., Hanus, D., & Tomasello, M. (2007). Spontaneous altruism by chimpanzees and young children. *Plos Biol*, **5**, e184.

Waters, E., Merrick, S., Treboux, D., Crowell, J., & Albersheim, L. (2000). Attachment security in infancy and early adulthood: a twenty-year longitudinal study. *Child Dev*, **71**, 684–89.

Watson, K.K., Werling, D.M., Zucker, N.L., & Platt, M.L. (2010). Altered social reward and attention in anorexia nervosa. *Front Psychol*, 1, 36.

Watson, P.J. & Andrews, P.W. (2002). Toward a revised evolutionary adaptationist analysis of depression: the social navigation hypothesis. *J Affect Disord*, **72**, 1–14.

Weaver, I.C., Cervoni, N., Champagne, F.A., et al. (2004). Epigenetic programming by maternal behavior. *Nat Neurosci*, 7, 847–54. DOI: 10.1038/nn1276 nn1276 [pii].

Wedekind, C. & Furi, S. (1997). Body odour preferences in men and women: do they aim for specific MHC combinations or simply heterozygosity? *Proc Biol Sci*, **264**, 1471–79.

Weekes-Shackelford, V.A. & Shackelford, T.K. (2004). Methods of filicide: stepparents and genetic parents kill differently. *Violence Vict*, **19**, 75–81.

Weeks, J.W. & Howell, A.N. (2012). The bivalent fear of evaluation model of social anxiety: further integrating findings on fears of positive and negative evaluation. *Cogn Behav Ther*, **41**, 83–95.

Weeks, J.W., Rodebaugh, T.L., Heimberg, R.G., Norton, P J., & Jakatdar, T.A. (2009). 'To avoid evaluation, withdraw': fears of evaluation and depressive cognitions lead to social anxiety and submissive withdrawal. *Cogn Ther Res*, **33**, 375–89.

Weiner, W.J. & Lang, A.E. (eds) (1995). *Behavioral Neurology of Movement Disorders. Advances in Neurology*. Raven Press, New York.

Weinfield, N.S., Sroufe, L.A., Egeland, B., & Carlson, E.A. (1999). The nature of individual differences in infant-cargiver attachment. In: Cassidy, J. & Shaver, P.R. (eds) *Handbook of Attachment. Theory, Research, and Clinical Applications*. Guilford Press, New York.

Weisman, O., Aderka, I.M., Marom, S., Hermesh, H., & Gilboa-Schechtman, E. (2011). Social rank and affiliation in social anxiety disorder. *Behav Res Ther*, **49**, 399–405.

Wells, A. & Cartwright-Hatton, S. (2004). A short form of the metacognitions questionnaire: properties of the MCQ-30. *Behav Res Ther*, **42**, 385–96.

Wells, J.C. (2000). Natural selection and sex differences in morbidity and mortality in early life. *J Theor Biol*, **202**, 65–76.

Wenegrat, B. (1984). *Sociobiology & Mental Disorder: A New View*. Addison/Wesley, Menlo Park.

Wenegrat, B. (1990). *Sociobiological Psychiatry: Normal Behavior and Psychopathology*. Lexington Books, Lexington.

Wentz, E., Gillberg, I.C., Gillberg, C., & Rastam, M. (2005). Fertility and history of sexual abuse at 10-year follow-up of adolescent-onset anorexia nervosa. *Int J Eat Disord*, **37**, 294–98.

Westermarck, E.A. (1889). *The History of Human Marriage. Part I, The Origin of Human Marriage*. Thesis. Printed by Frenckell & Son Helsingfors.

Wexler, B.E., Zhu, H., Bell, M.D., et al. (2009). Neuropsychological near normality and brain structure abnormality in schizophrenia. *Am J Psychiatry*, **166**, 189–95.

Wheelwright, S. & Baron-Cohen, S. (2001). The link between autism and skills such as engineering, maths, physics and computing: a reply to Jarrold and Routh. *Autism*, **5**, 223–27.

Whiten, A. (2000). Social complexity and social intelligence. *Novartis Found Symp*, **233**, 185–96; discussion 196–201.

Whiten, A. & Byrne, R.W. (1997). *Machiavellian Intelligence II: Extensions and Evaluations*. Cambridge University Press, Cambridge.

Wick, W.D., Gilbert, P.B., & Yang, O.O. (2009). Predicting the impact of blocking human immunodeficiency virus type 1 nef in vivo. *J Virol*, **83**, 2349–56.

Widom, C.S. & Brzustowicz, L.M. (2006). MAOA and the 'cycle of violence:' childhood abuse and neglect, MAOA genotype, and risk for violent and antisocial behavior. *Biol Psychiatry*, **60**, 684–89.

Wiederman, M.W. & Allgeier, E.R. (1993). Gender differences in sexual jealousy—adaptionist or social-learning explanation. *Ethol Sociobiol*, **14**, 115–40.

Wiederman, M.W. & Kendall, E. (1999). Evolution, sex, and jealousy: Investigation with a sample from Sweden. *Evol Hum Behav*, **20**, 121–28.

Williams, C.L. (2008). Food for thought: brain, genes, and nutrition Introduction. *Brain Res*, **1237**, 1–4.

Williams, G.C. (1957). Pleiotropy, natural-selection, and the evolution of senescence. *Evolution*, **11**, 398–411.

Williams, G.C. (1966). *Adaptation and Natural Selection; A Critique of Some Current Evolutionary Thought*. Princeton University Press, Princeton.

Williams, J.H. (1998). Using behavioural ecology to understand depression. *Br J Psychiatry*, **173**, 453–54.

Williams, J.H., Whiten, A., Suddendorf, T., & Perrett, D.I. (2001). Imitation, mirror neurons and autism. *Neurosci Biobehav Rev*, **25**, 287–95.

Williams, K.E. & Koran, L.M. (1997). Obsessive-compulsive disorder in pregnancy, the puerperium, and the premenstruum. *J Clin Psychiatry*, **58**, 330–34; quiz 335–36.

Wilson, D.R. (1998). Evolutionary epidemiology and manic depression. *Br J Med Psychol*, **71** (Pt 4), 375–95.

Wilson, D.S., Near, D., & Miller, R.R. (1996). Machiavellianism: a synthesis of the evolutionary and psychological literatures. *Psychol Bull*, **119**, 285–99.

Wilson, M. & Daly, M. (1985). Competitiveness, risk-taking, and violence—the young male syndrome. *Ethol Sociobiol*, **6**, 59–73.

Wilson, M. & Daly, M. (1993). An evolutionary psychological perspective on male sexual proprietariness and violence against wives. *Violence Vict*, **8**, 271–94.

Wilson, M. & Daly, M. (1994). Spousal homicide. *Juristat*, **14**, 1–14.

Wilson, M.I. & Daly, M. (1996). Male sexual proprietariness and violence against wives. *Curr Direction Psychol Sci*, **5**, 2–7.

Wilson, M. & Daly, M. (1997). Life expectancy, economic inequality, homicide, and reproductive timing in Chicago neighbourhoods. *BMJ*, **314**, 1271–74.

Wischniewski, J. & Brüne, M. (2013). How do people with borderline personality disorder respond to norm violations? Impact of personality factors on economic decision-making. *J Pers Disord*, **27**, 531–46.

Wischniewski, J., Windmann, S., Juckel, G., & Brüne, M. (2009). Rules of social exchange: game theory, individual differences and psychopathology. *Neurosci Biobehav Rev*, **33**, 305–13.

Wittchen, H.U. & Fehm, L. (2001). Epidemiology, patterns of comorbidity, and associated disabilities of social phobia. *Psychiatr Clin N Am*, **24**, 617–41.

Wittchen, H.U., Zhao, S., Kessler, R.C., & Eaton, W.W. (1994). DSM-III-R generalized anxiety disorder in the National Comorbidity Survey. *Arch Gen Psychiatry*, **51**, 355–64.

Wobrock, T., Sittinger, H., Behrendt, B., et al. (2007). Comorbid substance abuse and neurocognitive function in recent-onset schizophrenia. *Eur Arch Psychiatry Clin Neurosci*, **257**, 203–10.

Wohlschlager, A. & Bekkering, H. (2002). Is human imitation based on a mirror-neurone system? Some behavioural evidence. *Exp Brain Res*, **143**, 335–41.

Wolf, F.W. & Heberlein, U. (2003). Invertebrate models of drug abuse. *J Neurobiol*, **54**, 161–78.

Wolf, M., Van Doorn, G.S., Leimar, O., & Weissing, F.J. (2007). Life-history trade-offs favour the evolution of animal personalities. *Nature*, **447**, 581–84.

Wolf, M.E. (1999). Cocaine addiction: clues from Drosophila on drugs. *Curr Biol*, **9**, R770–72.

Wolf, R.C., Thomann, P.A., Sambataro, F., et al. (2012). Orbitofrontal cortex and impulsivity in borderline personality disorder: an MRI study of baseline brain perfusion. *Eur Arch Psychiatry Clin Neurosci*, **262**, 677–85.

Wood, G.K., Marcotte, E.R., Quirion, R., & Srivastava, L.K. (2001). Strain differences in the behavioural outcome of neonatal ventral hippocampal lesions are determined by the postnatal environment and not genetic factors. *Eur J Neurosci*, **14**, 1030-4.

Wood, P.B. (2005). Neuroimaging in functional somatic syndromes. *Int Rev Neurobiol*, **67**, 119–63.

Woody, E.Z. & Szechtman, H. (2011). Adaptation to potential threat: the evolution, neurobiology, and psychopathology of the security motivation system. *Neurosci Biobehav Rev*, **35**, 1019–33.

World Health Organization (WHO) (2004). *Prevention of Mental Disorders. Effective Interventions and Policy Options*. World Health Organization, Geneva.

Wrangham, R.W. (1999). Evolution of coalitionary killing. *Am J Phys Anthropol*, 29, 1–30.

Wrase, J., Schlagenhauf, F., Kienast, T., et al. (2007). Dysfunction of reward processing correlates with alcohol craving in detoxified alcoholics. *Neuroimage*, **35**, 787–94.

Wynne-Edwards, V.C. (1962). *Animal Dispersion in Relation to Social Behaviour*. Oliver and Boyd, Edinburgh.

Yanagi, M., Shirakawa, O., Kitamura, N., et al. (2005). Association of 14-13-3 epsilon gene haplotype with completed suicide in Japanese. *J Hum Genet*, **50**, 210–16.

Yang, B.Z., Zhang, H., Ge, W., et al. (2013). Child abuse and epigenetic mechanisms of disease risk. *Am J Prev Med*, **44**, 101–107.

Yang, Y., Raine, A., Colletti, P., Toga, A.W., & Narr, K.L. (2009). Abnormal temporal and prefrontal cortical gray matter thinning in psychopaths. *Mol Psychiatry*, **14**, 561–62, 555.

Yasumoto, F., Hayashi, A., Kamiya, A., et al. (2008). Genetic manipulation of brain cultures from the primates: a novel tool for molecular studies of neuropsychiatric disorders. *Mol Psychiatry*, **13**, 116–18.

Yehuda, R. (2000). Biology of posttraumatic stress disorder. *J Clin Psychiatry*, **61** (Suppl 7), 14–21.

Yehuda, R., McFarlane, A.C., & Shalev, A.Y. (1998). Predicting the development of posttraumatic stress disorder from the acute response to a traumatic event. *Biol Psychiatry*, **44**, 1305–13.

Yeniel, A.O. & Petri, E. (2014). Pregnancy, childbirth, and sexual function: perceptions and facts. *Int Urogynecol J*, **25**, 5–14.

Yeo, R.A., Gangestad, S.W., Edgar, C., & Thoma, R. (1999). The evolutionary genetic underpinnings of schizophrenia: the developmental instability model. *Schizophr Res*, **39**, 197–206.

Yoshida, M., Takayanagi, Y., Inoue, K., et al. (2009). Evidence that oxytocin exerts anxiolytic effects via oxytocin receptor expressed in serotonergic neurons in mice. *J Neurosci*, **29**, 2259–71.

Young, J.E., Klosko, J.S., & Weishaar, M.E. (2003). *Schema Therapy: A Practitioner's Guide*. Guildford Press, New York.

Young, L.J. (2007). Regulating the social brain: a new role for CD38. *Neuron*, **54**, 353–56.

Young, L.J. & Wang, Z. (2004). The neurobiology of pair bonding. *Nat Neurosci*, **7**, 1048–54.

Yovel, G., Sirota, P., Mazeh, D., et al. (2000). Higher natural killer cell activity in schizophrenic patients: the impact of serum factors, medication, and smoking. *Brain Behav Immun*, **14**, 153–69.

Yu, X., Zhang, S., Yan, Z., et al. (2014). Is interactional dissynchrony a clue to deception? Insights from automated analysis of nonverbal visual cues. *IEEE Trans Cybern*, **45**(3), 506–520.

Yun, K. (2013). On the same wavelength: face-to-face communication increases interpersonal neural synchronization. *J Neurosci*, **33**, 5081–82.

Yung, A.R., Yuen, H.P., McGorry, P.D., et al. (2005). Mapping the onset of psychosis: the comprehensive assessment of at-risk mental states. *Aust N Z J Psychiatry*, **39**, 964–71.

Zahl, D.L. & Hawton, K. (2004). Repetition of deliberate self-harm and subsequent suicide risk: long-term follow-up study of 11,583 patients. *Br J Psychiatry*, **185**, 70–75.

Zanarini, M.C., Frankenburg, F.R., Reich, D.B., et al. (2000). Biparental failure in the childhood experiences of borderline patients. *J Pers Disord*, **14**, 264–73.

Zeeman, E.C. (1980). *Population Dynamics from Game Theory*. Springer, Berlin.

Zeisel, S.H. (2008). Genetic polymorphisms in methyl-group metabolism and epigenetics: lessons from humans and mouse models. *Brain Res*, **1237**, 5–11.

Ziabreva, I., Schnabel, R., Poeggel, G., & Braun, K. (2003). Mother's voice 'buffers' separation-induced receptor changes in the prefrontal cortex of octodon degus. *Neuroscience*, **119**, 433–41.

Zilles, K. (1987). Graue und weiße Substanz des Hirnmantels. In: Leonhardt, H., Tillmann, B., Töndury, G., & Zilles, K. (eds) *Anatomie des Menschen. Band III. Nervensystem und Sinnesorgane*. Thieme, Stuttgart.

Zimbardo, P.G. & Boyd, J.N. (1999). Putting time in perspective: a valid, reliable individual-differences metric. *J Pers Soc Psychol*, **77**, 1271–88.

Zoia, S., Blason, L., D'ottavio, G., et al. (2007). Evidence of early development of action planning in the human foetus: a kinematic study. *Exp Brain Res*, **176**, 217–26.

Zolotova, J. & Brüne, M. (2006). Persecutory delusions: reminiscence of ancestral hostile threats? *Evol Hum Behav*, **27**, 185–92.

Zona, M.A., Sharma, K.K., & Lane, J. (1993). A comparative-study of erotomanic and obsessional subjects in a forensic sample. *J For Sci*, **38**, 894–903.

Author index

C

T

Subject index

T